Thomas E. Massey, PhD.
Dept. of Pharmacology & Toxicology
Queen's University
Kingston, Ontario K7L 3N6

D1217282

JOHN F. MURRAY, M.D., D. Sc. (hon.)

Professor of Medicine and Member of the Senior Staff
of the Cardiovascular Research Institute,
University of California School of Medicine,

Chief of Chest Division of the Medical Service,
San Francisco General Hospital, San Francisco

The
Normal
Lung

THE BASIS FOR DIAGNOSIS AND TREATMENT OF PULMONARY DISEASE

SECOND EDITION

W. B. Saunders Company   **1986**

Philadelphia   London   Toronto   Mexico City
Rio de Janiero   Sydney   Tokyo   Hong Kong

W. B. Saunders Company: West Washington Square
Philadelphia, PA 19105

Library of Congress Cataloging in Publication Data

Murray, John F. (John Frederic), 1927–

The normal lung.

Includes bibliographies and index.

1. Lungs.   I. Title.   [DNLM: 1. Lung.   2. Lung
   Diseases.   3. Microscopy, Electron. WF 600 M982n]

QP121.M87   1986   612′.2   85–11802

ISBN   0–7216–6613–2

The Normal Lung: The Basis for Diagnosis
and Treatment of Pulmonary Disease   ISBN   0–7216–6613–2

Last digit is the print number: 9   8   7   6   5   4   3   2   1

To Dinny,
with love and thanks

Preface

I began work on the first edition of *The Normal Lung* in 1972, while spending a sabbatical leave at the Brompton Hospital in London. Writing the book was a slow process, and it became even slower after I returned to my regular duties in San Francisco a year later. Because of this lengthy timetable, my review of the pertinent literature extended through 1974, and the manuscript was finally submitted in 1975. Because I enjoyed writing the first edition and it had proved relatively successful, I had planned for a long time to revise the book. A ten year interval between editions seemed just about right so I went back to the Brompton Hospital in early 1984 and started to work. This edition, then, includes material published through 1984 and references to a few key articles from the first three months of 1985.

When I started my review of the literature of the last decade, I quickly found out what is meant by the cliche "knowledge explosion," even in a field seemingly as restricted as the structure and function of the normal lung. Accordingly, I have had to be selective in my approach, and some may find reason to quarrel with my final choices. Although I have had help from many friends, the emphasis is my own. This, as before, has always been to include information that I considered to be new and important, particularly to physicians, therapists, and others who have an interest in patients with lung disease.

A medical text, like other literary works, can always be improved upon with more time and effort. Winston Churchill once said "you never finish a book, you finally abandon it." The second edition of *The Normal Lung* was abandoned in April 1985.

JOHN F. MURRAY

Acknowledgments

The second edition of *The Normal Lung,* like its predecessor, was born in the library of the Brompton Hospital in London. I am grateful to Professor Margaret Turner-Warwick for welcoming me back and providing facilities in which to work.

Chapters or sections of the manuscript in their particular field of interest were reviewed by Professor David Dennison, Drs. Ira M. Goldstein, Henry N. Hulter, H. Benfer Kaltreider, Steven J. Lai-Fook, Neil Pride, and Charis Roussos. Useful information was provided by Drs. A. Sonia Buist, Gordon Cumming, Ronald G. Crystal, Michael R. Flick, Lee V. Leak, Robert A. Mitchell, Lynne M. Reid, Norman C. Staub, and W. M. Thurlbeck.

Unpublished illustrations were generously supplied by Drs. Peter K. Jeffrey, Lauri and Annika Laitenen, Evelene Schneeberger, Norman C. Staub, Ewald R. Weibel, and Mary C. Williams. Prints of previously published photographs were provided by Drs. Kurt Albertine, John Bienenstock, Joan Gil, Jon M. Goerke, Professor Abraham Guz, Drs. Jay A. Nadel, John Richardson, Una Ryan, Ewald R. Weibel, and Kokichi Yoneda. Original art work was prepared by Wayne Emery.

Two persons deserve special recognition. Ms. Dorothy J. Ladd who expertly did virtually all of the typing and other secretarial chores, and Ms. Aja Lipavsky who carefully proofread and corrected the entire book at each step of its development.

J. F. M.

Contents

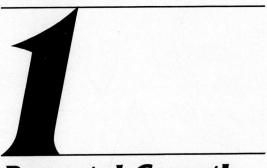

Chapter

1

Prenatal Growth and Development of the Lung

INTRODUCTION

Venus, goddess of love, was born by rising naked from the foam of the sea. She is usually depicted as being full grown at birth, and certainly her respiratory system was completely developed because she was able to ride a scallop shell through the waves and dance on the ocean immediately after her birth. Mortal man does not leave the aquatic environment in which he develops so well equipped, because his lungs must undergo a series of complex developmental changes both during embryogenesis and after birth, culminating ultimately in the structural organization and functional capabilities of the normal adult respiratory system.

The purpose of this and the next two chapters is to review the growth, development, and anatomy of the normal human lung, during fetal life (Chapter 1) and from birth to maturity (Chapters 2 and 3). Although emphasis in these three chapters is on morphology and in the remainder of the book on function, both structure and function are intimately interrelated, and it is impossible to ignore one or the other completely. Therefore, a functional interpretation has been applied to morphologic evi-

1

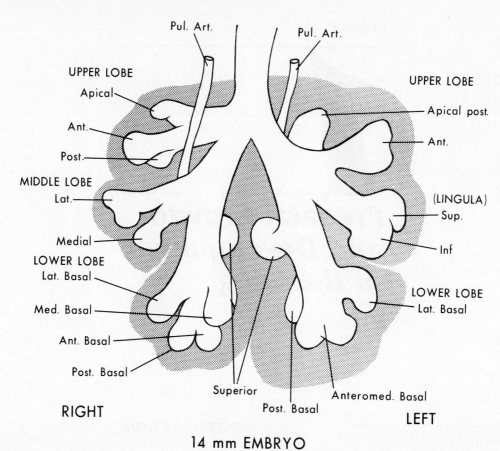

Figure 1–1. Schematic drawing of the lungs of a 14 mm (six week) human embryo. The tracheobronchial tree has subdivided so that the lobar and segmental branches that characterize the adult lung can be recognized. (Adapted and reprinted by permission from Krahl, V. E.: Anatomy of the mammalian lung. *In* Fenn, W. O., and Rahn, H. (eds.): Handbook of Physiology, Section 3. Respiration. Vol. I. Washington, D.C., American Physiological Society, 1964, pp. 213–284.)

dence, and a structural basis for physiologic phenomena has been derived, whenever possible. Clinical implications are introduced when they enhance an understanding of the normal lung and its behavior.

Knowledge about the pre- and postnatal growth and development of the lung provides important insights into pulmonary function in health and disease and an explanation for developmental anomalies; it also creates a wondrous appreciation of the ability of the lung to assume, within the few minutes that it takes for the placenta to separate during delivery, the complete role of providing gas exchange for the newborn baby. The heart, kidneys, liver, and other visceral organs begin functioning early in fetal life and increase their capabilities during gestation. This is not so with the lungs. Because the fetus develops in a completely aquatic environment, all O_2 uptake and CO_2 elimination are provided by the placenta,

and although the fetus makes breathing motions during gestation, the lung is not afforded any practice for its ultimate major role of gas exchange. Therefore, it must be carefully prepared to respond to the immediate demands of the transition from fetal to postnatal life.

EMBRYOLOGY

The entire epithelial structure of the human lung arises as a pouch from the primitive foregut and can be recognized about 22 to 26 days after fertilization (4 to 5 mm embryo); the single lung bud branches into primitive right and left lungs a few days later. By the sixth or seventh week (14 mm embryo), through a combination of monopodial (single budding) and irregular dichotomous (dividing) branching, ten principal branches can be discerned on the right and eight on the left (Fig. 1–1). The consistency of this early scheme provides the basis for the subsequent organization of the mature lung into its familiar lobar and segmental units.[1]

There is now substantial evidence to document an endodermal origin of the type I and type II cells of the alveolar epithelium. In contrast, the pleura, blood vessels, smooth muscle, and supporting tissues such as cartilage, collagen, and elastic fibers originate from the mesoderm. Although fundamentally distinct, an intimate and precise interaction between endoderm and mesoderm is necessary to ensure normal differentiation in the developing lung. The nature of the regulatory "growth factors" is unknown, but controlling influences between structures of endodermal and mesodermal origin are clearly evident.

The human lung develops and grows both during gestation and after birth; however, the order of maturation of the various structural components of the lung varies, as shown in Figure 1–2, and proceeds according to Reid's three "Laws of Development":

(1) The bronchial tree is developed by the sixteenth week of intrauterine life; (2) alveoli develop after birth, increasing in number until the age of eight years and in size until growth of the chest wall finishes with adulthood; and (3) the pre-acinar vessels (arteries and veins) follow the development of the airways, the intra-acinar that of the alveoli. Muscularization of the intra-

acinar arteries does not keep pace with the appearance of new arteries.[3]

It is perhaps artificial to divide lung growth into antenatal and postnatal periods, because growth and development follow a continuous, uninterrupted course that begins soon after conception and finishes when somatic growth ceases; however, there are important differences in extent of development and in functional demands between intrauterine and extrauterine existence. This division also conveniently allows special consideration of the momentous events that occur during the first few moments after birth.

AIRWAYS AND TERMINAL RESPIRATORY UNITS

In the simplest of structure-function classifications the lungs can be subdivided into two different portions: a conducting system of airways and blood vessels and a gas exchange system within the lung parenchyma. The former conducts blood and air into and out of the latter, where O_2 uptake and CO_2 elimination occur. As will be seen, however, there is considerable structural complexity to each of these systems that serves not only to enhance their contribution to gas exchange but also provides additional nonrespiratory functional capabilities.

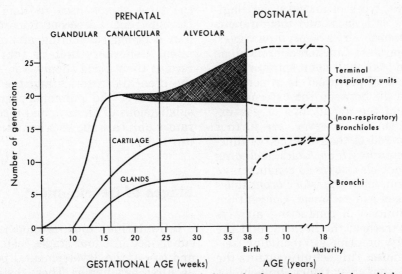

Figure 1–2. Sequence of development of bronchi (including glands and cartilage), bronchioles, and terminal respiratory units during gestation and postnatal growth. Generation number refers to an axial pathway beginning with the segmental bronchus. (Adapted and reprinted by permission from Reid, L.: The embryology of the lung. *In* De Reuck, A. V. S., and Porter, R. (eds.): Ciba Foundation Symposium: Development of the lung. Boston, Little, Brown and Company, 1967, pp. 109–124.)

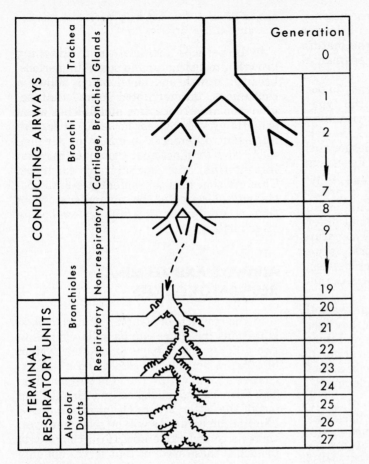

Figure 1–3. Schematic representation of the subdivisions of the conducting airways and terminal respiratory units. Note that generation number begins with the trachea. For details, see text. (Adapted and reprinted by permission from Weibel, E. R.: Morphometry of the Human Lung. Berlin, Springer-Verlag, 1963, p. 111.)

Definitions

The tracheobronchial system can be divided into two types of airways: cartilaginous airways or *bronchi* and membranous (noncartilaginous) airways or *bronchioles.* The only respiratory function of bronchi, as distinguished from their nonrespiratory role (e.g., clearance of particles), is to serve as conductors of air between the external environment and the distal sites of gas exchange. Bronchioles, however, are further subdivided to reflect their distinctive functions. *Nonrespiratory bronchioles,* including *terminal bronchioles,* serve as conductors of the gas stream, and *respiratory bronchioles* serve as sites of gas exchange. Conventionally, the definition of conducting airways includes the trachea, the bronchi, and the nonrespiratory bronchioles, including terminal bronchioles. This definition omits the obvious fact that respiratory bronchioles also conduct gas to more distal respiratory bronchioles, alveolar ducts, and alveoli, but because all these structures participate in

gas exchange they are designated collectively as the *terminal respiratory unit.* (The terminal respiratory unit is equivalent to the term acinus used in Reid's "Laws of Development.") A second important distinction between conducting airways and terminal respiratory units is that the former receive their blood supply from branches of the bronchial arteries and the latter from branches of the pulmonary arteries. The subdivisions of airways and terminal respiratory units are shown schematically in Figure 1–3.

Stages of Development

Intrauterine lung development is now subdivided into four stages instead of three, and two of the developmental periods have acquired new names. These distinctions are somewhat arbitrary because the processes of differentiation proceed from the hilus to the periphery of the developing lung and there is asynchrony between neighboring lobes.[5] A new term, the *embryonic period*, has been added to include the events during the first five to seven weeks after fertilization; at the end of this phase, the two lung primordia and their mainstem bronchi are present. Important developments during the last three stages are shown schematically in Figure 1–2, and representative histology is illustrated in Figure 1–4 (see also Plate I). The *pseudoglandular period* (formerly the glandular period), or extended lung bud period, occurs in the first 16 weeks of gestation; during this interval the lung structures consist of a loose collection of connective tissue with an actively proliferating central bronchial mass (see Fig. 1–4*A*). The progressive organization and differentiation of the cellular components that occurs during this period have two important outcomes: the formation of all branches of the conducting airways and the appearance of lobular outlines. The *canalicular period* occurs from 17 to 24 weeks of gestation. Even though all prospective conducting airways have formed, by further dichotomous branching primitive terminal bronchioles develop primitive respiratory bronchioles, the relative amount of connective tissue diminishes, a lobular pattern is clearly recognizable, and the lung mass becomes more highly vascularized (see Fig. 1–4*B*). The *terminal sac period* (formerly the alveolar period) starts at around the 24th week and extends until term. The duct system of the canalicular period becomes more extensive, and the surface area of the spaces increases through the formation of saccules. The close contact between surface epithelium and blood vessels occurs at this stage; many capillaries line the walls and may project into the lumen (see Fig. 1–4*C*).

At the outset of the canalicular period, the lobular architecture of the lung, which has just made its appearance, matures more completely, and the invasion of the peripheral structures by capillaries begins. Later during this period, a capillary network appears in a recognizable air-blood barrier that contains both type I and type II alveolar epithelial cells. During the terminal sac period, progressive thinning of the epithelium and protrusion of additional capillaries into the lining layer increase the total surface area available for gas exchange until, by the 28th week, the air-blood membrane is sufficiently mature to support life.

Airways

The primordial segmental airways undergo repeated ramifications until more than the number of generations found in the adult lung have been formed. This process is usually complete by the 16th week of intrauterine life, and thereafter no further formation of airways occurs.[6] In fact, the number of generations of conducting airways is actually reduced through the transformation of distal nonrespiratory bronchioles into respiratory bronchioles by a process of alveolarization, as shown by the crosshatched area in Figure 1–2.

Connective Tissue

The cluster of proliferating bronchi invades a mass of undifferentiated mesenchymal tissue near the midline (the future mediastinum) and expands into the pleural cavities, which have become delimited from the original coelomic tube. As the mass enlarges, it becomes invested with a mesothelial lining that is continuous with the mesothelial layer of the pleural spaces (the future visceral and parietal pleuras). The progressively branching bronchi become encircled by a mass of mesenchyme that gradually differentiates into sleeves of connective tissue, layers of smooth muscle, cartilaginous rings and plates, and other supporting structures.[1] The organization of cartilage begins centrally and extends peripherally with the formation of rings that are discernible by the seventh week of gestation. Although the formation of cartilage lags behind the formation of new bronchi, spreading of cartilaginous precursors ceases at around the 25th week (see Fig. 1–2). Thereafter, the number of bronchial generations that contain cartilage remains constant and is the same as that found in the adult lung.[6]

The connective tissue elements at the periphery of the proliferating lung become increasingly scanty as development proceeds. Finally, they form only a thin network of fibers. The appearance of elastic fibers in the terminal units of the newborn is said to resemble a fishnet; moreover, the elastic network, by forming the apertures of alveoli, may serve to partition existing saccules and to shape the formation of new alveoli.[7]

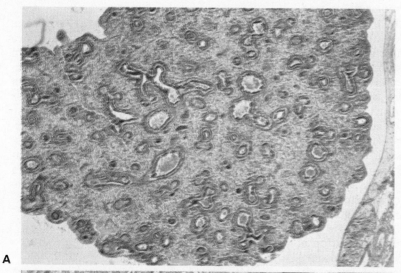

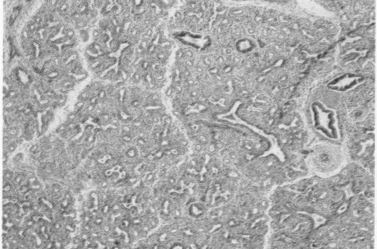

Figure 1–4. Micrographs of the lungs of the human fetuses showing: *A*, pseudoglandular period (transverse section of lung, surrounding pleural space and adjacent chest wall from about 8 weeks gestation); *B*, canalicular period (section of lung from about 20 weeks gestation); and *C*, terminal sac period (section of lung from 38 week [term] fetus). For details, see text and Plate I. (Hematoxylin and eosin stain; × 36. Courtesy of Dr. William Margaretten.)

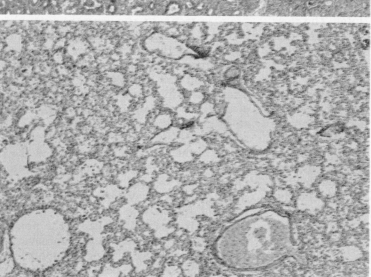

Mucus-secreting Structures

Goblet cells can be recognized in the epithelium of the trachea and proximal bronchi of the human fetus at the 13th week of intrauterine life.[8] Thereafter, they gradually appear toward the periphery, but even at term they are not found in proximal bronchioles. The origin of epithelial goblet cells is of practical importance because in chronic bronchitis and other hypersecretory diseases they increase in number throughout the airways and they are found in bronchioles, where they are normally sparse. The first evidences of bronchial gland formation are epithelial invaginations or buds that develop at about the 10th week of gestation. In bronchi the main growth period is between the 12th and 14th week of gestation, decreasing thereafter and virtually stopping in the 23rd week.[9] Few new glands are formed during infancy, and an increase in gland volume is the result of increased complexity. Mucin appears in the glands at an early stage, even before the lumen has appeared. Differentiation of the early cellular constituents of glands into mucus-secreting or serum-secreting cells and elaboration of secretions of characteristic chemical composition begin after the 26th week of fetal development and continue into the neonatal period.

Alveoli

The pattern of formation of conducting airways is such that they are complete by birth, when they may be viewed as miniature versions of their adult counterparts. In contrast, the development of alveoli follows a markedly different course. The morphology of neonatal airspaces in humans is sufficiently different from that of alveoli in adult lungs that some anatomists prefer to call them "saccules" to emphasize that morphologically recognizable alveoli do not develop until about two months after delivery.[10] Moreover, there are considerable differences in the extent of alveolar development at birth among various mammalian species.

Although true alveoli are not present at birth in some animals, such as the rat and mouse, lambs are born with well developed terminal respiratory units. As implied, the status of human beings appears to lie somewhere in between, but the extent of alveolar maturation is highly controversial. Clearly, the majority of alveoli develop after birth, although some are undoubtedly present in the newborn. Estimates of the number of alveoli vary widely—from none to 71 million—because counting them presents serious technical difficulties.[7]

The results of recent morphometric measurements in human neonates by Langston and coworkers[11] revealed a mean total alveolar number of about 50 million, with a wide normal range. Based on the observation that the formation of definite alveoli is an invariable feature of normal human fetal development, these investigators proposed adding a fifth period of intrauterine lung formation: the alveolar period, from 36 weeks to term. During this stage, true alveoli are uniformly acquired, and the alveolar surface area increases exponentially (Fig. 1–5). Between the onset of alveolar development at 30 to 32 weeks and term, the surface area increased from 1.0 to 2.0 m^2 to 3.0 to 4.0 m^2.[11] From these data and those to be presented concerning surfactant synthesis and release, it can easily be appreciated why premature birth is associated with such profound respiratory disadvantages.

BLOOD VESSELS AND CIRCULATION

The pattern of development of the pulmonary circulation in many respects follows that of the airways. Although there is obviously no movement of air in and out of the lungs during gestation, there is some perfusion of blood. However, the amount of pulmonary blood flow and the circulatory pathways differ considerably in the developing fetus from those in the newborn baby. This section will summarize prevailing concepts of normal structure and function of the fetal circulation and will introduce a few points about disturbances in disease (for review and additional references, see Reid[12]).

Pulmonary Arteries

While the lung bud is forming, primitive right and left pulmonary arteries grow caudally from the aortic sac to become associated with the developing respiratory primordium. A portion of the sixth aortic arch,

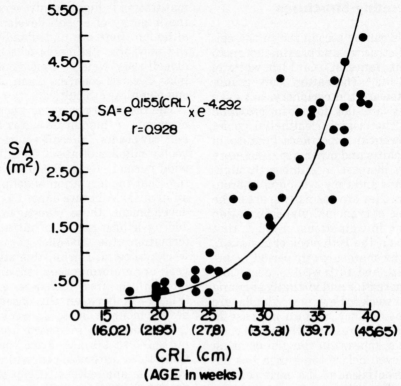

Figure 1–5. Internal surface area (SA) in square meters plotted against crown-rump length (CRL) in centimeters for lungs of 42 infants who died in late gestation or the neonatal period. Numbers in parentheses beneath those for CRL indicate the corresponding age (gestational plus chronologic) in weeks. (Reprinted by permission from Langston, C., et al.: Human lung growth in late gestation and in the neonate. Am. Rev. Respir. Dis., *129*:607–613, 1984.)

which originally joined the dorsal aorta to the roots of the pulmonary arteries, persists on the left as the ductus arteriosus.[1] Branches of the pulmonary arterial system assume a position next to branches of the bronchial system and maintain this partnership during subsequent ramifications of both airways and blood vessels, during the glandular and canalicular periods. Besides the "conventional" branches of the pulmonary arterial system (i.e., those accompanying bronchi), additional arterial vessels, the so-called "supernumerary" or "accessory" arteries, are evident by the 12th week of fetal maturation.[12] The full complement of all conventional and supernumerary arteries leading to the respiratory bronchioles, alveolar ducts, and saccules is complete in the fetus at about 16 weeks—in other words, at the same time that the adult pattern of conducting airways development is completed. In contrast to the arteries leading *to* the future gas exchange units, the arteries *within* the structures comprising the terminal units continue to proliferate, with new

ones being formed for several years after birth (see Chapter 2).

Pulmonary Veins

In early embryogenesis, the blood supply to the respiratory primordium drains into a venous plexus that empties into the heart through a single pulmonary vein. This vein becomes incorporated into the developing left atrium, and its principal tributaries on each side ultimately form the superior and inferior pulmonary veins.[1] The drainage pattern of the veins leading from the future gas exchange units to the hilus is complete about halfway through gestation and corresponds to the development of conducting airways and arteries; the fetal venous system is similar to the arterial system in that it also consists of "conventional" and "supernumerary" veins. More details about the pattern of branching, structure, and possible function of pulmonary veins are provided in the next chapter.

Pulmonary Circulation

The blood flow to the lungs during fetal development is only a small proportion of the total cardiac output. Studies in fetal lambs have revealed that mean blood flow to the lungs through the pulmonary artery is 3.7 per cent of the cardiac output in early gestation and rises to 7.0 per cent near term; expressed in another manner, the absolute magnitude of pulmonary blood flow increases from 38 ml/100 gm (lung)/min at 60 days gestation to 126 ml/100 gm (lung)/min in late gestation (140 to 150 days).[13] These values are compared with those of other organs in Table 1–1.

The increase in pulmonary blood flow with advancing gestation is accompanied by a reduction in pulmonary vascular resistance attributable to an increase in the total number of vessels, especially in the fifth and sixth generations. Although the cross-sectional area of the pulmonary vascular bed increases through the addition of new vessels, the amount of smooth muscle in each vessel is unchanged as compared with early gestation. By adding more vessels with the same amount of muscle, the total amount of smooth muscle in the lungs' vasculature increases steadily. This increase, in turn, is believed to account for the augmented fetal vasomotor reactivity to such vasoactive stimuli as hypoxia in late pregnancy.[14] It is also known that the increase in pulmonary blood flow in sheep after 120 days coincides with the appearance of increasing amounts of surface-active material in the lung,[15] and it is reasonable to infer that the change in blood flow is related to the metabolic demands associated with the production of surfactant (see section on Intrauterine Lung Function).

Blood flow in the pulmonary circulation in experimental animals is low, but the resistance to flow is high enough to maintain pulmonary arterial pressure at or even higher than the pressure in systemic arteries (Fig. 1–6). Although pulmonary vascular resistance has not been measured in human fetuses, it is probable that pressure and resistance are similar to those in other mammals. This hypothesis is believed to be true because hemodynamic conditions are reflected in the histologic appearance of blood vessels and because there is a similarity between human fetal pulmonary arteries and arteries of corresponding size in the systemic circulation. In fact, the muscle

Table 1–1. MEASUREMENT OF CARDIAC OUTPUT, DISTRIBUTION OF CARDIAC OUTPUT, AND ORGAN BLOOD FLOWS IN FETAL LAMBS OF VARIOUS ESTIMATED GESTATIONAL AGES*

Variable	Gestational Days, Estimated		
	60–85	**101–110**	**141–150**
Weight, gm	80–450	901–1500	>3600
Cardiac output			
ml/min/kg	485	549	548
% to placenta	47	45	40
Blood flow, ml/100 gm organ weight/min			
Myocardium	234	208	291
Brain	30	57	132
Lung	38	53	126
Kidney	122	117	173
Gut	40	42	69
Spleen	250	265	240

*Data from Rudolph, A. M., and Heymann, M. A.: Circulatory changes during growth in the fetal lamb. Circ. Res. 26:289–299, 1970.

layer of pulmonary arteries may be even greater than that of systemic arteries.[17] The structure of fetal pulmonary arteries undoubtedly contributes to and may in part result from the high resistance and high intravascular pressure in the pulmonary circulation. The amount of smooth muscle in the vessel walls and the pulmonary arterial pressure are interrelated, and this relationship is important in the induction or failure of changes to occur in both the structure of pulmonary arteries and the pulmonary arterial pressure following birth.

We can infer from the sudden and swift drop in pulmonary arterial pressure after birth that the high pulmonary vascular resistance does not have a purely anatomic origin. Active pulmonary arterial vasoconstriction has been demonstrated in fetal lambs through the experimental use of certain vasodilator drugs and appears to be primarily a local vasomotor response, part of which may be induced by the hypoxic condition of the fetus. Judging from the results in experimental animals, circulating catecholamines and sympathetic nervous system stimuli do not contribute to the reaction.[18]

Systemic Circulation

The major pathways of the fetal circulation are diagrammed schematically in Figure 1–7. Oxygenated blood (Po_2 28 to 30 mm Hg) from the placenta is returned to the fetus through the umbilical vein and flows

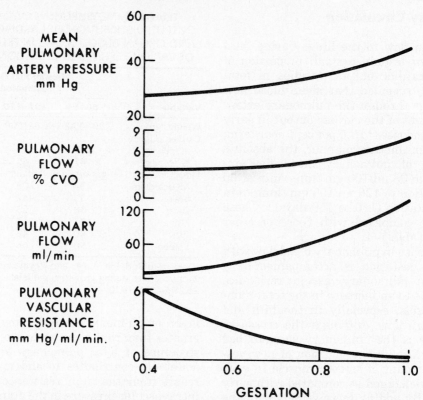

Figure 1–6. Diagrammatic representation of the changes in mean pulmonary arterial pressure, proportion of combined ventricular output (CVO) distributed to the lungs, actual pulmonary blood flow, and calculated pulmonary vascular resistance, in fetal lambs during gestational development from 0.4 of gestation to 1.0 (term). (Reprinted by permission from Rudolph, A. M.: Fetal and pulmonary circulation. Am. Rev. Respir. Dis. *115*(suppl.)11–18, 1977.)

through the ductus venosus and inferior vena cava into the right atrium; as most of the incoming blood from the placenta flows into the right atrium it is preferentially shunted through the foramen ovale into the left atrium and left ventricle, from which it is ejected into the ascending aorta for distribution to the organs supplied by the brachiocephalic vessels. Venous blood returning to the right atrium from the superior vena cava passes into the right ventricle and is injected into the pulmonary artery; from the pulmonary artery most of the incoming blood from the head and upper extremities is shunted through the ductus arteriosus into the descending aorta for distribution to the placenta and the lower part of the body. Thus, the fetal vascular system is elegantly designed for the useful purpose of distributing blood with the highest O_2 content to the heart and to the brain; conversely, blood with the least amount of O_2 is distributed to the placenta, where the O_2 supply is replenished. The lung, it should be pointed out, mainly receives poorly oxy-genated blood through the pulmonary artery, so it is among the relatively less favored (i.e., more hypoxic) fetal organs. A comparison between fetal and maternal blood gases in human beings just prior to birth is presented in Table 1–2.

Table 1–2. SYSTEMIC BLOOD GASES AND ACID-BASE VALUES IN MATERNAL (ARTERIAL) AND FETAL (UTERINE VEIN) BLOOD SPECIMENS OBTAINED DURING CESAREAN SECTION BEFORE SPONTANEOUS BREATHING BY THE FETUS OCCURRED*†

Variable	Maternal Blood	Fetal Blood
Arterial P_{O_2}, mm Hg	97 ± 3	29 ± 3
Arterial P_{CO_2}, mm Hg	26 ± 2	37 ± 7
Arterial pH, units	7.48 ± 0.06	7.31 ± 0.08
Buffer base, mEq/L	43 ± 5	35 ± 5
Base excess, mEq/L	−2 ± 3	−9 ± 3

*Data from Spackman et al.: Acid-base status of the fetus in human pregnancy. Obstet. Gynecol. *22*:785–791, 1963.
†Values are expressed as the mean ± standard deviation.

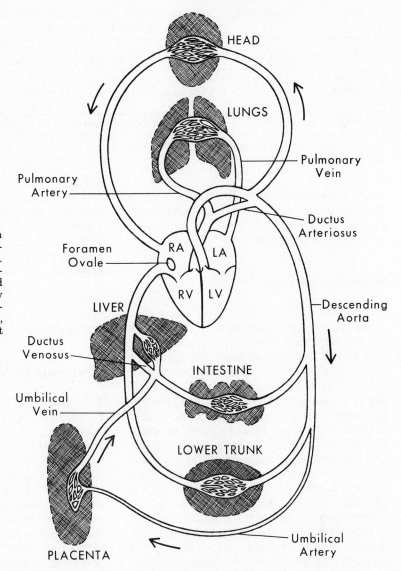

Figure 1–7. Schematic diagram of the human fetal circulation. Arrows show direction of blood flow. (Adapted and reprinted by permission from Rudolph, A. M., and Heymann, M. A.: Circulatory changes during growth in the fetal lamb. Circ. Res., *26*:289–299, 1970; and The American Heart Association, Inc.)

Labels in figure: HEAD, LUNGS, Pulmonary Vein, Pulmonary Artery, Ductus Arteriosus, Foramen Ovale, RA, LA, RV, LV, Descending Aorta, LIVER, Ductus Venosus, INTESTINE, Umbilical Vein, LOWER TRUNK, Umbilical Artery, PLACENTA

INTRAUTERINE LUNG FUNCTION

The fetal lung is not used as a gas exchange organ, and the question of whether it fulfills some of the nonrespiratory functions it provides in postnatal life, such as filtering and serving as a blood reservoir, providing host defenses, and activating and inactivating biologic substances, has not been thoroughly examined. There is limited evidence that the capacity of the fetal lung to inactivate angiotensin I and bradykinin (see Chapter 12) is much reduced compared with that of the adult lung; however, this capability increases remarkably during the postnatal period. Inactivation of prostaglandins E_1 and E_2 is well developed in the pulmonary circulations of fetal lambs and

fetal rabbits, and remains high for one week after birth (see Bakhle[19a] for review and additional references). It seems likely that the nonrespiratory functions of the fetal lung are quite different from those of mature lungs because of the different requirements between intrauterine and extrauterine life.

There are, however, three special features of prenatal lung function that deserve consideration: first, the secretory role of the developing lungs, because this contributes to the intrauterine environment in which the fetus matures; second, the synthesis of surface-active materials (surfactant), which are crucial to the function of the postnatal lung, beginning with the first breath and continuing thereafter; and third, the presence of intrauterine breathing movements,

Table 1–3. COMPOSITION OF LUNG LIQUID, LUNG LYMPH, AND
PLASMA IN MATURE FETAL LAMBS*

Source	Na⁺ mEq/kg†	K⁺ mEq/kg	Ca⁺⁺ mEq/kg	Cl⁻ mEq/kg	HCO₃⁻ mEq/kg	Protein g/100 ml
Lung liquid	150	6.3	0.86	157	2.8	0.03
Lung lymph	147	4.8	–	107	25	3.27
Plasma	150	4.8	2.49	107	24	4.09

*Data from Adamson, T. M., et al.: Composition of alveolar liquid in the foetal lamb. J. Physiol. (Lond.), *204*:159–169, 1969; and Olver, R. E., and Strang, L. B.: Ion fluxes across the pulmonary epithelium and the secretion of lung liquid in the foetal lamb. J. Physiol. (Lond.), *241*:327–357, 1974.
†kg water in each instance

which presumably serve the useful purpose of exercising the developing respiratory muscles and readying them for sustained ventilation after birth.

Secretion of Lung Liquid

A unique function of lungs *in utero*, compared with the postpartum state, is the constant secretion of a relatively large volume of liquid (2 to 3 ml/hr/kg in fetal lambs) by the transfer of solutes and water across the capillary endothelium and the epithelium of the developing lungs. Once formed, the liquid moves up the tracheobronchial system to the mouth, where it is swallowed or added to amniotic liquid.[20] Certain epithelial surfaces of postnatal lungs and airways have an important ongoing secretory role (see Chapter 2), but fetal lungs differ because of the requirements of the transition to air breathing: at or before birth liquid secretion must be switched off or markedly reduced, the liquid must be rapidly removed from the airways and airspaces, the lungs must remain aerated, and the new gas-blood barrier must become relatively impermeable to the passage of liquid from the blood vessels into the airspaces.

The compositions of lung liquid, lung lymph, and plasma in mature fetal lambs are shown in Table 1–3. The striking characteristics of lung liquid, in comparison with lymph and plasma, are its high Cl⁻ and K⁺ concentrations and its low HCO₃⁻, protein, and Ca⁺⁺ concentrations. The best explanation for these differences is that there is active transport of Cl⁻ in excess of a reverse flux of HCO₃⁻, with Na⁺ being transferred passively by the electrical gradient caused by Cl⁻ movement; net water flow is caused by the osmotic force of NaCl.[20] The extremely low protein concentration of alveolar liquid, which is 100 times less than the

concentration in lymph and plasma, means that the respiratory epithelium is virtually impermeable to macromolecules. No definitive studies have established either the location or the type of cells responsible for fetal ion transport and water flux. Late in gestation, surface active material, which is secreted by type II epithelial cells of the terminal sacs, can be identified in tracheal and amniotic liquids.

Synthesis of Surfactant

At about the 24th week of gestation, type II epithelial cells (granular pneumocytes) appear in the alveolar epithelium, and shortly afterward their characteristic osmiophilic *lamellar inclusion bodies* (Fig. 1–8) are detectable. These cells become more numerous until the 30th to 32nd week of human fetal development and are temporally related to the appearance of surface-active substances in the lungs and amniotic liquid (Fig. 1–9). The biochemical processes involved in the synthesis of surfactant have been studied carefully because of its vital role in maintaining postnatal lung function. If the production of surface-active substances is faulty or delayed or if a baby is born prematurely before adequate amounts have been synthesized and released, the neonatal respiratory distress syndrome (hyaline membrane disease) is likely to develop. These observations have led to the development of screening tests to detect the presence of pulmonary surface-active material in amniotic liquid.[24, 25] These tests have a high predictive value for the neonatal respiratory distress syndrome and are of considerable assistance in timing elective deliveries, in applying vigorous preventive therapeutic maneuvers to the newborn infant, and in deciding whether or not to treat the mother before delivery with a cortico-

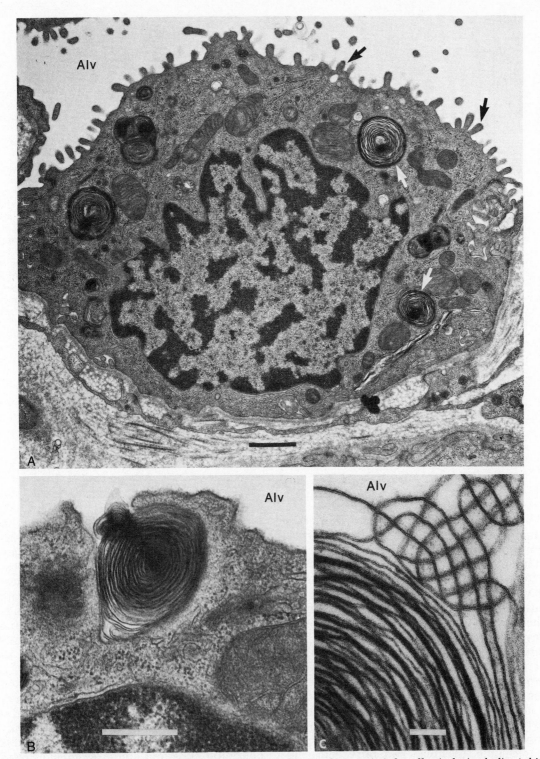

Figure 1–8. *A*, Type II epithelial cell from a human lung showing characteristic lamellar inclusion bodies (white arrows) within cell and microvilli (black arrows) projecting into alveolus (Alv). Horizontal line = 1μm. *B*, Beginning exocytosis of a lamellar body into the alveolar space of a human lung. Horizontal line = 0.5μm. *C*, Secreted lamellar body and newly formed tubular myelin in alveolar liquid in a fetal rat lung. Membrane continuities between outer lamellae and adjacent tubular myelin provide evidence of intraalveolar tubular myelin formation. Horizontal line = 0.1μm. (Courtesy of Dr. Mary C. Williams.)

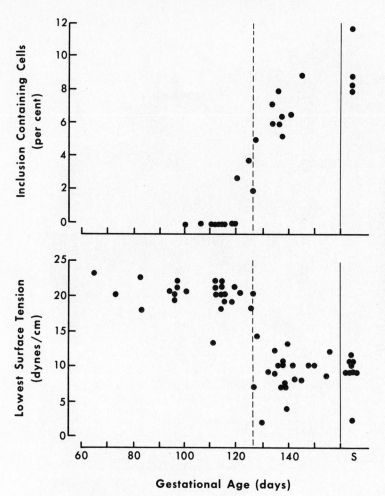

Figure 1–9. The number of alveolar cells containing osmiophilic inclusion bodies expressed as percentage of total lung tissue cells (upper panel) and the lowest surface tensions of lung extracts (lower panel) according to gestational age of fetal and spontaneously delivered (S) lambs. The interrupted vertical line at 126 days of gestation indicates the age after which surfactant is normally detectable. (Replotted and reprinted by permission from Orzalesi, M. A. et al.: The development of the lungs of lambs. Pediatrics, *35*:373–381, 1965.)

steroid (e.g., betamethasone) to accelerate functional maturation of the fetal surfactant-producing system.

Investigations by King and Clements[26] to determine the chemical composition of pulmonary surfactant have revealed four different surface-active fractions with similar chemical and physical properties. These investigators showed that surface active material is a complex mixture composed chiefly of lipids and a lesser amount of several proteins (Table 1–4). The protein most extensively studied, the surfactant apoprotein, appears on the basis of its immunoreactivity to be unique to the lung.[27] Among the lipids, the most important appears to be phosphatidylcholine, to which two fatty acids are added. As shown in Table 1–4, the most common fatty acid component is palmitate, which gives rise to dipalmitoylphosphatidylcholine (DPPC), a potent surface active substance. Because of the predominance of DPPC, the phosphatidylcholines in the

lungs differ from those in other organs in that approximately 35 per cent are disaturated. Recent data indicate that there may be a sequence of development of incorporation of different fatty acids into surface-active material during fetal maturation and that the presence of "immature" fatty acids correlates with the presence of hyaline membrane disease.[28] Further information about the synthesis of surfactant and of DPPC is provided in Chapter 12.

The sequence of intracellular storage and the subsequent release of surface-active material and its movement to the surface film is shown schematically in Figure 1–10. Surfactant is formed in the cytoplasm of type II epithelial cells and stored as folded layers in the lamellar bodies (see Fig. 1–8). How the newly synthesized phospholipid is transported to the lamellar bodies is unknown. After a lamellar body is completely formed, it migrates to the apical surface of the cell and is released, presumably by membrane

Table 1–4. COMPOSITION OF PULMONARY SURFACE–ACTIVE MATERIAL*

Chemical Components (%)		Lipid Fractions (%)		Phosphatidylcholine Fatty Acid Components (%)	
Lipid	85	Phosphatidylcholine	75	Palmitate(16:0)	71
Protein	13	Neutral lipid	9.1	Myristate(14:0)	6.1
Hexose	<1.7	Cholesterol	6.6	Stearate(18:0)	3.6
Nucleic acid	<0.7	Phosphatidylethanolamine	6.3	Palmitoleate(16:1)	11
Hexosamine	<0.5	Sphingomyelin	2.1	Oleate(18:1)	3.9
		Lysolecithin	0.9	Unidentified	3.6

*Data from King, R. J., and Clements, J. A.: Surface active materials from dog lung. II. Composition and physiological correlations. Am. J. Physiol., *223*:715–726, 1972.

fusion and exocytosis, into the overlying liquid subphase. After extrusion, many of the lamellar bodies seem to unravel, and the surfactant is transformed into a second form, *tubular myelin.* How tubular myelin and other precursors are finally incorporated into the monomolecular surface film is uncertain. Similarly, it is not known what happens to effete or inactivated surfactant, although the catabolism of the various lipid and protein constituents involves different turnover times; some surfactant has been identified after being phagocytosed by alveolar macrophages, and some appears to go back into and to be recycled by type II cells.[29]

Toward the end of gestation, the concentrations of endogenous corticosteriods increase in the blood stream and influence lung development in exactly the same manner as exogenously administered steroids. Glucocorticoid activity in the lungs, as in other organs, depends on the presence of cytoplasmic receptors with high affinity and specificity. The binding between steroid and

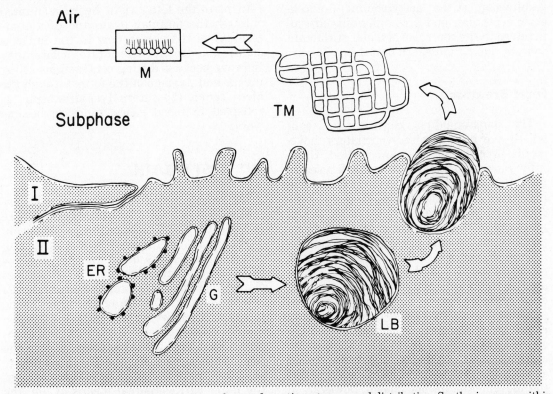

Figure 1–10. Presumed pathway of lung surfactant formation, storage, and distribution. Synthesis occurs within type II cell, beginning in the endoplasmic reticulum (ER) and progressing through the Golgi (G) to the lamellar bodies (LB) where it is stored. The lamellar bodies migrate to the apical surface of the cell and are ejected into the alveolar subphase, where they expand into tubular myelin (TM) figures, which, in turn, spread as a monolayer (M) at the air-liquid interface. (Compare with Fig. 1–6.) (Reprinted by permission from Goerke, J.: Lung Surfactant. Biochim. Biophys. Acta, *344*:241–261, 1974.)

receptor causes the complex to migrate into the nucleus, attach tightly to the components of chromatin, and influence the rate of synthesis of messenger ribonucleic acid for specific proteins. Administration of corticosteroids to pregnant rats has been shown to increase the activity of the enzyme phosphatidic acid phosphatase (PAPase), which stimulates choline incorporation into lecithin, one of the key steps in the synthesis of surfactant. Glucocorticoid activity has been detected in fetal and adult lungs from several mammalian species, including fetal and newborn humans.[30]

Although several other humoral substances, such as thyroid hormone, β-sympathetic agonists, acetylcholine, prostaglandins, and estradiol, are known to increase surfactant synthesis,[31] the constellation of factors that regulate its production and release in health and disease is poorly understood. Direct neural control is unlikely because the type II cells do not appear to be innervated. However, an increase in ventilation increased the content of alveolar surfactant in experimental animals, and the results suggest that acetylcholine, β-adrenergic receptors, and prostaglandins are all involved in the control of alveolar surfactant content during increased breathing.[32]

Fetal Breathing

The long-standing controversy about whether or not organized ventilatory movements precede birth is now settled. Carefully conducted studies in lamb fetuses *in utero* demonstrate fetal gasping or breathing activity, consisting of movements of the chest and diaphragm, that appear about midgestation and continue until term.[33] Respiratory movements are detectable approximately 45 per cent of the time during usual recording periods and appear to be associated with neural activity within the medulla, phrenic nerves, or intercostal nerves; movements are invariably present during rapid eye movements (a phase of sleep described in Chapter 10) but do not appear to correlate with changes in arterial blood gases.[33] The factors that control fetal breathing movements are not known; however, in fetal sheep they are profoundly inhibited by prostaglandins.[34]

Furthermore, episodic chest wall movements, similar to those observed in fetal lambs, have been recorded in human fetuses. Using ultrasonic techniques, investigators found these movements to be present about 65 per cent of the time.[35] Thus it is incontrovertible that the maturing human fetus can generate spontaneous activity in its neural pathways and muscles concerned with breathing. Although these movements are brief and weak (they are insufficient to cause tidal flow of amniotic liquid), they reflect to some extent how healthy the fetus will be at birth.[36] It is tempting to speculate that antenatal breathing affords practice to the ventilatory system of the fetus to help ready it for the formidable task of breathing during the transition to extrauterine life.

And so the time of birth finally arrives. The fetus, accustomed to a warm but hypoxic, hypercarbic, and acidotic medium, all alien to its future extrauterine environment, lies submerged in amniotic fluid. Its liquid-filled lungs have never served as a gas exchanger, and although episodic respiratory movements have occurred, they are probably considerably weaker than those required after birth. Most of the blood that returns to the fetus' right heart is shunted through the foramen ovale and ductus arteriosus so that blood flow to the lungs is small. Conditions deteriorate before they improve because during contractions of the uterus and passage of the fetus through the birth canal, the internal environment, as reflected in blood gases, tends to become worse.

THE FIRST BREATH

The events of delivery and birth are dominated by the legacy of nature because there is little that can be done by participating parties that will influence the multitude of changes that must occur in the first few minutes of extrauterine life. The traditional slap, aspiration of the oropharynx, and even attempts at insufflation of the lungs made to assist the newborn are minuscule external efforts compared with the extensive internal adjustments taking place. Within the few minutes required for the placenta to separate from the uterus, which removes the fetus' extracorporeal means of life, the newborn must "turn on" his central and autonomic nervous systems, replace the liquid in his lungs with air, establish a substantial pulmonary circulation, and markedly revise the direction of blood flow through his cardiac chambers and great vessels. These processes should not be considered separate but rather as interdependent events essential to the development of a cardiorespiratory system capable of maintaining an adequate supply of O_2 to the infant's body. That these complex requirements are met seems miraculous, but they are met—usually perfectly—thousands of times a day and more often, in fact, if one considers that all mammals presumably undergo the same fundamental physiologic transformations at birth.

The climax of delivery is the first breath, an event that can also be viewed as the ending of fetal existence and the beginning of postnatal life. However, before the first breath is taken, the respiratory center of the central nervous system must integrate incoming afferent impulses and initiate efferent signals to the respiratory muscles. The factors that control breathing in children and adults are reasonably well understood and are described in Chapter 10. In contrast, exact knowledge of the mechanisms that underlie the onset of rhythmic ventilation during the transition from fetal to neonatal life does not exist. Although the mature fetus makes frequent respiratory movements, the responses of its control systems behave as if they were relatively suppressed. Thus, in the fetus the carotid chemoreceptors seem inactive, and central responses to hypoxia and hypercapnia appear to be present but blunted; some vagally mediated reflexes are intact, but the importance of these is problematic. Breathing in the newborn, therefore, must be the result of either removing inhibitory influences or actuating previously inactive systems, or both.[37]

A plausible hypothesis, which includes the interacting and compounding influences of the multiple stimuli associated with delivery and removal of the newborn from its former "buffered" environment, can be proposed to explain the onset and persistence of breathing after birth. A profound drive to breathe must accompany the hypoxia and hypercapnia that follow clamping of the cord or separation of the placenta. Sensory stimuli, which may result at birth from new thermal, tactile, and other exteroceptive and proprioceptive stimuli, in the absence of changes in blood gases, can initiate rhythmic breathing.[38] However, we must acknowledge ignorance about the relative importance of these various complex neurologic contributions to the first breath.

After the first breath, the newborn breathes rapidly and shallowly for about 90 minutes with frequent interruptions of expiration. Probably one of the most important stimuli to sustain neonatal breathing comes from the carotid chemoreceptors, which are inactive or nearly so in the fetus. Activation occurs soon after birth, and the newly established chemosensitivity appears to provide a crucial excitatory input to the reticular formation that offsets the inhibitory response to hypoxia that characterized the fetal state.[39] Further information about the maturation of respiratory control appears in Chapter 14.

Expansion of the Lungs

Once initiated, the contractions of the respiratory muscles must generate sufficient force to (1) move air and a column of liquid (that is 100 times more viscous than air) ahead of it into the lungs, (2) overcome the forces of surface tension at the interface of the contiguous columns of air and liquid moving through small airways, and (3) distend the lung tissues. Measurements made using an esophageal balloon have revealed that human infants produce extreme negative intrathoracic pressures of 40 to 80 cm H_2O during the first few breaths.[40] Figure 1–11 depicts the pressure-volume curves of the first three breaths of a normal newborn infant. High distending pressures from muscular contraction during inspiration are followed by vigorous expiratory efforts associated with positive or collapsing pressures during expiration. All the air that is taken in during the first inspiration is usually not completely exhaled, because if it were, either the lung would collapse or the liquid that had been displaced would return again. Some air is retained with each of the first few breaths so that a functional residual capacity (FRC) is gradually established. (The FRC is the amount of air left in the lungs at the end of passive expiration; normally, FRC is the lung volume at which the forces tending to expand the chest wall are balanced by the forces tending to retract the lung.) At 10 minutes of age, the FRC of a newborn human is about 17 ml/kg body weight. At 30 minutes of age, the volume

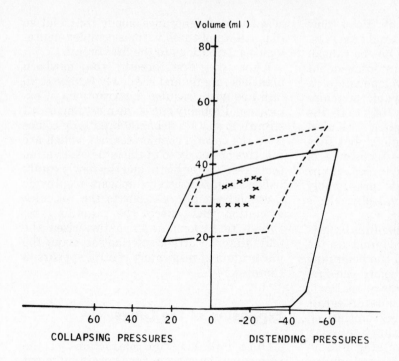

Volume (ml)

COLLAPSING PRESSURES   DISTENDING PRESSURES

Figure 1–11. Schematic representation of the relationships between the distending and collapsing pressures and the resulting volumes during the first (——), second (----), and third (xxxxx) breaths. (Reprinted by permission from Avery, M. E. et al.: The Lung and Its Disorders in the Newborn Infant. 4th ed. Philadelphia, W. B. Saunders Co., 1981, p. 33.)

has increased to 25 to 35 ml/kg, a value that does not change further during the next four days.[41]

Removal of Lung Liquid

The amount of liquid in the lungs at birth has never been measured in humans; in fetal lambs the lungs contain about 50 ml of liquid, which is approximately equal to the volume of the air-filled lungs at their resting position (FRC) a few hours after birth. The FRC might be expected to decrease in the newborn period because of the inward recoil forces exerted by the film of surfactant at the newly formed air-liquid interface. The constancy of FRC is probably attributable to the offsetting outward recoil of the chest wall due to progressive recruitment and tone of skeletal muscles.

Several factors act in concert and serve to promote removal of liquid from fetal lungs. Formerly, it was believed that some of the liquid was removed during labor, but most was removed after delivery. New data indicate that the process actually begins late in gestation (i.e., well before labor begins), when approximately one-third of the liquid leaves the lungs; another 19 per cent is removed during delivery, and the remaining 40 to 50 per cent is cleared during the 24 hours after birth.[42] Furthermore, previous

notions about the respective contributions of the pulmonary circulation and the pulmonary lymphatics to the removal of the excess fetal lung liquid have been revised and clarified. Although most of this information has been obtained from studies of experimental animals, it is likely that the same general phenomena occur in humans as well.

It is now well established that the rate of secretion of lung liquid decreases for several days before spontaneous delivery.[43] The factors controlling the decrease in secretion are unknown, but they presumably depend on the hormonal changes that accompany late gestation in mother and fetus. During labor, there is a further decrease in the amount of liquid in the lungs from increased reabsorption, which causes the volume of the potential airspaces to decrease;[44] again, the mechanisms underlying this phenomenon are unknown. Infusion of β-adrenergic agonists causes an increase in reabsorption of fetal lung liquid in experimental animals,[45] but endogenous release of epinephrine during spontaneous delivery of lambs could not be established.[44] Because pulmonary lymphatic drainage does not increase during labor, the liquid must be removed by the bloodstream, a process that is facilitated by the concomitant increase in plasma protein concentration that occurs. After delivery, as the lungs are inflated, the remaining liquid is displaced from the aerating saccules to the interstitial spaces surrounding the conducting airways and blood vessels (discussed more fully in Chapters 2 and 12). From these new locations, where it has little or no effect on gas exchange, the liquid is slowly cleared from the lungs. Lymph drainage from the lungs increases slightly and transiently after delivery, and accounts for removal of only about 10 per cent of the residual liquid present in the lungs at birth.[44] Another important and desirable consequence of the removal of lung liquid is that the suspended surfactant is concentrated and deposited on the alveolar epithelial surface, thus equipping the newborn with an "instant" surface film.

Immediately after the start of respiration, in the newborn, the volume within the saccules consists of both displaced lung liquid and air. A few hours are required before all the residual liquid is replaced by air, and even though the infant no longer generates such high negative intrathoracic pressures as it did during the first few breaths, a negative interstitial pressure is maintained by the recoil characteristics of the lungs, including that contributed by the newly deposited layer of surfactant on the alveolar surface. Because surfactant serves to stabilize small airspaces, it is of special importance in determining the mechanical properties of the tiny saccules in the lungs of infants.[46] Furthermore, it has recently been shown that the presence of surfactant at the air-liquid interface serves to maintain the normal impermeability of the alveolar epithelium to protein.[47]

Pulmonary Vascular Resistance Changes

An important concomitant of the first breath is the decrease in pulmonary vascular resistance and the increase in flow of blood to the lungs through the pulmonary circulation. At least three mechanisms contribute to the fall in pulmonary vascular resistance: (1) replacement of the liquid in the lungs by air and establishment of an air-liquid interface at the alveolar surface—these phenomena change the geometry of the alveolus and the newly produced surface forces "pull open" capillaries and other small vessels exposed to alveolar pressure; (2) increase of the Po_2 within the alveoli—this process alleviates alveolar hypoxia and in turn relieves a pulmonary arterial vasoconstrictor stimulus acting upon intensely reactive blood vessels; and (3) decrease of Pco_2 within the alveoli—this also decreases pulmonary arterial vasoconstriction, although it has not been established whether the response is a direct effect of changing Pco_2 or an indirect effect of pH.

Administration of both α- and β-adrenergic agonists and cholinergic and vagal stimuli elicit vasomotor responses in the fetal pulmonary circulation; however, it appears that neither parasympathetic nor sympathetic nerves exert a significant tonic effect on pulmonary blood vessels in the intact fetus.[48] Experiments with blocking drugs and surgical denervation have shown that the vasodilatation in the newborn is a local phenomenon and not dependent on neurohumoral mechanisms. Thus, it seems clear that of all the possible influences, the major cause of the remarkable decrease in pulmonary vascular resistance immediately after birth is locally mediated vasodilatation from the greatly increased Po_2 to which pulmonary vessels are exposed. Recruitment of new, previously poorly perfused vessels probably also contributes, by increasing the cross-sectional area of the pulmonary circulation, to the decrease in vascular resistance.[20]

Distending the pulmonary vessels with blood helps slightly to inflate the lung with air. However, it seems certain that this is of secondary importance compared with the beneficial effects on pulmonary vascular resistance of replacing the liquid with air and raising alveolar Po_2.

Other Circulatory Adjustments

Another important consequence of the phenomena of the first breath is the alteration of the patterns of blood flow that existed during gestation. Accompanying the fall in pulmonary vascular resistance is a reversal of blood flow through the ductus arteriosus from right to left (fetal state) to left to right (newborn state); flow through the ductus arteriosus, which is labile the first few days of life, gradually ceases as the ductus closes. The shunt of blood from right atrium to left atrium through the foramen ovale, another hallmark of the fetal circulation, also ceases soon after birth. The distensibility characteristics of the left atrium do not allow it to accommodate the extra volume of blood that it must receive after pulmonary vascular resistance decreases—and essentially the entire cardiac output flows through the lungs—without a pressure increase sufficient to close the foramen.

It has been suggested that generation of kinins, potent vasoactive substances, may play a role in some of the immediate postnatal hemodynamic adjustments such as pulmonary vasodilatation, constriction of the umbilical circulation, and closure of the ductus arteriosus.[49] Although the first two possibilities have not been excluded, recent evidence suggests that other factors contribute to ductus closure. Two mechanisms have been identified: (1) a functional closure, which usually occurs within a few hours to days after birth, and then (2) an anatomic closure that is usually complete by the second week of life. The functional significance of an open ductus to the fetal circulation has already been stressed. A widely patent state is attributable to the smooth muscle relaxant effects of prostaglandins of the E series,[50] which are produced in response to the low P_{O_2} in the fetal circulation. After birth, with its accompanying increase in arterial P_{O_2}, the hypoxic stimulus is removed, the prostaglandin level decreases, and the ductus constricts. The ductus can be made to dilate again, at least during the first three to four days after delivery, by administration of prostaglandin E_2; advantage is taken of this responsiveness in newborn babies with ductus arteriosus–dependent congenital heart disease.[51]

The respiratory and circulatory systems of the fetus are thus well prepared to adapt immediately to the strenuous requirements of neonatal life. However, once the severe tests of the newborn period have been surmounted, the lungs must continue to grow in order to meet the demands for increased gas exchange of the adult. Postnatal growth and development of the lung will be considered in the next chapter.

REFERENCES

1. Krahl, V. E.: Anatomy of the mammalian lung. In Fenn, W. O., and Rahn, H. (eds.): Handbook of Physiology, Section 3. Respiration. Vol. I. Washington, D.C., American Physiological Society, 1964, pp. 213–284.
2. Reid, L.: The embryology of the lung. In De Reuck, A. V. S., and Porter, R. (eds.): Ciba Foundation Symposium: Development of the Lung. Boston, Little, Brown and Company, 1967, pp. 109–124.
3. Hislop, A., and Reid, L.: Growth and development of the respiratory system. In Davis, J. A., and Dopping, J. (eds.): Scientific Foundations of Paediatrics. London, Heineman, 1974, pp. 214–254.
4. Weibel, E. R.: Morphometry of the Human Lung. Berlin, Springer-Verlag, 1963, p. 111.
5. Burri, P. H.: Fetal and postnatal development of the lung. Annu. Rev. Physiol., 46:617–628, 1984.
6. Bucher, U., and Reid, L. M.: Development of the intrasegmental bronchial tree: The pattern of branching and development of cartilage at various stages of intra-uterine life. Thorax, 16:207–218, 1961.
7. Thurlbeck, W. M.: State of the Art Review. Postnatal growth and development of the lung. Am. Rev. Respir. Dis., 111:803–844, 1975.
8. Bucher, U., and Reid, L.: Development of the mucus-secreting elements in human lung. Thorax, 16:216–225, 1961.
9. Jeffrey, P. K., and Reid, M.: Ultrastructure of airway epithelium and submucosal gland during development. In Hodson, W. A. (ed): Development of the Lung. New York, Marcel Dekker, Inc., 1977, pp. 87–134.
10. Boyden, E. A., and Tompsett, D. H.: The changing patterns in the developing lungs of infants. Acta Anat. (Basel), 61:164–192, 1965.
11. Langston, C., Kida, K., Reed, L. M., and Thurlbeck, W. M.: Human lung growth in late gestation and in the neonate. Am. Rev. Respir. Dis., 129:607–613, 1984.
12. Reid, L. M.: The 1978 J. Burns Amberson Lecture. The pulmonary circulation: Remodeling in growth and disease. Am. Rev. Respir. Dis., 119:531–546, 1979.
13. Rudolph, A. M., and Heymann, M. A.: Circulatory changes during growth in the fetal lamb. Circ. Res., 26:289–299, 1970.
14. Levin, D. L., Rudolph, A. M., Heymann, M. A., and Phibbs, R. H.: Morphological development of the pulmonary vascular bed in fetal lambs. Circulation, 53:144–151, 1976.
15. Howatt, W. F., Avery, M. E., Humphreys, P. W., Normand, I. C. S., Reid, L., and Strang, L. B.: Factors affecting pulmonary surface properties in the foetal lamb. Clin. Sci., 29:239–248, 1965.
16. Rudolph, A. M.: Fetal and neonatal pulmonary circulation. Am. Rev. Respir. Dis., 115(Suppl.): 11–18, 1977.
17. Naeye, R. L.: Arterial changes during the perinatal period. Arch. Pathol., 71:121–128, 1961.
18. Dawes, G. S.: Pulmonary circulation in the foetus and the newborn. In De Reuck, A. V. S., and Porter, R. (eds.): Ciba Foundation Symposium: Development of the Lung. Boston, Little, Brown and Company, 1967, pp. 332–347.
19. Spackman, T., Fuchs, F., and Assali, N. S.: Acid-base status of the fetus in human pregnancy. Obstet. Gynecol., 22:785–791, 1963.
19a. Bakhle, Y. S.: Pulmonary metabolism of arachidonic acid. An endocrine function of lung. In Becker, K. L., and Gazdar, A. F. (eds.): The Endocrine Lung in Health and Disease. Philadelphia, W. B. Saunders Co., 1984, pp. 98–119.
20. Strang, L. B.: Growth and development of the lung: fetal and postnatal. Annu. Rev. Physiol., 39:253–276, 1977.
21. Adamson, T. M., Boyd, R. D. H., Platt, H. S., and

Strang, L. B.: Composition of alveolar liquid in the foetal lamb. J. Physiol. (Lond.), *204*:159–169, 1969.

22. Olver, R. E., and Strang, L. B.: Ion fluxes across the pulmonary epithelium and the secretion of lung liquid in the foetal lamb. J. Physiol. (Lond.), *241*:327–357, 1974.

23. Orzalesi, M. A., Motoyama, E. K., Jacobson, H. N., Kikkawa, Y., Reynolds, O. R., and Cook, C. D.: The development of the lungs of lambs. Pediatrics, *35*:373–381, 1965.

24. Gluck, L., Kulovich, M. V., Borer, R. C., Jr., Brenner, P. H., Anderson, G. G., and Spellacy, W. N.: Diagnosis of the respiratory distress syndrome by amniocentesis. Am. J. Obstet. Gynecol., *109*:440–445, 1971.

25. Clements, J. A., Platzker, A. C. G., Tierney, D. F., Hobel, C. J., Creasy, R. K., Margolis, A. J., Thibeault, D. W., Tooley, W. H., and Oh, W.: Assessment of the risk of the respiratory-distress syndrome by a rapid test for surfactant in amniotic fluid. New Engl. J. Med., *286*:1077–1081, 1972.

26. King, R. J., and Clements, J. A.: Surface active materials from dog lung. II Composition and physiological correlations. Am. J. Physiol., *223*:715–726, 1972.

27. King, R. J.: Pulmonary surfactant. J. Appl. Physiol., *53*:1–8, 1982.

28. Shelley, S. A., Kovacevic, M., Paciga, J. E., and Balis, J. U.: Sequential changes of surfactant phosphatidylcholine in hyaline-membrane disease of the newborn. New Engl. J. Med., *300*:112–116, 1979.

29. Goerke, J.: Lung surfactant. Biochim. Biophys. Acta, *344*:241–261, 1974.

30. Ballard, P. L.: Glucocorticoid effects in the fetal lung. Am. Rev. Respir. Dis., *115*(Suppl.):29–36, 1977.

31. Rooney, S. A.: The surfactant system and lung phospholipid biochemistry. Am. Rev. Respir. Dis., *131*:439–460, 1985.

32. Oyarzun, M. J., and Clements, J. A.: Control of lung surfactant by ventilation, adrenergic mediators, and prostaglandins in the rabbit. Am. Rev. Respir. Dis., *117*:879–891, 1981.

33. Dawes, G. S., Fox, H. E., Leduc, B. M., Liggins, G. C., and Richards, R. T.: Respiratory movements and rapid eye movement sleep in the foetal lamb. J. Physiol. (Lond.), *220*:119–143, 1972.

34. Kitterman, J. A., Liggins, G. C., Fewell, J. E., and Tooley, W. H.: Inhibition of breathing movements in fetal sheep by prostaglandins. J. Appl. Physiol., *54*:687–692, 1983.

35. Boddy, K., and Mantell, C. D.: Observations of fetal breathing movements transmitted through maternal abdominal wall. Lancet, *2*:1219–1220, 1972.

36. Platt, L. D., Manning, F. A., Lemay, M., and Sipos, L.: Human fetal breathing: relationship to fetal condition. Am. J. Obstet. Gynecol., *1322*:514–518, 1978.

37. Woodrum, D. R., Guthrie, R. D., and Hodson, W. A.: Development of respiratory control mechanisms in the fetus and newborn. *In* Hodson, W. A. (ed): Development of the Lung. New York, Marcel Dekker, Inc., 1977, pp. 561–585.

38. Jansen, A. H., and Chernick, V.: Development of respiratory control. Physiol. Rev., *63*:437–483, 1983.

39. Walker, D. W.: Peripheral and central chemoreceptors in the fetus and newborn. Annu. Rev. Physiol., *46*:687–703, 1984.

40. Karlberg, P.: The adaptive changes in the immediate postnatal period, with particular reference to respiration. J. Pediatr., *56*:585–604, 1960.

41. Avery, M. E., Fletcher, B. D., and Williams, R. G.: The Lung and Its Disorders in the Newborn Infant. 4th Ed. Philadelphia, W. B. Saunders Co., 1981, p. 33.

42. Bland, R. D.: Dynamics of pulmonary water before and after birth. Acta Paediatr. Scand. (Suppl), *305*:12–20, 1983.

43. Kitterman, J. A., Ballard, P. L., Clements, J. A., Mescher, E. J., and Tooley, W. H.: Tracheal fluid in fetal lambs: spontaneous decrease prior to birth. J. Appl. Physiol., *47*:985–989, 1979.

44. Bland, R. D., Hansen, T. N., Haberkern, C. M., Bressack, M. A., Hazinski, T. A., Raj, J. U., and Goldberg, R. B.: Lung fluid balance in lambs before and after birth. J. Appl. Physiol., *53*:992–1004, 1982.

45. Walters, D. W., and Olver, R. E.: The role of catecholamines in lung liquid absorption at birth. Pediatr. Res., *12*:239–242, 1978.

46. Clements, J. A.: Editorial: Pulmonary surfactant. Am. Rev. Respir. Dis., *101*:984–990, 1970.

47. Jobe, A., Ikegame, M., Jacobs, H., Jones, S., and Conaway, D.: Permeability of premature lamb to protein and the effect of surfactant on that permeability. J. Appl. Physiol., *55*:169–176, 1983.

48. Rudolph, A. M.: Fetal and neonatal pulmonary circulation. Annu. Rev. Physiol., *41*:383–395, 1979.

49. Melmon, K. L., Cline, M. J., Hughes, T., and Nies, A. S.: Kinins: possible mediators of neonatal circulatory changes in man. J. Clin. Invest., *47*:1295–1302, 1968.

50. Coceani, F., and Olley, P. M.: The response of the ductus arteriosus to prostaglandins. Can. J. Physiol. Pharmacol., *51*:220–225, 1973.

51. Olley, P. M., Coceani, F., and Bocach, E.: E-type prostaglandins: a new emergency therapy for certain cyanotic congenital heart malformations. Circulation, *53*:228–231, 1976.

Chapter

2

Postnatal Growth and Development of the Lung

INTRODUCTION

The neonatal lung undergoes remarkable immediate functional transformations so that by the end of the first few minutes of life it is serving as an adequate organ of gas exchange. Measurements of arterial blood gases one to four hours after birth reveal a P_{O_2} of about 62 mm Hg and a P_{CO_2} of about 38 mm Hg.[1] To achieve these values, the newborn breathes at an average respiratory rate of 37 breaths/min and has a tidal volume of 21 ml.[2] This means that the baby has a minute ventilation of 777 ml/min (37 × 21 = 777).

Moreover, within a day or two of birth the intrathoracic pressure changes, and the ratios of wasted ventilation (i.e., physiologic dead space) to tidal volume, tidal volume to FRC, O_2 consumption to minute ventilation, and diffusing capacity to O_2 consumption are similar to those in adults. However, neonatal pulmonary function is carried out in lungs that obviously still retain their fetal structure. Although some histologic changes can be recognized in the caliber of the newborn's pulmonary blood vessels and the geometry of its alveoli (presumably related to inflation), the development of the human lung to its adult state continues long

23

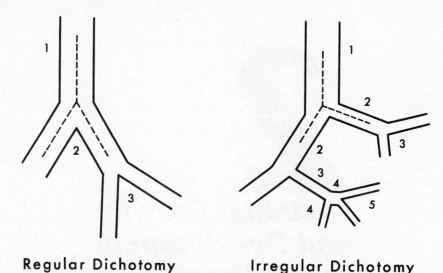

Regular Dichotomy   **Irregular Dichotomy**

Figure 2–1. Schematic representation of regular and irregular dichotomous patterns of airway branching. Apparent monopody shown in first and apparent trichotomy in third generation. (Adapted and reprinted by permission from Weibel, E. R.: Morphometry of the Human Lung. Berlin, Springer-Verlag, 1963, p. 111.)

after birth. However, the rate at which the different structural components of the lung mature after birth, as well as before birth, varies considerably. This chapter reviews the postnatal growth and development of human lungs, with emphasis on the structural findings in normal adults. Additional details and references are provided in excellent reviews.[3, 4, 4a]

TRACHEOBRONCHIAL SYSTEM

At birth, the basic formation of cartilaginous airways is complete, and additional division does not occur. In fact, the number of generations of conducting airways may actually decrease through the conversion by alveolarization of usually one to two, or at times three or more, generations of nonrespiratory bronchioles into respiratory bronchioles. The data concerning the presence and extent of alveolarization are controversial.[3] However, the sum of the evidence indicates that alveolarization, which extends centrally (toward the hilus), continues until about three years of age; thereafter, the system of branches remains constant. Growth of each segment of the conducting airways appears to occur mainly in a symmetric fashion, both in length and in diameter, until growth of the thorax ceases. Conflicting evidence also exists about the relative rates of growth of the different generations of intrapulmonary airways. Some

investigators believe that in the first five years of life the growth of small airways (those distal to the 12th to the 15th generation) may lag behind the growth of larger airways.[5]

Airways

The number of bronchial divisions varies markedly *within* the lungs, depending on the length of pathways from segmental bronchi to the various gas exchange units throughout the lung. For example, respiratory bronchioles near the hilus may be reached from a segmental bronchus with only ten bronchial branches, whereas more than 25 branches may be required to reach respiratory bronchioles in the most peripheral basal parts of the lung.[6]

The asymmetry in pathway lengths derives from the pattern of irregular dichotomous branching (Fig. 2–1) and has considerable effect on local resistances to airflow and on the transit times from mouth to gas exchange sites.[8] The engineering of the airways is also complicated by variations in the size and angulation of each pair of branches; the branch serving the longer pathway is straighter and has a larger cross-sectional area than the smaller, more angulated branch leading to the closer gas exchange units. This arrangement may serve in part to equalize the distribution of resistances among the various pathways.

As seen in Figure 2–2, the diameter of each new generation of airways decreases progressively from the trachea outward. However, the change in caliber is such that the cross-sectional area of the airway lumen steadily increases at successive levels throughout the tracheobronchial system; this increase is especially marked distal to the origin of the bronchioles, where branching is accompanied by practically no decrease in diameter of new generations. The increase in cross-sectional area means that the velocity of airflow must be sharply reduced as the airstream moves peripherally through the airways. Accordingly, resistance to airflow differs substantially in central and peripheral airways (see Chapter 4), and mixing in terminal respiratory units of newly inspired fresh air with gas remaining from the previous breath takes place by diffusion not by bulk flow (see Chapter 7).

The conducting airways are not merely rigid tubes through which air flows between the outside environment and the gas exchange units. They are structures with secretory capabilities, and they dilate and contract passively in response to influences such as lung inflation and actively in response to a variety of neurohumoral and chemical stimuli. The active reactions are mediated by the elements that compose the walls of airways: epithelium, smooth muscles, glands, nerves, and cells with tiny cachets of potent pharmacologic substances—each of which is a functioning unit that is described separately in the subsequent pages. Additional details are available in recent reviews.[9, 10, 11]

Bronchial Epithelium

The entire system of airways, from the trachea to the respiratory bronchioles, is covered with an epithelial lining that rests on a thin basement membrane overlying the lamina propria, a loose network of fibers containing cells, a rich capillary plexus, and unmyelinated nerves. In large airways, the epithelium is of the ciliated pseudostratified columnar type; however, the thickness of the lining layer gradually decreases as the airways become smaller so that in the terminal bronchioles, the epithelium consists

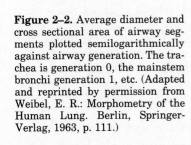

Figure 2–2. Average diameter and cross sectional area of airway segments plotted semilogarithmically against airway generation. The trachea is generation 0, the mainstem bronchi generation 1, etc. (Adapted and reprinted by permission from Weibel, E. R.: Morphometry of the Human Lung. Berlin, Springer-Verlag, 1963, p. 111.)

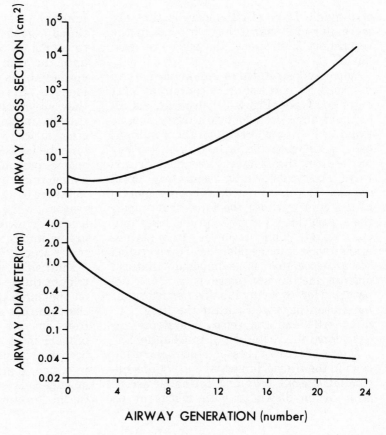

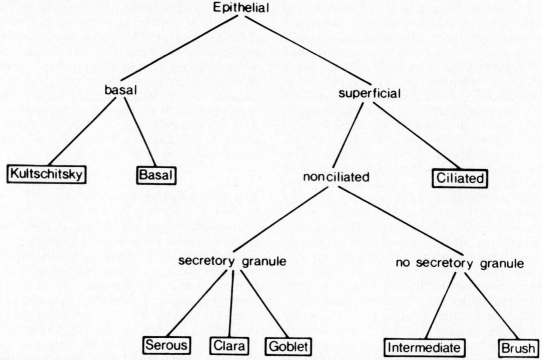

Figure 2–3. Eight cell types identified in the surface epithelium of airways. Of the secretory cells, the serous cell is normally present in the proximal airways and the Clara cell in the distal airways (Reprinted by permission from Reid, L. M., and Jones, R.: Mucous membrane of respiratory epithelium. Environ. Health Perspect., *35*:113–120, 1980.)

of a single layer of ciliated cells that are more cuboidal than columnar, and in the respiratory bronchioles the cells are even flatter.

The pseudostratified columnar epithelium of bronchi is now known to contain at least eight cell types (Fig. 2–3), although not all of them have been found in every species examined. *Ciliated cells* are the dominant cells of the epithelial layer (Fig. 2–4); they are present throughout all conducting airways and extend into respiratory bronchioles. The coordinated, sweeping motion of the cilia provides the force that impels the superficial layer of secretions (the "mucus blanket") along its journey from peripheral airways into the pharynx. This so-called "ciliary escalator" is an important natural defense mechanism, since it is the chief pathway for removing inhaled particles that have been deposited within the lung. Ciliated cells and the removal systems are considered in greater detail in Chapter 13.

There are two types of mucus-secreting cells in the tracheobronchial epithelium: epithelial *mucous cells* and epithelial *serous cells*. When distended with mucus at its luminal pole, the bulging mucous cell is called a *goblet cell* (Fig. 2–5); however, because not all cells present a similar appearance, the term mucous cell is preferred. Both epithelial mucous and serous cells can be identified in the human fetus and newborn; they are relatively more numerous in the trachea and large airways than in medium-sized airways, and they are infrequent in bronchioles. In adults, serous cells are sparse, presumably because they have been transformed into mucous cells under the influence of air pollutants. Mucous cells also respond to the chronic stimulus of cigarette smoke by increasing in number and propagating into bronchioles, where they are normally scarce.[12]

Epithelial mucous and serous cells contribute their secretions to the mucus layer on the surface of the epithelium, although the principal sources of this material vary from one set of airways to the next. In bronchi most of the mucus is produced by bronchial glands. In most of the bronchioles, in which glands are absent, the epithelial mucous cells are normally the sole suppliers. In the terminal bronchioles, in which all

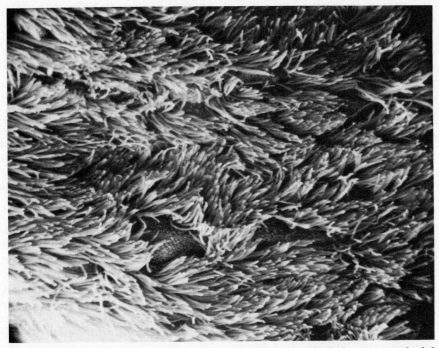

Figure 2–4. Scanning electron micrograph of the luminal surface of a bronchiole from a normal adult man; many cilia are evident surrounding a nonciliated cell. (× 2000. Reprinted by permission from Ebert, R. V., and Terracio, M. J.: Am. Rev. Resp. Dis., *111*:4, 1975.)

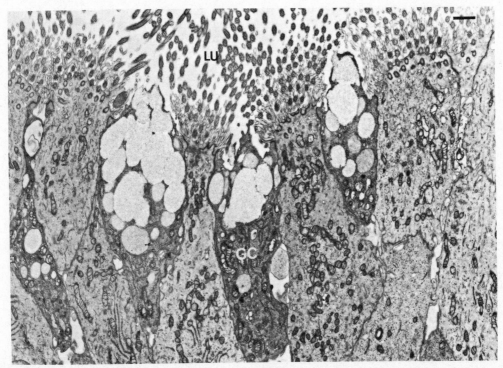

Figure 2–5. Electron micrograph of normal bronchial epithelium showing ciliated cells with numerous cilia projecting into the lumen (LU) of the airway and goblet cells (GC) containing mucous droplets. Horizontal bar = 1 μm. (× 6000. Courtesy of Dr. Donald McKay.)

mucous cells are normally the sole suppliers. In the terminal bronchioles, in which all mucus-secreting cells are sparse, the scant mucus layer may come from Clara cells or type II epithelial cells.

Basal cells are found in the epithelium as far as the bronchioles, although they are most numerous in the trachea and extra-pulmonary bronchi. The single row of ovoid basal cells along the basement membrane gives the epithelium its pseudostratified appearance. Basal cells are not known to have a special function of their own, but they serve the important purpose of differentiating as needed to replace superficial ciliated and mucous cells. Thus, they constitute a reserve population of cells that replenishes the surface layer.

Intermediate cells form a poorly defined layer above the basal cells, from which they are derived. As the intermediate cells extend toward the lumen, they elongate and change their electron density as they differentiate into epithelial mucous cells or ciliated cells.

Brush cells are rare and their function remains unknown. The presence of microvilli and other similarities between brush cells of the bronchial epithelium and those in the gastrointestinal tract have suggested similar roles in liquid absorption.

During the past decade, it has become clear that the tracheobronchial epithelium contains *endocrine cells,* which are also called *argyrophil* or *Kultschitsky cells* (Fig. 2–6), and which are similar to endocrine cells found in other organs. Those in the lungs have been included in the APUD series of cells, so named because of their cytochemical characteristics (i.e., *A*mine and amine-*P*recursor, *U*ptake, and *D*ecarboxylation) and because they are known to secrete several different hormones.[11] Pulmonary endocrine cells are much more impressive in the epithelium of newborns than in that of either children or adults. Electron microscopy has demonstrated a characteristic ultrastructure and has provided suggestive evidence that the cells are innervated.[13] On the basis of granular morphology, several types of endocrine cells have been described in human lungs. Whether these morphologic differences have functional significance is not known. Details about the endocrine substances produced by Kultschitsky and other cells are provided in Chapter 12. The Kultschitsky cells are also important as the precursors of carcinoids and small cell bronchogenic carcinomas.

Clumps of 10 to 30 Kultschitsky argyrophilic cells have been described in the bronchial, bronchiolar, and even alveolar epithelium of various mammals, including humans. These *neuroepithelial bodies,* which appear to be innervated, are of considerable interest because of their strategic locations and the possibility that they may regulate airway or pulmonary blood vessel caliber (see Fig. 3–17). The cells within neuroendothelial bodies of fetal rabbits have recently been shown to contain serotonin[14]. and to alter their morphology in response to acute hypoxia.[15]

The cellular components of the terminal and respiratory bronchiolar epithelium are remarkably different from those of larger airways. Ciliated cells are still present, although they are less numerous. Nonciliated *Clara cells* (Fig. 2–7) are conspicuous and abundant. Some can be readily recognized by their plump protoplasmic extensions that protrude into the lumen of the air passage; the remainder do not project beyond the luminal surface. In respiratory bronchioles, the epithelium between the interstices of the outpouching alveoli consists of low cuboidal cells with diminutive cilia and nonciliated Clara cells.

It is generally believed that Clara cells have a secretory function because they are furnished with numerous ovoid membrane-bound bodies, which are presumably secretory granules. But the nature and function of the granules are poorly understood. The most tenable explanation for a secretory role of Clara cells, at least for the moment, is that they contribute their secretions to the extracellular liquid lining of the bronchioles and possibly to the subphase of the alveolar lining layer.[16] Clara cells are known to contain enzymes that presumably serve to detoxify inhaled toxic substances; the cells also have an important progenitor function after bronchiolar epithelial injury in that they may differentiate into ciliated cells and possibly brush cells.[11]

Bronchial Glands

The bronchial glands (Fig. 2–8) are one of the characteristic features of the submucosal layer beneath the lamina propria. Each gland typically consists of four distinct regions (Fig. 2–9): (1) a short funnel-shaped ciliated duct that is a continuation of the

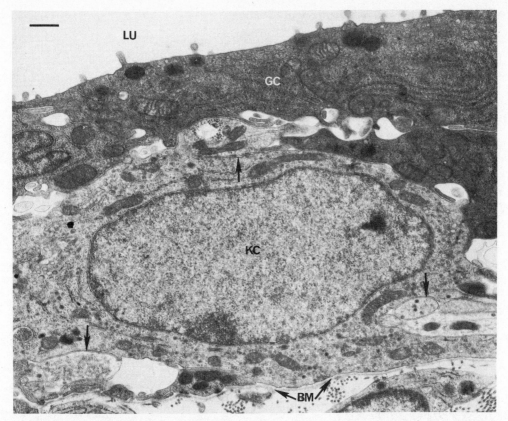

Figure 2–6. Electron micrograph showing a Kultschitsky cell (KC) in the tracheal epithelium of the rat. Intraepithelial nerves make contact with the cell at arrows. Horizontal bar = 1 μm; LU = tracheal lumen; GC = goblet cell; BM = epithelial basement membrane. (× 8000. Reprinted by permission from Jeffery, P., and Reid, L.: Intra-epithelial nerves in normal rat airways: A quantitative electron microscope study. J. Anat., *114*:35–45, 1973.)

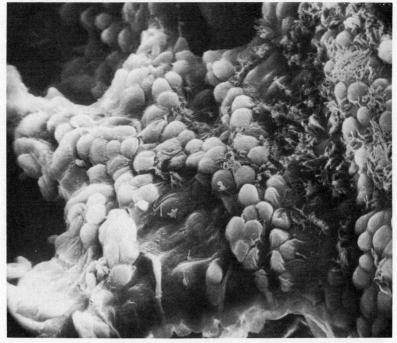

Figure 2–7. Scanning electron micrograph of a terminal bronchiole opening into several respiratory bronchioles. Epithelial surface is composed chiefly of Clara cells and ciliated cells. (× 900. Courtesy of Dr. Richard V. Ebert.)

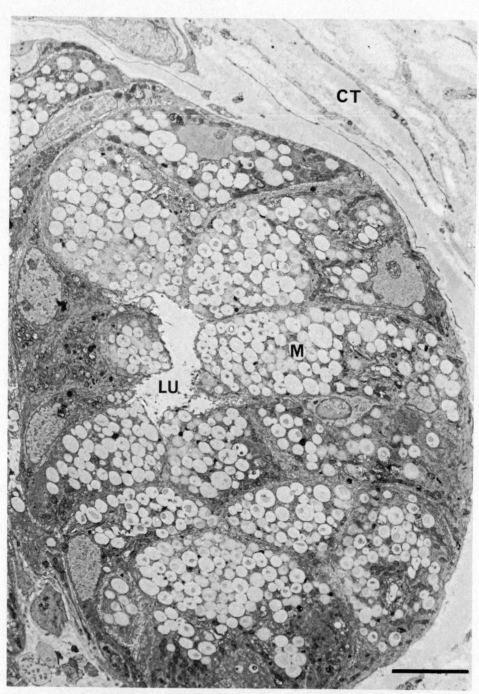

Figure 2–8. Electron micrograph of a transverse section through a normal bronchial gland surrounded by conective tissue (CT). Mucous droplets within mucous cells (M) are concentrated toward the lumen (LU) of the gland. Horizontal bar = 10 μm. (× 2100. Courtesy of Dr. Donald McKay.)

surface epithelium, (2) a nonciliated collecting duct, (3) tubules lined with mucous secreting cells that open into the collecting duct, and (4) tubules lined with serous secreting cells that open into the mucous tubules.[17] Among the cellular constituents are serous cells, mucous cells, collecting duct cells, clear cells (probably lymphocytes), and myoepithelial cells, which can be identified regularly, and mast cells and Kultschitsky cells, which are observed occasionally.[18] The myoepithelial cells, which are closely apposed to the secretory cells, may aid the movement of secretions along the tubules by contracting and squeezing the cells.[17] The glands are innervated by nerve fibers, which, on the basis of their ultrastructural characteristics, are believed to be parasympathetic efferent nerves.[19] Evidence for sympathetic innervation varies among the different species that have been studied but is absent in humans.[20] Bronchial glands are especially numerous in medium-sized bronchi, less prevalent in smaller bronchi, and absent in bronchioles.

It can be inferred from morphologic studies that mucous cells produce secretory granules continuously but release them into the glandular lumen intermittently; serous cells probably follow the same sequence but the evidence is less convincing. There are both morphologic and histochemical differences between mucous and serous cells, but the chemical composition of their respective secretions is unknown. The material that reaches the airway lumen, therefore, represents a mixture of the products of both cell types and any chemical reactions that result from the combination. (There is a possibility that secretions from serous cells may be

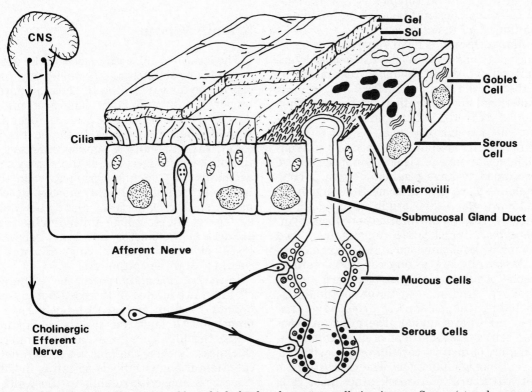

Figure 2–9. Schematic illustration of bronchial gland and secretory cells in airways. Serous (•) and mucus (○) secretions from the appropriate cells in the submucosal gland combine with water to form the submucosal gland secretion, which is discharged via the gland duct onto the airway luminal surface. This secretion mixes with the mucous and serous secretions from the epithelial goblet and serous cells to coat the epithelial surface with an upper gel and a lower more fluid sol in which the cilia beat and propel the gel toward the mouth. The apical surface of some cells is covered by microvilli whose function is unknown. Golgi apparatus (≋) of the secretory epithelial cells, nuclei (🖋), endoplasmic reticulum (𝄁), and mitochondria (⬯) in the other surface cells are shown. Endings of cholinergic afferent nerves in the lateral intercellular spaces close to the junctions between epithelial cells send impulses to the central nervous system and by reflex action stimulate secretion from the serous and mucous cells of the submucosal glands via cholinergic efferent nerves. (From Nadel, J. A., et al.: Control of mucus secretion and ion transport in airways. Ann. Rev. Physiol., *41*:369–381, 1979. Reprinted by permission from Annual Reviews, Inc.)

enzymatic and alter the physical properties of secretions from mucous cells.) The factors that control the basal rate of secretion are not well understood. Increased rates of mucous gland secretion can be provoked through a direct chemical effect or by a vagally mediated reflex (see next chapter).

Irritants, upon reaching the mucosa, initiate a reflex via the parasympathetic nervous system that causes the subject to cough and the submucosal glands to evacuate their contents rapidly; the discharged mucus isolates, dilutes, and may chemically alter the noxious substance. Thickening of the mucous layer overlying the epithelium facilitates removal of the added mucus and the offending substance by cough. In chronic bronchitis, which may occur in response to chronic irritation of the airways from cigarette smoking or inhalation of chemicals, the submucosal glands increase markedly in their structural complexity and number of cells and constitute one of the histologic hallmarks of the disease.[21]

Many observers have reported the presence of *lymphocytes* in the tracheobronchial epithelium. Some lymphocytes must be either on the luminal surface or extremely superficial in the epithelium because they can be recovered in large numbers by washing out a relatively small region of lung through its attendant bronchus by bronchoalveolar lavage. These lymphocytes are presumed to have originated from a bone marrow–blood pool at some time, but little is known about their origin, traffic, and life history. Additional information about lymphocytes, lymphocytic aggregates, and lymph nodes is provided in the next chapter.

Mast cells are a functionally heterogeneous population of cells of diverse origin that are found in many tissues of the lungs, including the submucosa, connective tissues, and parenchyma. There are at least two separate populations of mast cells, presumably of distinct cellular origin, with different biologic functions. The characteristic ultrastructural feature of intact mast cells is their cytoplasmic granules (Fig. 2–10); however, mast cells that have degranulated are difficult to recognize in tissue preparations, a fact that complicates the use of histologic techniques to assess mast cell function. Mast cells in various mammalian species have been found to release both preformed and newly generated biologically active substances. Among the preformed mediators are histamine, serotonin, eosino-phil chemotactic factor of anaphylaxis (ECF-A), ECF-oligopeptides, high molecular weight neutrophil chemotactic factor, chymase, and macromolecular heparin. The newly formed mediators include the following: slow-reacting substance of anaphylaxis (now known as sulfidopeptide leukotrienes LTC_4, LTD_4, and LTE_4), a platelet-activating factor, and a lipid chemotactic factor (for review and references, see Lewis and Austen[22]). The chemical content of human mast cells is not fully known, but they can elaborate histamine, ECF-A, leukotrienes, and one or more neutrophil chemotactic factors. It is clear that mast cells mediate important physiologic and pathologic events, particularly IgE-induced type I immediate hypersensitivity responses, including asthma and anaphylaxis. Further details about mast cell function, leukotrienes, and histamine are provided in Chapter 12.

Smooth Muscle

The location of smooth muscle in the walls of the tracheobronchial tree varies with the size of the airway. In the trachea and large bronchi (main and lower lobe bronchi), a band of muscle bridges the posterior opening of the U-shaped cartilages. In the next largest airways, the muscle bundle connects the tips of the cartilages, but as the airway size decreases (i.e., moving peripherally in the tracheobronchial tree), the muscle attachments shift progressively along the inner surface of the cartilage until finally they are detached completely and form a separate layer between the partial rings of plates of cartilage and the epithelium.

In the trachea and bronchi, the only muscle fibers are located in the posterior muscle bundle. Medium and small bronchi have a proper muscle layer, but it does not circumscribe the airway with a band of uniform thickness. Rather, the muscles have a helical orientation, with fibers spiraling in both directions and crisscrossing in the walls.[23] Thus, the effect of muscle contraction depends upon the location and density of fibers. In the large airways, muscle contraction serves to oppose or even overlap the tips of the U-shaped cartilages. In medium and small bronchi, owing to the geodesic distribution of muscle elements, contraction reduces both the caliber and length of the bronchus. Muscle contraction, therefore, leads to greater rigidity in all airways.

Smooth muscle does not end in the terminal bronchioles, but spirals of muscle form part of the walls of respiratory bronchioles, and muscle fibers have been identified in the openings of alveolar ducts;[24] contraction of these elements will affect significantly the mechanical properties of the gas exchange units. The important role of changes in airways resistance and the distensibility of terminal respiratory units in governing the partition of inspired air within the lung is discussed in Chapter 4.

Tracheobronchial smooth muscle and its innervation vary in structure and function among different species, and generalizations are hazardous. In the extrapulmonary airways of humans the smooth muscle has numerous cell-to-cell connections of the nexus or gap junction type (Fig. 2–11), suggesting that the complex of muscle fibers is electrically coupled. The principal innervation of these muscles is from parasympathetic (excitatory) and nonadrenergic (inhibitory) nervous pathways,[25] which are described in more detail in the next chapter. A recent workshop report summarizes what

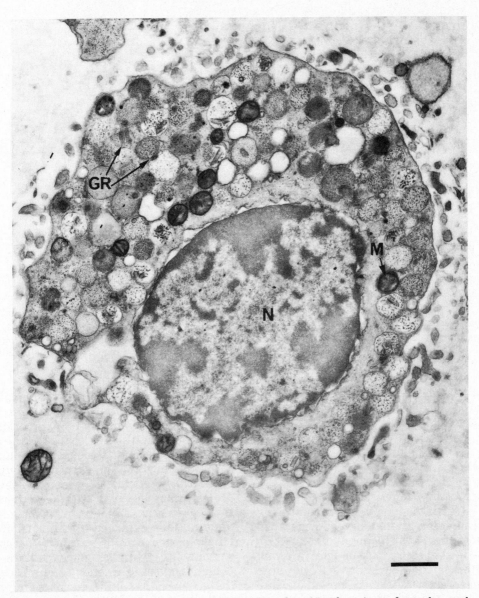

Figure 2–10. Electron micrograph of a normal mast cell in the adventitia of an airway from a human lung. Note the numerous granules (GR) with variable staining characteristics and mitochondria (M) in the cytoplasm surrounding the nucleus (N). Horizontal bar = 1 μm. (× 12, 750. Courtesy of Dr. Donald McKay.)

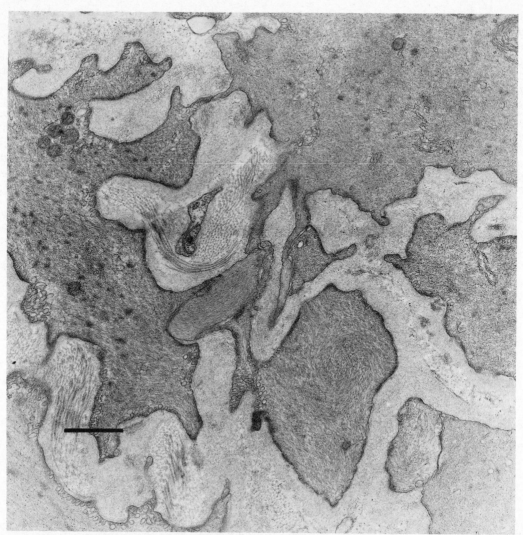

Figure 2–11. Electron micrograph of human trachealis muscle. The smooth muscle cells show frequent cell-to-cell connections. A nerve is situated between the cells but does not contact them. Horizontal bar = 1 μm. (Reprinted by permission from Richardson, J. B., and Ferguson, C. C.: Neuromuscular structure and function in the airways. Fed. Proc., *38*:202–208, 1978.)

is known as well as many of the uncertainties concerning airway smooth muscle structure and function.[25a]

Connective Tissue

During embryogenesis, as the developing bronchial buds penetrate the neighboring mass of undifferentiated mesenchyme, they carry with them an investment of connective tissue. By the 16th week of fetal life and thereafter, cartilaginous airways and large pulmonary arteries, which travel in close partnership through the substance of the lung, are surrounded by a sleeve of loose connective tissue that contains lymphatic vessels and a potential space. The *peribronchovascular interstitial space* is a site at which liquid and solute localize in the early stages of pulmonary edema accumulation (see Chapter 12). The sheath surrounding conducting bronchioles ends at the level of the terminal bronchioles, where they lose their connective tissue investment and become directly attached to the surrounding lung parenchyma. In contrast, the sheath surrounding arterioles and venules accompanies the vessels as they extend deep into the gas exchange units before giving off or arising from alveolar capillaries.

The elastic tissue network of the lungs

not only plays an important role in the pre- and postnatal development of alveoli, but the continuum of connective tissue fibers, both elastin and collagen, provides part of the structural support for the enormous surface area of the extremely delicate lung parenchyma. The remarkable ways in which the engineering requirements for support of the alveoli are satisfied are considered later in this chapter.

Contractile Tissue

The presence of abundant smooth muscle in airways, blood vessels, and even the lung parenchyma is well known and has already been described. The extent to which these contractile elements affect the regional distributions of ventilation and blood flow is by no means clear, and it is even conceivable that they have some different, as yet unrecognized, function. The presence of other cells with contractile properties, the *capillary pericyte* and *contractile interstitial cell*,[26] whose physiologic roles are totally unknown, adds to the mystery about the purpose of the lungs' inherent contractability.

BLOOD VESSELS

Generation counts have established that the number of pulmonary arteries and veins leading *to* the terminal respiratory units, both conventional and supernumerary branches, is completely formed at birth.[27] However, even at birth there are very few vessels *within* the incompletely developed gas exchange units; both arteries and veins increase enormously in number within lobules during the first decade of life, and their development accompanies the formation of new respiratory bronchioles, alveolar ducts, and alveoli.

Pulmonary Arteries

During gestation, all branches of the arterial system are relatively thick walled owing to their medial layer of smooth muscle. However, after birth the vessels rapidly become thinner, so that by four months of age, they show nearly the same relationship between wall thickness and external diameter that is observed in adult lungs (Fig. 2–12).[28] While this change is occurring, the

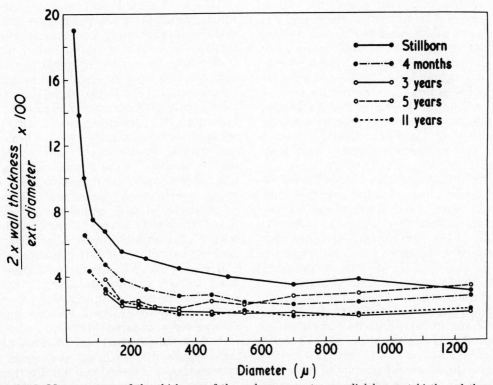

Figure 2–12. Measurements of the thickness of the pulmonary artery medial layer at birth and throughout childhood. Adult values are reached at four months of age. (Reprinted by permission from Davies, G., and Reid, L.: Growth of the alveoli and pulmonary arteries in childhood. Thorax, *25*:669–681, 1970.)

amount of smooth muscle appears to diminish in small vessels, a process that continues for several years because many new arteries without muscle are formed during the phase of rapid multiplication of alveoli. After five years of age, the multiplication of both alveoli and arteries has slowed, but new arteries continue to be formed and old ones continue to grow without muscle appearing in their walls. Smooth muscle begins to extend peripherally in the medial layer of small arteries after they are formed.[28] At birth, about half the arteries accompanying terminal bronchioles are muscular, and the rest are partially muscular; by the age of five years, all have reached the adult form of complete muscular development. In contrast, almost no muscular arteries are encountered within the terminal respiratory units at birth. Furthermore, during infancy and childhood, the process of muscularization proceeds slowly; muscle reaches arterioles at the level of respiratory bronchioles at four months of age, alveolar ducts at three years, some alveoli at ten years, and the process is not complete until 19 years of age.[3]

It is of interest that elastic arteries extend from the hilus to nearly halfway in the bronchial tree of newborns and that this is the same level as in adults. Moreover, the pattern of development of elastic arteries, like that of the bronchi that accompany them, is complete by the 16th week of gestation and is another example of adult morphology being formed in miniature well in advance of maturity. During growth, length and diameter of pulmonary arteries increase proportionately, and pulmonary arterial (blood) volume changes directly with lung volume.

The postnatal evolution of both the abundant elastic elements in elastic arteries and the thick layer of smooth muscle in muscular arteries, from their appearance during fetal life to their final adult structure, can proceed only if pulmonary arterial pressure falls to the normal low values found in infants living near sea level. If pulmonary hypertension is maintained after birth, for example, either because of hypoxia induced by residence at high altitude or because of congenital cardiac anomalies such as a large ventricular septal defect or truncus arteriosus, then thinning and atrophy of the muscular and elastic elements fail to occur.

Three types of pulmonary arteries can be identified in the normal adult human lung (Fig. 2–13; see also Plate II).[29] However, it must be recognized that this classification is arbitrary, and because the pulmonary arterial system is a continuous one, transitional forms occur in regions where one type of artery gradually merges into another type. (1) The *elastic pulmonary arteries* (> 1000 µm external diameter) contain distinctive layers of elastic fibers embedded in a coat of muscle cells. The pulmonary artery trunk, its main branches, and all extralobular pulmonary arteries are of the elastic type. (2) The *muscular pulmonary arteries* (100 to 1000 µm external diameter) have a thin medial layer of muscle sandwiched between well-delimited internal and external elastic laminae. Muscular pulmonary arteries lie within lung lobules and, hence, accompany bronchioles. Although these vessels are designated by their muscular elements, the thickness of the muscle layer does not exceed about 5 per cent of the external diameter of the vessel; any increase above this value connotes a pathologic state and is found in well-defined conditions usually associated with pulmonary arterial hypertension. (3) The *pulmonary arterioles* (<100 µm external diameter) are the terminal branches of the pulmonary arterial system; at their origin from muscular arteries they contain a partial layer of muscle that gradually disappears until the vessel wall consists only of endothelium and an elastic lamina (Fig. 2–14). Pulmonary arterioles supply alveolar ducts and alveoli.

Functional Considerations. The partnership between branches of the bronchial and arterial systems as they course through both connective tissue boundaries and the lung parenchyma, in contrast to pulmonary veins, which are as far removed from the bronchoarterial pair as possible, indicates that factors that affect the regional distribution of ventilation will also affect the distribution of blood flow to the same region, and vice versa. When both ventilation and blood flow are impaired similarly, compared with disproportionate involvement of one or the other, optimum conditions for gas exchange are maintained. It is easy to appreciate how this might occur in gross pathologic conditions, such as atelectasis and tumors, but the functional implications of the anatomic arrangement can be extended to include a much more delicate control mechanism, one that confers a high degree of autonomous regulation of blood flow and ventilation to maintain optimum gas exchange. Experiments in which either blood flow or ventilation is impaired suggest that autoregulation exists, but the site of and mechanisms governing the response are not fully understood.

The location of thin-walled muscular arteries and arterioles within lobules means that the vessels are exposed to the same gas tensions that prevail in the adjacent alveolar spaces. The intimate relationship be-tween a pulmonary arteriole and its surrounding alveolar air spaces is evident from Figure 2–15.

Experiments have demonstrated that pulmonary arterial vasoconstriction occurs in a lung or lobe ventilated with low concentrations of O_2 or, to a lesser extent, perfused with blood that has a low Po_2.[30] It is also known that the effect is mediated locally and does not require systemic neural or humoral responses.[31] Anatomic studies under conditions of unilobar hypoxia in cats have shown vasoconstriction in small muscular arteries and arterioles.[32] We can sur-

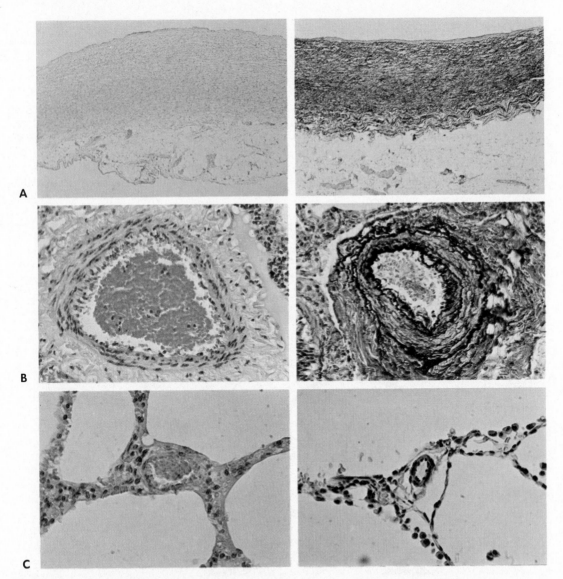

Figure 2–13. Micrographs of A, elastic (main) pulmonary artery (× 15); B, muscular pulmonary artery (× 60); and C, pulmonary arteriole (× 150). Left panels, hematoxylin and eosin stain; right panels, elastic stain. (Courtesy of Dr. Robert Wright.) See also Plate II.

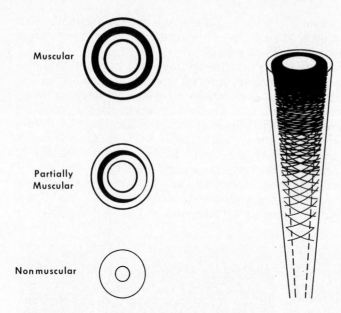

Figure 2–14. Schematic representation of the changes in the amount and thickness of the smooth muscle layer in muscular, partially muscular, and nonmuscular pulmonary arteries.

mise, therefore, that even though small pulmonary arteries contain relatively little muscle (compared with their systemic analogues), they are capable of constricting; moreover, there must be some sort of extraluminal (e.g., adventitial) receptor system that responds to alveolar hypoxia and, to some extent, to pulmonary arterial hypoxemia. Obviously, it would be desirable for the lung to reduce blood flow to a gas exchange unit(s) within which the P_{O_2} is low or the P_{CO_2} is high. Because autonomous

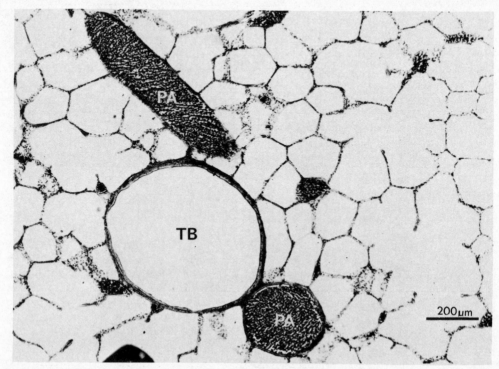

Figure 2–15. Fixed frozen section of cat lung showing terminal bronchiole (TB) and its associated pulmonary artery (PA) in a thin section. Note that the vessels and airway are completely surrounded by alveolar spaces that are usually part of the same terminal respiratory unit that the vessels and airway are supplying. Horizontal bar = 200 μm. (× 70. Courtesy of Dr. Norman Staub.)

regulation has been shown to occur in whole lungs or lobes, we can infer that smaller regions are probably also capable of demonstrating similar responses. Indeed, the results of studies in mammals such as the coatimundi, which have well developed connective tissue barriers surrounding lobules, indicate that blood flow to small regions of the lung is adjustable when inspired gas composition to these units is altered.[33]

Supernumerary Arteries

The pulmonary arterial circulation has two sets of branches: "conventional" arteries, which accompany airways, and "supernumerary" arteries, which travel alone and which are usually smaller than the others. Supernumerary arteries appear at the hilus and emerge from the main arterial channels at right angles as far peripherally as the end of the respiratory bronchioles. The extra branches outnumber the conventional ones and provide about 25 per cent of the total cross-sectional area of the pulmonary arterial bed near the hilus and about 40 per cent of the total toward the periphery. Supernumerary arteries are present at birth but mainly those that lead to the terminal respiratory unit;[27] there is extensive growth of new conventional and supernumerary branches, the latter outnumbering the former, accompanying the development of alveolar ducts and alveoli during the first 18 months of childhood.[34] The appearance of new conventional arteries virtually ceases at 18 months, whereas supernumerary arteries continue to increase in number up to about eight years of age, while new alveoli are being formed.

Supernumerary vessels undoubtedly serve as an auxiliary arterial supply to the capillary beds of the terminal respiratory units, and thus they constitute an important source of collateral blood flow to the sites of gas exchange. Of interest is the observation that neither supernumerary branches nor many conventional branches fill during routine angiography; whether this is a technical artifact or of functional significance is unknown.

Functional Considerations. There is no known reason to believe that the lung was accidentally equipped with "extra" pulmonary arteries. Blood undoubtedly has access to the entire arterial circulation, even though local changes in vascular resistance

probably determine which pathways are utilized at any given moment. Whether or not the network was designed for filtering the bloodstream is unknown, but the extensive arterial system is well suited to carry out this important nonrespiratory function of the lungs.[35]

Pulmonary blood vessels trap particles, depending on their size and physical characteristics. Some intravascular coagulation probably goes on in normal persons at all times, and the lung serves as a sieve for the aggregates of red blood cells, platelets, and fibrin. The anatomic orientation of the arterial system means that several collateral channels are available to the terminal gas exchange units in case one or more vessels become temporarily obstructed.

Besides the normal physiologic functions of trapping and removing particles that circulate in the venous blood stream, the lung serves as a filter of materials formed in the evolution of a variety of pathologic processes. Blood clots, fat particles, tissue fragments, tumor cells, and amniotic fluid all may enter into or be formed within the venous circulation and cause pulmonary arterial embolization; collateral pathways are obviously useful in these conditions, not only to maintain gas exchange but also to preserve the viability of the lung subserved by the obstructed vessel.

The endothelium of the pulmonary arterial circulation, presumably in both conventional and supernumerary vessels, is known to be the site of transformation of several different biochemical substances (see Chapter 12). The pulmonary circulation has also been shown to affect the concentration of circulating leukocytes and platelets by releasing them into the systemic circulation of humans following the injection of epinephrine.[36] Subsequent studies revealed that the lungs of sheep contain a large marginated pool of neutrophilic leukocytes; nearly three times as many neutrophils were present in the lungs as in the bloodstream.[36a] Surprisingly, the cells were marginated along the walls of small pulmonary arteries and not along the veins, which is exactly opposite of the pattern of margination of neutrophils in the systemic circulation. Very few neutrophils were found in the pulmonary interstitium and even fewer in the alveolar spaces.[36a] There also appeared to be a small marginated pool of platelets in the lungs of dogs, although its location was not determined. When blood flow through the lungs was decreased, pulmonary sequestration of platelets inceased.[36b] It seems logical to expect that platelets would be governed by the same hemodynamic forces as neutrophils and, accordingly, would also marginate in pulmonary arterioles.

Pulmonary Veins

The pulmonary veins are usually considered to be simple tubes that conduct arterialized blood from the pulmonary capillaries to the left atrium. Drainage of blood is certainly the main function of veins, and the design of the system is well suited for this purpose. However, other structure-function relationships can be inferred from considerations of the extent of the venous network and the morphology of veins themselves.

There are both similarities and differences between pulmonary veins on the one hand and pulmonary arteries on the other. The development of the adult pattern of venous drainage from the terminal respiratory units to the hilus is completed, like that of the corresponding arteries, by about mid-gestation. The venous system is also similar to the arterial system because both have conventional and supernumerary branches. Both arteries and veins increase in number as new alveoli are formed, and all vessels increase in size as the volume of lung increases with age.[37]

The important differences between veins and arteries, besides the anatomy of the extrapulmonary branches leading into and away from the heart, lie chiefly in the number of vessels and the structure of their walls, both of which have important functional implications.

Functional Considerations. First, there are more veins than arteries, and because the number of conventional branches of both systems is equal, the increased density of veins per unit area of lung is accounted for by a larger number of supernumerary veins than arteries. Second, veins have thinner walls than arteries, owing to a less developed muscular layer in veins at all ages.[37] During early fetal life, pulmonary arteries are considerably more muscular than pulmonary veins; however, this discrepancy becomes less marked late in gestation as the venous muscular layer thickens. During in-

fancy, the attrition of arterial smooth muscle makes the thickness of the layers in arteries and veins of corresponding size even more uniform. These morphologic alterations appear to be related to the intravascular pressure changes that take place within the respective vessels. Moreover, in patients with congenital or acquired heart diseases the thickness of the smooth muscle layer of pulmonary arteries and veins has been observed to vary with corresponding changes in intravascular pressures, and medial hypertrophy in the walls of veins is believed to be pathognomonic of pulmonary venous hypertension.[38]

Although no information is available on the cross-sectional area of the pulmonary venous bed, the large number of thin-walled veins implies a low resistance to blood flow, which confers the ability to accommodate large increases in cardiac output with negligible changes in pressure (see Chapter 6). The pulmonary arterial system is also a low-resistance vascular bed but *not as low as* the pulmonary venous system.

Pulmonary veins serve, with the left atrium, as a reservoir of blood for the left ventricle. As shown in Figure 2–16, if pulmonary arterial inflow is suddenly interrupted, the left ventricle will continue to fill with blood from pulmonary veins and to eject a substantial stroke volume for several beats.[39] Gross disturbances in right ventricular output are ultimately reflected in left ventricular output, but minor variations, such as might occur during respiration, are probably partially "absorbed" by the pulmonary venous reservoir.

Bronchial Circulation

The lung receives blood from two different vascular systems, the pulmonary circulation and the bronchial circulation. There are substantial differences between the amount of blood flow, the composition of the blood, and the functional importance of these two circulations. The pulmonary circulation consists of virtually the entire cardiac output; it contains venous blood, and the "arterialization" of this blood is essential for life. In contrast, the bronchial circulation consists of only a small proportion of the cardiac output; it contains systemic arterial blood, and the normal adult lung remains viable without it. However, this statement oversimplifies the role of the bronchial circulation because it does not recognize the possible importance of bronchial blood flow to lung development in the fetus and its crucial contributions to gas exchange in many varieties of congenital cardiac anomalies. Furthermore, there is a striking increase in the size and number of bronchial arteries in certain kinds of lung diseases, especially chronic inflammation and neoplasms.

Morphologic studies have shown that the caliber of bronchial arteries of a human fetus is nearly the same as that of an adult.[40] This observation suggests that the lung might receive proportionately more blood flow, O_2, and nutrients from the bronchial circulation during fetal life than it does in adult life. However, studies in fetal lambs have revealed that the bronchial blood supply to the lungs is extremely low, 0.1 to 0.2 per cent of total cardiac output.[41] It should be pointed out that the bronchial arteries of fetal lambs are not as large as they appear

to be in human fetuses, so it is possible that there may be an important species difference in the contribution of the bronchial circulation to the metabolic needs of the developing lung.

The bronchial arteries in the human adult vary considerably in number and origin.[23] There is usually a single artery to the right lung that arises from an upper right intercostal artery or from the right subclavian or internal mammary artery. The two arteries supplying the left lung arise as direct branches from the upper thoracic aorta. Variable numbers of smaller arterial branches emerge from vessels in and near the mediastinum and cross into the lung. As soon as the bronchial arteries enter the lung, they become invested in the layer of connective tissue surrounding the bronchi and begin branching. Ordinarily, two or three bronchial arterial branches, which anastomose with each other to form a peribronchial plexus with an elongated and irregular

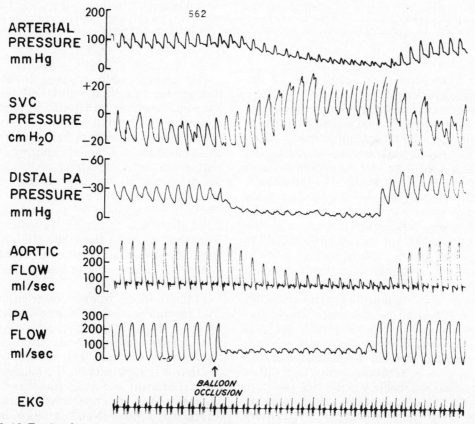

Figure 2–16. Tracing from an experiment in which sudden occlusion (arrow) of the main pulmonary artery (PA) of a dog by inflating a balloon caused an immediate cessation in pulmonary blood flow but a gradual decrease in aortic blood flow. SVC = superior vena cava. (Reprinted by permission from Hoffman, J. I. E. et al.: Stroke volume in conscious dogs; effect of respiration, posture, and vascular occlusion. J. Appl. Physiol., *20*:865–877, 1965.)

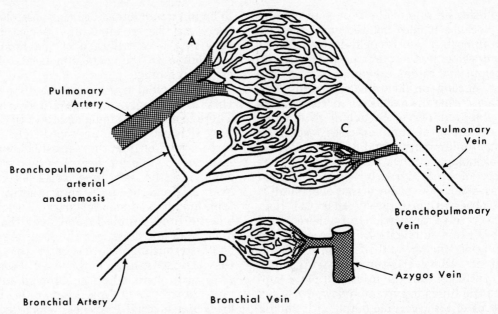

Figure 2–17. Schematic representation of the relationships between the bronchial and pulmonary circulations. The pulmonary artery supplies the pulmonary capillary network A. The bronchial artery supplies capillary networks B, C, and D. Network B represents the bronchial capillary supply to bronchioles that anastomoses with pulmonary capillaries and drains through pulmonary veins. Network C represents the bronchial capillary supply to most bronchi; these vessels form bronchopulmonary veins that empty into pulmonary veins. Network D represents the bronchial capillary supply to lobar and segmental bronchi; these vessels form true bronchial veins that drain into the azygos, hemiazygos, or intercostal veins. Shaded areas represent blood of low O_2 content.

mesh, accompany each subdivision of the conducting airways.

In most mammalian species, the bronchial arteries are the principal source of nutrient blood to virtually all intrapulmonary structures except the parenchyma, including the bronchial tree from the mainstem bronchi to the terminal bronchioles, the pulmonary nerves and ganglia, the elastic and some muscular pulmonary arteries and veins, the lymph nodes and lymph tissue, and the connective tissue septa. The blood supply to the visceral pleura varies among different mammals;[42] in humans the visceral pleura is supplied by the bronchial circulation, a feature of some importance when considering the sites and magnitude of liquid formation and removal by the pleural surfaces (see Chapter 12). Near the end of the terminal bronchioles, the bronchial arterioles terminate in a network of capillaries that anastomose extensively with the capillary plexus in the alveoli of the adjoining respiratory bronchioles. Because respiratory bronchioles are supplied by branches of the pulmonary artery, communication between the two blood supplies to the lung occurs at the junction of the conducting airways and the terminal respiratory units.

The amount of blood flow to the lung through the bronchial arterial circulation is low and, therefore, quite difficult to measure accurately in normal humans. The results of recent studies in dogs indicate that bronchial blood flow to the left lung was 0.4 per cent of the cardiac output; of this flow, 55 per cent went to the lung parenchyma and the remainder to the trachea and bronchi.[43] There is no reason to believe that bronchial blood flow in humans differs substantially from that in dogs; therefore, the estimates that total bronchial blood flow to both lungs is about 1 to 2 per cent of the cardiac output are probably correct.[44]

Effluent blood from capillaries supplied by bronchial arteries returns to the heart by two different venous pathways (Fig. 2–17). True *bronchial veins* are found only at the hilus; they are formed from tributaries that originate around the lobar and segmental bronchi and from branches from the pleura in the neighborhood of the hilus. Bronchial venous blood empties into the azygos, hemiazygos, or intercostal veins and then flows into the right atrium. Veins that originate from bronchial capillaries within the lungs unite to form venous tributaries that join the pulmonary veins; these communicating vessels are sometimes called *bronchopulmonary veins.* Blood leaving the capillary bed around terminal bronchioles flows through anastomoses with the alveolar capillaries, and the mixture of blood returns to the left atrium through pulmonary veins.

The distribution of bronchial arterial inflow between the two available venous outflow pathways has never been determined in humans, and only tentative conclusions can be drawn from the technically difficult studies in experimental animals. These indicate that about 25 to 33 per cent of the bronchial arterial supply returns ultimately to the right atrium via bronchial veins, and 67 to 75 per cent flows into the left atrium via pulmonary veins.[45]

The controversy still exists concerning the presence and significance of *bronchopulmonary arterial anastomoses,* direct vascular connections between pulmonary arteries and bronchial arteries. The available evidence suggests that bronchopulmonary arterial anastomoses do exist, that they occur sporadically and infrequently in normal lungs, that they are more easily demonstrable in the lungs of infants than of adults, and that they may increase considerably in number in certain pathologic disorders. It is of interest that functional bronchopulmonary arterial anastomoses have been identified in dogs, a species in which the communications have not been demonstrated anatomically.[46]

Although the magnitude of the bronchial arterial inflow, the partition of its venous outflow, and the identity of bronchopulmonary arterial anastomoses are all uncertain, reliable experimental data are available concerning the physiology of the bronchial circulation, especially the functional interrelationships between the bronchial and the pulmonary circulations. Blood flow to the lung through its two circulations, even though the amount supplied by each differs markedly, is balanced, so that if the perfusing pressure in one system increases or decreases, there is a change in the opposite direction in the amount of blood supplied by the other system.[47] This means that if pressure falls in part of the pulmonary arterial circulation (e.g., distal to the site of a pulmonary embolus), blood flow to that part of the lung through the bronchial circulation will increase. And conversely, if pressure in the bronchial system falls (e.g., in autotransplantation, which deprives the lung of all its bronchial blood flow), blood flow in

the pulmonary circulation will increase and supply those tissues that formerly received blood through the bronchial circulation.

This reciprocal relationship is obviously of great benefit in preserving viability of pulmonary structures when one or the other circulation is impaired. The adequacy of the mechanism depends on the presence of functioning anastomoses between the two circulations that are capable of accommodating an increase in blood flow. When circumstances prevent the increase in collateral flow from occurring, lung damage develops. Pulmonary infarction will follow pulmonary embolism when the bronchial circulation is compromised, or necrosis of the airways will follow lung transplantation when the pulmonary circulation is affected.

TERMINAL RESPIRATORY UNITS

A terminal respiratory unit consists of the structures distal to the end of a terminal bronchiole. A typical unit, shown schematically in Figure 2–18, contains a characteristically variable branching pattern. There are usually two to five orders of respiratory bronchioles (indicated by Roman numerals in Fig. 2–18), the last of which leads into the first of two to five orders of alveolar ducts (indicated by Arabic numerals). Alveolar ducts are relatively short (with lengths only one to one and one-half times the diameter) and they branch in rapid sequence; each duct has openings for 10 to 16 alveoli.[48] The last in the series of alveolar ducts empties through what used to be called the atrium (now an obsolete term) into one to three dome-shaped alveolar sacs from which the terminal alveoli project.

As indicated in Figure 2–18, the extent of alveolarization of respiratory bronchioles increases, proceeding from the terminal bronchiole toward the periphery. The chief difference between alveolar ducts and respiratory bronchioles is that the ducts are completely alveolarized and ciliated respiratory epithelium is absent. Alveolar ducts can be viewed mainly as a supporting framework of delicate connective tissue fibers and slender smooth muscle cells interspersed between a continuous succession of alveoli.

The terminal respiratory unit shown in Figure 2–18 is displayed in only one plane; a "complete" unit can be visualized by rotating the structures within the hatched line through 360 degrees. Furthermore, it should

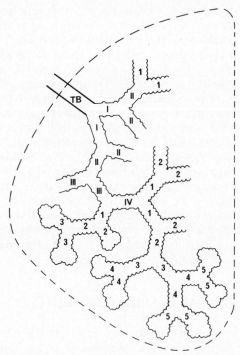

Figure 2–18. Schematic representation of the anatomic subdivisions in a single plane through a terminal respiratory unit (i.e., those structures distal to a terminal bronchiole, TB). Roman numerals indicate respiratory bronchioles; arabic numerals indicate alveolar ducts. The entire unit can be visualized by rotating the structures within the hatched boundary through 360 degrees.

be emphasized that adjacent terminal respiratory units are not separated by spaces or by well-defined anatomic boundaries and that they interdigitate to some extent with each other like a three-dimensional jigsaw puzzle.

A cluster of three to five terminal bronchioles, each with its appended terminal respiratory unit, is usually referred to as a *lobule*; a typical lobule is shown schematically in Figure 2–19. Contiguous lobules in human lungs are partly but incompletely delimited by connective tissue septa; in other mammals, such as the cow, the septal barriers between adjacent lobules are structurally complete. The lobular architecture of the lung is important in determining whether or not collateral ventilation occurs (see next section).

The blood supply of several adjacent lobules is shown in Figure 2–20. The lobular architecture in a lung specimen of a dog in which the pulmonary artery was injected with opaque material is shown in *A*; branches of both pulmonary arterial and

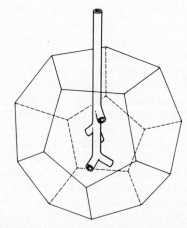

Figure 2–19. Schematic representation of a pulmonary lobule, in this instance composed of five terminal bronchioles. The five terminal respiratory units (not shown) occupy the space within the boundaries of the lobule.

bronchial systems travel together and supply the terminal respiratory units within a single lobule. In contrast, as shown in *B*, a pulmonary vein drains blood from *many* lobules that can be identified by their parent bronchioles.

The modern terminology used by various authors to describe the gas exchange regions of the lung differs from that advocated by the great lung anatomist Miller[23] and needs to be standardized. Equivalent terms are listed in Table 2–1. The terminal unit as just defined is equivalent to the *acinus* used by many authors; the term acinus literally means grape and is preferred by morphologists in view of its obvious descriptive connotation. The acinus (or primary lobule) is sometimes designated by pathologists as the anatomic basis for differentiating emphysema into either "centriacinar" (centrilobu-

Table 2–1. PARTIAL LIST OF COMMON SYNONYMS AND THEIR DEFINITIONS USED TO DESCRIBE THE GAS EXCHANGE REGIONS OF THE LUNG*

Synonyms	Definition
Terminal respiratory unit Acinus[50] Primary lobule[23]	Those structures distal to the end of a terminal bronchiole
Lobule Secondary lobule[23]	A cluster of a variable number of terminal respiratory units that are separated from adjacent clusters by connective tissue septa

*The terms employed in this text are *italicized*.

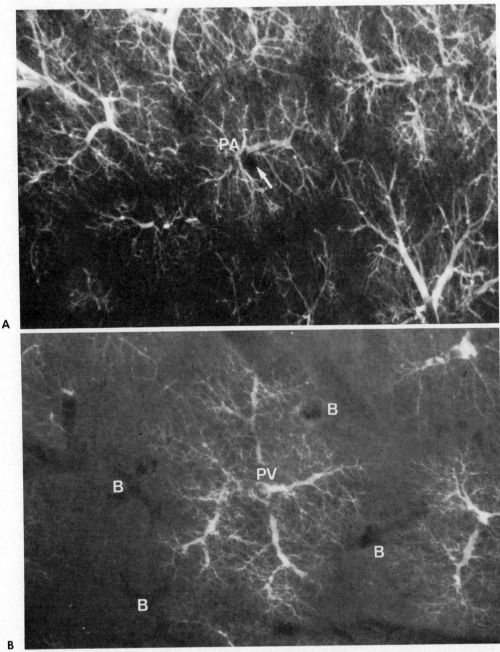

Figure 2–20. *A*, Section of a dog lung showing pulmonary arteries injected with a barium sulfate suspension. A branch of the pulmonary artery (PA) lies next to a radiolucent bronchiole (arrow). The architecture of several adjacent lobules is distinctly outlined. *B*, Injected specimen of dog lung showing how pulmonary veins (PV) receive blood from several lobules that can be identified by the location of their parent bronchioles (B). (*A* × 7.0; *B* × 6.3. Reprinted by permission from Lauweryns, J. M.: The blood and lymphatic microcirculation of the lung. *In* Sommers, S. C. (ed.): Pathology Annual 1971. New York, Appleton-Century-Crofts, 1971, pp. 365–415.)

lar) or "panacinar" (panlobular) emphysema. As shown in Table 2–1, the term "terminal respiratory unit" will be used throughout this text in recognition of its role as the anatomic site of gas exchange.

Alveoli

Alveoli in newborns are fewer in number and less complex in anatomic detail than their counterparts in adults; this dissimilarity has led some morphologists to call them "saccules" rather than alveoli.[50] However, neonatal alveoli, even though primitive, correspond to Macklin's definition of alveoli as "the ultimate respiratory chamber."[51] They contain numerous capillaries in their walls and thus serve as the site of gas exchange.

According to Thurlbeck,[3] alveoli are "obviously" present in the lungs of newborn babies, but there are formidable technical problems in trying to count them. Accordingly, the number of alveoli reported in neonates has varied from none to 71 million.[52] As discussed in Chapter 1, the results of recent morphometric studies of 42 premature or term babies who died at or shortly after birth revealed an average total number of 50 million alveoli at the end of normal gestation.[53] Furthermore, the range of normality that was observed was sufficiently wide to include the results of all previously reported alveolar counts in full-term newborns. Thus, the conclusion now seems firm that the normal human fetus is born with considerable numbers of alveoli.

Although virtually everyone seems to agree that the majority of alveoli appear in the postnatal period, there is considerable dispute over when alveolar multiplication stops, and estimates vary markedly. The results of Dunnill's careful studies suggested that formation of new alveoli ceases at about 8 years of age.[50] However, more recent data from Angus and Thurlbeck,[54] shown in comparison with Dunnill's[50] and other investigators[7, 28, 55, 56] in Figure 2–21, has opened this question once again; Angus' data also cast doubt on the prevailing notion that the number of alveoli, said to be about 300 million, is constant in normal adult human lungs. Clearly, all the answers are not available concerning the number of alveoli and the rate and cessation of their development in pre- and postnatal human lungs. On a more positive note, there does

seem to be agreement that lung volume always increases more than alveolar number during the period of body growth; this means that individual alveoli, once formed, must progressively enlarge. Alveoli of an adult human are about 250 μm in diameter and relatively uniform in size (± 10 per cent of the mean).[48]

The pre- and postnatal development of saccules/alveoli by septation is intimately related to the elastic tissue network in the lung parenchyma. Each new septum begins as a crest that is demarcated by an elastic fiber. The meshwork of fibers in the developing lungs can be viewed as shaping alveolar formation by establishing the boundaries of the interstices through which new alveoli emerge.

In contrast to previous beliefs, recent observations indicate that (1) the size of conducting airways is related to stature, (2) the number of bronchioles is constant, regardless of stature, and (3) the total number of alveoli in the lungs is proportional to height.[3] Thus, a tall person has the same number of bronchi and bronchioles as a short person, but these airways are larger in diameter and lead to more alveoli that are probably of the same size. To date, no firm morphologic basis has been found in normal lungs for so-called dysanapsis, a term used for the postulated mismatch between lung volume and airway size that would explain the remarkable variability of maximal expiratory flow rates (see Chapter 4) among healthy adults of comparable body size.[57]

Not only do alveoli increase in number by multiplication and alveolarization of bronchioles, but also alveolar surface area increases more rapidly than can be accounted for by the addition of new alveoli *per se*. This change in surface area suggests that alveoli become more complex in shape as they grow, and thus present more alveolar surface area for a given proportion of lung volume. Enlargement of alveolar surface area during growth from infancy to adulthood is closely related to increasing O_2 requirements.

The lessons from studies of comparative morphology are clear concerning lung volume on the one hand and alveolar surface area on the other. Lung volume correlates with body size, but alveolar surface area correlates with metabolic activity, regardless of body size.[58] This is illustrated by comparing two animals that are similar in size but that have different metabolic rates; the lungs of both will be equal in volume, but the alveolar surface area of the one with the higher metabolism will be greater than that of the other. The difference in area can only be attained by increased compartmentalization, which is evidenced by a change in size and number of alveoli. These features are another example of the interdependence of structure and function based upon an optimum design for functional requirements. Although the basic structure of the lung is undoubtedly fixed genetically, there is good evidence that, at least in some circumstances, morphologic adaptations may in fact take place in response to changing physiologic conditions (see section on Adaptation).

Recent morphometric studies of normal adult human lungs using electron microscopy instead of light microscopy have shown that the dimensions of the lung parenchyma are considerably larger than previously thought.[59] The mean total alveolar surface area of a normal human adult is about 143 ± 4 (standard error) m^2, of which nearly 85 to 95 per cent is covered with pulmonary capillaries; thus, the alveolar capillary interface has a surface area of approximately 126 ± 12 m^2 and provides an area of contact between the body and its external environment that is more than 70 times greater than that provided by the skin. To protect itself and the rest of the body from the numerous potentially noxious substances and infectious agents that are inhaled and may be deposited within the lung, the air-

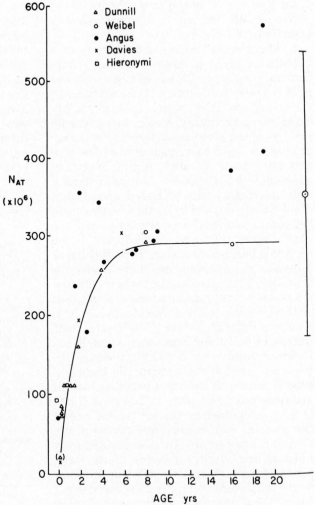

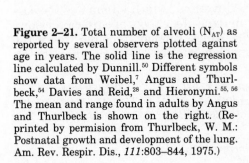

Figure 2–21. Total number of alveoli (N_{AT}) as reported by several observers plotted against age in years. The solid line is the regression line calculated by Dunnill.[50] Different symbols show data from Weibel,[7] Angus and Thurlbeck,[54] Davies and Reid,[28] and Hieronymi.[55, 56] The mean and range found in adults by Angus and Thurlbeck is shown on the right. (Reprinted by permision from Thurlbeck, W. M.: Postnatal growth and development of the lung. Am. Rev. Respir. Dis., *111*:803–844, 1975.)

ways and alveolar surfaces are equipped with elaborate defense mechanisms, which are considered in detail in Chapter 13.

Alveolar-Capillary Membrane

The old controversy regarding how many tissue layers compose the interalveolar septum was unequivocally settled shortly after the introduction of electron microscopic techniques for histologic examination in the 1950's. It is now agreed that the alveolar-capillary membrane (Fig. 2–22) consists of (1) alveolar epithelium and its basement membrane, (2) capillary endothelium and its basement membrane, (3) contiguous tissue elements in the intercalated interstitial space, and (4) surfactant lining. Another, but inconsistent, cellular component of the terminal respiratory unit is the alveolar macrophage. The proportions of the cell types that comprise the parenchyma of the normal adult human lung have recently been analyzed (Table 2–2).[60]

1. The alveolar epithelium consists of a continuous layer of tissue made up of two principal cell types: type I cells, or *squamous pneumocytes*, have broad, thin extensions, 0.1 to 0.3 μm thick, which contain mainly cytoplasmic ground substance and cover 93 per cent of the alveolar surface. Cytoplasmic organelles, such as mitochondria, are rare and are usually located in the cytoplasm surrounding the nucleus. Alveolar type I cells are highly differentiated and do not divide; their large thin surface, with sparse cytoplasm, makes them extremely susceptible to injury from a variety of blood-borne or inhaled/aspirated toxins. Type II cells, or *granular pneumocytes*, are more numerous than type I cells, but owing to their cuboidal shape they occupy approximately 7 per cent of the alveolar surface. The electron microscopic hallmarks of type II cells are their microvilli and their osmiophilic lamellated inclusion bodies (see Fig. 1–8); the convincing data linking the osmiophilic bodies of type II cells with storage sites of surfactant are reviewed in Chapter 1. The type II cell is now recognized as the progenitor cell of the alveolar epithelium, both during gestation and after a variety of experimentally induced and clinical injuries of the lung parenchyma.[11] Type III cells, or *alveolar brush cells*, were originally discovered in rat lungs,[61] but they also occur, though very rarely, in human lungs.[48] Alveolar brush cells bear a striking resemblance to brush cells found in the epithelium of large airways.

2. The capillary endothelium is composed chiefly of the cytoplasmic extension of the *endothelial cells*, which by their contiguous arrangement form a thin vascular tube. These extensions, like those of the squamous epithelial cells lining alveoli, rarely contain organelles. Besides its important but passive role in gas and liquid exchange, the capillary endothelium is now known to be the major site of liquid and solute exchange in the lungs, and the locus of a variety of active biochemical processes; these important nonrespiratory functions of the pulmonary microcirculation and the structural features that presumably underlie them are considered in detail in Chapter 12.

3. The alveolar epithelium and the capillary endothelium both rest on separate *basement membranes,* but because of the presence of structural differences that have important functional implications, the alveolar-capillary membrane has been subdivided into two separate regions. (1) The "thin portion" of the septum, or the *air-blood barrier,* occurs over the convex half of the capillary surface that bulges into the alveolus (see Fig. 2–22) and over which the two basement membranes appear to be fused. (As will be explained, the bulging is an artefact attributable to the use of intratracheal fixation, which eliminates the surface film and the effects of surface tension.) (2) The "thick portion" is found where the basement membranes are separated by an

Table 2–2. RESULTS OF STUDIES (mean ± standard error) OF THE DIFFERENT CELL TYPES IN THE PARENCHYMA OF THE NORMAL ADULT HUMAN LUNGS*

Total Number of Cells (per cent)	
Type I	8.3 ± 0.6
Type II	15.9 ± 0.8
Endothelial	30.2 ± 2.4
Interstitial	36.1 ± 1.0
Macrophage	9.4 ± 2.2
Alveolar Suface Covered (per cent)	
Type I	92.9 ± 1.0
Type II	7.1 ± 1.0
Alveolar Surface Area (μm²/cell)	
Type I	5,098 ± 659
Type II	183 ± 14
Endothelial	1,353 ± 67

*Data from Crapo, J. D., et al.: Cell number and cell characteristics of the normal human lung. Am. Rev. Respir. Dis., *125:*740–745, 1982.

interstitial space containing fine elastic fibers, small bundles of collagen fibrils, and an occasional fibroblast. Pulmonary capillaries weave their way back and forth through the interstitial space of the interalveolar septum, first facing one alveolus and then the other. Thus, the interstitial space is perforated by capillaries and should be thought of as a communicating mesh-work, not a continuous sheet. The interstitial space of the interalveolar septum extends directly into the connective tissue sheath and the interstitial space surrounding airways and blood vessels.[48] Diffusion of gases takes place mainly across the thin portion (see Chapter 7), and liquid and solute exchange occurs mainly across the thick portion (see Chapter 12).

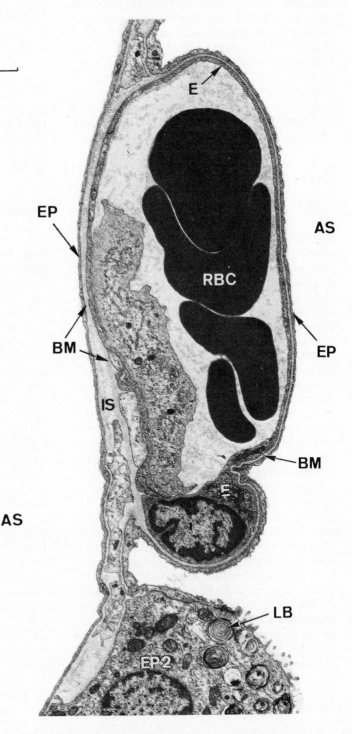

Figure 2–22. Electron micrograph of a transverse section through a capillary in the interalveolar septum of a normal human lung. The surface of the septum facing the two alveolar spaces (AS) is mainly lined by thin squamous extensions of type I epithelial cells (EP). The lower right-hand portion of the septum is covered by a type II epithelial cell (EP2) containing osmiophilic lamellar bodies (LB). The capillary, containing red blood cells (RBC), is lined by endothelium (E). Both epithelium and endothelium rest on basement membranes (BM) that are fused over the "thin" portion of the septum and that are separated by an interstitial space (IS) over the "thick" portion of the septum. Horizontal bar = 1 μm. (Courtesy of Dr. Ewald R. Weibel.) (Reprinted by permission from Murray, J. F.: Respiration. *In* Smith, L. H., and Thier, S. (eds.): *Pathophysiology*. Philadelphia, W. B. Saunders Company, 1985, pp. 753–854.)

4. Surfactant can be recovered easily in lung extracts and washes, and its anatomic location is well defined (Fig. 2–23).[62] A great deal is known about the metabolic pathways of surfactant synthesis, its storage in lamellar bodies of type II cells, its release into the overlying subphase, and the constituents of the monomolecular film of active surfactant at the air-liquid interface (see Chapters 1 and 12 for further details). Although little is known about the physiologic factors that regulate the formation and removal of surfactant, they appear to be linked, at least in part, to ventilatory requirements. This is fortuitous because, as will be pointed out, surfactant not only contributes to the recoil properties of the lung but plays an important role in stabilizing and supporting the lung parenchyma.

Other Cells

Alveolar macrophages are phagocytic cells that are found in varying numbers lying submerged in the extracellular lining of the alveolar surface (Fig. 2–24). There is general agreement that alveolar macrophages originate from stem cell precursors in the bone marrow and reach the lung through the bloodstream, presumably as circulating monocytes. However, because the enzyme profile of alveolar macrophages differs considerably from that of monocytes, immediate transcapillary migration from blood to alveolus is untenable and differentiation must occur. Transformation of blood monocytes to alveolar macrophages occurs within a few hours after arrival in the lungs and entry into the interstitium. Alveolar macrophages that can be recovered by bronchopulmonary lavage from experimental animals are highly variable in bactericidal capacity, metabolic activity, lysosomal enzyme content, surface receptors, cytoplasmic morphology, and size.[63] These and other properties may be expressions of a continuum of differentiation.[64] Functional heterogeneity is further augmented after exposure of alveolar macrophages to such diverse stimuli as bacteria, toxins, particulate matter, or immunologic challenge. The turnover time of alveolar macrophages in the mouse was recently shown to be 5.5 days.[65] Alveolar macrophages are of considerable interest because they elaborate a large variety of potent chemical substances, because they constitute the chief mechanism of clearance of bacteria and other particles that are deposited in the terminal respiratory units, and because deficiencies in their function undoubtedly contribute to the pathogenesis of pulmonary infections. For these reasons, alveolar macrophages are reviewed further in the chapter on pulmonary defense mechanisms (see Chapter 13).

STRUCTURAL SUPPORT

The important and difficult question of how the lungs are able to maintain such a thin parenchyma over so large a surface area has been largely answered by the careful anatomic studies of Weibel.[66] The essential features are an interconnected system of connective tissue fibers and a film of surfactant that exerts surface forces at the air-liquid interface of the alveoli.

Fibrous Networks

A complicated system of connective tissue forms and maintains the architecture of the lungs at the gross and microscopic levels. The primary fibrous elements of this system are collagen and elastin, which are closely associated in three interconnecting but anatomically distinct networks throughout the lung (Fig. 2–25; see also Plate III).

1. The *peripheral fiber system* begins in the connective tissue sheets that are part of the visceral pleura. Thus, each lobe of the lungs is invested in a fibrous envelope from which additional connective tissue sheets radiate *inward* to subdivide the lobe into segments, and to varying degrees into lobules.

2. The *central fiber system* consists of three axial, parallel interdigitating networks that invest airways, pulmonary arteries, and pulmonary veins, beginning at the hilus. As these structures branch within each lobe, their accompanying axial fibers radiate *outward* toward the lung parenchyma.

3. The *septal fiber system* is the network of short, extremely fine fibers that are found in the alveolar walls themselves. As mentioned, alveoli are formed in the meshes of this delicate connective tissue latticework so that these fibers form, in their terminal boundaries, the reinforced entrance rings of individual alveoli.

Both the peripheral and central fiber systems begin as relatively thick sheets or

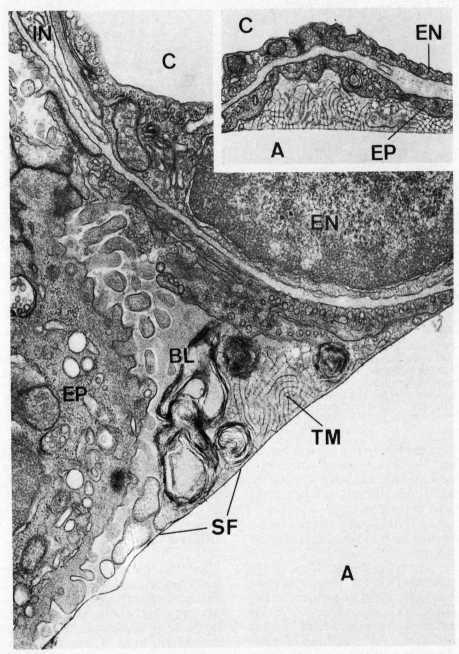

Figure 2–23. Electron micrograph of a thin section of rat lung fixed by vascular perfusion. The depression in the surface of the alveolar epithelium (EP) is smoothed out with extracellular material. Its base layer (BL) contains globular and tubular myelin figures (TM) with some of the osmiophilic lamellae reaching and connecting with the surface film (SF). (× 26,400). The inset shows similar structures in a region where the alveolar-capillary tissue barrier is thin (× 23,010). A = alveolar space; C = capillary; EN = endothelium; IN = interstitial space. (Reprinted by permission from Untersee, P. et al.: Visualization of extracellular lining layer of lung alveoli by freeze-etching. Respir. Physiol., *13*:171–185, 1971.)

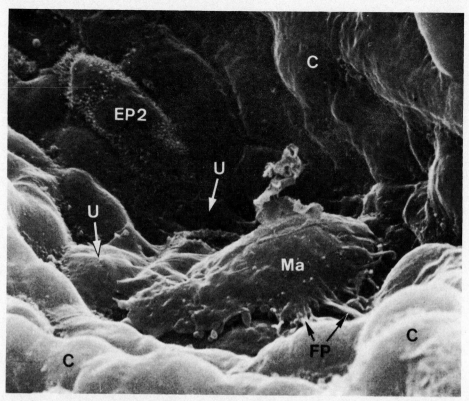

Figure 2–24. Scanning electron micrograph of a normal human lung showing an alveolar macrophage (Ma) attached to the epithelium partly by filopodia (FP) and forming an undulating membrane (U) in the direction of forward movement to the left. Several capillaries (C) are evident, and a type II epithelial cell (EP2) can be seen in the background. (Original magnification × 3700). (Reprinted by permission from Gehr, P., et al.: The normal human lung: Ultrastructure and morphometric estimation of diffusion capacity. Respir. Physiol., *32*:121–140, © 1978, The Williams & Wilkins Company, Baltimore.)

layers of connective tissue, which become thinner and less dense as each meshwork radiates toward its ramifications into the septal system. A continuity is established, whereby the lung parenchyma is supported by a fibrous network, albeit delicate, that is firmly anchored both at the pleural surface and at the hilus.

The fine connective tissue fibers of the lung parenchyma lie in the interstitial space of the thick portion of the interalveolar septum. This space is continuous in the sense that liquid that enters it at one end can flow to the other end, but it is perforated by the pulmonary capillaries as they weave their way from one side of the septum to the other. The interweaving capillary network of the interalveolar septum is itself interwoven by the septal fiber network (Fig. 2–26; see also Plate III). The arrangement is such that at any point along the length of an individual capillary, approximately half of the perimeter of the capillary comprises part of the thin air-blood barrier for

gas exchange, and the other half faces the thick portion of the septum where liquid and solute filtration occur and where the connective tissue fibers lie (see Fig. 2–22).

Surface Film

The anatomic arrangement just described gives rise to a highly corrugated surface, with pits and crevices formed by the capillary network bulging above and below the flat plane of the septum. This configuration can be seen in the lungs fixed by vascular perfusion after filling them with saline to eliminate the effects of surface forces (Fig. 2–27, *C* and *D*); the protruding capillaries, the irregularly shaped alveoli, and the resulting high surface curvatures at both 40 and 80 per cent of full inflation are readily apparent. In contrast, examination of air-filled lungs, in other words those in which surface forces are still present, reveals a very different appearance at comparable

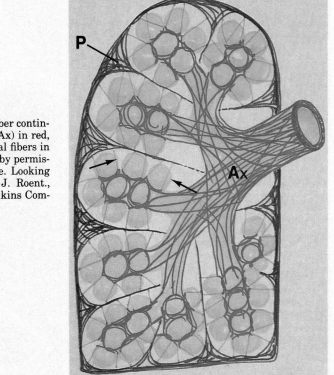

Figure 2–25. Schematic illustration of the fiber continuum of the lung parenchyma. Axial fibers (Ax) in red, peripheral fibers (P) in brown, and fine septal fibers in alveolar walls (arrows) in green. (Reprinted by permission from Weibel, E. R.: Fleischner Lecture. Looking into the lung: What can it tell us? Am. J. Roent., *133*:1021–1031, © 1979, The William & Wilkins Company, Baltimore.) See also Plate III.

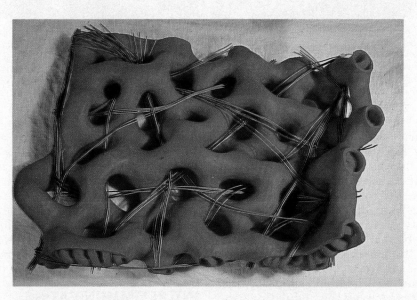

Figure 2–26. Reconstruction of a capillary network in the alveolar septum interwoven with the network of septal fibers. (Reprinted by permission from Weibel, E. R.: Fleischner Lecture. Looking into the lung: What can it tell us? Am. J. Roent., *133*:1021–1031, © 1979, The Williams & Wilkins Company, Baltimore.) See also Plate III.

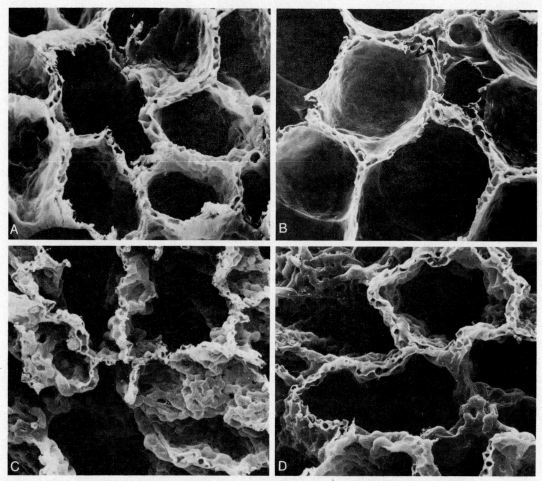

Figure 2–27. Scanning electron micrographs of air- and saline-filled lungs, both fixed by vascular perfusion. *A* and *B*, Air-filled lungs at 40 and 80 per cent of total lung capacity (TLC), respectively. Note crumpled surface of the lung deflated to 40 per cent TLC but smooth surface of the lung at 80 per cent TLC. *C* and *D,* Saline-filled lungs at 40 and 80 per cent TLC, respectively. Note undulating alveolar septa, especially at the lower lung volume, and protruding capillaries at both degrees of inflation. (Reprinted by permission from Gil, J., et al.: Alveolar volume-surface area relation in air- and saline-filled lungs fixed by vascular perfusion. J. Appl. Physiol., *47*:990–1001, 1979.)

lung volumes (Fig. 2–27, *A* and *B*). At 80 per cent of full inflation the alveolar surfaces are smooth; at 40 per cent inflation the alveolar surfaces have a more wrinkled appearance, but not nearly as irregular as that seen in saline-filled lungs.[67]

The relatively smooth alveolar surface geometry of normal air-filled lungs is explained by the presence of the two components of the surface layer, each fulfilling a different function. The liquid subphase fills the interstices between the undulating capillary network, thus smoothing the surface to some extent (see Fig. 2–23). The interfacial tension of the surface film itself creates a smooth surface by pushing in on the capillaries from one side or the other; this pressure causes the septum to buckle and to

lose the planar configuration observed in saline-filled lungs. Because the interalveolar septum becomes deformed in air-filled lungs, a relative slackness in the septal connective tissue network is suggested. In any case, the tendency of the air-liquid interface to round up into the smallest surface area possible clearly prevails over any tensions exerted by the septal fibers.

INTERCOMMUNICATING CHANNELS

One of the important developments in pulmonary physiology during the last decade has been the resurgence of experimental activity concerning the structural basis and functional consequences of collateral ventilation. The increased interest is related to observations that the physiologic effects of airways obstruction, both in patients with various forms of obstructive lung disease and in laboratory animals, are critically dependent upon the magnitude of collateral ventilation.[68] Despite the compelling physiologic evidence that has underscored the importance of intercommunicating channels to normal respiratory function and to the pathogenesis of common lung diseases, only limited descriptive anatomic information is available about the possible pathways involved. However, some recent progress has been made that adds to our understanding of the subject.

Alveolar Pores of Kohn

Originally, considerable doubt existed as to whether the alveolar pores of Kohn were normal structures or fixation artefacts. Now, however, there is general agreement that these pores are anatomic entities and that they occur in the interalveolar septa of nearly all mammalian species, including humans. Alveolar pores (Fig. 2–28) are openings in alveolar walls that are located in intercapillary spaces and are often bordered by a capillary loop. They are lined with alveolar epithelial cells that usually abut adjacent cells in the alveolar wall on each side of the opening.[68]

Alveolar pores can be viewed as short cylinders whose dimensions, although they have not been measured directly, probably vary with lung volume. This conclusion is based on the response to lung inflation of microholes that were punctured in the alveolar walls of experimental animals.[69] The diameter of alveolar pores varies from 3 to 12 μm, and their width, which is the thickness of the alveolar septum (between capillaries), is about 2 μm. During inflation of the lung, the diameter presumably increases and the width decreases as the alveolar wall stretches.

The results of studies using lung fixation techniques that preserve the surface layer have revealed that most pores of Kohn are covered—hence closed—by a film of surfactant; the pores that were found to be open may well have been closed during life.[70] Thus, it appears that alveolar pores contribute little, if at all, to collateral ventilation. Interalveolar openings greater than 12 μm are too large always to be covered by the surface lining layer and may serve as collateral pathways; such channels, which are properly called "fenestrae," probably represent degeneration or a pathologic process because they appear to increase in number with age.

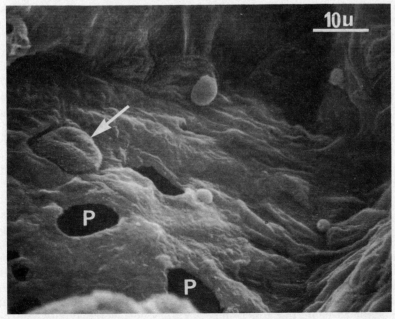

Figure 2–28. Scanning electron micrograph of the surface of a human alveolus showing pores of Kohn (P) and a macrophage (arrow). (× 1500. Courtesy of Dr. N. S. Wang.)

Canals of Lambert

Lambert and coworkers[71, 72] have demonstrated the presence of accessory pathways from respiratory bronchioles, terminal bronchioles, and even larger airways to airspaces supplied by other airways—in other words alternate channels for gas movement to distal respiratory units. Details about the number, location, and extent of Lambert's canals are lacking. Although they have been identified in infants, virtually nothing is known about the factors that influence the development of the communications other than that they may be increased in the lungs of patients with various lung diseases such as emphysema and honeycombing. Lambert's canals may well prove to be important pathways for collateral ventilation in normal subjects and in patients with lung diseases. It is regrettable that so little is known about them.

Other Pathways

Physiologic studies have revealed that polystyrene spheres 64 μm in diameter can pass through collateral pathways in excised human lungs.[73] Even larger spheres (120 μm in diameter) can traverse collateral channels in dog lungs.[74] Anatomic pathways even larger than these dimensions were convincingly demonstrated in human lungs by Raskin and Herman,[75] using micropuncture and injection techniques; these investigators discovered short tubular structures, 200 μm or more in diameter, that connected respiratory bronchioles and alveolar ducts of adjacent terminal respiratory units. Studies were possible only in the subpleural regions of the lung, where such communications were "common." Further information is needed concerning the structural and functional interrelationships of collateral ventilation in normal subjects and how these factors are changed by diseases of the lung.

ADAPTATION AND AGING

Most organs of the body thrive on work and languish without it; the prototype is skeletal muscle but included also is the brain (especially the mind). The capacity of the lungs to adapt to changing functional demands has been disputed until recently. Other continuously working organs, such as the heart and the kidney, increase their functional mass when an additional chronic work load must be dealt with. Because the main function of the lungs is to supply O_2 to the cells of the body at the rate they need it to sustain metabolism, most studies of pulmonary adaptation have examined the extent to which the structural design of the lungs can change in response to imposed disturbances of O_2 supply or O_2 demand. Basically, the lungs can respond to new gas exchange needs by changing their size or by changing their compartmentalization; in either case, more or less surface area for O_2 uptake results.

Adaptation

There is now unequivocal evidence that the lungs are adaptable to altered functional demands, at least while certain experimental animals are growing (see Weibel[76] for review and references). In response to increased O_2 consumption, environmental hypoxia, or partial lung resection, rodents developed an increase in their lungs' maximal capacity to transfer O_2 from inspired gas to blood as assessed both morphometrically and functionally. Opposite changes occurred in animals given increased concentration of O_2 to breathe.

The usual way of determining the capacity of the human respiratory system to adapt to unusual conditions of O_2 supply or demand has been to examine the lungs of persons living in the hypoxic environment of high altitude. It is well known that long-term residents of high altitude, especially natives, are capable of astonishing physical feats that require large amounts of O_2, and it is clear that changes in the respiratory system contribute to exercise capacity by enhancing the uptake of O_2 by the lungs. But it is still not fully established, especially in humans, how much of the improvement in gas exchange that occurs at high altitude is the result of functional changes (e.g., polycythemia) and how much is attributable to actual structural adaptations (e.g., increased number of alveoli).

Although the lungs of natives of high altitudes are slightly larger than those of residents at sea level or acclimatized sojourners, the most striking difference in respiratory performance between these groups of subjects is in their pulmonary diffusing capacities, a measurement of the alveolar-capillary surface area and blood volume available for gas exchange.[77] Natives of high altitudes are favored with a diffusing capacity 20 to 30 per cent higher than that of their counterparts at sea level. This difference cannot be explained on the basis of an elevated pulmonary arterial pressure or polycythemia, both of which increase the diffusing capacity by increasing the number of red blood cells in pulmonary capillaries, because both natives and acclimatized sojourners have similar values for these altitude-dependent variables. These observations raise the possibility that either adaptive responses or genetic factors account for the fact that natives have an increased ability to transfer O_2.

Morphometric studies performed on lungs of five natives of high altitude who died accidentally revealed an increase in number and size of alveoli; both factors contributed to an increase in alveolar surface area as compared with the alveolar surface area of matched control subjects who lived at sea level.[78] Further evidence in favor of pulmonary adaptation comes from studies of pulmonary mechanics in Peruvian natives living at sea level or high altitude.[79] The findings suggest that the large lungs of the highlanders result from hypoxic stimulation to growth of the lung parenchyma but not of the airways. Similarly, it is becoming clear that true lung growth can occur in infants after pulmonary resection,[80] a phenomenon that has been well documented in experimental animals.[3] Recent experimental data also indicate that after pneumonectomy central and peripheral airways in the remaining lung increase in cross-sectional area but that airway growth is less than the compensatory increase in lung volume.[81] It now seems clear that growing children, like other young mammals, adapt to environmental hypoxia and lung resection by forming increased numbers of alveoli. In contrast, the effects of hormonal stimulation on lung growth in both experimental animals and humans are poorly documented and need further study.

Aging

Growth and development of the lungs cease in normal human beings when somatic growth stops. The lung shares with the rest of the body the consequences of advancing years, and as in other organs, aging causes changes in the lungs' morphometry and chemical composition as well as in its function. Because the effects of aging are expressed in deterioration of specific aspects of lung function that have not yet been explained, complete discussion of age-related changes is deferred until the last chapter of this book.

REFERENCES

1. Polgar, G., and Promadhat, V.: Pulmonary Function Testing in Children: Techniques and Standards. Philadelphia, W. B. Saunders Company, 1971, p. 207.
2. Swyer, P. R., Reiman, R. C., and Wright, J. J.: Ventilation and ventilatory mechanics in the newborn. J. Pediatr., *56*:612–622, 1960.
3. Thurlbeck, W. M.: Postnatal growth and development of the lung. Am. Rev. Respir. Dis., *111*:803–844, 1975.
4. Polgar, G., and Weng, T. R.: The functional development of the respiratory system: from the period of gestation to adulthood. Am. Rev. Respir. Dis., *120*:625–695, 1979.
4a. Weibel, E. R.: The Pathway for Oxygen. Structure and Function in the Mammalian Respiratory System. Cambridge, Harvard University Press, 1984, pp. 1–425.
5. Hogg, J. C., Williams, J., Richardson, J. B., Macklem, P. T., and Thurlbeck, W. M.: Age as a factor in the distribution of lower-airway conductance and in the pathologic anatomy of obstructive lung disease. New Engl. J. Med., *282*:1283–1287, 1970.
6. Horsfield, K., and Cumming, G.: Morphology of the bronchial tree in man. J. Appl. Physiol., *24*:373–383, 1968.
7. Weibel, E. R.: Morphometry of the Human Lung. Berlin, Springer-Verlag, 1963, p. 111.
8. Horsfield, K., and Cumming, G.: Functional consequences of airway morphology. J. Appl. Physiol., *24*:384–390, 1968.
9. Breeze, R. G., and Wheeldon, E. B.: The cells of the pulmonary airways. Am. Rev. Respir. Dis., *116*:705–777, 1977.
10. Reid, L. M., and Jones, R.: Mucous membrane of respiratory epithelium. Environ. Health Perspect., *35*:113–120, 1980.
11. Gail, D. B., and Lenfant, C. J. M.: Cells of the lung; biology and clinical implications. Am. Rev. Respir. Dis., *127*:366–367, 1983.
12. Cosio, M. G., Hale, K. A., and Niewoehner, D. E.: Morphologic and morphometric effects of prolonged cigarette smoking on the small airways. Am. Rev. Respir. Dis., *122*:265–271, 1980.
13. Jeffery, P., and Reid, L.: Intra-epithelial nerves in normal rat airways: A quantitative electron microscope study. J. Anat., *114*:35–45, 1973.
14. Lauweryns, J. M., DeBock, V., Verhofstad, A. A. J., and Steinbusch, H. W. M.: Immunohistochemical localization of serotonin in intrapulmonary neuro-epithelial bodies. Cell Tissue Res., *226*:215–223, 1982.
15. Lauweryns, J. M., and Van Lommel, A.: Morphometric analysis of hypoxia-induced synaptic activity in intrapulmonary neuro-epithelial bodies. Cell Tissue Res., *226*:201–214, 1982.

16. Widdicombe, J. G., and Pack, R. J.: The Clara cell. Eur. J. Respir. Dis., 63:202–220, 1982.
17. Nadel, J. A., Davis, B., and Phipps, R. J.: Control of mucus secretion and ion transport in airways. Annu. Rev. Physiol., 41:369–381, 1979.
18. Meyrick, B., and Reid, L.: Ultrastructure of cells in the human bronchial submucosal glands. J. Anat., 107:281–299, 1970.
19. Bensch, K. G., Gordon, G. B., and Miller, L. R.: Studies on the bronchial counterpart of the Kultschitzky (argentaffin) cell and innervation of bronchial glands. J. Ultrastruct. Res., 12:668–686, 1965.
20. Richardson, J. B.: Nerve supply to the lungs. Am. Rev. Respir. Dis., 119:785–802, 1979.
21. Reid, L.: Measurement of the bronchial mucous gland layer: a diagnostic yardstick in chronic bronchitis. Thorax, 15:132–141, 1960.
22. Lewis, R. A., and Austen, K. F.: Nonrespiratory functions of pulmonary cells: the mast cell. Fed. Proc., 36:2676–2683, 1977.
23. Miller, W. S.: The Lung. Springfield, Illinois, Charles C Thomas, 1937, pp. 27–37.
24. von Hayek, H.: The Human Lung. New York, Hafner Publishing Company, Inc., 1960, pp. 206–212.
25. Richardson, J. B., and Ferguson, C. C.: Neuromuscular structure and function in the airways. Fed. Proc., 38:202–208, 1978.
25a. Workshop Report: Workshop on airway smooth muscle. Am Rev. Respir. Dis., 131:159–162, 1985.
26. Kapanci, Y., Assimacopoulos, A., Irle, C., Zwahlen, A., and Gabbiani, G.: "Contractile interstitial cells" in pulmonary alveolar septa: a possible regulator of ventilation-perfusion ratio? Ultrastructural, immunofluorescence, and in vitro studies. J. Cell. Biol., 60:375–392, 1974.
27. Hislop, A., and Reid, L.: Intra-pulmonary arterial development during fetal life—branching pattern and structure. J. Anat., 113:35–48, 1972.
28. Davies, G., and Reid, L.: Growth of the alveoli and pulmonary arteries in childhood. Thorax, 25:669–681, 1970.
29. Heath, D.: Pulmonary vasculature in postnatal life and pulmonary hemodynamics. In Emery, J. (ed.): The Anatomy of the Developing Lung. Suffolk, W. Heinmann Ltd., 1969, pp. 147–169.
30. Marshall, C., and Marshall, B.: Site and sensitivity for stimulation of hypoxic pulmonary vasoconstriction. J. Appl. Physiol., 55:711–716, 1983.
31. Fishman, A. P.: Vasomotor regulation of the pulmonary circulation. Annu. Rev. Physiol., 42:211–220, 1980.
32. Kato, M., and Staub, N. C.: Response of small pulmonary arteries to unilobar hypoxia and hypercapnia. Circ. Res., 19:426–440, 1966.
33. Hughes, J. M. B., Grant, B. J. B., Jones, H. A., and Davies, E. E.: Relationship between blood flow and alveolar gas tensions in lung lobules. Scand. J. Respir. Dis. (Suppl)., 85:17–21, 1974.
34. Hislop, A., and Reid, L.: Pulmonary arterial development during childhood: Branching pattern and structure. Thorax, 28:129–135, 1973.
35. Heinemann, H. O., and Fishman, A. P.: Nonrespiratory functions of mammalian lung. Physiol. Rev., 49:1–47, 1969.
36. Bierman, H. R., Kelly, K. H., Cordes, F. L., Byron, R. L., Jr., Polhemus, J. A., and Rappoport, S.: The release of leukocytes and platelets from the pulmonary circulation by epinephrine. Blood, 7:683–692, 1952.
36a. Staub, N. C., Schultz, E. L., and Albertine, K. H.: Leukocytes and pulmonary vascular injury. In Malik, A. B., and Staub, N. C. (eds.): Mechanisms of Lung Microvascular Injury. New York, New York Academy of Sciences, 1982, pp. 332–342.
36b. Martin, B. A., Dahlby, R., Nicholls, I., and Hogg, J. C.: Platelet sequestration in lung with hemorrhagic shock and reinfusion in dogs. J. Appl. Physiol., 50:1306–1312, 1981.
37. Hislop, A., and Reid, L.: Fetal and childhood development of the intrapulmonary veins in man—branching pattern and structure. Thorax, 28:313–319, 1973.
38. Heath, D., and Edwards, J. E.: Histological changes in the lung in diseases associated with pulmonary venous hypertension. Br. J. Dis. Chest, 53:8–18, 1959.
39. Hoffman, J. I. E., Guz, A., Charlier, A. A., and Wilken, D. E. L.: Stroke volume in conscious dogs; effect of respiration, posture, and vascular occlusion. J. Appl. Physiol., 20:865–877, 1965.
40. Marchand, P., Gilroy, J. C., and Wilson, V. H.: An anatomical study of the bronchial vascular system and its variations in disease. Thorax, 5:207–221, 1950.
41. Heymann, M. A., Creasy, R. K., and Rudolph, A. M.: Quantitation of blood flow pattern in the foetal lamb in utero. In Proceedings of the Sixth Joseph Barcroft Centenary Symposium: Foetal and Neonatal Physiology. Cambridge, Cambridge University Press, 1973, pp. 129–135.
42. McLaughlin, R. F., Jr.: Bronchial artery distribution in various mammals and in humans. Am. Rev. Resp. Dis., 128(suppl):557–558, 1983.
43. Baile, E. M., Nelems, J. M., Schulzer, M., and Paré, P. D.: Measurement of regional bronchial arterial blood flow and bronchovascular resistance in dogs. J. Appl. Physiol., 53:1044–1049, 1982.
44. Cudkowicz, L., Abelmann, W. H., Levinson, G. E., Katznelson, G., and Jreissaty, R. M.: Bronchial arterial blood flow. Clin. Sci., 19:1–15, 1960.
45. Aviado, D. M.: The Lung Circulation. Vol. 1. Oxford, Pergamon Press Ltd., 1965, pp. 185–254.
46. Modell, H. I., Beck, K., and Butler, J.: Functional aspects of canine bronchial-pulmonary vascular communications. J. Appl. Physiol., 50:1045–1051, 1981.
47. Auld, P. A., Rudolph, A. M., and Golinko, R. J.: Factors affecting bronchial collateral flow in the dog. Am. J. Physiol., 198:1166–1170, 1960.
48. Weibel, E. R.: Morphological basis of alveolar-capillary gas exchange. Physiol. Rev., 53:419–495, 1973.
49. Lauweryns, J. M.: The blood and lymphatic microcirculation of the lung. In Sommers, S. C. (ed.): Pathology Annual 1971. New York, Appleton-Century-Crofts, 1971, pp. 365–415.
50. Dunnill, M. S.: Postnatal growth of the lung. Thorax, 17:329–333, 1962.
51. Macklin, C. C.: Musculature of bronchi and lungs. Physiol. Rev., 9:1–60, 1929.
52. Thurlbeck, W. M., and Angus, G. E.: Growth and aging of the normal human lung. Chest, 67:3S–7S, 1975.
53. Langston, C., Kida, K., Reed, M., and Thurlbeck, W. M.: Human lung growth in late gestation and in the neonate. Am. Rev. Respir. Dis., 129:607–613, 1984.
54. Angus, G. E., and Thurlbeck, W. M.: Number of alveoli in the human lung. J. Appl. Physiol., 32:483–485, 1972.

55. Hieronymi, G.: Über den durch das Alter bedingten Formwandel menschlicher Lungen. Ergebn. Allg. Pathol., *41*:1–62, 1961.

56. Hieronymi, G.: Veränderungen der Lungenstruktur in verschiendenen Lebensaltern. Verh. Deutsch. Ges. Pathol., *44*:129–130, 1960.

57. Mead, J.: Dysanapsis in normal lungs assessed by the relationship between maximal flow, static recoil, and vital capacity. Am. Rev. Respir. Dis., *121*:339–342, 1980.

58. Taylor, C. R., Maloiy, G. M. O., Weibel, E. R., Langman, V. A., Kamau, J. M., Seeherman, H. J., and Heglund, N. C.: Design of the mammalian respiratory system. III. Scaling maximum aerobic capacity to body mass: wild and domestic mammals. Respir. Physiol., *44*:25–37, 1981.

59. Gehr, P., Bachofen, M., and Weibel, E. R.: The normal human lung: ultrastructure and morphometric estimation of diffusion capacity. Respir. Physiol., *32*:121–140, 1978.

60. Crapo, J. D., Barry, B. E., Gehr, P., Bachofen, M., and Weibel, E. R.: Cell number and cell characteristics of the normal human lung. Am. Rev. Respir. Dis., *125*:740–745, 1982.

61. Meyrick, B., and Reid, L.: The alveolar brush cell in rat lung—a third pneumonocyte. J. Ultrastruct. Res., *23*:71–80, 1968.

62. Untersee, P., Gil, J., and Weibel, E. R.: Visualization of extracellular lining layer of lung alveoli by freeze-etching. Respir. Physiol., *13*:171–185, 1971.

63. Dauber, J. H., Holian, A. H., Rosemiller, M. A., and Daniele, R. P.: Separation of bronchoalveolar cells from guinea pig on continuous density gradients of Percoll: Morphology and cytochemical properties of fractionated lung macrophages. J. Reticuloendothel. Soc., *33*:119–126, 1983.

64. Zwilling, B. S., Campolito, L. B., and Reiches, N. A.: Alveolar macrophage subpopulations identified by differential centrifugation on a discontinuous albumin density gradient. Am. Rev. Respir. Dis., *125*:448–452, 1982.

65. Blusse, A., Van Oud, A., and Van Furth, R.: The origin of pulmonary macrophages. Immunobiology, *161*:186–192, 1982.

66. Weibel, E. R.: Fleischner Lecture. Looking into the lung: what can it tell us? Am. J. Roentgenol., *133*:1021–1031, 1979.

67. Gil, J., Bachofen, H., Gehr, P., and Weibel, E. R.: Alveolar volume-surface area relation in air- and saline-filled lungs fixed by vascular perfusion. J. Appl. Physiol., *47*:990–1001, 1979.

68. Macklem, P. T.: Airway obstruction and collateral ventilation. Physiol. Rev., *51*:368–436, 1971.

69. Kuno, K., and Staub, N. C.: Acute mechanical effects of lung volume changes on artificial microholes in alveolar walls. J. Appl. Physiol., *24*:83–92, 1968.

70. Takaro, T., Price, H. P., and Parra, S. C.: Ultrastructural studies of apertures in the interalveolar septum of the adult human lung. Am. Rev. Respir. Dis., *119*:425–434, 1979.

71. Lambert, M. W.: Accessory bronchiole-alveolar communications. J. Pathol. Bacteriol., *70*:311–314, 1955.

72. Duguid, J. B., and Lambert, M. W.: The pathogenesis of coal miner's pneumoconiosis. J. Pathol. Bacteriol., *88*:389–403, 1964.

73. Henderson, R., Horsfield, K., and Cumming, G.: Intersegmental collateral ventilation in the human lung. Respir. Physiol., *6*:128–134, 1968.

74. Martin, H. B.: Respiratory bronchioles as the pathway for collateral ventilation. J. Appl. Physiol., *21*:1443–1447, 1966.

75. Raskin, S. P., and Herman, P. G.: Interacinar pathways in the human lung. Am. Rev. Respir. Dis., *119*:425–434, 1979.

76. Weibel, E. R.: Is the lung built reasonably? Am. Rev. Respir. Dis., *128*:752–760, 1983.

77. Lenfant, C., and Sullivan, K.: Adaptation to high altitude. New Engl. J. Med., *284*:1298–1309, 1971.

78. Saldana, M., and Garcia Oyola, E.: Morphometry of the high altitude lung. Lab. Invest., *22*:509, 1970.

79. Brody, J. S., Lahira, S., Simpser, M., Motoyama, E. K., and Velasquez, T.: Lung elasticity and airway dynamics in Peruvian natives to high altitude. J. Appl. Physiol., *42*:245–251, 1977.

80. McBride, J. T., Wohl, M. E. B., Strieder, D. J., Jackson, A. C., Morton, J. R., Zwerdling, R. G., Griscom, N. T., Treves, S., Williams, A. J., and Schuster, S.: Lung growth and airway function after lobectomy in infancy for congenital lobar emphysema. J. Clin. Invest., *66*:962–970, 1980.

81. McBride, J. T.: Postpneumonectomy airway growth in the ferret. J. Appl. Physiol. *58*:1010–1014, 1985.

Chapter

3

Lymphatic and Nervous Systems

ences among various species. But it is also clear that there are many unifying anatomic and physiologic generalities that apply to humans, even though some of the details are lacking. The purpose of this chapter is to review the structure–function relationships of the lymphatic drainage pathways, the lymphatic aggregates, and the innervation of the lung. Additional details about the contribution of these structures to normal function and in disease states are provided later in this book.

INTRODUCTION

During the last 10 years, a considerable amount of new information has been obtained about the pulmonary lymphatic and nervous systems. Of necessity, much of the experimental data has been acquired from studies of mammals other than humans, and it is clear that there are important differ-

LYMPHATIC VESSELS AND LYMPH NODES

Compared with most other organs, the lungs have an unusually extensive lymphatic system. Contrary to the old opinion that the lungs are a "dry organ," it is now well established that there is constant filtration of liquid from the microcirculation and

61

that there must be removal of an equal amount through the lymphatics (see Chapter 12). When filtration exceeds removal for very long, pulmonary edema occurs. The lungs are also richly supplied with lymphatic tissue, which plays an important role in pulmonary defenses (see Chapter 13). Thus, the lungs' lymphatic system is vital both in homeostasis and in protection against disease.

Lymphatic Vessels

The pulmonary lymphatics, like those of other organs, are situated in connective tissue spaces: the pleura, interlobular septa, and peribronchovascular sheath.[1] The pulmonary lymphatic system in humans is organized into two main sets of vessels: the superficial or *pleural network* and the deep or *peribronchovascular network* (Fig. 3–1; see also Plate IV).[2] Although the principal routes of lymph flow to the hilus are through the lung, the superficial network is continuous, and it is possible for lymph to flow around the surface of the lung to reach the hilus.

Lymphatic capillaries form extensive plexuses within the connective tissue sheaths that surround both large and small airways and blood vessels; the network of vessels extends to the level of terminal and respiratory bronchioles, where the lymphatic capillaries begin as blind-end tubes or saccules.[3] Lymphatic vessels are not found in the interalveolar walls at the site where most of the filtration of liquid occurs. The lymphatic capillaries of the lungs are similar to those of other organs in that they lack a continuous basal lamina and they contain many anchoring filaments that connect the outer endothelial surface to the neighboring interstitium.[3] The capillary tubes are formed by endothelial cells with thin cytoplasmic extensions that are characterized by their numerous filaments, some of which, because they can be made to form so-called arrowhead complexes, are believed to be actin; these may contribute to rhythmic contractions or to the regulation of intercellular gaps or clefts.[4] The margins of adjacent endothelial cells overlap considerably with an intercellular cleft of varying width and complexity in between (Fig. 3–2). The lymphatic endothelial cells also contain the usual cytoplasmic organelles, which are concentrated in the perinuclear regions and scattered elsewhere, and numerous plasmalemmal invaginations and pinocytic vesicles, which participate in the removal of particulate substances from both luminal and connective tissue sides of the cell wall.

The lymphatic capillaries in the connective tissue sheaths around the larger conducting airways and blood vessels have been called *juxtaalveolar lymphatics* by Lauweryns[5] and Leak.[6] The term indicates that even though lymphatic capillaries are not located within the interalveolar system, they are not very far from the sites of liquid and solute filtration (Fig. 3–3). Judging from the dimensions of terminal respiratory units, most pulmonary capillaries are within a few 100 μm or, at most, 1 mm of the nearest juxtaalveolar lymphatic.

The networks of lymphatic capillaries drain into collecting vessels, which are characterized by their larger diameter, thicker walls, and numerous valves. The walls of pulmonary collecting vessels contain three layers: an intima composed of endothelial cells that rest on a continuous basal lamina, a media that contains several layers of spiraling smooth muscle cells, and an adventitia made up chiefly of bundles of collagen and fibroblasts.[3]

Lymph flow within the collecting vessels is directed toward the hilus by regularly distributed valves, which are nearly all bicuspid.[7] The two semilunar cusps arise from the vessel wall and are oriented so that their free edges fit together like a miter joint (Fig. 3–4). The presence of cytoplasmic filaments suggestive of actin has raised the possibility that contraction of the endothelial cells lining the valve leaflets opens the orifice to the passage of lymph and, conversely, that relaxation of these cells restricts the flow.

As discussed in detail in Chapter 12, liquid flows from its site of filtration in the interstitial spaces surrounding capillaries and other small vessels to its site of removal through the lymphatics located in the peribronchovascular interstitial spaces. Liquid presumably enters the lymphatics through the intercellular clefts, a process that is facilitated by the anchoring filaments.[8] As the interstitium becomes distended by liquid, the delicate lymphatic capillaries are prevented from collapsing by the anchoring

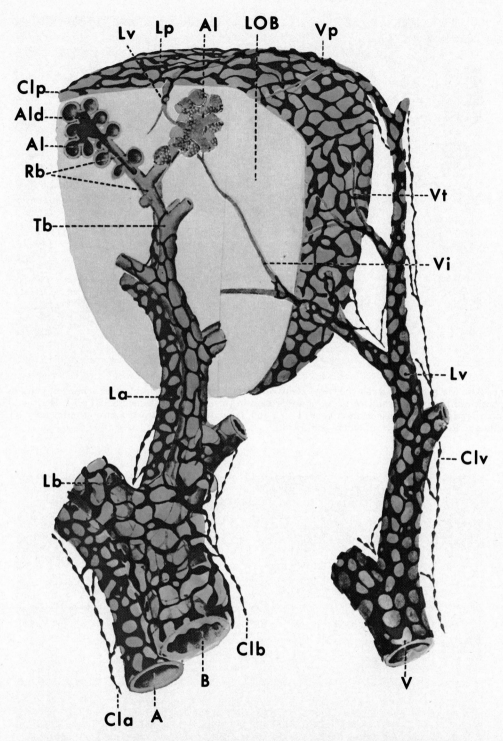

Figure 3–1. Schematic representation of the distribution of the pulmonary lymphatics. A = pulmonary artery; Al = alveolus; Ald = alveolar duct; B = bronchus; Cla = collecting lymph vessel accompanying pulmonary artery; Clb = collecting lymph vessel accompanying bronchus; Clp = subpleural collecting lymph vessel; Clv = collecting lymph vessel accompanying pulmonary vein; La = periarterial lymphatic plexus; Lb = peribronchial lymphatic plexus; LOB = lobule; Lp = subpleural lymph vessel; Lv = perivenous lymphatic plexus; Rb = respiratory bronchiole; Tb = terminal bronchiole; V = pulmonary vein; Vi = intralobular branch of pulmonary vein; Vp = subpleural branch of pulmonary vein; Vt = interlobular branch of pulmonary vein. (Reprinted by permission from Nagaishi, C.: Functional Anatomy and Histology of the Lung. Baltimore, University Park Press, 1972, p. 148.) See also Plate IV.

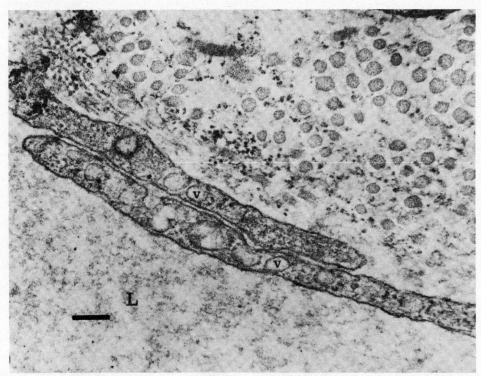

Figure 3–2. Electron micrograph showing extensive overlapping of the adjacent endothelial cell margins of the lymphatic capillary (L). Several vesicles (V) are present in this region of the endothelial cells. Horizontal bar = 10 μm. (Reprinted by permision from Leak, L. V., and Jamuar, M. P.: Ultrastructure of pulmonary lymphatic vessels. Am. Rev. Respir. Dis., *128*:S59–S65, 1983.)

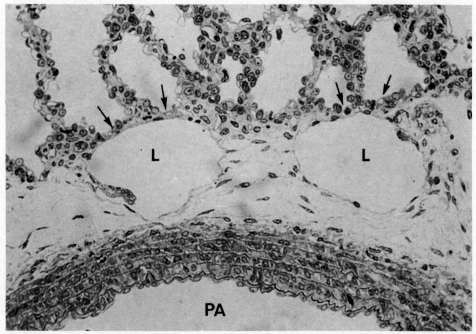

Figure 3–3. Juxtaalveolar lymphatic capillaries (L) located between the alveolar wall (arrows) and the adventitial connective tissue of a large pulmonary artery (PA) in a newborn rabbit. (× 634. Reprinted by permission from Lauweryns, J. M.: The blood and lymphatic microcirculation of the lung. *In* Sommers, S. C. (ed.): Pathology Annual 1971. New York, Appleton-Century-Crofts, 1971, pp. 365–415.)

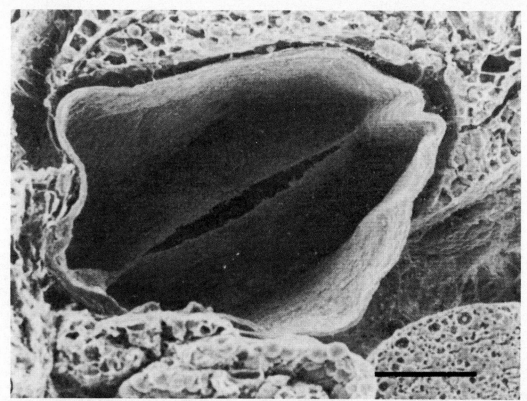

Figure 3–4. Scanning electron micrograph showing the appearance of a valve in a cross section of a lymphatic duct. A pair of leaflets extend from the wall in a circumferential fashion and project into the lumen of the vessel at such an angle that their free edges fit together like a miter joint. Horizontal bar = 1 mm. (Reprinted by permission from Leak, L. V.: Lymphatic removal of fluids and particles in the mammalian lung. Environ. Health Persp., *35*:55–76, 1980.)

filaments, and the overlapping flaps are pulled wider apart, making it easier for liquid to enter the lumen (Fig. 3–5).

The results of studies using histologic tracers suggest that the major pathway for liquid and particulate uptake by pulmonary lymphatic capillaries is through the patent clefts of intercellular junctions.[3, 9] There is also evidence that vesicular uptake (endocytosis) may occur from either the connective tissue or the luminal surface of the lymphatic endothelial cell. Endocytosis is undoubtedly more important in the handling of particles than of liquid. Moreover, in addition to providing a pathway for shuttling particles across the cell wall for subsequent removal through the lumen, much of the material that has been taken up by endocytosis is degraded locally by lytic enzymes.[9, 10] Thus, the pulmonary lymphatic system serves the dual roles of removing excess liquids and particles by luminal flow and of breaking down certain substances in the endothelial cells themselves.

The forces that cause lymph to flow centrally in the lungs are poorly understood. Pulsations from active contraction of smooth muscles in the walls of lymphatic collecting vessels and major trunks have been shown to propel lymph in experimental animals.[11, 12] Because the pulsatile pressures (1 to 25 mm Hg) and the pulse frequencies (1 to 30/min) are related to the rate of lymph formation, it has been concluded that the contractile mechanism causes the removal of lymph in proportion to its rate of formation.[11] The major lymphatic trunks contain numerous nerve filaments and alter their propulsive activity in response to various pharmacologic agents.[12] But the extent of neurohumoral control in lymphatic collecting vessels under ordinary physiologic conditions is completely unknown. Similarly, it is uncertain whether or not pulsatile contractions occur in tiny pulmonary lymphatic capillaries, although the fact that the capillaries contain smooth muscle in their walls favors this possibility. Moreover, contractions have been observed in lymphatic capillaries in other organs. Flow of lymph toward the hilus may depend on, or at least be facilitated by, the massaging effects of

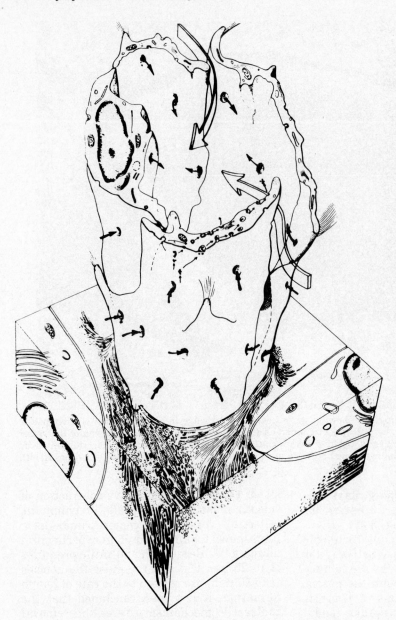

Figure 3–5. Schematic three-dimensional diagram, that was reconstructed from collated electron micrographs, showing a portion of a lymphatic capillary. The major passageway for transport of fluids and large molecules from the interstitium into the lymphatic lumen is the intercellular cleft (long white arrow). The uptake of large molecules from both the connective tissue and luminal fronts may occur within vesicles (small arrows). The vesicles move toward the central cytoplasm where they merge to form heterophagic vacuoles in which intercellular digestion occurs, and in which the products of digestion are held for subsequent utilization or discharge. However, inert particles such as carbon and colloidal thorium are not digested by the cell and remain aggregated into large vacuoles. (Reprinted by permission from Leak, L. V.: Studies on the permeability of lymphatic capillaries. J. Cell. Biol., *50*:300–323, 1971. By copyright permission of the Rockefeller University Press.)

inflation and deflation of the lungs, cardiovascular pulsations, and movements of the thorax and abdomen. A gradient of hydrostatic pressure in the peribronchovascular interstitial space that would promote the flow of lymph from the periphery toward the hilus has recently been measured by Bhattacharya and coworkers.[13]

Lymphoid Tissue

Scattered lymphocytes and plasma cells are found in the wall of the entire tracheobronchial tree and, to a lesser extent, surrounding the blood vessels. Lymphocytes are particularly noticeable in the lamina propria of the mucosa and are more numerous and appear to form small clusters at the points of airways branching. Collections of lymphoid tissue in intimate relationship with the mucous membrane of bronchi and bronchioles have been described by von Hayek.[14] More recent histologic and tracer studies have attempted to differentiate among lymphoepithelial nodules, lymphoid aggregates, and lymph nodes, depending on their location, the presence of germinal centers, and the appearance of the overlying epithelium.[15]

The lymphoid nodules in the bronchial wall, which are covered with mainly nonciliated lymphoepithelium (Fig. 3–6), bear a

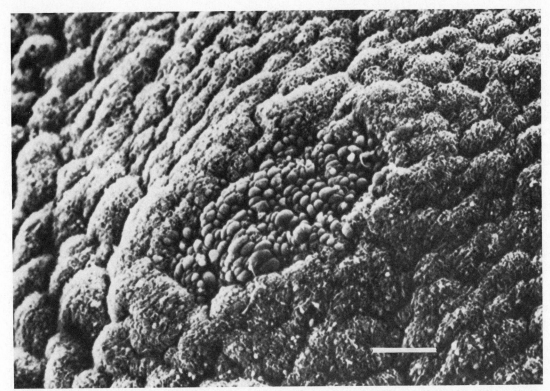

Figure 3–6. Scanning electron micrograph of rabbit bronchial epithelium showing island of lymphoepithelium surrounded by a carpet of ciliated epithelium. Horizontal bar = 1 mm. (Reprinted by permission from Bienenstock, J., and Johnston, N.: A morphologic study of rabbit bronchial lymphoid aggregates and lymphoepithelium. Lab. Invest., 35:343–348, 1976, © 1976, The Williams & Wilkins Company, Baltimore.)

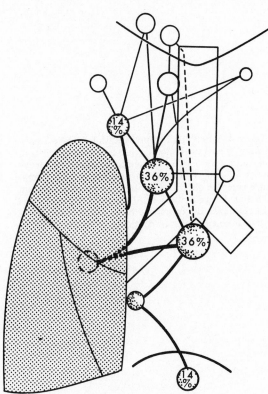

Figure 3–7. Schematic representation of the primary (heavy lines and shaded circles) and secondary (thin lines and open circles) lymphatic drainage pathways of the right lung following injection of the lobar lymph node complex shown. (Reprinted by permission from Dyon, J. F.: Contribution à l'étude du drainages des lymphatiques du poumon. Ph. D. dissertation, Université Scientifique et Médicale de Grenoble, 1973, p. 199.)

striking morphologic resemblance to Peyer's patches of the intestine.[16] Collectively, the system in the tracheobronchial tree is known as *bronchus-associated lymphoid tissue* (BALT), and is believed to play an important role in immunologic defenses, both antibody-mediated and cell-mediated, as a principal site for antigen sampling and processing.[17] Furthermore, the lymphatic aggregations in bronchioles are situated where they appear to favor the traffic of alveolar macrophages during their journey from interstitial tissue to airway lumen. The roles of lymphoid structures in pulmonary defense mechanisms are considered in greater detail in Chapter 13.

Bronchopulmonary lymphoid tissue is present, albeit sparse, at birth and increases afterward. The proliferation is likely to represent an adaptive response to cumulative antigenic challenge during the person's lifetime.

Lymph Nodes

Formed lymph nodes, with germinal centers and a definite sinusoidal structure, ap-

pear in the lung at birth or during infancy. Because they usually contain only a small number of cells, lymph nodes are difficult to identify within the lung except when they are enlarged owing to a pathologic process.

According to Dyon,[18] the extrapulmonary lymph drainage of the human lungs occurs through a maze of interconnecting mediastinal, paratracheal, and subdiaphragmatic lymph nodes and channels. The principal and secondary drainage pathways of the right and left lungs are depicted schematically in Figures 3–7 and 3–8. The main right lymphatic ducts follow the right side of the trachea and join the venous system at the junction of the right jugular and subclavian veins; the left lymphatic ducts, which are usually smaller than those on the right, lie along the left side of the trachea until they empty into the thoracic duct as it terminates in the confluence of veins in the left side of the neck. It is no longer believed that the right lymphatic duct drains about 80 per cent of the total pulmonary lymph and that the remaining 20 per cent, mainly from the left upper lobe, is drained through the left lymphatic duct; it is now agreed that pulmonary lymph drainage patterns are

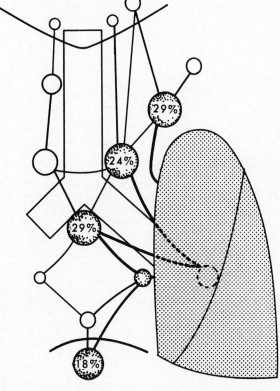

Figure 3–8. Schematic representation of the primary (heavy lines and shaded circles) and secondary (thin lines and open circles) lymphatic drainage pathways of the left lung following injection of the lobar lymph node complex shown. (Reprinted by permission from Dyon, J. F.: Contribution à l'étude du drainages des lymphatiques du poumon. Ph. D. disertation, Université Scientifique et Médicale de Grenoble, 1973, p. 199.)

complex and variable, a fact that has important clinical implications concerning the diagnosis and prognosis of bronchogenic cancer.

NERVE SUPPLY OF THE LUNG

The lungs are richly supplied with nerve fibers and specialized receptors, which are organized into afferent and efferent systems. As will be described, these networks contribute to a variety of neural events that, in general, serve to protect the lungs or to influence the rate and depth of breathing. The innervation of the lungs and the most important pulmonary reflexes are considered in this section. The role of afferent signals from the lungs in the control of breathing is reviewed in Chapter 10.

Afferent and Efferent Pathways

The general patterns of innervation and physiologic responses of mammalian lungs have been recently reviewed and updated.[19, 20] Preganglionic fibers from the vagal nuclei descend in the vagus nerves to ganglia situated around airways and blood vessels; ramifying postganglionic fibers innervate the smooth muscle of airways and blood vessels and the epithelium of the bronchial glands and epithelial mucous (goblet) cells. To a large extent, the same structures are innervated by postganglionic fibers from the sympathetic ganglia. The double innervation explains the two opposing types of neurophysiologic responses, which are characterized as excitatory or inhibitory. Stimulation of the vagus nerves causes airway constriction, dilatation of the pulmonary circulation, and increased glandular secretion; these responses are blocked by atropine, which indicates that the neurotransmitter acetylcholine is acting on muscarinic receptors. Stimulation of the sympathetic nerves causes bronchial relaxation, constriction of pulmonary blood vessels, and inhibition of glandular secretions.[19] There are, however, some important variations on these general themes in humans that warrant emphasis, although many important details are missing.

The innervation of the human lung, diaphragm, and chest wall is illustrated in Figure 3–9 (see also Plate V). The vagus

nerves and the upper four or five thoracic sympathetic ganglia contribute fibers to the anterior and posterior pulmonary plexuses at the roots of the lungs. As the bronchi, arteries, and veins enter the lung at the hilus, they carry with them extensions of the plexus; the largest branches accompany the bronchi and the smallest accompany the veins. The bronchial fibers are subdivided into an extrachondrial plexus and a subchondrial plexus, depending on whether the network is external or internal (respectively) to the cartilaginous plates. Ramifying nerve fibers continue to invest airways and blood vessels as they subdivide within the lung.[21] Efferent parasympathetic fibers terminate in clumps of ganglion cells, which are situated in the intrabronchial, peribronchial, and perivenous regions.

Unmyelinated postganglionic efferent fibers (Fig. 3–10) have been followed to the smooth musculature of all divisions of conducting airways, respiratory bronchioles, and alveolar ducts. Postganglionic fibers, which are presumably mainly parasympathetic in origin, innervate bronchial glands. The location and role of postganglionic sympathetic fibers are controversial. According to Richardson,[19, 22] sympathetic postganglionic fibers, which have been observed to terminate on the ganglia in lungs from humans, have not been demonstrated to extend to the glands or smooth muscle. Thus, despite the presence of β-adrenergic and α-adrenergic receptors in human airway smooth muscle, adrenergic innervation is questionable. This view is contrary to the results of recent studies of human lungs, which revealed nerve endings near to bronchial glands and smooth muscles that contained vesicles characteristic of adrenergic nerves.[23] The prevailing concept of the autonomic innervation of the airways is shown schematically in Figure 3–11.

As indicated previously, the ultrastructure of the Kulchitsky cells and the neuroepithelial bodies of the epithelium suggests that they are also innervated, but this has not been definitely proved. The motor innervation of pulmonary blood vessels and the functional consequences of stimulation of the components of the autonomic nervous system need to be clarified. There seems little doubt, however, that the vasculature is innervated. Although less dense than the plexus around airways, the periarterial plexus reduces to a single fiber at the level

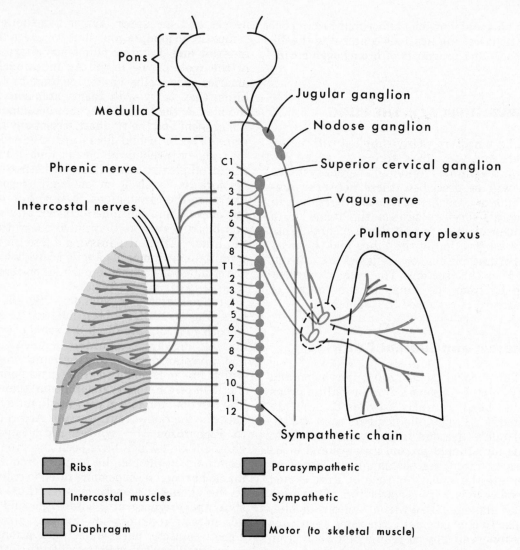

Pons

Medulla

Phrenic nerve

Intercostal nerves

Jugular ganglion

Nodose ganglion

Superior cervical ganglion

Vagus nerve

Pulmonary plexus

C 1
2
3
4
5
6
7
8
T 1
2
3
4
5
6
7
8
9
10
11
12

Sympathetic chain

Ribs

Intercostal muscles

Diaphragm

Parasympathetic

Sympathetic

Motor (to skeletal muscle)

Figure 3–9. Schematic depiction of the autonomic innervation (motor and sensory) of the lung and the somatic (motor) nerve supply to the intercostal muscles and diaphragm. See also Plate V.

of arterioles and continues to the level of the capillaries.[24] Sympathetic vasoconstrictor activity has been observed in the pulmonary circulation of dogs[25] but has not been demonstrated in humans. The effect of vagal stimulation on pulmonary blood vessels is difficult to document, and although vasodilator responses have been reported, they are too feeble to be of physiologic importance. Certainly, it has not been possible to demonstrate any influences mediated by the autonomic nervous system on the pulmonary circulation of spontaneously breathing, normal human adults.[26]

In addition to parasympathetic (cholinergic) and sympathetic (adrenergic) nerve fibers, there is increasing evidence that the lungs of several mammalian species, includ-

ing humans, are also innervated by a third component of the autonomic nervous system.[27] For want of a better name, this network is called the *nonadrenergic-noncholinergic* system to indicate that other, as yet unidentified, neurotransmitters are involved. Burnstock[28] has presented evidence that a purine compound is the sought-after agent and, therefore, the term "purinergic" is often used to identify the system. Furthermore, Burnstock[29] has also attempted to subdivide the receptors of the purinergic system into two types; this chemical characterization is based on the actions of the putative agonists, adenosine for P1 receptors and adenosine triphosphate for P2 receptors, and the response to certain selective antagonists. However, these efforts to categorize the pharmacologic properties of the nonadrenergic system were not supported by the results of recent experiments in cats.[30]

Other possible neurotransmitters of the nonadrenergic-noncholinergic system are substance P and vasoactive intestinal peptide (VIP). Substance P has not been consistently identified in human lungs but recent studies have demonstrated VIP-immuno-

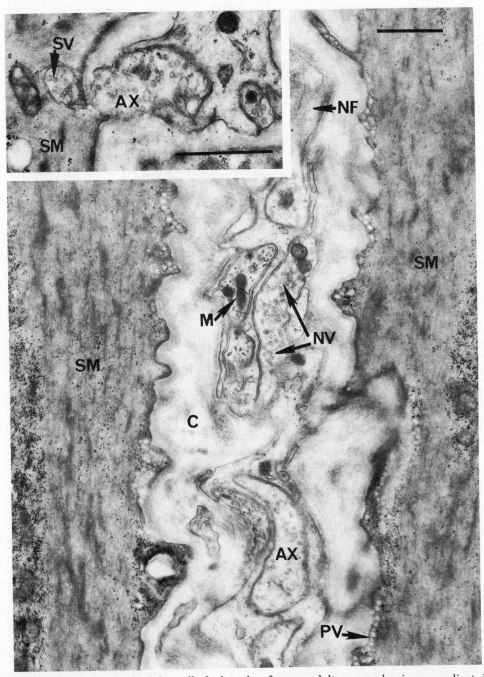

Figure 3–10. Electron micrograph of the wall of a bronchus from an adult woman showing unmyelinated axons (AX) (probably motor) lying in a connective tissue space containing collagen (C) between two smooth muscle cells (SM). Within the axons are mitochondria (M), clear and dense cord vesicles (NV), and neurofilaments (NF). Pinocytotic vesicles (PV) are evident in the cytoplasmic membrane of the muscle cell. The inset shows a nerve terminal containing synaptic vesicles (SV) located at the junction between an axon and muscle cell. Horizontal bar = 1 μm. (× 18,225 and × 26,000 [inset]. Courtesy of Dr. Donald McKay.)

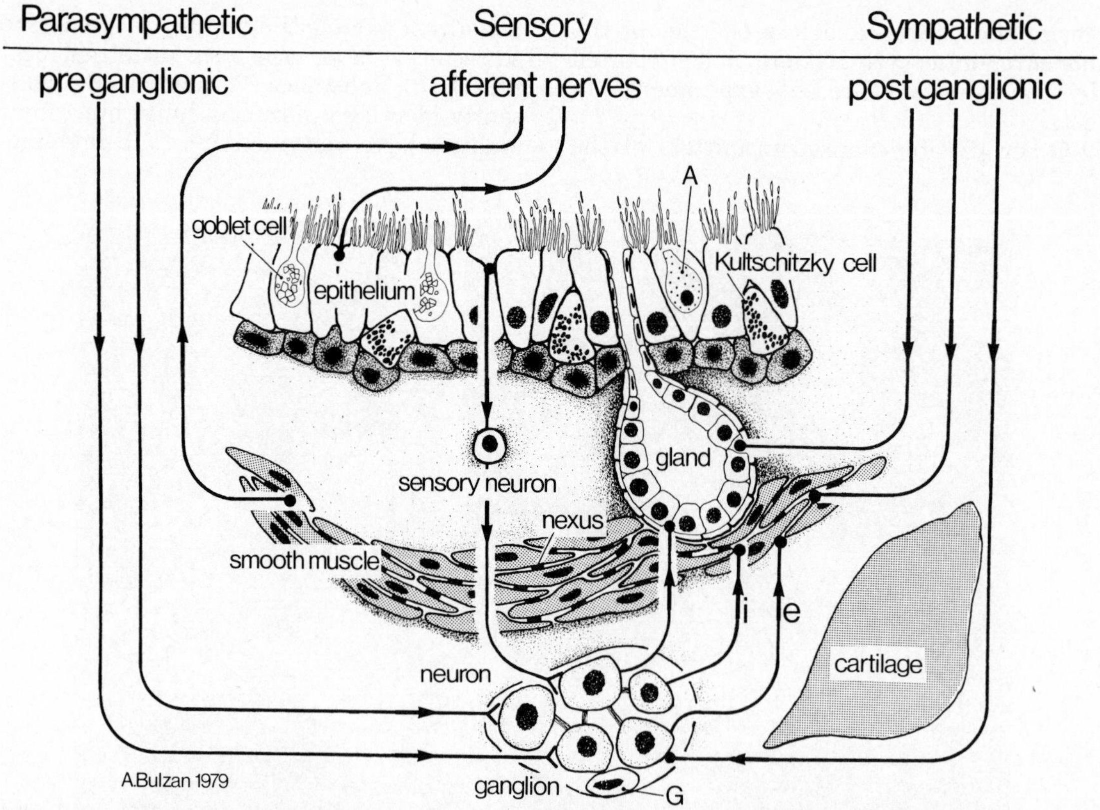

Parasympathetic Sensory Sympathetic

pre ganglionic afferent nerves post ganglionic

A.Bulzan 1979

Figure 3–11. Schematic summary of the innervation of the airways. In the human lung, parasympathetic, preganglionic fibers descend into the vagus and terminate in the ganglia. The ganglia contain excitatory neurons that are cholinergic and inhibitory neurons that are nonadrenergic. Other neurons with an integrative function are probably also present. Glial cells (G) are present in the ganglia. Blood vessels and collagen are excluded from the neuropil. Postganglionic fibers to the smooth muscle are excitatory (e) or inhibitory (i). Excitatory fibers may also terminate in the glands. Sensory afferent endings are present in the epithelium and the smooth muscle. The neurons associated with these endings may be in the vagus or the vagal nuclei. Sensory neurons may also be present in the mucosa, and fibers from these neurons may terminate in the ganglia, as in the gastrointestinal tract. Sympathetic, postganglionic fibers terminate on the ganglia, in humans and in other species, but adrenergic fibers to the glands or smooth muscle, although found in some mammals, have not been demonstrated in humans. In the epithelium, there are cells, such as the Kultschitsky type cell and the granular cell (A), found only in the chicken, whose functions are unknown. Nerves may be related to these cells. The human airway smooth muscle cells are connected by low resistance junctions, such as the nexus (see Fig. 2–11), and these connections may permit the muscle mass to act as a syncytium. (Reprinted by permission from Richardson, J. B.: Nerve supply to the lungs. Am. Rev. Respir. Dis., *119*:785–802, 1978.)

reactivity in nerve fibers associated with human bronchial smooth muscle and bronchial glands.[23]

The nonadrenergic-noncholinergic nervous system is important in the intestine, in which it is believed to modulate peristalsis. In the lungs, the system seems clearly to cause bronchial smooth muscle relaxation, and thus is inhibitory. If Richardson's view that adrenergic nerves do not have a function in human airways is correct, the nonadrenergic-noncholinergic system may be the normal source of inhibitory activity and thus may provide the expected recipro-

cal neural balance to the excitatory activity of the cholinergic system.

It is generally accepted that the vast majority of afferent nerve fibers to the central nervous system from the lungs travel in the vagus nerves. The remaining pulmonary afferent fibers have been identified in the sympathetic nerves and dorsal roots. However, judging from the results of neurophysiologic investigations, including vagotomy, the contribution of nonvagal afferent pathways to reflexes has yet to be established.

Numerous other signals that affect respiration are transmitted to the central nervous system by means of afferent nerves that serve receptors located in parts of the body other than the lungs and respiratory tract. The structure and function of the most important of these, the chemoreceptors and skeletal muscle proprioceptors, are considered in Chapter 10.

Receptors

There are three groups of well-defined vagal sensory receptors in the lungs:[31] the bronchopulmonary stretch receptors, the irritant receptors, and the C-fiber receptors. These receptors and their reflex effects have been differentiated by neurophysiologic studies in experimental animals and are characterized by the features listed in Table 3–1. Although the neural pathways and the effector responses are well established, there is still uncertainty about the precise location and morphology of the receptors that detect the appropriate stimuli because it is extremely difficult to integrate the results of the three classic methods of study: histologic examinations, nerve fiber recording, and reflex assessment. There is, however, anatomic and physiologic evidence in support of the receptors included in Table 3–1. In addition, chemoreceptors have been proposed as a fourth set of intrapulmonary sensory elements, but convincing demonstration of their presence and physiologic function is lacking.

1. Slowly adapting pulmonary *stretch receptors* are believed to be the nerve filaments that are closely associated with smooth muscles throughout the conducting airways. According to general agreement, there is a much higher concentration of stretch receptors in extrapulmonary airways (trachea and main bronchi) than in intrapulmonary airways, and whether they occur at all in bronchioles is uncertain and seems unlikely. The receptors appear to be stimulated by deformation of the endings when changes occur in the caliber of the bronchial wall; therefore, changes in the distending pressure "across" the airways, as well as the actual volume of air entering the lung, are the chief stimuli. Stretch receptors also respond to an increased PCO_2 in the airways (not the bloodstream), but the physiologic significance of this reflex is not known.[32]

Pulmonary stretch receptors respond in phase during normal breathing to terminate inspiration. After inspiration begins, the rate of firing from the receptors progressively increases and new receptors are recruited; finally the crescendo of neural activity signals the end of inspiration, and expiration ensues.[33] In most mammalian species, the threshold for stretch receptor activity is within the range of tidal volumes that occur during ordinary breathing. The inhibitory effect of lung inflation on respiratory rate is one component of the Hering-Breuer reflex; the other mediates, in part,

Table 3–1. CHARACTERISTICS OF THE THREE PULMONARY VAGAL SENSORY REFLEXES

Receptor	Location	Fiber Type	Stimulus	Response
Pulmonary stretch, slowly adapting	Associated with smooth muscle of intrapulmonary airways	Medullated	1. Lung inflation 2. Increased transpulmonary pressure	1. Hering-Breuer inflation reflex 2. Bronchodilation 3. Increased heart rate 4. Decreased peripheral vascular resistance
Irritant, rapidly adapting	Epithelium of (mainly) extrapulmonary airways	Medullated	1. Irritants 2. Mechanical stimulation 3. Anaphylaxis 4. Lung inflation or deflation 5. Hyperpnea 6. Pulmonary congestion	1. Bronchoconstriction 2. Hyperpnea 3. Expiratory constriction of larynx 4. Cough 5. Mucous secretion
C-fibers pulmonary (type J) bronchial	Alveolar wall Airways and blood vessels	Nonmedullated	1. Increased interstitial volume (congestion) 2. Chemical injury 3. Microembolism	1. Rapid shallow breathing 2. Laryngeal and tracheobronchial constriction 3. Bradycardia 4. Spinal reflex inhibition 5. Mucous secretion

the adjustments of respiratory muscles to transient mechanical loads. However, it is now known that the contribution of vagal reflexes to respiratory load-compensation, which is important in some experimental animals, is weak or absent in humans.[34] Additional reflex effects from stimulating stretch receptors are laryngeal and bronchial dilatation, an increase in heart rate, and a fall in peripheral vascular resistance.

Recording from afferent nerves subserving stretch receptors in experimental animals reveal that about 60 per cent of the fibers have detectable activity during the pause between breaths; the remainder of the nerves are progressively recruited as inflation proceeds. Section or blockade of the vagus in most mammalian species causes a low frequency–large tidal volume pattern of breathing without changing the level of arterial CO_2 tension. These observations led to speculation that pulmonary stretch receptors may regulate the rate and depth of breathing and that they adjust the pattern to achieve the optimal combination at which mechanical work, inspiratory force or both are minimal.[35] But this attractive hypothesis does not appear to apply to humans, because the Hering-Breuer reflex is very weak or absent during normal quiet breathing in healthy adults.[36] At large tidal volumes, however, an inflation reflex can be demonstrated in anesthetized humans and a brisk inflation reflex has been reported in newborn babies.[37]

2. Rapidly adapting *irritant receptors* are not active in normal breathing but respond to a variety of stimuli, including inhalation of gaseous irritants, mechanical stimulation of the larynx and airways, histamine-induced bronchoconstriction, anaphylactic reactions in the lung, pulmonary arterial microembolism, mechanical stimulation by large inflations and deflations, pneumothorax, hyperpnea due to asphyxia or hypercapnia or to an increase in artificial ventilation, and pulmonary congestion due to left atrial obstruction.[26] Most of these diverse stimuli produce an increase in the distending force on the bronchial wall and, accordingly, probably activate pulmonary stretch receptors as well.

Although analysis is complicated when

more than one receptor is involved,* the reflex responses from the stimulation of irritant receptors are bronchoconstriction, hyperpnea, constriction of the larynx during expiration, cough, and increased mucous secretion. It has also been postulated that (1) irritant receptors are responsible for the periodic deep breaths that punctuate normal human breathing and that (2) these receptors, by redistributing the film of surfactant, may reverse the continuous tendency of alveoli to collapse.[38] It is noteworthy that the threshold for bronchoconstriction and laryngeal constriction appears to be considerably lower than that for cough.

The actual receptor sites are unknown, but persuasive evidence points to the free unmyelinated nerve filaments that have been demonstrated in the superficial epithelium of the airways;[31] the endings in turn are attached to myelinated vagal nerve fibers (Fig. 3–12). Axons that resemble free sensory endings located elsewhere in the body have been identified among and below ciliated cells, goblet cells, and basal cells in humans and experimental animals (Fig. 3–13). Judging from physiologic studies, irritant receptors are mainly concentrated in the larynx, trachea, and extrapulmonary bronchi, but intrapulmonary receptor activity has also been demonstrated in some animals.[26] There are differences between intra- and extrapulmonary irritant receptors in that stimulation of the intrapulmonary fibers does not appear to cause cough. No one knows how irritant receptors in central airways are stimulated by events, such as microembolism, that affect the lung parenchyma; the best explanation is that stimulation occurs through the peripheral release of mediators, such as prostaglandins, that act centrally.

3. *C-Fiber Receptors* are the terminal branches of an extensive network of unmyelinated afferent nerve fibers that are located in the lung parenchyma, conducting airways, and blood vessels. C-fibers differ from A-fibers, the axons of stretch and irritant receptors, in being unmyelinated, in having a much slower conduction velocity, and in being accessible to chemicals injected into the bloodstream. Two groups of C-fiber receptors have been identified.[39] *Pulmonary* C-fibers innervate the lung parenchyma and are located sufficiently close to the capillaries to be stimulated by chemicals injected into the pulmonary artery. The network of parenchymal C-fiber receptors includes

---

*Multiple receptors are nearly always involved because any primary response actuated by a single receptor system usually evokes secondary responses from other receptors.

Paintal's juxtacapillary (or simply J) receptors, which were so named because of their accessibility to stimuli in and around pulmonary capillaries.[40] Small unmyelinated axons, with the structural characteristics of sensory nerve endings, have been observed within the interalveolar septum of the rat lung; although scarce and difficult to demonstrate, these terminals are appropriately located to serve as pulmonary C-fibers.[41] Recently, similar nerve endings have been identified in lungs from humans. (Fig. 3–14).[42]

Bronchial C-fibers are distinguished from pulmonary C-fibers by their accessibility to chemical substances injected into the bronchial arterial circulation, which supplies conducting airways and blood vessels. Bronchial C-fiber receptors differ from pulmonary C-fiber receptors not only in their blood supply but in being less susceptible to mechanical stimuli and more susceptible to certain chemicals (e.g., bradykinin).[43] When the two groups are stimulated separately, bronchial C-fibers cause more airway constriction and less cardiac slowing than pulmonary C-fibers.

C-fiber receptors probably do not play a role in normal breathing. It has been pro-posed that pulmonary C-fibers may contribute to the sensation of dyspnea that accompanies clinical conditions in which they are likely to be excited: pulmonary edema, pneumonia, and inhalation of noxious chemicals.[44] Similarly, in view of the fact that bradykinin is released in asthma and anaphylaxis, some of the respiratory sensations and physiologic consequences of those disorders may be explained by the remarkable chemosensitivity of bronchial C-fibers.[43]

Physiologic Role

Receptors located throughout the respiratory tract play an important role in the nervous control of breathing; in the production of cough; and in the regulation of the smooth muscle tone in airways, the caliber of the larynx, and the quantity and composition of the mucous secretions in the respiratory tract. Several reflexes arising in the lungs also affect the cardiovascular system. The control of breathing is considered in detail later (see Chapter 10). The discussion that follows will consider the reflex mechanisms that control cough, mucous secretion, and changes in heart rate. In addi-

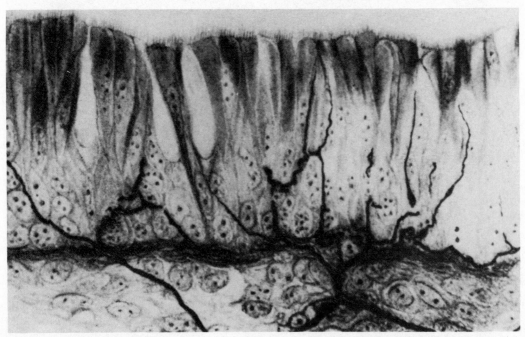

Figure 3–12. Drawing of a light microscopic picture of a nerve complex in airway columnar cell epithelium. Note the ramification of nerve terminals between the columnar and mucus cells of the epithelium, and the thick fiber connections at the base. Such nerve complexes are thought to be epithelial irritant receptors. (Reprinted from Widdicombe, J. G.: Nervous receptors in the respiratory tract and lungs. *In* Hornbein, T. F. (ed.): Regulation of Breathing. 1981, pp 429–472, by courtesy of Marcel Dekker, Inc.)

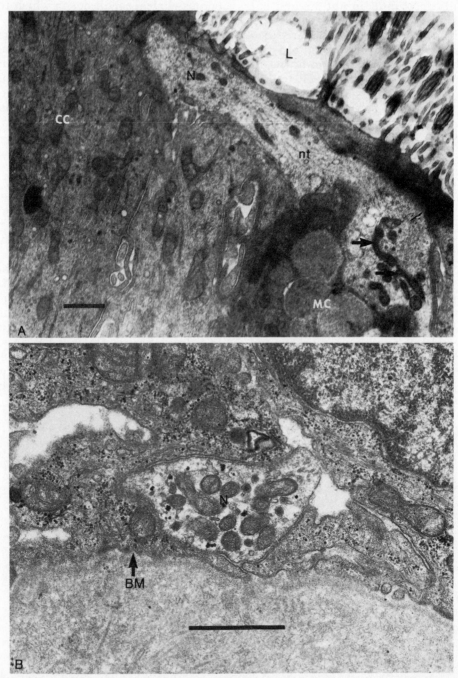

Figure 3–13. Electron micrographs of human airway surface epithelium, showing intraepithelial nerve fibers (N) lying near the airway lumen (L) in *A* and near basement membrane (BM) in *B. A,* The nerve terminal contains characteristic pale cytoplasm with neurotubules (nt) and thin condensed mitochondria (arrows). Note the ciliated cell (CC) and mucous cell (MC). (Courtesy of Dr. Peter K. Jeffrey.) *B,* The nerve profile contains granular vesicles, neurotubuli, and many mitochondria. (Courtesy of Dr. Annika Laitinen and Dr. Lauri A. Laitinen.) Both horizontal bars = 1 μm.

tion, the elusive pulmonary chemoreceptors will be briefly reviewed.

Cough. Receptors subserving cough are located in many parts of the respiratory tract, such as the oropharynx, larynx, trachea, and large bronchi; this correspondence seems functionally obvious because these are the air passages from which cough is effective in clearing secretions and particles. However, cough receptors are also found occasionally in an unexpected location such as the external auditory canal. In humans and other animals, coughing can be provoked by mechanical or chemical stimuli of the mucosa of the larynx, carina, trachea, and central bronchi, in descending order of sensitivity. These sites, as already pointed out, are the locations of the greatest densities of the intra- and subepithelial nerve filaments that are almost certainly rapidly adapting irritant receptors.[45] Thus, these receptors cause coughing in addition to their other reflex effects. Cough, however, is not invariably associated with other reflex consequences of stimulating irritant receptors, particularly bronchospasm. It is not known whether cough is a threshold effect in a single system of receptors or whether it depends on the number of receptors recruited and their discharge frequencies.

The afferent pathways depend on the location of the receptors. Impulses from the larynx travel in the various branches of the laryngeal nerves; those from the tracheobronchial system travel in the vagus nerves. There is considerable uncertainty about the central nervous system structures that coordinate coughing, but it is known that there are several efferent neural pathways. The most important outflows are to the expiratory muscles of respiration (see Chapter 5), the larynx, the tracheobronchial smooth muscle, and the airway mucus-secreting system.[46]

In response to stimulation of suitable receptors, cough usually consists of a deep

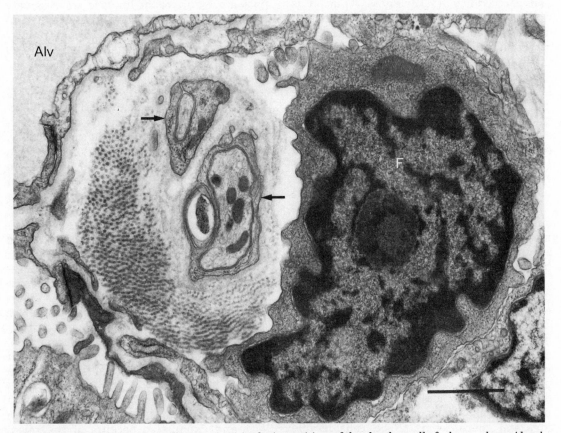

Figure 3–14. Two separate nerve fibers (arrows) in the interstitium of the alveolar wall of a human lung. Alveolar space (Alv) is on the left. The microvilli of a type II pneumocyte can be seen in the lower left hand corner and a fibroblast (F) lies to the right. Horizontal bar = 1 μm. (Reprinted by permission from Fox, B., et al.: Innervation of alveolar walls in the human lung: an electron microscopic study. J. Anat., *131*:683–692, 1980.)

inspiration followed by constriction of laryngeal smooth muscles and contraction of the skeletal muscles of expiration. Sudden opening of the closed glottis allows rapid ejection of air; frequently, there is a series of four to six coughs during the same expiration. As will be explained in detail in the next chapter, the airflow out of the lungs during cough only transiently exceeds the maximum flow during ordinary forced expiration at that lung volume. Cough is effective in clearing secretions because the extra pressure of the vigorous expiratory effort causes central airways to be markedly compressed. By this means, the velocity of airflow is increased sufficiently to generate a shearing force that dislodges mucus and particles from the luminal surface of the narrowed airways.

Mucous Secretion. Whether or not the mucous layer of the airways is sheared off the surface during cough depends not only on the velocity of airflow but also on the properties of the mucus itself, its viscosity, and particularly its thickness. Thus, it is not surprising that the same irritating stimuli that provoke cough also cause increased secretion of mucus, partly by a direct effect of the toxin and partly by a reflex action from stimulation of irritant receptors. There is also good evidence that stimulation of the C-fiber network, of both pulmonary and bronchial receptors, causes reflex increase of airway secretion.[46a] The combination of cough and increased mucus output constitutes an important defense mechanism for ridding the respiratory tract of inhaled noxious substances. Although it is possible that the reflex pathways for certain chemical stimuli are different from those for dust-mediated responses, in nearly all cases, stimuli that cause coughing also consistently increase mucus output.[46]

Release of secretions from the airway submucosal glands is clearly regulated by vagal efferent nerves. Evidence in humans for direct sympathetic innervation is lacking; however, submucosal gland secretions increase in response to adrenergic agonists, indicating that adrenergic receptors are present in the secretory cells. However, evidence for innervation of epithelial secretory cells (mucous, serous, and Clara) is conflicting, and there seems to be considerable species variation.

Changes in Heart Rate. In 1871 Hering demonstrated that moderate inflation of the lungs caused a vagally mediated reflex increase in heart rate and that insufflation to larger volumes provoked a decrease in heart rate.[47] Although there have been some inconsistencies in subsequent attempts to reproduce these changes, for the most part they are repeatable and the reflex pathways subserving them appear to have been worked out.

The vagal afferent fibers responsible for cardioacceleration at moderate increases in lung volume are believed to originate mainly from slowly adapting pulmonary stretch receptors, but there is also a contribution from rapidly adapting irritant receptors, which, as pointed out, respond to lung inflation as well as to irritating stimuli. In contrast, the afferent fibers responsible for slowing of the heart rate at greater increases in lung volume arise from both pulmonary and bronchial C-fibers. However, at least in dogs, the firing rates of these four sets of fibers varies considerably as the inflation pressure of the lungs is progressively increased (Fig. 3–15); slowly adapting receptors are always more active than rapidly adapting receptors, and pulmonary C-fibers are always more active than bronchial C-fibers at any given inflation pressure.[48]

Inflation of the lung with 30 cm H_2O pressure (i.e., virtually to total lung capacity) has other reflex effects on cardiovascular function. Left ventricular contractility, stroke volume, peripheral vasomotor tone, and systemic arterial pressure in addition to heart rate are all depressed after sudden lung inflation. The vagus nerve is the common afferent pathway for each effect. In contrast, the efferent responses require participation of cholinergic, α-adrenergic, and β-adrenergic mechanims.[48a]

Chemoreceptors. Pulmonary stretch receptors, irritant receptors, and C-fiber receptors can all be stimulated by various suitable chemicals. In this sense, they are "chemosensitive." However, chemosensitivity to test substances does not prove chemoreceptor sensitivity to physiologic stimuli such as changes in the gaseous composition of blood or air.

The search for pulmonary chemoreceptors in the airways and blood vessels has been long and exhaustive because of the teleologic attractiveness of sensors that would "taste" the blood and "smell" the air. Al-

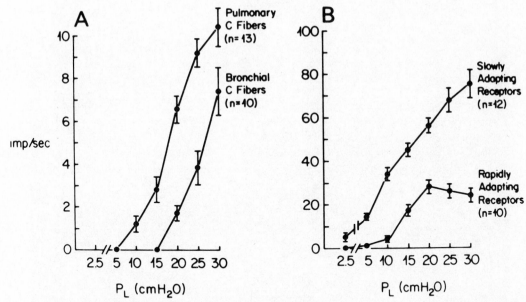

Figure 3–15. Graph showing rates of impulses (imp/sec) of pulmonary and bronchial C-fibers *(A)* and rapidly and slowly adapting receptors with A-fibers *(B)* in response to increasing transpulmonary pressure (P_L) from 2.5 to 30 cm H_2O. Solid circles = means; vertical bars = standard errors. (From Kaufman, M. P., et al.: Response to inflation of vagal afferents with endings in the lung of dogs. Circ. Res., *51*:525–531, 1981, by permission of the American Heart Association, Inc.)

though the reports of studies thus far have indicated far more negative than positive results, the quest nevertheless continues. The most promising clues are (1) the nests of cells that are found occasionally at autopsy and are believed to be tumors or hyperplasias of normal cellular constituents; because these cells resemble chemoreceptor cells elsewhere in the body, appear to be heavily innervated, and are invariably situated in close relationship to pulmonary veins (Fig. 3–16), they are in a perfect location to monitor the composition of blood leaving the lung;[49] and (2) the neuroepithelial bodies found in airways (Fig. 3–17) have an abundant nerve supply and are strategically located to sample and respond to changes in the composition of gas entering and leaving regions of the lung.[50] Lauweryns and Van Lommel[51] concluded from recent denervation experiments that the neuroepithelial bodies are neuroreceptor structures and that they are innervated by sensory neurons whose cell bodies lie in the nodose ganglion of the vagus nerve. Additional studies indicate that the neuroepithelial bodies respond to the administration of a hypoxic gas mixture by secreting serotonin or peptides into the neighboring lung tissue.[52] However, much experimental work remains to be done before the nervous pathways and reflex roles for these structures are established. They remain a physiologic enigma.[31]

The current state of knowledge about pulmonary vagal receptors and their responses can be summarized succinctly. Pulmonary stretch receptors are mainly important in controlling the pattern of breathing but are weakly active in humans after the newborn period; irritant receptors and C-fiber receptors are mainly activated in lung disease and abnormal conditions and may interact with many reflex responses; the presence of pulmonary chemoreceptors that respond to changes in inspired air or blood gas composition has not been demonstrated convincingly, although some recently identified structures have been suggested as possible candidates for the role.

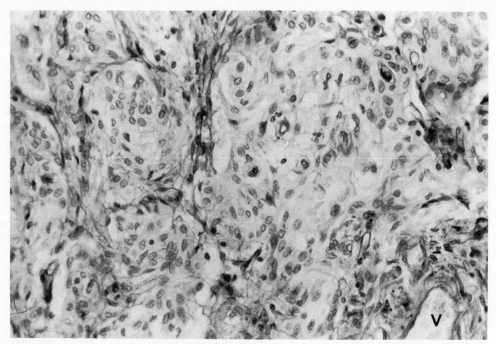

Figure 3–16. Pulmonary chemodectoma. Nests of chemoreceptor-like cells in the interstitium of the lung adjacent to a pulmonary vein (V). (× 420. Courtesy of Dr. Averill Liebow.)

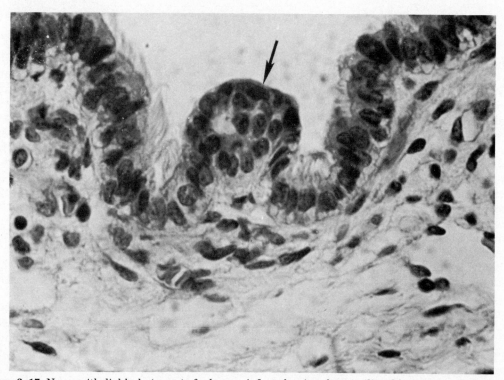

Figure 3–17. Neuroepithelial body (arrow) of a human infant showing the nonciliated lining on the luminal side and the protrusion slightly above the level of the surrounding ciliated epithelium. (× 1040. Reprinted by permission from Lauweryns, J. M., and Peuskens, J. C.: Neuroepithelial bodies (neuroreceptor or secretory organs?) in human infant bronchial and bronchiolar epithelium. Anat. Rec., *172*:471–482, 1972.)

REFERENCES

1. Nagaishi, C.: Functional Anatomy and Histology of the Lung. Baltimore, University Park Press, 1972, p. 148.
2. Lauweryns, J. M.: The juxta-alveolar lymphatics in the human adult lung. Histologic studies in 15 cases of drowning. Am. Rev. Respir. Dis., 102:877–885, 1970.
3. Leak, L. V., and Jamuar, M. P.: Ultrastructure of pulmonary lymphatic vessels. Am. Rev. Respir. Dis., 128:S59–S65, 1983.
4. Lauweryns, J. M., Baert, J., and DeLoecker, W.: Intracytoplasmic filaments in pulmonary endothelial cells. Cell Tiss. Res., 163:111–124, 1975.
5. Lauweryns, J. M.: The blood and lymphatic microcirculation of the lung. In Sommers, S. C. (ed.): Pathology Annual 1971. New York, Appleton-Century-Crofts, 1971, pp. 365–415.
6. Leak, L. V.: Lymphatic removal of fluids and particles in the mammalian lung. Environ. Health Perspect., 35:55–76, 1980.
7. Albertine, K. H., Fox, L. M., O'Morchoe, C. C. C.: The morphology of canine lymphatic valves. Anat. Rec., 202:453–461, 1982.
8. Leak, L. V.: Studies on the permeability of lymphatic capillaries. J. Cell Biol., 50:300–323, 1971.
9. Lauweryns, J. M., and Baert, J. M.: The role of the pulmonary lymphatics in the defenses of the distal lung: morphological and experimental studies of the transport mechanisms of intratracheally instilled particles. Ann. N.Y. Acad. Sci., 221:244–275, 1974.
10. Lauweryns, J. M., and Baert, J. M.: Alveolar clearance and the role of pulmonary lymphatics. Am. Rev. Respir. Dis., 115:625–683, 1977.
11. Hall, J. G., Morris, B., and Woolley, G.: Intrinsic rhythmic propulsion of lymph in unanesthetized sheep. J. Physiol. (Lond.), 180:336–349, 1965.
12. Reddy, N. P., and Staub, N. C.: Intrinsic propulsive activity of thoracic duct perfused in anesthetized dogs. Microvasc. Res., 21:183–192, 1981.
13. Bhattacharya, J., Gropper, M. A., and Staub, N. C.: Interstitial fluid pressure gradient measured by micropuncture in excised dog lung. J. Appl. Physiol., 56:271–277, 1984.
14. von Hayek, H.: The Human Lung. New York, Hafner Publishing Company, Inc., 1960, pp. 298–314.
15. Fournier, M., Vai, F., Derenne, J. P., and Pariente, R.: Bronchial lymphoepithelial nodules in the rat. Morphologic features and uptake and transport of exogenous proteins. Am. Rev. Respir. Dis., 116:685–694, 1977.
16. Bienenstock, J., and Johnston, N.: A morphologic study of rabbit bronchial lymphoid aggregates and lymphoepithelium. Lab. Invest., 35:343–348, 1976.
17. Bienenstock, J., McDermott, M. R., and Befus, A. D.: The significance of bronchus-associated lymphoid tissue. Bull. Eur. Physiopathol. Respir., 18:153–177, 1982.
18. Dyon, J. F.: Contribution à l'étude du drainages des lymphatiques du poumon. PhD dissertation, Université Scientifique et Médicale de Grenoble, 1973, p. 199.
19. Richardson, J. B.: Nerve supply to the lungs. Am. Rev. Respir. Dis., 119:785–802, 1979.
20. Richardson, J. B.: Recent progress in pulmonary innervation. Am. Rev. Respir. Dis., 128:S65–S68, 1983.
21. Spencer, H., and Leof, D.: The innervation of the human lung. J. Anat., 98:599–609, 1964.
22. Zorychta, E., and Richardson, J. B.: Control of smooth muscle of human airways. Bull. Eur. Physiopathol. Respir., 16:581–586, 1980.
23. Laitinen, A.: Autonomic innervation of the human respiratory tract as revealed by histochemical and ultrastructural methods. Eur. J. Respir. Dis., 66(Suppl. 140):1–42, 1985.
24. Larsell, G., and Dow, R. S.: The innervation of the human lung. Am. J. Anat., 52:125–135, 1933.
25. Daly, I. DeB.: Intrinsic mechanisms of the lung. Q. J. Exp. Physiol., 43:2–26, 1958.
26. Widdicombe, J. G., and Sterling, G. M.: The autonomic nervous system and breathing. Arch. Intern. Med., 126:311–329, 1970.
27. Richardson, J., and Beland, J.: Nonadrenergic inhibitory nervous system in human airways. J. Appl. Physiol., 41:764–771, 1976.
28. Burnstock, G.: Purinergic receptors. J. Theor. Biol., 62:491–503, 1976.
29. Burnstock, G.: A basis for distinguishing two types of purinergic receptor. In Straub, R. W., and Bolis, L. (eds.): Cell Membrane Receptors for Drugs and Hormones. A Multidisciplinary Approach. New York, Raven Press, 1978, pp. 107–118.
30. Irvin, C. G., Martin, R. R., and Macklem, P. T.: Nonpurinergic nature and efficacy of nonadrenergic bronchodilatation. J. Appl. Physiol., 52:562–569, 1982.
31. Widdicombe, J. G.: Nervous receptors in the respiratory tract and lungs. In Hornbein, T. F. (ed.): Regulation of Breathing. New York, Marcel Dekker, Inc., 1981, pp. 429–472.
32. Coleridge, H. M., Coleridge, J. C. G., and Banzett, R. B.: Effect of CO_2 on afferent vagal endings in the canine lung. Respir. Physiol., 24:135–151, 1978.
33. Clark, F. J., and von Euler, C.: On the regulation of depth and rate of breathing. J. Physiol. (Lond.), 222:267–295, 1972.
34. Margaria, E. E., Iscoe, S., Pengelly, L. D., Couture, J., Don, H., and Milic-Emili, J.: Immediate ventilatory response to elastic loads and positive pressure in man. Respir. Physiol., 18:347–369, 1973.
35. Mead, J.: Control of respiratory frequency. J. Appl. Physiol., 15:325–326, 1960.
36. Guz, A., Noble, M. I. M., Widdicombe, J. G., Trenchard, D., Mushin, W. W., and Makey, A. R.: The role of vagal and glossopharyngeal afferent nerves in respiratory sensation, control of breathing and arterial pressure regulation in conscious man. Clin. Sci., 30:161–170, 1969.
37. Cross, K. W., Klaus, M., Tooley, W. H., and Weisser, K.: The response of the newborn to inflation of the lungs. J. Physiol. (Lond.), 151:551–565, 1960.
38. Thach, B. T., and Taeusch, H. W.: Sighing in newborn human infants: role of inflation augmenting reflex. J. Appl. Physiol., 41:502–507, 1976.
39. Coleridge, H. M., and Coleridge, J. C. G.: Impulse activity in afferent vagal C-Fibers with endings in the intrapulmonary airways of dogs. Respir. Physiol., 29:125–142, 1977.
40. Paintal, A. S.: Vagal sensory receptors and their reflex effects. Physiol. Rev., 53:159–227, 1973.
41. Meyrick, B., and Reid, L.: Nerves in rat intra-

acinar alveoli: An electron microscopic study. Respir. Physiol., *11*:367–377, 1971.

42. Fox, B., Bull, T. B., and Guz, A.: Innervation of alveolar walls in the human lung: An electron microscopic study. J. Anat., *131*:683–692, 1980.

43. Roberts, A. M., Kaufman, M. P., Baker, D. G., Brown, J. K., Coleridge, H. M., and Coleridge, J. C. G.: Reflex tracheal contraction induced by stimulation of bronchial C-Fibers in dogs. J. Appl. Physiol., *51*:485–493, 1981.

44. Paintal, A. S.: The mechanism of excitation of type J receptors, and the J reflex. *In* Porter, R. (ed.): Ciba Foundation Symposium: Breathing: Hering-Breuer Centenary Symposium. London, J. & A. Churchill, 1970, pp. 59–71.

45. Widdicombe, J. G.: Respiratory reflexes and defense. *In* Brain, J. D., Proctor, D. F., and Reid, L. M. (eds.): Respiratory Defense Mechanisms, Part II. New York, Marcel Dekker, Inc., 1977, pp. 593–630.

46. Richardson, P. S., and Peatfield, A. C.: Reflexes concerned in the defense of the lungs. Bull. Eur. Physiopathol. Respir., *17*:979–1012, 1981.

46a. Schultz, H. D., Roberts, A. M., Bratcher, C., Coleridge, H. M., Coleridge, J. C. G., and Davis, B.: Pulmonary C-fibers reflexly increase secretion by tracheal submucosal glands in dogs. J. Appl. Physiol., *58*:907–910, 1985.

47. Shepherd, J. T.: The lungs as receptor sites for cardiovascular regulation. Circulation, *63*:1–19, 1981.

48. Kaufman, M. P., Iwamoto, G. A., Ashton, J. H., and Cassidy, S. S.: Responses to inflation of vagal afferents with endings in the lung of dogs. Circ. Res., *51*:525–531, 1982.

48a. Ashton, J. H., and Cassidy, S. S.: Reflex depression of cardiovascular function during lung inflation. J. Appl. Physiol., *58*:137–145, 1985.

49. Liebow, A. A.: New concepts and entities in pulmonary disease. *In* Liebow, A. A. (ed.): The Lung. International Academy of Pathology Monograph No. 8, Baltimore, The William & Wilkins Company, 1967, pp. 332–365.

50. Lauweryns, J. M., and Peuskens, J. C.: Neuroepithelial bodies (neuroreceptor or secretory organs?) in human infant bronchial and bronchiolar epithelium. Anat. Rec., *172*:471–482, 1972.

51. Lauweryns, J. M., and Van Lommel, A.: The intrapulmonary neuroepithelial bodies after vagotomy: demonstration of their sensory neuroreceptor–like innervation. Experientia, *39*:1123–1124, 1983.

52. Lauweryns, J. M., de Bock, V., Guelincky, P., and Decramer, M.: Effects of unilateral hypoxia on neuroepithelial bodies in rabbit lungs. J. Appl. Physiol., *55*:1665–1668, 1983.

Chapter

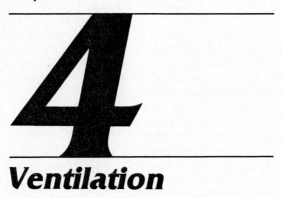

4

Ventilation

INTRODUCTION

Respiration can be defined as "those processes that contribute to gas exchange—the uptake of O_2 and the elimination of CO_2—between an organism and its environment." The previous chapters demonstrated that the structure of the mammalian lung, which evolved over eons, is elegantly designed for the efficient transfer of O_2 and CO_2 between gas in the alveoli and blood in the pulmonary capillaries. Moreover, it should be apparent that the lung is also elaborately furnished to carry out its non-respiratory functions, such as filtering the bloodstream, transforming biochemical substances, and serving as a reservoir of blood.

Gas exchange in humans can be subdivided into four principal, but interdependent, functional components: (1) those concerned with the volume and distribution of *ventilation* within the lungs (present chapter), (2) those concerned with the volume and distribution of *blood flow* through the pulmonary circulation (Chapter 6), (3) those concerned with the *diffusion* of O_2 and CO_2 across the air-blood barrier (Chapter 7), and (4) those concerned with the *regulation of breathing* (Chapter 10), usually in accordance with the metabolic need of the moment. Thus, O_2 uptake and CO_2 elimination (diffusion) occur in the terminal respiratory units, the sites at which inspired fresh air (ventilation) is brought into apposition with the film of blood flowing through the pulmonary capillaries (circulation), in quantities sufficient to satisfy metabolic demands (regulation).

Ventilation consists of the bulk movement of air from outside the body through the upper air passages and the subdivisions of the conducting airways into the terminal respiratory units. The amount of inspired air that reaches the sites of gas exchange is determined by the distensibility of the lung parenchyma and the factors that govern the movement of air as it flows through the tracheobronchial tree. Muscular effort (or force from a mechanical ventilator) is required to enlarge the lungs and thorax and to cause air to flow through the system. In other words, ventilation depends upon the capabilities of the respiratory muscles, which are described in the next chapter, and the mechanical properties of the conducting airways and distal respiratory units.

This chapter will consider certain basic aspects of ventilation and the mechanics of respiration to provide a background for analysis of most of the commonly used tests of ventilatory function and of the principles on which they are based. Excellent review articles are available, if additional details are desired.[1-5]

STATIC PROPERTIES

Everyone who has witnessed an autopsy has had the opportunity to notice that when the thorax is incised it enlarges and the lungs collapse. This simple observation vividly displays two fundamental static properties of the respiratory system: (1) the lungs tend to recoil inward, and (2) the chest wall tends to recoil outward. Movement in opposite directions by the lungs and chest wall is possible when the force that ordinarily couples them into a functioning unit, the pleural pressure, is removed.

Compliance

The recoil properties of both the lungs and the chest wall, which include not only the rib cage but also the diaphragm and abdominal contents, are displayed in the static volume-pressure diagrams of the two component structures. Volume-pressure curves may be determined experimentally by measuring the pressure change that results from adding or subtracting a given volume to the

system or by determining the volume change that results from the application of a known amount of pressure to the system. The relationship between change in volume and change in pressure defines the compliance of a structure, and is expressed as follows:

$$\text{Compliance} = \frac{\text{Change in volume}}{\text{Change in pressure}}. \quad (1)$$

Under ordinary conditions, any change in volume of the lungs must be equaled by a corresponding change in volume of the chest wall, assuming no change in intrapulmonary blood volume.* In other words, changes in volumes are equal throughout the respiratory system, which in reference to pulmonary mechanics means the lungs and chest wall combined. Because changes in volume are similar, the compliances of the respiratory system and its lung and chest wall components vary according to the change in the pressure differences "across" (i.e., from the inside to the outside) the various structures. These pressures are referred to as distending pressures and are shown schematically in Figure 4–1. Under static relaxed conditions, the distending pressures for the lung (P_l), chest wall (P_w), and respiratory system (P_{rs}) can be written as follows:

pressure difference across lung (transpulmonary pressure) = alveolar pressure (P_{alv}) minus pleural pressure (P_{pl}),

$$P_l = P_{alv} - P_{pl}; \quad (2)$$

pressure difference across the chest wall = pleural pressure minus body surface pressure (P_{bs}),

$$P_w = P_{pl} - P_{bs}; \quad (3)$$

pressure difference across the respiratory system = alveolar pressure minus body surface pressure,

$$P_{rs} = P_{alv} - P_{bs}; \quad (4)$$

or transpulmonary pressure plus pressure difference across chest wall,

$$P_{rs} = P_l + P_w. \quad (5)$$

---

*This is not true in pathologic disturbances such as pneumothorax or pleural effusion.

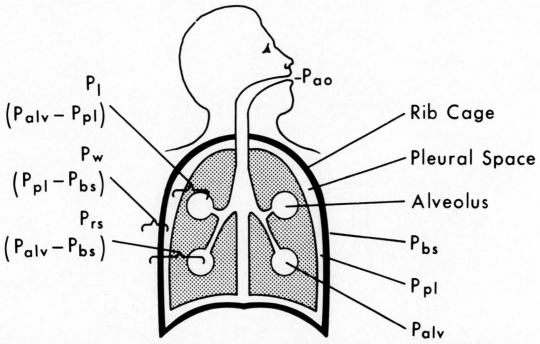

Figure 4–1. Schematic representation of the pressures and pressure differences that determine ventilation. P_{ao} = pressure at the airway opening; P_{bs} = pressure at the body surface; P_{pl} = pressure at the pleural surface; P_{alv} = pressure within the alveoli; P_l = pressure difference across the lung; P_w = pressure difference across the chest wall; and P_{rs} = pressure difference across the respiratory system.

It follows that the compliance of the lungs (C_l), chest wall (C_w), and respiratory system (C_{rs}) relate the change in volume (ΔVol), which is the same throughout, to the appropriate static distending pressure so that

$$C_l = \frac{\Delta\text{Vol, L}}{\Delta P_l, \text{ cm H}_2\text{O}}, \quad (6)$$

$$C_w = \frac{\Delta\text{Vol, L}}{\Delta P_w, \text{ cm H}_2\text{O}}, \quad (7)$$

$$C_{rs} = \frac{\Delta\text{Vol, L}}{\Delta P_{rs}, \text{ cm H}_2\text{O}}, \quad (8) \text{ or}$$

$$C_{rs} = \frac{\Delta\text{Vol, L}}{\Delta(P_l + P_w), \text{ cm H}_2\text{O}}. \quad (9)$$

A single value for compliance of the respiratory system or either of its components is of limited value for three reasons. (1) Volume-pressure curves for the separate structures and the structures combined are alinear. For example, the volume-pressure curve of the lung (Fig. 4–2) is steepest at its origin and becomes flatter as inflation progresses; therefore, compliance will have a higher value if it is derived from the lower part rather than from the upper part of the curve. (2) Conditions of measurement may affect the resulting values of compliance markedly. For example, volume-pressure curves of the lung obtained during inflation differ from those obtained during deflation owing to hysteresis; similarly, the "volume history" of the lungs (i.e., the pattern of ventilation) before the breathing sequence, when volume and pressure are recorded, will influence the measurements. In excised lungs, the temperature and the timing are also important in obtaining accurate measurements. (3) Total lung volume influences the absolute value of compliance. For example, a person with a large lung volume will have a higher lung compliance than a person with a small lung volume even though the lungs of both may be perfectly normal and have exactly the same distensibilities. The latter phenomenon has led to the use of the term *specific compliance*, or compliance divided by the lung volume at which it is measured, usually FRC. Values of specific compliance for normal persons are the same, regardless of body build.

In the discussion that follows, the volume-pressure curves, through the entire range of

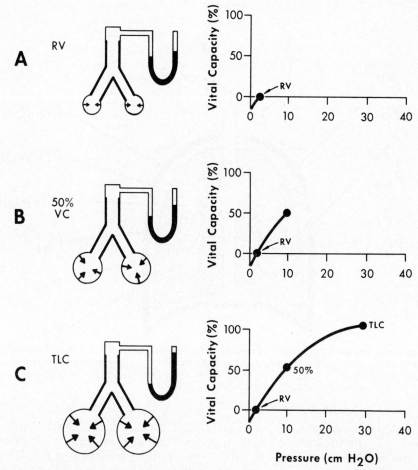

Figure 4–2. Schematic representation of the volume-pressure relationships of isolated lungs. *A*, Because excised lungs collapse to less than residual volume (RV), at RV a small recoil pressure (small arrows facing inward) is evident; this pressure is reflected in the slight deflection of the column in the manometer and the value on the horizontal (pressure) axis. *B*, At 50 per cent vital capacity (VC), the recoil pressure is increased (more and larger arrows than in *A*); thus more pressure is reflected in the manometer and on the horizontal axis. *C*, At total lung capacity (TLC), recoil pressure is maximal (normally about 30 cm H_2O).

vital capacity, are shown; it can be assumed that these are deflation curves (more reproducible than inflation curves), and that they were obtained after inflating the lung fully several times to ensure a constant volume history.

Elastic Recoil of the Lung

Because compliance is an expression of the distensibility of the elastic respiratory system, measured values of compliance depend upon the elastic recoil properties of the lungs and chest wall. The lungs can be depicted, for schematic purposes, as two completely collapsible elastic balloons sup-

ported by a rigid Y-shaped tube (see Fig. 4–2A). As volume is added in increments through the tube to expand the collapsed lungs, pressure is generated within the system owing to the tendency for the elastic walls to recoil inward (see Fig. 4–2B). The magnitude and direction of the recoil forces are represented by the size and direction of the arrows and by the deflection of the black column in the manometers in the figures. As more volume is added, the lungs continue to expand, but finally the volume-pressure curve begins to flatten as the elastic elements reach the limits of their distensibility (Fig. 4–2C). At this pressure, the volume of the lung is maximal, and attempts to increase the volume further cause a huge rise in pressure due to the flatness of the volume-pressure curve, and the lungs are apt to rupture.

It can be seen from Figure 4–2 that under static conditions the pressure generated by the lung is determined solely by its elastic recoil pressure (P_{stl}). This means that when the airways are open and there is no airflow, static elastic recoil pressure is equal to transpulmonary pressure ($P_{stl} = P_l = P_{alv} - P_{pl}$). It follows that under static conditions, when $P_{alv} = 0$, both P_{stl} and P_l are equal and opposite to P_{pl}. This is easy to understand by considering the situation of the subject holding his breath at any lung volume, with his glottis open (so that $P_{alv} = 0$). Because the tendency of the lungs to recoil inward establishes the transpulmonary pressure, to keep the lungs inflated to that volume pleural pressure must be equal and opposite to recoil pressure ($- P_{pl} = P_l = P_{stl}$).

The relationship between elastic recoil and compliance is also depicted in Figure 4–2. Because compliance is defined as a change in volume resulting from a change in pressure, it is derived from the volume-pressure curves as the *slope* of the line ($\Delta Vol/\Delta P$) at any point along the line. The *position* of the line depends upon the elastic recoil of the lungs.

The lungs of patients with emphysema are more distensible and the lungs of patients with diffuse interstitial fibrosis or other infiltrative diseases are less distensible, or stiffer, than normal lungs. Representative volume-pressure curves from adults with normal lungs, with emphysema, and with pulmonary fibrosis are shown in Figure 4–3; the curves were compiled assuming that the three persons were similar in age and body build, so that they would have lungs with similar vital capacities and volume-pressure relationships. The curve from

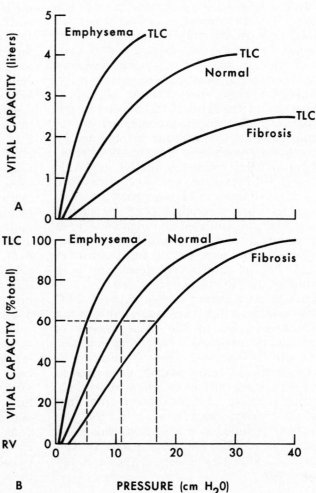

Figure 4–3. Representative volume-pressure curves from adult subjects of the same age, sex, and body size, showing changes caused by emphysema and pulmonary fibrosis compared with normal lungs. *A,* depicts volume-pressure relations in terms of measured (i.e., observed) vital capacity and demonstrates that emphysematous lungs are larger and fibrotic lungs smaller than normal. *B,* When expressed in terms of percentage of measured vital capacity, at any given vital capacity (e.g., 60 per cent, shown by dashed lines), elastic recoil pressure is less than normal in emphysema and greater than normal in fibrosis. TLC = total lung capacity; RV = residual volume.

the patient with emphysema is steeper and is shifted above the normal curve, whereas the curve from the patient with fibrosis is flatter and is shifted below. When expressed at any given lung volume or per cent of vital capacity (e.g., 60 per cent, as shown in Fig. 4–3), elastic recoil is lower with fibrosis. Thus, values of elastic recoil can be used to describe the static properties of normal and abnormal lungs; but, as will be described subsequently, elastic recoil also is an important determinant of the dynamic behavior of the lungs.

Measurement of Pleural Pressure

A measurement of pleural pressure is obviously necessary for the assessment of the pulmonary elastic recoil properties both of normal subjects and of patients with pulmonary diseases. Although it is difficult and dangerous to measure pressure directly from the pleural space in human beings, the problem has largely been overcome through the use of pressure recordings from a balloon positioned in the subject's esophagus. Because the esophagus is located between the two pleural spaces, esophageal pressure measurements, when carried out correctly, provide a close approximation of pleural pressure at the level of the balloon in the thorax.[6] Static volume-pressure (elastic recoil) curves of the lung can be obtained by measuring esophageal pressure at different lung volumes while the subject holds his breath with his glottis open to eliminate the effect of changes in alveolar pressure. Values are usually recorded after the subject has maximally inflated his lungs a few times to ensure a constant volume history. Measurements are made first at full inspiration and then at successively decreasing lung volumes to FRC to provide a deflation volume-pressure curve; studies between FRC and residual volume are less reliable owing to inaccuracies in the measurement of esophageal pressure at low lung volumes. As will be discussed, there is uncertainty concerning the actual magnitude of what is called pleural surface pressure and its regional distribution in the intact thorax. Part of the problem stems from the fact that the various techniques of measuring this pressure, including the esophageal balloon method, often yield different values at the same site.

Origin of Lung Elastic Recoil

The total force causing the inflated human lung to recoil inward has two different origins. Part arises from the elastic properties of the lung tissue itself, and part arises from the film of surface-active material that lines the terminal respiratory units. The two components of elastic recoil were first deduced by von Neergaard[7] over 50 years ago, and their separate influences can be demonstrated by repeating his classic experiment of comparing the volume-pressure relationships of the air-filled lung with those of the saline-filled lung. It can be seen in Figure 4–4 that less pressure is required to inflate the lung to a given volume and that hysteresis is nearly absent when saline is used instead of air. Filling with saline eliminates the effect of surface forces at the air-liquid interfaces in the lungs and demonstrates the effect of surface forces on pulmonary compliance and hysteresis.

Surface Forces. The surface forces at the air-liquid interfaces are determined by the surface tension of the thin film of surfactant that covers the surface of terminal respiratory units and probably also lines the luminal surface of terminal bronchioles. (The cellular origin, metabolism, and anatomic location of the surface-active material are described in Chapters 1 and 2.) The important property of pulmonary surfactant is that its surface tension decreases remarkably as the area of the surface layer is reduced, as shown in Figure 4–5. Surfactant from normal lungs is unique in its behavior, and it has the lowest surface tension of any biologic substance ever measured. Furthermore, when studied *in vitro*, lung surfactant displays a striking hysteresis loop (see Fig. 4–5) that is qualitatively similar to and presumably accounts for most of the hysteresis encountered when filling the normal lung with air and then emptying it (see Fig. 4–4).

Recent evidence suggests that surfactant is absorbed into the film at the alveolar interface as a complex quasi-*liquid* during lung inflation; in contrast, as the surface area decreases during deflation, most of the lipid components other than dipalmitoyl phosphatidylcholine are extruded, leaving a quasi-*crystalline* film that is highly stable at 37°C and can maintain a low surface tension for a long period.[9] The net effect of these physicochemical properties is that the

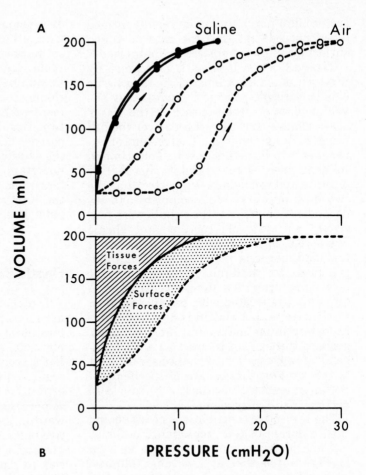

Figure 4–4. A, Volume-pressure curves of lungs filled with saline and with air. B, The use of saline eliminates the effect of surface forces at the air-liquid interface and allows subdivision of the total pressure required to inflate the lung into the amounts necessary to overcome tissue forces and surface forces. The arrows indicate whether the lung is being inflated or deflated; note than when using saline, hysteresis (i.e., the difference between inflation and deflation limbs of the curve) is virtually eliminated. (Adapted and reprinted by permission from Clements, J. A., and Tierney, D. F.: Alveolar instability associated with altered surface tensions. *In* Fenn, W. O., and Rahn, H. (eds.): Handbook of Physiology, Section 3. Respiration. Vol. II. Washington, D.C., American Physiological Society, 1964, pp. 1565–1583.)

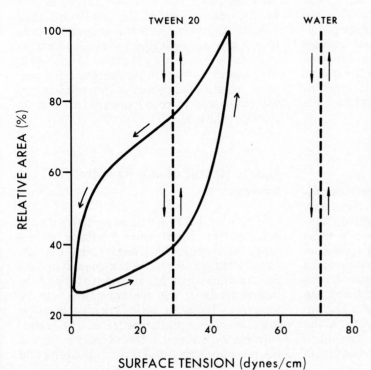

Figure 4–5. Surface area-surface tension relationships for lung washings containing normal surfactant (solid lines) and for Tween 20 (a detergent) and for water (dashed lines). Note that when the surface film containing surfactant is reduced in area, its surface tension decreases nearly to 0 dynes/cm. The arrows indicate expansion (upward) or compression (downward) of the material. Note the similarity between the hysteresis loops in lung washings and normal lungs (see Fig. 4–4). (Adapted and reprinted by permission from Clements, J. A., and Tierney, D. F.: Alveolar instability associated with altered surface tensions. *In* Fenn, W. O., and Rahn, H. (eds.): Handbook of Physiology, Section 3. Respiration. Vol. II. Washington, D.C., American Physiological Society, 1964, pp. 1565–1583.)

surface film normally can be rapidly formed when needed, but that the rate at which surfactant must be replaced is diminished.[10]

Tissue Forces. It is not known precisely in which structural elements the lung tissue elasticity resides, nor is it known why the volume-pressure relationship of the tissue components is smoothly curved over the full range of lung deflation. The results of experiments in hamsters in which elastin and collagen fibers were separately digested by elastase and collagenase suggested that the two fiber networks were complete and independent;[11] moreover, the results were consistent with the old concept that elastic fibers contribute to tissue recoil forces at low- and mid-lung volumes and that collagen fibers set the limit of distensibility at high lung volumes.[1] More recent observations in dogs treated with papain (an elastase) indicate that elastin is also important in determining maximum lung volumes, perhaps through an interaction with collagen.[12] However, all such studies are difficult to interpret because of lack of specificity of the enzymes used to attack a certain connective tissue component.

The respective contributions of tissue and surface forces to total compliance differ at low and high lung volumes; it can be seen in Figure 4–4 that at low lung volumes, surface forces are the chief determinant of the lung's distensibility and at high lung volumes, tissue forces predominate. This difference is attributable to the changing volume-pressure relations of the elastic structures and to the augmented effects of surface tensions (T) on pressure (P) when the radius of curvature (r) is small. These relationships are expressed in the Laplace equation for a spherical structure:

$$P = \frac{2T}{r}. \qquad (10)$$

This analysis obviously assumes that alveoli are idealized spheres and that they inflate and deflate uniformly, notions that are no longer supportable. There is little doubt, however, that the surface tension of the surfactant film decreases strikingly as lung volume is reduced;[13] however, the actual values encountered throughout the full range of lung inflation are not known. Furthermore, the "classic" concepts of the volume-pressure behavior of the lung parenchyma, which were derived from

experiments in which the lungs were filled with either air or liquid, are now recognized as marked oversimplifications. Because alveolar geometry varies greatly in the air- or liquid-filled lung (see Fig. 2–27), the mechanical contributions of the tissue elements, which are aligned differently in the two situations, cannot be directly compared.[14] (The interested reader is referred to the detailed analysis of the complexities and uncertainties concerning the mechanical interactions of the structural components of the lung parenchyma, which was recently published.[10])

Elastic Recoil of the Chest Wall

The chest wall can be depicted for schematic purposes as a compressible and distensible structure that contains an appreciable volume in its resting state (Fig. 4–6A). If the volume of the thorax-diaphragm is reduced by contraction of the muscles of expiration, the chest wall tends to resist compression and, by tending to recoil outward to its resting volume, creates a negative pressure within the system (Fig. 4–6B). The pressure exerted by the expiratory muscles to empty the thorax a given volume from its resting state must, therefore, overcome the outward recoil pressure generated by the chest wall at the newly attained volume. Conversely, if the thorax is made to accommodate a larger volume by contraction of the inspiratory muscles (Fig. 4–6C), the muscular effort must overcome the positive pressure generated by the tendency of the chest wall to recoil inward, back to its resting position.

Elastic Recoil of the Respiratory System

It is useful for introductory purposes to describe the recoil characteristics of the lungs and chest wall separately, but obviously they have to be considered in concert, because their physiologic functions are interdependent. The two structures can be viewed as being in series with each other, and therefore, the pressure of the (total) respiratory system is the algebraic sum of the pressure generated by both the lung and

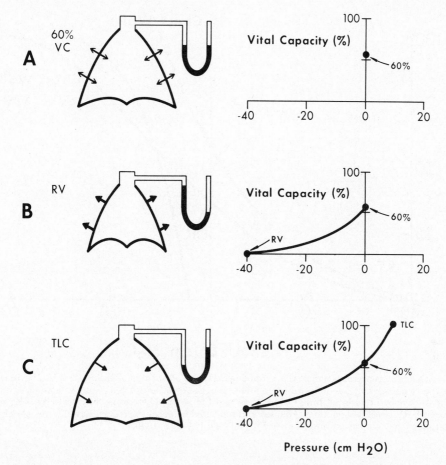

Figure 4–6. Schematic representation of the volume-pressure relationships of the isolated chest wall. *A*, The chest wall in the relaxed position (zero pressure) has a volume approximately 60 per cent of vital capacity (VC). *B*, When the chest wall is compressed to residual volume (RV), it tends to recoil outward to its resting position and thus generates the negative pressure shown on the manometer and horizontal axis. *C*, When the chest wall is expanded to total lung capacity (TLC), the chest wall tends to recoil inward and thereby generates the positive pressure shown on the manometer and horizontal axis.

chest wall: $P_{rs} = P_l + P_w$. Because any given volume change is equal throughout the respiratory system, the lungs and the chest wall, the separate volume-pressure curves shown in Figures 4–2 and 4–6 can be combined into one for the total respiratory system by simply adding the pressures at a chosen volume (Fig. 4–7). The resulting curve indicates the pressure that must be applied by contraction of the respiratory muscles, or by a mechanical respirator, to achieve a volume change throughout the respiratory system; under static conditions, the total pressure must equal the sum of the pressures required to offset the elastic recoil pressures of the lungs and chest wall at that volume.

Lung Volumes

The volume-pressure diagram of the respiratory system and its components also provides an easily understood explanation about the determinants of normal lung volumes. Moreover, abnormalities in these relationships account for the characteristic lung volume changes in various diseases such as pulmonary emphysema and interstitial fibrosis. It can be seen in Figure 4–7 that FRC occurs normally at the volume of the total system at which the inward recoil force of the lung is equal and opposite to the outward recoil force of the chest wall; in other words, the resting volume (FRC) is that volume at which the net force in the

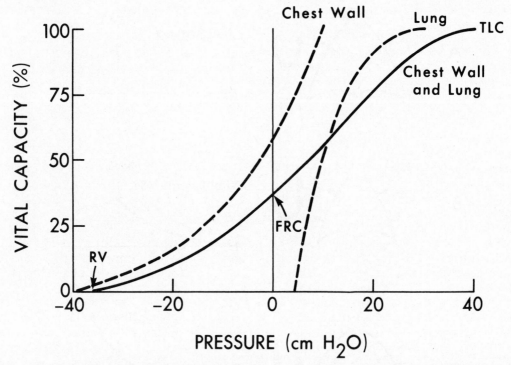

Figure 4–7. Schematic representation of the volume-pressure relationships of the chest wall and lung combined (solid line). The combined curve is obtained by summation of the recoil pressures of the isolated chest wall (dashed line and Fig. 4–6) and the isolated lung (dashed line and Fig. 4–2). TLC = total lung capacity; FRC = functional residual capacity; RV = residual volume. (Adapted and reprinted by permission from Rahn, H., et al.: The pressure-volume diagram of the thorax and lung. Am. J. Physiol. *146*:161–178, 1946.)

respiratory system is zero. This is true of normal persons when they are supine, but as discussed in more detail in the next chapter, in the erect and sitting positions, the end-expiratory lung volume is slightly smaller than the relaxed FRC because of expiratory muscle contraction.

During a continuous inspiration, the net force developed by the contracting muscles of respiration (agonist and antagonist groups) meets progressively increasing recoil forces from the combined expansion of the lungs and chest wall. Furthermore, as the contracting muscle fibers shorten, they generate progressively less force. Finally, *total lung capacity* (TLC) is reached at the volume at which inspiration must cease, because the opposing forces are balanced (i.e., the weakening forces of inspiration can no longer overcome the increasing force required to distend the lungs and chest wall).

Similarly, during a continuous expiration the net force developed by the contracting muscles encounters increasing opposition from the recoil force in the system, which originates chiefly from the chest wall (see Fig. 4–7). In children and young adults,

expiration ceases at the volume at which the opposing forces are equal (i.e., expiratory muscle force is insufficient to cause a further reduction in chest wall volume); *residual volume* (RV), therefore, in young subjects is determined by the balance of forces operating in the chest wall. In older persons, however, RV appears to be governed increasingly by the factors that regulate the caliber and patency of small airways; this means that even though the respiratory muscles are capable of compressing the chest wall and emptying the lungs further, they are prevented from doing so by airway closure and the trapping of gas in the lungs.[16]

The *vital capacity* (VC) is the maximum amount of gas that can be exhaled in a single effort, after fully inflating the lungs. Measurements of VC, which are simple and accurate, are the most common and widely used tests of pulmonary function. But as is evident in Figure 4–7, VC is not a unique volume but the difference between TLC and RV; thus, a given value of VC can be influenced by all of the factors that affect both TLC and RV.

Forces Holding Lung Against Chest Wall

As just described, at FRC the lungs and chest wall tend to recoil in opposite directions, creating forces that operate to separate the visceral from the parietal pleura; if the layers were allowed to part, a space would form that would need to be filled with either liquid or gas. The lungs and chest wall do *not* separate from each other but remain apposed throughout their ventilatory excursions owing to the mechanisms that prevent gas and liquid from collecting in the pleural space. Moreover, the same mechanisms operate to cause the removal of gas from a pneumothorax or liquid from a pleural effusion, if either is formed as part of a pathologic process.

The pleural space, though an anatomically delimited cavity, is otherwise analogous to a tissue space and is therefore governed by the same mechanisms that regulate the pressure of gases everywhere in the body. This subject is treated more fully in the section on Gas Exchange (see Chapter 7), because tissue gas pressure depends upon the respective shapes of the oxyhemoglobin and the CO_2 dissociation curves. The net result of the exchange of respiratory gases between blood and cells determines that the sum of the partial pressures of all the individual gases in capillaries and venous blood (O_2, CO_2, N_2, H_2O) will be about 700 mm Hg and that interstitial tissues will be exposed to a gas pressure that is nearly 60 mm Hg subatmospheric (760 − 700 mm Hg). The high negative pressure serves to keep the pleural space free of gas and to cause the absorption of gases once they are introduced into any closed-off part of the body.

The pleural cavity normally contains a small amount of liquid, which has proved difficult to measure accurately, especially in healthy humans. Original estimates for most mammals were in the range of 0.1 to 0.2 ml pleural liquid per kg body weight;[17] new data indicate that pleural liquid has a low protein concentration and that both liquid and protein turnover may be much slower than previously estimated.[18] The sites of pleural liquid formation and removal and the forces that govern these processes are considered in detail in the section on Liquid and Solute Exchange (see Chapter 12). The pleural space and the liquid it contains have both a static and a dynamic function. The static effect is to couple the lungs to the chest wall and to permit the transmission of forces between the two structures. The dynamic effect is to provide a lubricated system in which the lungs can move rapidly and freely, with respect to the chest wall.

Everyone agrees that the pressure in the pleural space at FRC in most mammalian species that have been studied, including humans, is negative with respect to atmospheric pressure and that there is a gradient of pleural pressure within the intact thorax. But the regional distribution of pleural expansive force (*pleural surface pressure*) and the extent of differences between this pressure and the pressure in the liquid film surrounding the lungs (*pleural liquid pressure*) are the subjects of considerable controversy. Because the distribution of pleural surface pressure is the principal factor affecting the distribution of inspired air within normal lungs, detailed discussion of pleural pressure is deferred until later in this chapter.

DYNAMIC PROPERTIES

To cause air to move from outside the body into the terminal respiratory units, a force must be applied to the respiratory system that is sufficient to overcome three opposing forces: (1) the *elastic recoil* of the lungs and chest wall, (2) the *frictional resistance* afforded by the airways and by the tissues of the lungs and thorax, and (3) the *inertance* (impedance of acceleration) of the entire system. The elastic forces of the lungs and chest wall, as discussed in the previous section, depend upon the volume introduced into the system and are not affected by motion (i.e., rate of deformation) within the system. In contrast, frictional resistance is determined by the *rate* of change of volume (i.e., flow) and not by the magnitude of the change in volume *per se*. Inertance depends upon the rate of change of flow (i.e., acceleration) of the gas and of the tissues that compose the system.

Analysis of the mechanical properties of the respiratory system can be simplified because inertance has been found to be a negligible quantity during normal breathing and because the contributions of elastic forces and flow-resistance forces can be separated by studying the system under static and dynamic conditions, respectively.

Frictional Resistance

Resistance to airflow in the respiratory system is computed from simultaneous measurements of the airflow and the pressure difference causing the airflow. Resistance is calculated according to the general equation:

$$\text{Resistance} = \frac{\text{pressure difference}}{\text{rate of flow}}. \quad (11)$$

Airflow is easy to measure, but measuring the pressure differences that cause air to flow requires specialized recording equipment. However, by measuring the appropriate individual pressure differences that are described subsequently, the flow-resistance properties of individual components of the respiratory system can be analyzed separately, i.e., the airways, the tissues of lung parenchyma, and the tissues of the thorax and abdomen that surround the respiratory tract and are deformed by its movements. The various resistances that can be calculated by measurement of different "driving pressures" are as follows:

1. *Airway resistance* (R_{aw}) is defined as the frictional resistance afforded by the entire system of air passages to airflow from outside the body to within the alveoli. Airway resistance is determined from the simultaneous measurements of the flow and the pressure difference between the airway opening (P_{ao}) and the alveoli. These variables can all be measured accurately in the body plethysmograph;[19] accordingly,

$$R_{aw} = \frac{P_{ao} - P_{alv}, \text{ cm } H_2O}{\text{flow, L/sec}}. \quad (12)$$

2. *Pulmonary resistance* (R_l) is defined as the frictional resistance afforded by the lungs and air passages combined. Hence, pulmonary resistance is the sum of lung-tissue resistance and airway resistance and is determined from the simultaneous measurements of the flow and the pressure difference between the airway opening and the pleural surface. The total pleural pressure must be corrected by subtracting, either graphically or electronically, the lung elastic pressure to obtain the lung resistive pressure ($P_{pl(cor)}$). Given these variables,

$$R_l = \frac{P_{ao} - P_{pl(cor)}, \text{ cm } H_2O}{\text{flow, L/sec}}. \quad (13)$$

Because pulmonary resistance consists of both the frictional resistance of the airways (R_{aw}) and the frictional (viscous) resistance of lung tissue (R_{lt}), the latter, which cannot be measured separately, may be derived by subtraction:

$$R_{lt} = R_l - R_{aw}, \text{ cm } H_2O \text{ per L/sec.} \quad (14)$$

3. *Chest wall tissue resistance* (R_w) is defined as the frictional resistance of the chest wall and abdominal structures. Chest wall tissue resistance is determined from the simultaneous measurements of the flow and the pressure difference from the pleura to the body surface, after subtracting from the total pressure difference the amount required to overcome the elastic recoil of the chest, leaving a corrected value ($P_{bs(cor)}$):

$$R_w = \frac{P_{pl} - P_{bs(cor)}, \text{ cm } H_2O}{\text{flow, L/sec}}. \quad (15)$$

Chest wall resistance can be measured by using a respirator or the oscillation technique[20] and an esophageal balloon to record the appropriate pressure difference across the chest wall; by either method, however, it is difficult to avoid the spurious effects from respiratory muscle contractions.

Partitioning of Frictional Resistance

Only a limited number of complete studies have been performed on normal subjects to assess the total frictional resistance of the entire respiratory system and to subdivide the total into the parts contributed by the various components of the system.[2] A graphic representation of how frictional resistance is partitioned is given in Figure 4–8. The flow-resistance contributions of the various components vary, depending upon the flow rate. For reference purposes it should be pointed out that the peak flow rates achieved during quiet breathing are about 0.4 L/sec, and between 1.25 and 1.50 L/sec during mild exercise (minute volume 25 to 30 L/min). Figure 4–8 also shows that the resistance offered by the nose is the largest single component, comprising one-half to two-thirds of the airway resistance during nasal breathing at low flow rates. The resistance of the nose, which is markedly nonlinear, increases proportionately

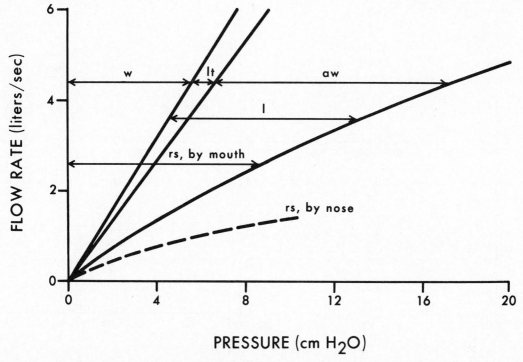

Figure 4–8. Schematic representation of the flow-pressure relationships of the respiratory system (rs) of normal man breathing through the nose or mouth. The distance from the vertical axis to the curves or between one curve and another indicates the pressure necessary to overcome the frictional resistance imposed by the various components of the respiratory system at a given flow (e.g., the horizontal lines). w = chest wall; lt = lung tissue; aw = airway; l = pulmonary (lung tissue + airway). (Adapted and reprinted by permission from Mead and Agostoni, Chapter 14. *In* Fenn, W. O., and Rahn, H. (eds.): Handbook of Physiology, Section 3. Respiration. Vol. I. Washington, D.C., American Physiological Society, 1964, pp. 357–476.)

much more than flow as flow increases and must become prohibitively large during heavy exercise. The transition from nose to mouth breathing presumably occurs for this reason, when flow through the nasal passages requires pressures of 6 to 8 cm H_2O.[21]

The resistance offered by the oropharynx and larynx is also nonlinear and accounts for about 40 per cent of the resistance offered by all the air passages during quiet mouth breathing. As flow rate increases, the partition of frictional resistance becomes weighted toward an increased contribution of either the nose or the oropharynx owing to their nonlinear flow-resistance characteristics. The contribution of the larynx is minimized by the widening that occurs from reflex activity during deep breathing.

Resistance in the tracheobronchial tree is nearly linear up to flow rates of 2 L/sec, and during quiet mouth breathing it accounts for about 60 per cent of total airway resistance. Lung tissue resistance is small compared with airway resistance; of the total pulmonary resistance (tissue plus airway),

lung tissue resistance accounts for about one-sixth (or less) and airway resistance for about five-sixths of the total.[22] Chest wall resistance is also approximately linear up to flow rates of 2 L/sec and contributes about 40 per cent and 19 per cent of the total respiratory resistance during mouth and nose breathing, respectively, at flow rates of 1 L/sec.[21]

By the technique of measuring pressures simultaneously in the trachea and small airways, the latter through a catheter that has been passed retrograde and wedged into a small bronchus, resistance of the tracheobronchial tree can be partitioned into contributions from the large or central airways (trachea and all branches out to about 2 mm diameter) and from the small or peripheral airways (< about 2 mm diameter). The results of the original studies of excised human lungs and of both living and excised animal lungs revealed that peripheral airways resistance was only a small proportion of the total resistance afforded by the entire tracheobronchial tree.[23, 24] In addition, as

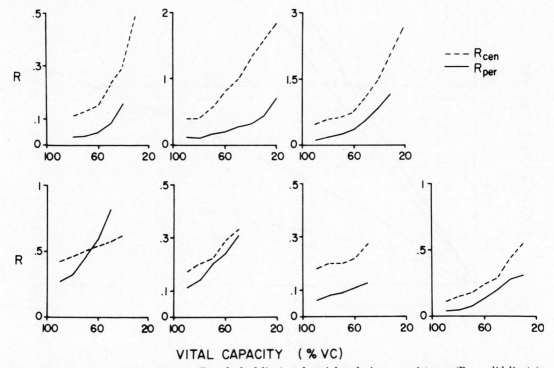

Figure 4–9. Central airway resistance (R_{cen}, dashed line) and peripheral airway resistance (R_{per}, solid line) (cm $H_2O \cdot L^{-1} \cdot S$) plotted against lung volumes (% VC) for seven dogs. Interpolated values at intervals of 10 per cent VC were averaged for three to eight runs with vagi intact. Note consistent volume dependency and roughly proportional slopes for R_{per} and R_{cen}. (Reprinted by permission from Hoppin, F. G., Jr., et al.: Relationship of central and peripheral airway resistance to lung volume in dogs. J. Appl. Physiol., *44*:728–737, 1978.)

lung volume was changed in the same studies, total resistance apparently increased near TLC. Because these observations, particularly the second, were at variance with conclusions derived from studies of airway dimensions using tantalum bronchography[25, 26] and morphometry,[27] the measurements were repeated using a different technique to partition airflow resistance into its peripheral and central components; the newer data indicated that the resistances of airways proximal and distal to a 2 to 3 mm diameter bronchus are about the same (Fig. 4–9).[28] Furthermore, in contrast to the results of previous studies, (1) when lung volume was decreased with the vagus nerves intact, the increase in peripheral resistance was at least as great as the increase in central resistance, (2) the lung volume dependencies of central and peripheral resistances were not abolished by vagotomy, and (3) neither resistance increased systematically at high lung volumes. These findings are consonant with the behavior of airways when they are examined by bronchography.

Thus, the peripheral airways are not as "quiet" as originally believed, but the notion that they contribute only slightly to total airways resistance had important consequences: It encouraged the development of new pulmonary function tests designed to examine the behavior of "small" airways, and it led to studies of pathologic abnormalities located in peripheral airways in an effort to document their role in the evolution of chronic obstructive airways disorders.[29] As a result of these investigations, we now know considerably more about the structure-function relationships of this important, previously unappreciated, part of the lungs.

Factors Affecting Airway Resistance

Airway resistance depends upon the number, length, and cross-sectional area of the conducting airways. The number of airways in the normal lung is determined by the pattern of branching that is established by the 16th week of fetal life. Airways do not form thereafter, and in fact, the total number of small airways becomes reduced during the first few years of life by the transformation of conducting bronchioles into respiratory bronchioles. At times, the number of airways may be reduced further by surgical resection and pulmonary diseases. The length of airways varies considerably from person to person, depending upon age and body size; airway length also varies in an individual depending upon the phase of ventilation, lengthening during inspiration as lung volume increases and shortening during expiration. Because resistance to airflow in a given airway changes according to the fourth power of the radius of the airway, the cross-sectional area within the tracheobronchial tree is by far the most important, as well as potentially the most variable, determinant of airway resistance.

The cross-sectional area of any given intrathoracic airway must be determined by the balance between two opposing forces: Those tending to contract the walls, primarily tension of airway smooth muscle and elastic elements, and those forces tending to distend the walls. Outward traction is provided either from the attached lung parenchyma in the case of terminal brochioles, which are directly enmeshed in the structural framework of the terminal respiratory unit they serve, or from the indirect effects of pleural pressure (discussed subsequently) in the case of intrapulmonary conducting airways that are surrounded by an interstitial space and bronchovascular sheath. In addition to the pattern of breathing before measurements are made (i.e., the volume history, which must always be taken into account), airway resistance is governed by the following interacting factors:

Lung Volume. Many years ago, Macklin[30] observed that if the tracheobronchial tree were rigid, the lungs could not inflate and deflate. That airways do change their length and diameter during breathing has been verified many times and, in general, both dimensions change in proportion to lung volume. Studies of airway resistance at different lung volumes have revealed the relationship shown in Figure 4–10A. Changes in lung volume above FRC have little effect on airway resistance, but between FRC and RV airway resistance increases rapidly and approaches infinity (no airflow) at RV. The curvilinear relationship between changes in airway resistance and lung volume can be transformed into a nearly linear diagram by plotting the reciprocal of airway resistance, airway conductance ($G_{aw} = 1/R_{aw}$), against lung volume (Fig. 4–10B). Furthermore, the marked variations in individual values of airway resistance and conductance among children and adults of both sexes, primarily the result of differences in body size, can be reduced if conductance is related to lung volume.[31] This relationship has led to the use of the term *specific airway conductance,* which is airway conductance divided by the lung volume at which it was measured, usually FRC. Although it is useful to relate measurements of airway conductance to those of lung volume, the determinant of the relationship between lung volume and airway resistance is the elastic recoil at the given lung volume. When elastic recoil and lung volume are made to vary independently (e.g., by chest strapping), it can be shown that elastic recoil and not lung volume is the variable that determines airway resistance.[32]

Elastic Recoil. The elastic recoil properties of the lung affect the caliber of both bronchioles and bronchi but by different mechanisms: first, by providing direct traction on small intrapulmonary airways, and second, by being one of the two determinants (alveolar pressure being the other) of intrapleural pressure, which provides the pressure surrounding bronchi and extrapulmonary airways and thereby distends them.* Therefore, elastic recoil establishes airway size and becomes the chief determinant of intrathoracic airway resistance in normal subjects breathing under conditions in which flow is not limited by airway compression (see subsequent section on Flow-Volume Relationships).

Geometry of Airways. Changes in the geometry of normal bronchi depend not only on the transmural pressure across their walls but also on the distensibility of the elements composing the walls. These phenomena are reflected in the diameter-pressure and length-pressure relationships of the airways. The results of previous studies of airway geometry during lung inflation fall into two general categories: (1) one in which most of the changes occur at relatively low distending pressures (e.g., 6 to 10 cm H_2O),[34] and (2) one in which both length and diameter change continuously over the full range of pressures.[25] These apparently

---

*Intrapulmonary peribronchial pressure is at least as negative as, and probably slightly more negative than, pleural pressure.[33]

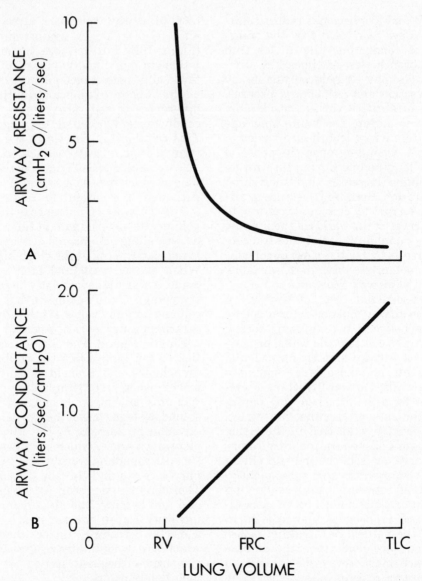

Figure 4–10. Schematic illustrations of the relationship between airway resistance *(A)* and airway conductance *(B)* and lung volume. The hyperbolic resistance-volume curve becomes a straight line when the same data are expressed as conductance-volume. (Reprinted by permission from Murray, J. F.: Respiration. *In* Smith, L. H., and Thier, S. (eds.): Pathophysiology. Philadelphia, W. B. Saunders Company, 1985, pp. 753–854.)

discrepant findings can now be explained by differences in bronchial smooth muscle tone at the time the experiments were conducted.[26] When bronchomotor tone is absent, the airways become relatively floppy and distend almost fully at low pressures. In contrast, when tone is present, the airways distend more slowly and continuously during inflation. Smooth muscle tone also accounts for the presence and magnitude of hysteresis in the dimensions of the airways as the lungs are inflated and deflated; there

is little or no hysteresis when bronchomotor tone is lacking, and hysteresis progressively develops as tone is augmented.[26]

It is of interest that, under apparently normal conditions of airway tone, the percentage change in diameter along the length of intrapulmonary airways is so consistent because the distending pressure differs from one segment to another. The small bronchioles are directly tethered by the lung parenchyma and are thus stretched by the elastic recoil of the lungs,[27] whereas the airways surrounded by a connective tissue sheath are exposed to a pressure that is about the same as pleural pressure at FRC but becomes increasingly more negative during lung inflation.[35] Thus, the distensibilities of various segments must differ to offset the differences in distending pressures; this means that bronchi should be stiffer than bronchioles, a prediction for which there is experimental support.[36]

In the walls of normal human airways there is a small amount of resting smooth muscle tone that serves to narrow the lumen and to decrease distensibility. Administration of bronchodilator drugs to healthy subjects causes bronchial smooth muscle to relax and produces a corresponding decrease in airway resistance. An increase in smooth muscle tone (i.e., bronchospasm) not only narrows the lumen of the airway but also decreases the distensibility of the walls. In addition to bronchospasm, a variety of other pathologic processes can affect the geometry of airways by causing thickening of the walls, secretions in the lumen, or narrowing from external compression.

Flow-Volume Relationships

It has long been recognized that there is a maximum limit to the flow rate that can be attained during expiration and that once this limit is achieved, greater muscular effort does not further augment flow. The key

documentation of what is now called expiratory flow limitation was made by Fry and coworkers,[37, 38] in a series of experiments carried out in the mid-1950s and early 1960s concerning isovolumic pressure-flow relationships. The best explanation of an isovolumic pressure-flow curve lies in understanding how one is constructed. Flow, volume, and esophageal (i.e., pleural) pressure are measured simultaneously during the performance of repeated expiratory vital capacity maneuvers by a subject seated in a volume plethysmograph, which corrects for gas compression. The subject is instructed to exhale with varying amounts of effort that are reflected by changes in pleural pressure. From these data, it is possible to plot flow rate against pleural pressure at any given lung volume, for example, at 60 per cent of vital capacity, as shown in Figure 4-11. It is apparent from the figure that flow rate reached a plateau at a relatively low positive pleural pressure and that once maximum flow for that lung volume was reached, it remained constant despite increasing pleural pressure to substantially higher values. The observation that expiratory flow was limited over most of the range of vital capacity provided the solution to the longstanding dilemma concerning why simple measurements during a forced expiratory maneuver, like the forced expiratory volume in 1 sec (FEV_1), were such useful tests of pulmonary function. The answer lay in the fact that some intrinsic property of the

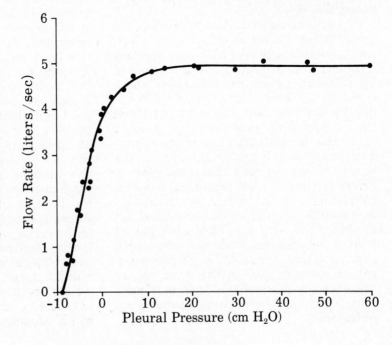

Figure 4-11. An example of an isovolume flow-pressure curve at 60 per cent vital capacity from an idealized series of measurements. The points depict the relationship between flow rate and pleural pressure at 60 per cent vital capacity during a series of vital capacity maneuvers with varying amounts of expiratory effort. It is evident that after a certain flow is reached, increasing effort, reflected by increasing pleural pressure, does *not* cause flow rate to increase.

ISOVOLUME FLOW—PRESSURE CURVES

MAXIMUM FLOW—VOLUME CURVE

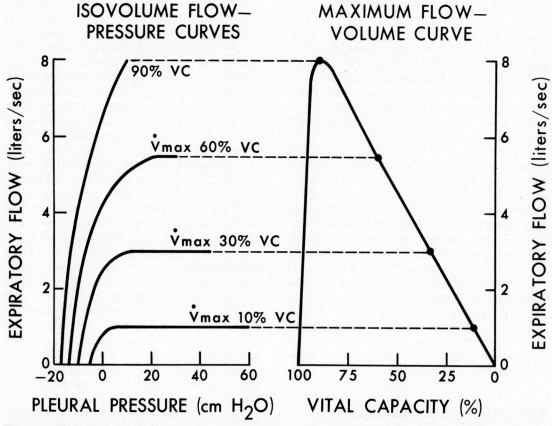

Figure 4–12. From a series of isovolume flow-pressure curves at varying vital capacities (VC) (left part of diagram), it is possible to construct a maximum flow-volume curve (right part of diagram). $\dot{V}max$ = maximum expiratory flow.

lungs, not effort, determines maximal expiratory flow.[39]

Figure 4–12 depicts a family of isovolumic pressure-flow curves at different lung volumes; they show that at high lung volumes (i.e., near TLC) expiratory flow is not limited by a flow maximum but that below about 80 to 85 per cent vital capacity, plateaus develop and maximum flow is limited. From the left part of the panel in Figure 4–12, it is possible to construct a maximum expiratory flow-volume curve (right part of the panel). It can be seen that peak flow is achieved shortly after beginning a forced exhalation from full inspiration; thereafter, flow declines as lung volume is reduced but is always the *maximum* attainable flow at a given lung volume. Peak flow varies with effort, and thus is regarded as *effort dependent;* in contrast, flow on the downslope of the curve is maximal for that particular lung volume and hence is considered *effort independent.*

Carrying out the measurements necessary to construct isovolumic pressure-flow curves is cumbersome and requires specialized equipment. However, it is now easy to obtain flow-volume curves by using a suitable X-Y recorder and plotting the flow signal on the Y-axis and the volume signal on the X-axis. A typical curve is shown in Figure 4–13 and differs only slightly from one recorded using a plethysmograph. The overall appearance of the curve is important, as are the instantaneous values of maximal flow after exhaling one-half ($\dot{V}max_{50}$) and three-quarters ($\dot{V}max_{75}$) of the vital capacity. Because interpretation of flow-volume curves is based primarily on the downslope of the curve—in other words, on the effort-independent portion—a high degree of patient cooperation is not necessary to obtain a satisfactory tracing. Patient effort is paramount in determining the results of such tests as the maximum expiratory flow rate, which depends completely on performance in the early, or effort-dependent, part of the forced vital capacity (FVC) maneuver. Even the FEV_1, because it includes the volumes exhaled during both effort-dependent and effort-independent phases, depends to some extent on subjective participation. Despite this inherent problem, measurements of FVC and FEV_1 by conventional spirometry have stood the test of time, and there is no evidence that—for routine clinical purposes—recordings of maximum expiratory flow-volume relationships have any more to offer.

When the test is properly carried out, maximum expiratory flow-volume curves are extremely reproducible in the same person. However, there is considerable variation among different persons, even among those of the same body build. To explain this variation, Green and associates[40] proposed the term *dysanapsis*, or a dissociation between airway size on the one hand and lung size on the other. More recently, Mead[41]

has provided further functional evidence for dysanapsis by identifying previously unrecognized differences in airway-parenchymal relationships between men and women and between men and boys. But the associations, if any, between these characteristics and exercise capacity or predisposition to diseases are unknown.

Flow Limitation

The basic mechanism of maximal expiratory airflow limitation has been conceptually recognized as a coupling between airway compression and the pressure drop that occurs along the airways during forced expiration. In 1967, two theoretical models were proposed to explain flow limitation that embodied this concept: the *equal pressure point* theory of Mead and coworkers[42] and the *Starling resistor* theory of Pride and coworkers.[43] According to the equal pressure

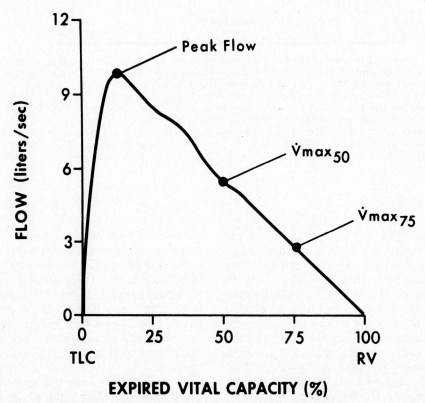

Figure 4–13. Representative forced expiratory flow-volume tracing of a normal adult man showing points of peak flow, maximal flow at 50 per cent expired vital capacity ($\dot{V}max_{50}$), and maximal flow at 75 per cent expired vital capacity ($\dot{V}max_{75}$). (Reprinted by permission from Murray, J. F.: Respiration. *In* Smith, L. H., and Thier, S. (eds.): Pathophysiology. Philadelphia, W. B. Saunders Company, 1985, pp. 753–854.)

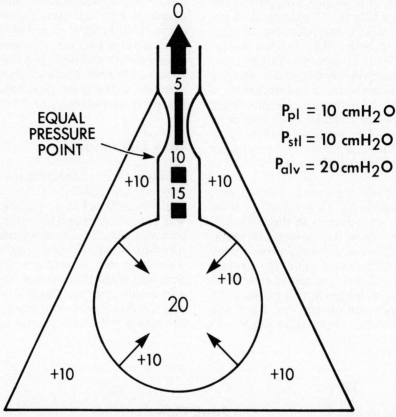

Figure 4–14. Schematic diagram of the equal pressure point concept. At a particular lung volume during forced expiration, pleural pressure (Ppl) = 10 cm H₂O, and static recoil pressure (Pstl) = 10 cm H₂O. The sum of these pressures, alveolar pressure (Palv) = 20 cm H₂O, is the driving pressure that must be dissipated as air flows along the airway to the mouth, where the pressure is zero. Accordingly, there must be a pressure along the airway at which the pressures inside and outside the wall are the same: the equal pressure point. Downstream (toward the mouth) from the equal pressure point, the airway is compressed because the pressure surrounding it is greater than the pressure in the lumen. (Reprinted by permission from Murray, J. F.: Respiration. *In* Smith, L. H., and Thier, S. (eds.): Pathophysiology. Philadelphia, W. B. Saunders Company, 1985, pp. 753–854.)

point theory (Fig. 4–14), during forced expiration alveolar pressure is augmented to the extent that pleural pressure becomes positive (remember that $P_l = P_{alv} - P_{pl}$, or in this instance, $P_{alv} = P_l + P_{pl}$). The heightened alveolar pressure provides the total pressure that must be dissipated—overcoming flow-resistance—along the airways from the alveoli to the mouth, where the pressure is zero. Bearing in mind that peribronchial pressure is approximately the same as pleural pressure, it follows, as shown in Figure 4–14, that there must be a point or points somewhere along the intrathoracic airway at which the pressure within the lumen of the airway equals the pressure

surrounding the wall. The site at which the intraluminal and extraluminal (i.e., pleural) pressures are equal, and hence the pressure difference across the wall is zero, is called the *equal pressure point*. "Downstream" (i.e., toward the mouth) from the equal pressure point, lateral pressure within the lumen is less than the external pressure around the walls, and compression of the airway develops.

It can be seen from the model in Figure 4–14 that as effort and pleural pressure increase, the equal pressure point moves "upstream" (i.e., toward the alveolus) but becomes fixed at any given lung volume when maximum flow rate occurs. Further increases of pleural pressure only augment the degree of compression of the downstream segment.

Because the transmural pressure at the equal pressure point is zero, the pressure inside and outside the wall at that point must be equal to pleural pressure. Under these conditions (i.e., maximum flow at a given lung volume), the driving pressure of the upstream segment from the alveolus (where $P_{alv} = P_{pl} + P_l$) to the equal pressure point (where the intraluminal pressure = P_{pl}) is the elastic recoil pressure of the lung ($P_l = P_{stl}$); furthermore the resistance to flow is that offered by the airways between the alveoli and only as far as the equal pressure point, which defines the junction of the upstream and downstream segments. Therefore, both driving pressure (i.e., elastic recoil) and resistance (i.e., caliber of airways of the upstream segment) are fixed.[37]

The Starling resistor model differs from the equal pressure point model in that it postulates a critical transmural pressure beyond which downstream airways would narrow sufficiently to limit flow.[43] This means that driving pressure for maximal expiratory flow is alveolar pressure minus the critical transmural pressure. Thus both theories incorporated two similar concepts: that the intrathoracic airways toward the mouth become narrowed distal to certain points according to the transmural pressure compressing them, and that the sole or principal driving pressure at maximal flow is the lungs' intrinsic elastic recoil.

Recently, new insights have been obtained as well as the ability to test predictions mathematically by applying the concepts of wave-speed limitation to the physiological determinants of maximal expiratory airflow.[44, 45] According to the *wave-speed theory,* which is derived from the principles of fluid mechanics, the tracheobronchial tree, like other systems carrying flowing fluid, cannot accommodate an airflow faster than the speed at which pressures will propagate along the airways. The velocity at which pressures will propagate in a given system is called the wave speed, and can be thought of as the velocity at which a small disturbance will travel in a compliant tube filled with fluid. In the circulation, for example, this is the speed at which the pulse propagates in arteries. In the airways, wave speed is faster than in the circulation because air is less dense than blood. Wave

speed decreases with an increase in the density of the fluid, a decrease in the cross-sectional area of the tubes, and an increase in the compliance of their walls.

According to Mead's recent analysis,[46] there are three features that contribute to a gradient of decreasing wave-speed flows during expiration, as the expirate flows from the alveoli to the thoracic outlet: (1) decreasing transmural pressure, (2) decreasing cross-sectional area, and (3) mechanical interdependence that stiffens the intrapulmonary airways in comparison to extrapulmonary airways. The continuum of decreasing wave-speed flow is offset to some extent by the increasing mechanical rigidity of the airway walls, which serves to increase wave speed. But now it is easy to understand that because the velocity of exhaled gas increases as it moves toward the mouth and because wave speed decreases in the same direction, the former can "catch up" to the latter and, once it does, flow is limited; the location at which limitation occurs is called the *choke point.* Further increases in driving pressure serve only to narrow the airways downstream from the choke point(s) and thus have no influence on the velocity of airflow.

When these considerations of wave speed theory are used to model the behavior of the respiratory system, maximal expiratory airflow limitation can be described quite accurately, especially at high and midlung volumes. At low lung volumes, predicted airflow velocities are higher than those observed, presumably because viscosity-dependent forces begin to prevail over density-dependent forces.[39]

The obvious value of flow limitation with its attendant compression of central airways is to improve the effectiveness of cough. The increased linear velocity of flow that occurs in compressed airways generates the force necessary to dislodge secretions and particles from the luminal surface. Thus, cough is most effective in the compressed segments mouthward from the choke point(s). At high lung volumes the choke point is believed to be near the carina;[46] as lung volumes decrease, the choke points move outward, but how far out no one knows. A good guess would be that choke points extend peripherally only as far as the epithelial irritant receptors, which when stimulated, initiate the cough reflex.

Inspiratory flow is not normally limited

by effort because compression does not occur. As greater inspiratory efforts are made, intrathoracic airways become progressively distended, and flow is enhanced.

Density Dependence

Reference has already been made to viscosity-dependent and density-dependent forces. Advantage can be taken of these phenomena, because they occur in different segments of the tracheobronchial system, to study the characteristics of airflow. Furthermore, tests have been devised using these principles to detect the presence of early structural abnormalities in peripheral airways. The most commonly used maneuver is to compare two maximal expiratory flow-volume curves, one recorded while the subject is breathing room air (79 per cent N_2 and 21 per cent O_2), and the other after a few breaths of 79 per cent helium and 21 per cent O_2 (He-O_2).[47] Helium is a less dense but more viscous gas than nitrogen, so any differences in the two curves must be attributable to density- and viscosity-dependent factors.

During forced expiration, pressure is lost in the airways overcoming frictional opposition to airflow and producing convective acceleration. *Frictional losses* can be subdivided into those attributable to laminar flow and those attributable to turbulent flow. Laminar flow occurs in the peripheral airways, where the velocity of the airstream is low because of the large cross-sectional area, whereas turbulent flow occurs in the more central airways, where the velocities are high because the cross-sectional area is small. Losses of pressure in laminar flow are independent of the density but dependent on the viscosity of the gas. In contrast, losses of pressure in turbulent flow are dependent on the density and largely independent of the viscosity of the gas breathed. *Convective acceleration* refers to the necessary acceleration of gas molecules as they flow from the peripheral branches of the tracheobronchial tree, in which the total cross-sectional area is large and the velocity of flow is low, through the more central airways, in which the cross-sectional area is much smaller and the velocity considerably higher. The pressure losses required to produce convective acceleration are, like losses from turbulence, dependent on the density, not the viscosity, of the gas involved.

Thus, during maximal expiratory airflow, the total pressure dissipated between the alveoli and the airways in which flow limitation occurs is the sum of pressure losses from three separate mechanisms: (1) viscosity-dependent losses in the peripheral airways where laminar flow occurs, (2) density-dependent losses in more central airways where turbulent flow exists, and (3) density-dependent losses from convective acceleration as the velocity of flow increases from alveoli to central airways. Accordingly, maximal expiratory flow-volume curves after breathing room air or He-O_2 (Fig. 4–15) differ from each other in normal persons because of differences in the densities and viscosities of the two gas mixtures. Thus, higher flow rates are achieved with He-O_2 during the early and middle portions of a forced expiratory maneuver, during which density-dependent turbulence and convective acceleration occur; later, when slower laminar flow develops, viscous effects prevail and the He-O_2 curve is identical with or even lower than the room air curve. The derivatives that are used to compare He-O_2 with room air maximal expiratory flow-volume curves are also shown in Figure 4–15. Normally, as indicated, flow rates are higher breathing He-O_2 than room air throughout most of expiration; differences in flows are measured at 50 per cent ($\dot{V}max_{50}$) and 75 per cent ($\dot{V}max_{75}$) of expired VC. The volume at which the two curves intersect is the $Viso_{\dot{v}}$.

In the presence of narrowing of peripheral airways, turbulence and convective acceleration are less prominent, so the He-O_2 curve is closer to the room air curve than it should be; this means that $\dot{V}max_{50}$ and $\dot{V}max_{75}$ decrease and $Viso_{\dot{v}}$ increases. However, responsiveness to helium must be governed by the distributions of small and large airway dimensions, which apparently differ considerably in normal subjects and account for the wide range of variability of $\dot{V}max_{50}$, $\dot{V}max_{75}$, and $Viso_{\dot{v}}$. Except for one study,[48] functional disturbances detectable by He-O_2 and room air maximal expiratory flow-volume curves did not correlate with morphologic evidence of abnormalities in peripheral airways.[49, 50]

Frequency Dependence of Compliance

The sustained interest in frequency dependence of compliance, like the interest in

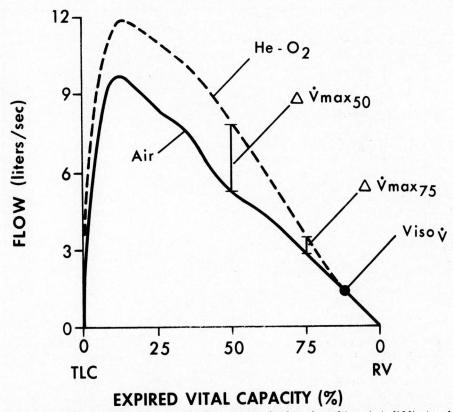

Figure 4–15. Forced expiratory flow-volume curves from a normal subject breathing air (solid line) and a mixture of 79 per cent He and 21 per cent O_2 (He-O_2, dashed line). The difference at expired vital capacity values of 50 per cent ($\Delta \dot{V}max_{50}$) and 75 per cent ($\Delta \dot{V}max_{75}$) and the volume at which the curves converge (Viso$_v$) are shown. TLC = total lung capacity; RV = residual volume. (Reprinted by permission from Hinshaw, H. C., and Murray, J. F.: Diseases of the Chest 4th ed. Philadelphia, W. B. Saunders Company, 1979, p. 88.)

maximum expiratory flow-volume relationships, derives from the potential usefulness of both these tests of ventilatory function in the early recognition of certain lung diseases.[51] In contrast with the testing procedure for recording maximum expiratory flow-volume relationships, measurement of frequency dependence of compliance is complicated and extremely difficult to perform accurately. However, knowledge of the physiologic principles that underlie normal or abnormal tests of frequency dependence of compliance provides insight into the pathogenesis of the disturbances in the mechanics of ventilation and in the distribution of inspired gas.[52] Static compliance of the lung, as described previously, is used to define the static volume-pressure relationships of the lungs and is determined while the subject holds his breath. Lung compliance can also be determined during a normal breathing cycle without breath holding from measurements of lung volumes and esophageal pres-

sures at the end of inspiration and expiration; in other words, at the instants when flow at the mouth has ceased. These values may be obtained at varying breathing frequencies and under these conditions yield a measurement of *dynamic compliance*.

In normal subjects, dynamic compliance is approximately equal to static compliance, even at high breathing frequencies; but in patients with various bronchopulmonary disorders, dynamic compliance falls as respiratory rate increases.[51] These two patterns of response are depicted in Figure 4–16. Dynamic compliance in normal subjects can be seen to be relatively independent of respiratory frequency; in contrast, the patients with bronchial asthma demonstrated a fall of compliance to less than 80 per cent of the extrapolated value at zero frequency; this reduction signifies abnormal frequency dependence of compliance.

The origin of frequency dependence of compliance can be displayed in the three

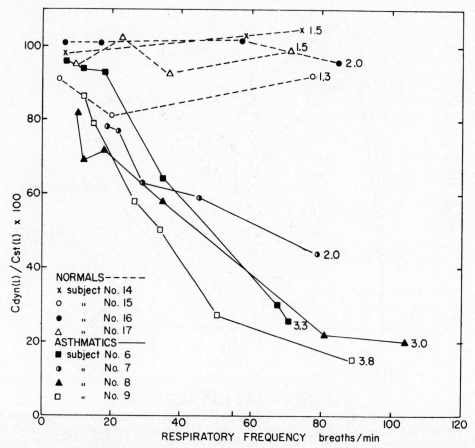

Figure 4–16. Dynamic compliance [Cdyn(l)] as a percentage of static compliance [Cst(l)] at different breathing frequencies in four normal subjects (dashed lines) and four patients of similar age with asthma (solid lines). The number to the right of each person's graph is the value of pulmonary resistance obtained at the time of the study. (Reprinted by permission from Woolcock, A. J., et al.: Frequency dependence of compliance as a test for obstruction in the small airways. J. Clin. Invest. *48*:1097–1106, 1969.)

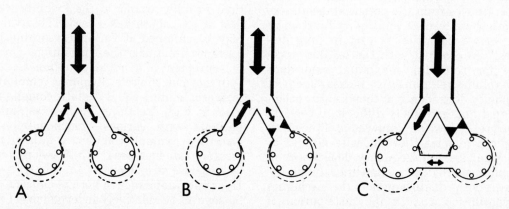

Figure 4–17. Three models of the lung showing the origin of frequency dependence of compliance. *A,* Because resistance in the two peripheral airways and compliance of the two distensible alveoli are equal, the amount of gas distributed to the two units at constant tidal volumes (shown by the size of the arrows) is equal at all breathing frequencies. *B* and *C,* There is a high resistance pathway to one of the units. At low breathing frequencies, the effects of increased resistance are trivial, and the distribution of inspired air is equal; however, at increasing frequencies, the effects of resistance become progressively important, and the distribution of inspired air shifts from the partially obstructed alveolus to the nonobstructed unit. Thus a phase lag and frequency dependence of compliance occur. For details, see text.

lung models shown in Figure 4–17. In normal subjects, model A, about half of the flow resistance in the tracheobronchial tree resides in the central airways (shown by the thick wall), and the remaining half is equally distributed between the two peripheral airways (shown by their thin walls); furthermore, both alveoli are equally distensible (shown by similar springs). In this system, one of the major sources of flow resistance is common to both peripheral pathways and the other source is evenly partitioned between the two peripheral pathways, which also have similar distensibility characteristics. Another way of expressing the equality of the mechanical properties of the peripheral units is to say that their "time constants"* are the same. If "subject A" breathes at a given tidal volume and a slow respiratory rate, both alveoli will expand and contract the same amount and at the same time (i.e., there is no phase lag between them). If the subject now breathes at the same tidal volume but increases his respiratory rate, both alveoli will continue to respond identically.

Model B simulates the condition of partial obstruction of a peripheral bronchus. When the same tidal volume as in model A is applied to this system at low breathing frequencies so that the flow rate of air within the peripheral airways is very low, both alveoli will expand and contract identically. When respiratory frequency and flow rate begin to increase, there will be a progressively increasing pressure drop across the resistance in the partially obstructed airway, which causes a corresponding decrease in the pressure "available" to fill the alveolus distal to the obstruction. Because tidal volume is constant, at increased breathing frequencies the unobstructed alveolus will fill more than it does in model A, and the partially obstructed alveolus will fill less than it did at slower frequencies of breathing; this means that the system is showing frequency dependence of compliance.

Exactly the same argument pertains to model C, in which the peripheral airway to one alveolus is completely obstructed but the unit does not become atelectatic owing to the presence of a collateral ventilatory pathway from the unobstructed alveolus. At low respiratory rates, both units will fill and empty equally and synchronously. When respiratory frequency increases, frequency dependence of compliance occurs because, owing to the resistance offered by the collateral channel, the distal alveolus will fill less and less and the proximal "normal" alveolus will fill more and more.

One might expect some frequency dependence of compliance in normal lungs because, as already pointed out, the terminal respiratory units at the top and bottom of the lungs are operating on different portions of the same volume-pressure curve (i.e., their compliances differ), and the airways leading to these units are of different dimensions (i.e., their resistances differ). The stability of compliance at high breathing frequencies in normal lungs is a useful attribute that is explained by the fact that regional time constants can vary up to fourfold before frequency dependence occurs.[53]

It can be inferred from the models that when frequency dependence of compliance occurs, unevenness in the distribution of inspired gas must also occur. Moreover, as in model B, whenever the time constants of parallel pathways differ sufficiently to produce a phase shift in the time course of gas flow, the slowly ventilating unit will receive part of its inspired volume from the rapidly ventilating unit ("pendelluft") because the former is still inspiring while the latter is exhaling. A unit dependent upon collateral ventilation, as in model C, is in series with its proximal alveolus and is totally parasitic upon it for inspired air.

Although the use of models considerably oversimplifies the complexity of pathophysiologic abnormalities, such models realistically depict the disturbances in distribution of ventilation that may be produced by numerous common lung diseases.[54] The consequences of these events are important because any change in the distribution of ventilation is likely to lead to an abnormality of gas exchange.

DISTRIBUTION OF VENTILATION

As already stated, the regional distribution of inspired air within normal lungs depends chiefly on the regional distribution of pleural surface pressure. Other mecha-

---

*The term "time constant" derives from the use of an electrical analogue of the condition in which a resistance (resistor) and a compliance (capacitor) are in series with each other. Time constants can be used to calculate the phase shift in current that will occur when a phasic voltage is applied to the circuit.[52]

nisms affecting the distribution of ventilation during inspiration are the distensibilities of the individual terminal respiratory units and the resistance of the airways leading to them. In other words, regional pleural surface pressure is an expression of the force tending to cause inflation of that part of the lung; how much inspired air actually reaches the region depends on local compliance and airflow resistance. Additional factors that must be considered, because each may influence regional ventilation, are (1) the magnitude of the differences in compliance and resistance in the uppermost and lowermost regions of the lungs, (2) the interdependence that exists between adjacent lung units and between the lungs and chest wall, and (3) the presence of collateral pathways for ventilation.

Pleural Pressure Gradient

The principle of transpulmonary pressure, which is the difference between alveolar pressure and pleural surface pressure, has already been introduced: (1) transpulmonary pressure is the pressure that keeps the lungs inflated, and (2) it is the pressure that must change to cause inflation and deflation. Despite the fundamental importance of pleural surface pressure as the chief determinant of transpulmonary pressure, there is no unanimity about the magnitude or the regional distribution of surface pressure in the intact thorax.

Until recently, most workers accepted the analysis of Agostoni[17] that there was a difference between pleural liquid and pleural surface pressures attributable to pressure losses from the forces of deformation at points of contact or the intermolecular forces of adhesion and cohesion. Indeed, the results of studies using methods that presumably measured pleural liquid pressure revealed a vertical gradient of 0.6 to 0.7 cm H_2O per cm vertical distance (height), whereas values for the gradient of pleural surface pressure were only 0.2 to 0.5 cm H_2O per cm distance (see Hoffman, E. A., et al.[55] for additional references). More recently, however, values for the gradient of pleural surface pressure have been reported that are not only higher than those observed previously, but are the same as simultaneously measured pleural liquid pressures.[56] Even though it is too early to predict how this controversy will be reconciled, there remains no doubt that there is a vertical gradient in the distribution of pleural surface pressure such that the pressure is lower (more negative) in the uppermost compared with that in the lowermost regions of the lungs. At the extreme apex of the lungs of upright dogs, highly negative pressures (-30 cm H_2O) have been reported at FRC; these pressures are presumably related to the unusual stresses and strains that occur in that region.[57, 58]

The factors that contribute to the vertical gradient of pleural pressure are complex and appear to vary among species. In small animals that have a compliant rib cage the effects of gravity on the shape of the chest wall appear to be the major determinant; in contrast, in larger animals with relatively less compliant rib cages the weight of the lungs is the major factor causing the regional gradient of pleural pressure and, consequently, the regional variation in transpulmonary pressure.[59] Persuasive evidence concerning the importance of gravity on the regional distribution of ventilation in humans has been obtained by showing that Phase 3 of the single breath O_2 test becomes horizontal and closing volume (described in the next section) disappears during periods of weightlessness.[60] However, one must be careful not to generalize too much from studies of this sort because other factors can clearly affect the regional distribution of pleural pressure, at least in humans and dogs. For example, the vertical gradient of pleural pressure that was evident in dogs when they were studied in the supine position disappeared when they were turned to the prone position.[61] These findings were interpreted as showing that the effects of gravity were predominant when supine, but that these were overcome by changes in the shape of the thorax when prone. As will be discussed in more detail subsequently, voluntary breathing with different groups of respiratory muscles will also affect the distribution of pleural pressure and regional ventilation.

Under ordinary circumstances of quiet breathing while sitting or standing, the functional implications of the higher transpulmonary pressure at the top compared with that at the bottom of the lung are the following.

1. Regional differences in lung volumes are created, such that alveoli at the top of

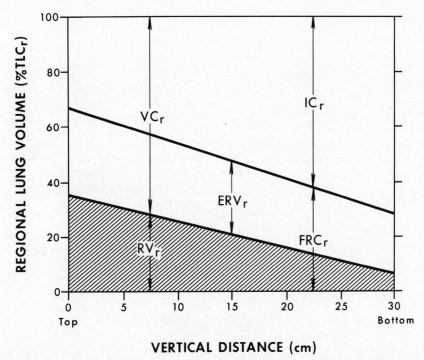

Figure 4–18. Schematic representation of the changes in regional lung volumes, expressed as a percentage of regional total lung capacity (% TLC$_r$), at varying distances from the top to the bottom of the vertical lungs of healthy men. Measurements were made at full expiration (lower heavy line) and at resting end-expiratory lung volume (upper heavy line). VC$_r$ = regional vital capacity; RV$_r$ = regional residual volume; ERV$_r$ = regional expiratory reserve volume; IC$_r$ = regional inspiratory capacity; FRC$_r$ = regional functional residual capacity. (Adapted and reprinted by permission from Milic-Emili, J., et al.: Regional distribution of inspired gas in the lung. J. Appl. Physiol., *21*:749–759, 1966.)

the lung are more fully expanded at FRC than those at the bottom; these differences have been thoroughly documented in studies of both humans[62] and experimental animals.[63] Functional evidence for the presence of regional differences in lung volumes in humans is reproduced in Figure 4–18, and morphometric evidence from experimental animals is presented in Figure 4–19.

2. Because the volume-pressure curve is believed to be the same for different regions regardless of their location within the normal lung, the higher distending pressure at the top compared with that at the bottom means that alveoli in the two regions are operating on different portions of the same curve (Fig. 4–20A). This causes them to expand differently when a given change in distending pressure, which is uniformly distributed throughout the lung, is added to the different initial values. For this reason, when inspiration begins at FRC, alveoli at the bottom expand considerably more than do those at the top. Accordingly, during

normal breathing at rest, the lowermost regions ordinarily ventilate more than the uppermost regions; this difference increases the efficiency of gas exchange because, under these same conditions, there is also more blood flow to the bottom of the lungs than to the top (see Chapter 6).

3. When inspiration is continued to TLC, alveoli at the top and bottom of the lungs inflate to nearly the same size because, even though the pleural pressure difference persists, both regions are now functioning on the flat portion of the volume-pressure curve (Fig. 4–20B).

4. During expiration to RV, when plural pressure in the lowermost lung regions becomes positive, or, in other words, transpulmonary pressure becomes negative, there is a compressing force that begins to close airways (Fig. 4–20C). As exhalation continues, closure moves progressively up the lungs and involves more and more airways.

If blood flow continues to the terminal respiratory units distal to the site of airway

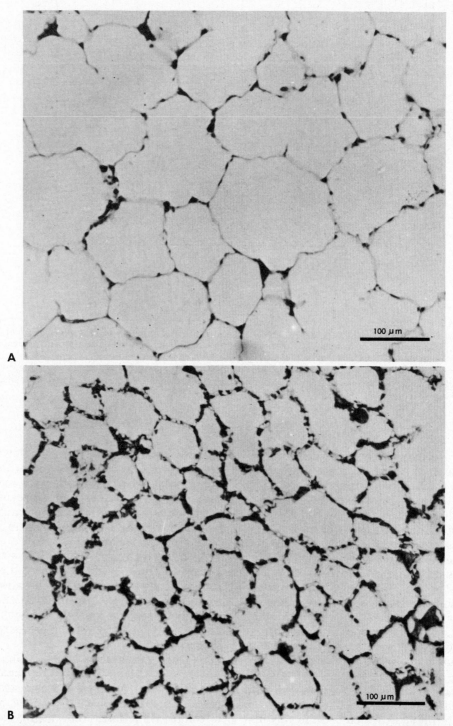

Figure 4–19. Sections of lung from the apex (A) and 20 cm below the apex (B) obtained from a greyhound dog frozen in the vertical position. At functional residual capacity it is obvious that the alvoelar spaces are larger at the apex than near the base. Horizontal bar = 100 μm. (× 188. Courtesy of Dr. Jon B. Glazier.)

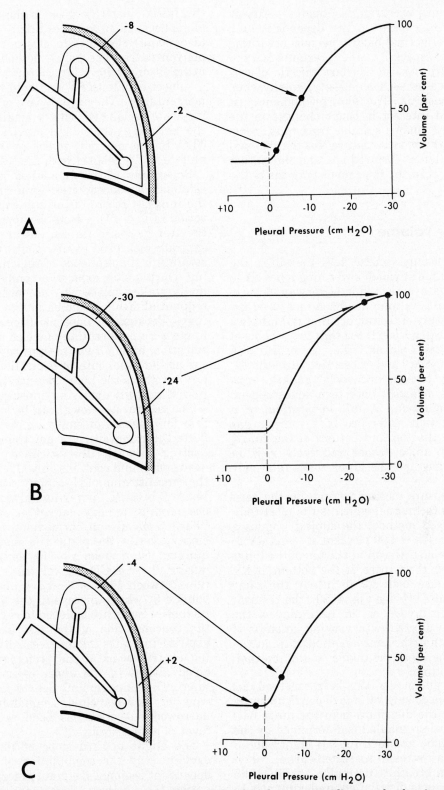

Figure 4–20. Schematic representation of the effects of the pleural pressure gradient on alveolar size and airway caliber at functional residual capacity *(A)*, total lung capacity *(B)*, and residual volume *(C)*. The right portion of each panel shows a normal volume-pressure curve and the points on the curve at which the various lung units are operating. For further discussion, see text. (Reprinted by permission from Hinshaw, H. C., and Murray, J. F.: Diseases of the Chest, 4th ed. Philadelphia, W. B. Saunders Company, 1979, p. 90.)

closure, gas exchange is impaired. Airway closure may occur in the dependent lung regions of normal elderly persons breathing at FRC, especially when recumbent, and premature closure is characteristic of certain diseases such as obesity, emphysema, and bronchitis. The four phenomena just described interact to cause changes in the concentration of a suitable tracer gas, measured at the mouth, that reflect the regional distribution of inspired gas and the caliber of airways in the dependent portions of the lungs.

Closing Volume

The closing volume test measures the lung volume at which lower lung zones cease to ventilate as a result of airway closure. The closing volume has been measured using a variety of techniques that fall into two general categories: those that use a bolus of foreign gas such as ^{133}Xe, Ar, or He (the *bolus method*) and those that use the N_2 normally present in alveolar gas (the *resident gas method*). Both techniques depend on the creation, at full inspiration, of a concentration difference of a marker gas between the top and bottom of the lungs, with the upper zones relatively rich in marker gas and the lower zones relatively poor.

To measure closing volume by the resident gas technique, which is the most commonly used method, the subject inhales a single breath of 100 per cent O_2 from RV to TLC. Because alveoli at the top of the lungs are larger than those at the bottom at RV and because both fill to nearly the same volume at TLC (see Fig. 4–20), the resident N_2 within alveoli at the beginning of the breath is diluted with varying amounts of O_2 such that the concentration of N_2 at the end of the breath is higher at the top than at the bottom.

The principle of the bolus method for measuring closing volume depends upon the fact that the distribution in the lungs of a test gas when inhaled is determined by the lung volume at which the gas is introduced into the air stream. As stated earlier, when a subject breathes normally at FRC, the inspired air is distributed predominantly to the dependent lung regions. However, when inspiration begins at or near RV, the usual pattern of distribution is reversed. Most of the initial inspirate goes to the upper regions because airways leading to the lower (dependent) regions are closed and hence nonventilated. The bolus method of measuring closing volume is performed by having a subject exhale to RV and hold his breath momentarily. The initial part of the next inspirate is labeled with a small bolus of the test gas as the subject inhales slowly to TLC. In this manner, alveoli at the top are preferentially labeled with the test gas.

Regardless of which method is used to establish a concentration gradient within the lungs, a record of the subsequent expiration (Fig. 4–21) reflects the appearance of the test gas, and its concentration in the expirate measured at the mouth varies according to the sequence of regional emptying. During slow expiration, emptying normally takes place in an orderly and sequential fashion from bottom to top of the lungs. Because the uppermost regions of the lungs were preferentially labeled during inspiration, after airway closure begins to occur at the bases late in expiration, the expirate reflects the high concentration of gas from the slowly emptying upper regions.

The record, as shown, can be subdivided into four phases of emptying: Phase 1 reflects the composition of gas from the conducting airways (the so-called anatomic dead space) and contains only O_2 and no N_2; the concentration of N_2 rapidly rises during Phase 2 because airway and alveolar gases are mixing; a near-plateau is evident in Phase 3 as alveoli throughout the lungs empty; finally, the plateau is abruptly terminated by a steep rise in concentration during Phase 4. Closing volume is the junction between Phases 3 and 4 and is that volume at which airways in the dependent regions of lungs are believed to close so that the concentration of the test gas in the expirate indicates the progressively increasing contributions of the preferentially labeled alveoli in the upper regions of the lungs. The long-standing debate concerning whether airways close completely or are narrowed but open has been resolved in favor of actual closure.[64]

The slight upward slope of Phase 3 is explained by the combination of gravity-dependent regional inequality of gas distribution (i.e., between lobes) and stratified inhomogeneity of gas mixing within lung units (i.e., within lobes; see subsequent section for additional details).

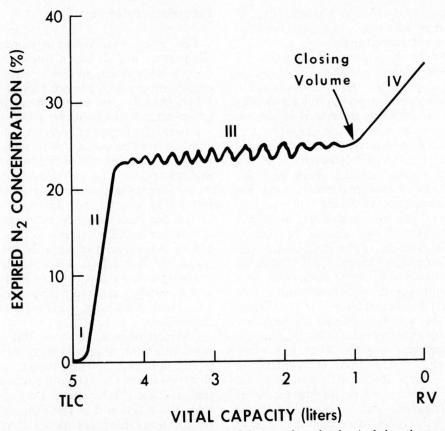

Figure 4–21. Representative tracing of the measurement of closing volume by the single breath oxygen (resident gas) method. Measurement of expired N_2 concentration at the mouth during exhalation from total lung capacity (TLC) to residual volume (RV) yields a tracing with four phases (I to IV) that are described in the text. Closing volume is at the junction of phases III and IV. Cardiogenic oscillations are shown during phase III (the alveolar plateau). (Reprinted by permission from Murray, J. F.: Respiration. *In* Smith, L. H., and Thier, S. (eds.): Pathophysiology. Philadelphia, W. B. Saunders Company, 1985, pp. 753–854.)

Closing volume is usually expressed as a percentage of vital capacity (CV/VC, %). The term *closing capacity* (CC) is used to express the combination of closing volume and RV (CC = CV + RV) and is usually expressed as a percentage of TCL (CC/TLC, %). Because the CC/TLC ratio has less variability than the CV/VC ratio and because closing capacity includes RV, which itself changes early in diseases causing airway obstruction, the CC/TLC ratio is the better measurement of the two.

Closure is believed to occur in small (<1 mm) airways whose patency is determined normally by the transpulmonary pressure across them and by the compliance of their walls; in addition, the stability of small airways at low lung volumes may depend, in part, on the surface tension of the liquid layer overlying the epithelium. Because the distending pressure acting on airways is known to be low in young children, to increase during maturation, and to diminish with advancing age, the airways of a child and an old person will not be "held open" as well as those of a young adult. Therefore, closing volume, as a percentage of vital capacity, is high in infancy, decreases during growth to maturation, and increases again during senescence.[65, 66] Although closing volume remains relatively constant despite variations in body position, FRC decreases upon changing from the upright to the supine position and under these conditions may be less than closing volume. When closing volume exceeds FRC (as in young and old persons, and especially in the recumbent position), dependent regions of the lung are poorly ventilated and abnormalities of gas exchange may result (see Chapter 7 for discussion of mechanisms).

It is now well established that closing volume and closing capacity increase, as expected, in patients with lung disorders in which the patency of peripheral airways is compromised by either decreased elastic recoil (e.g., in emphysema) or abnormalities of the airways themselves (e.g., in bronchitis or asthma). Furthermore, changes in closing volume or closing capacity have been observed as early manifestations of lung disease in asymptomatic patients.[48] In addition, the slope of Phase 3 is also useful in the early detection of lung disease because it provides a measure of the evenness of the distribution of ventilation. Well ventilated units fill and empty more completely and rapidly than poorly ventilated units; this means that the concentration of N_2 will be lower in the better ventilated regions that empty earlier during exhalation than in the poorly ventilated regions. Thus the more uneven the distribution of ventilation within the lungs, the steeper is the slope of Phase 3; in this context, interpretation of Phase 3 is exactly the same as that of the single breath O_2 test described by Comroe and Fowler[67] many years ago.

Regional Compliance and Resistance

The vertical gradient of pleural pressure means that airways and alveoli at the top of the lung are more distended than those at the bottom; this in turn implies that there must be time-constant differences among units throughout the lung. The reason why these variations do not cause frequency dependence of compliance in normal lungs has already been explained. Furthermore, because regional gravity-dependent unevenness of ventilation can be demonstrated by analyzing the washout of inhaled boluses of inert gases or by examining changes in the slope of the alveolar nitrogen plateau (Phase 3), these tests are more sensitive methods of detecting asynchronous behavior than are tests of frequency dependence or the external detection of the distribution of inhaled radioactive gases.

Interdependence

The lung parenchyma, as pointed out in Chapters 1 and 2, has a connective tissue framework containing elastic elements. Because contiguous units are attached to each other, they are not free to move independently; instead, the behavior of one unit must influence the behavior of its neighbors. This summarizes the concept of interdependence among peripheral units introduced by Mead and coworkers[33] and now generally accepted as an important mechanism promoting uniformity of ventilation. The magnitude of interdependence depends upon the number of elastic elements and the forces transmitted by each and the area of the surface involved. The effect, however, is always unifying because it serves to offset (in part) any coexisting tendency that would otherwise make units larger or smaller than they should be.

Interdependence between the lung parenchyma and neighboring airways serves to stiffen intrapulmonary bronchi and bronchioles but not the extrapulmonary bronchi and trachea; this is one of the factors that may affect the site of the choke point(s).[46] In addition, interdependence between the lungs and the chest wall provides a mechanism that preserves uniformity of distribution of ventilation among regions.[68]

Collateral Ventilation

The presence of pathways for collateral ventilation between adjacent alveoli (pores of Kohn, although these are probably closed by a layer of surfactant), neighboring terminal units, and contiguous lobules (Lambert's canals) is well established (see Chapter 2 for details); furthermore, the factors affecting flow through and the resistance offered by collateral pathways have been studied in several species of experimental animals (for a summary of these results, see Menkes and Traystman[69]). Studies are limited in humans, but those that are available indicate that in supine normal subjects holding their breaths near FRC, resistance in collateral channels is so high that very little flow occurs.[70] This does not mean that collateral flow never takes place, because studies were not carried out at high lung volumes at which, in virtually all experimental animals, resistance to collateral flow decreases markedly, presumably through enlargement of partially open collateral pathways or recruitment of previously closed channels, or both. There is also abundant evidence from studies in both humans and experimental animals that collateral ventilation is of considerable importance in determining the mechanical behavior and distribution of ventilation of lungs with airway obstruction.[68, 70]

Table 4–1. REPRESENTATIVE PLEURAL PRESSURES (P_{pl}) AND TRANSPULMONARY PRESSURES (P_l) IN CM H_2O AT THE TOP AND BOTTOM OF THE LUNG IN A NORMAL MAN AT FRC*

Position	Top		Bottom	
	P_{pl}	P_l	P_{pl}	P_l
Sitting	−8	8	−2	2
Lateral	−6	6	0	0
Supine	−4	4	0	0
Prone	−3.5	3.5	0	0

Data from Agostoni, E.: Mechanics of the pleural space. Physiol. Rev., 52:57–128, 1972.

Regional Inhomogeneity

Regional inhomogeneity derives from the anatomy of the tracheobronchial tree and the vertical gradient of pleural pressure. It has already been pointed out that the length of various pathways within the tracheobronchial tree varies considerably, depending upon whether the pathways lead to a central or a peripheral gas exchange unit. Because the bronchial tree is asymmetric, so is the volume of gas occupying different pathways, the so-called *anatomic dead space*; this means that the amount of dead space gas that precedes inspired fresh air into central and peripheral gas exhange units during inhalation must also vary. Consequently, unequal alveolar gas concentrations must result from the mixing of the incoming boluses of fresh air with varying volumes of dead space gas.

The vertical gradient of pleural pressure (see section on Pleural Pressure Gradient) causes regional changes in alveolar geometry and airway caliber. Accordingly, topographic variations in the distribution of inspired gas result; these vary with the lung volume at which inspiration begins. Furthermore, because body position influences the magnitude of the difference in pleural and transmural pressures between the top and bottom of the lung (Table 4–1), the subject's position during breathing also affects the regional distribution of the inspired fresh air. More recently, by analyzing the pattern of washout of inert gases or the slope of the nitrogen plateau (see Fig. 4–21), it has become clear that the distribution of inspired air and the sequence of subsequent lung emptying can be voluntarily altered by

contracting different groups of respiratory muscles (described more fully in the next chapter). Contraction of the diaphragm causes preferential ventilation of the lung bases, whereas contraction of the intercostal/accessory muscles shifts ventilation toward the apices (Fig. 4–22).[72]

During breathing at slow respiratory frequencies from FRC, it has been demonstrated that each breath is distributed according to regional compliances.[71] In other words, the lowermost regions receive more of the inspirate because they are functioning on a steeper, more compliant part of the lungs' volume-pressure curve than the uppermost regions (see Fig. 4–10). However, of considerable importance is the additional observation that when breathing frequency increases, the distribution of the inspirate becomes more uniform.[73] At inspiratory flows beginning at 0.2 L/sec and increasing up to 1.5 L/sec, there is a progressive redistribution of ventilation until the apex and base receive approximately equal shares. The most important mechanism serving to redistribute newly inspired air from the bases to the apices—when inspiratory flow rate is increased in the upright position—is the pattern of muscle contraction. When ventilation increases during exercise, the intercostal/accessory muscles are progressively recruited. As just pointed out, contraction of these muscle groups favors ventilation of the apex. Redistribution of inspired air could also be caused by interdependence between the lungs and the chest wall. During inspiration, to the extent that a region of lung lags behind its neighbors and produces a deformity of the contiguous chest wall, the overlying pleural surface

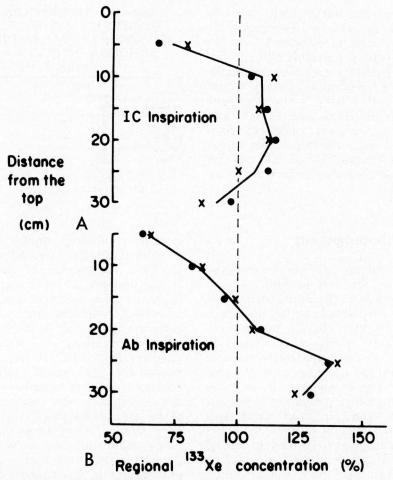

Figure 4–22. Regional distribution of a bolus of ^{133}xenon inhaled at 0.4 l/sec from functional residual capacity in a seated subject. *A,* Inspiration using predominantly intercostal and accessory muscles (IC). *B,* Inspiration with enhanced abdominal motion (Ab). Different symbols indicate duplicate measures. Abscissa is normalized alveolar ^{133}xenon concentration. Note preferential distribution of ^{133}xenon to basal regions after abdominal inspiration and to upper mid-zones after intercostal inspiration. (Reprinted by permission from Roussos, C. S., et al.: Voluntary factors affecting the distribution of inspired gas. Am. Rev. Respir. Dis., *116*:457–467, 1977.)

pressure will be amplified, which will tend to minimize the nonuniformity.[59]

The changes in the distribution of pleural pressure should be viewed as homeostatic mechanisms that produce uniformity of regional ventilation during exercise. Thus, the "wisdom of the body" is again apparent. Ventilation is distributed to those regions of the lung where it can be most useful in maintaining a balance with the distribution of blood flow. Thus, while the body is at rest, both blood and inspired air flow chiefly to the lung bases, but during exercise, blood flow becomes more uniformly distributed as pulmonary artery pressure increases, and

the factors just described cause ventilation to be redistributed similarly.

Stratified Inhomogeneity

Because the total cross-sectional area of conducting airways becomes progressively larger from the trachea to the terminal bronchioles and because the cross-sectional area of respiratory bronchioles increases proportionately more (because several orders of branching occur with virtually no change in the diameter of the component bronchioles), the forward velocity of the inspired airstream moving peripherally through the airways slows markedly. Finally, in the neighborhood of the alveolar ducts, forward velocity is probably so slow that it becomes superseded by movement of gas molecules owing to thermal agitation. Thus, inspired gas reaches alveolar ducts by mass flow (sometimes called convection or bulk flow) through the airways, but alveoli are "ventilated" because of movement of molecules by gaseous diffusion. The completeness of mixing determines whether or not stratified inhomogeneity will occur.[74]

Diffusion of molecules within a mixture of gases depends upon the physical properties of the gases involved, the volume through which they have to move, and the time available for carrying out the process. The distance for gas-phase diffusion between alveolar ducts and their adjacent alveoli is sufficiently small that in normal subjects breathing at slow (resting) rates, stratified inhomogeneity is barely discernible. During the determination of closing volume, for example, the procedure is such that the slope of the alveolar plateau (Phase 3, Fig. 4–21) is mainly influenced by sequential emptying of regions owing to the vertical gradient of pleural pressure; stratified inhomogeneity contributes very little to the changing alveolar gas concentration, primarily because the breathing maneuver is a slow one, and gas-phase mixing is complete. However, the presence of stratified inhomogeneity can be demonstrated in normal subjects by varying the pattern of breathing, especially by using high inspiratory flow rates and beginning inspiration above FRC.[75] Furthermore, incompleteness of gas mixing has been shown to be an important factor in determining the distribution, and hence the adequacy of gas exchange, in patients with various forms of lung diseases. However, as emphasized in a recent review by Piiper,[76] more studies are needed to define the physiologic importance of stratified inhomogeneity in gas exchange.

REFERENCES

1. Mead, J.: Mechanical properties of lungs. Physiol. Rev., *41*:281–330, 1961.
2. Fenn, W. O., and Rahn, H. (eds.): Handbook of Physiology, Section 3. Respiration. Vol. I. Washington, D.C., American Physiological Society, 1964, pp. 357–476.
3. Campbell, E. J. M., Agostoni, E., and Davis, J. N.: The Respiratory Muscle: Mechanics and Neural Control. 2nd Ed. London, Lloyd-Luke (Medical Books) Ltd., 1970.
4. Hoppin, F. G., Jr., and Hildebrandt, J.: Mechanical properties of the lung. *In* West, J. B. (ed.): Bioengineering Aspects of the Lung. New York, Marcel Dekker, Inc., 1977, pp. 83–162.
5. McFadden, E. R., Jr., and Ingram, R. H., Jr.: Clinical application and interpretation of airway physiology. *In* Nadel, J. A. (ed.): Physiology and Pharmacology of the Airways. New York, Marcel Dekker, Inc. 1980, pp. 297–324.
6. Milic-Emili, J., Mead, J., Turner, J. M., and Glauser, E. M.: Improved technique for estimating pleural pressure from esophageal balloons. J. Appl. Physiol., *19*:207–211, 1964.
7. von Neergaard, K.: Neue Auffassungen über einen Grundbegriff der Atemmechanik. Die Retraktions-Kraft der Lunge, abhängig von der Oberflächenspannung in den Alveolen. Z. Ges. Exp. Med., *66*:373–394, 1929.
8. Clements, J. A., and Tierney, D. F.: Alveolar instability associated with altered surface tension. *In* Fenn, W. O., and Rahn, H. (eds.): Handbook of Physiology, Section 3. Respiration. Vol. II. Washington, D.C., American Physiological Society, 1964, pp. 1565–1583.
9. Hildebran, J. N., Goerke, J., and Clements, J. A.: Pulmonary surface film stability and composition. J. Appl. Physiol., *47*:604–611, 1979.
10. Report of Workshop on Mechanics of Lung Parenchyma. U.S. Department of Health and Human Services, NIH Publication No. 80–2109, 1980, pp. 1–32.
11. Karlinsky, J. B., Synder, G. L., Franzblau, C., Stone, P. J., and Hoppin, F. G., Jr.: In vitro effects of elastase and collagenase on mechanical properties of hamster lungs. Am. Rev. Respir. Dis., *113*:769–777, 1976.
12. Klassen, T., Thurlbeck, W. M., and Berend, N.: Correlation between lung structure and function in a canine model of emphysema. J. Appl. Physiol., *51*:321–326, 1981.
13. Schurch, S., Goerke, J., and Clements, J. A.: Direct determination of surface tension in the lung. Proc. Natl. Acad. Sci. USA, *73*:4698–4708, 1976.
14. Bachofen, H., Hildebrandt, J., and Bachofen, M.: Pressure-volume curves of air- and liquid-filled excised lungs—surface tension in situ. J. Appl. Physiol., *29*:422–431, 1970.
15. Rahn, H., Otis, A. B., Chadwick, L. E., and Fenn, W. O.: The pressure-volume diagram of the thorax and lung. Am. J. Physiol., *146*:161–178, 1946.
16. Leith, D. E., and Mead, J.: Mechanisms determining residual volume of the lungs in normal subjects. J. Appl. Physiol., *23*:221–227, 1967.
17. Agostoni, E.: Mechanics of the pleural space. Physiol. Rev., *52*:57–128, 1972.
18. Wiener-Kronish, J. P., Albertine, K. H., Licko, V., and Staub, N. C.: Protein egress and entry rates in pleural fluid and plasma in sheep. J. Appl. Physiol., *56*:459–463, 1984.
19. DuBois, A. B., Botelho, S. Y., and Comroe, J. H., Jr.: A new method for measuring airway resistance in man using a body plethysmograph: values in normal subjects and in patients with respiratory disease. J. Clin. Invest., *35*:327–335, 1956.
20. DuBois, A. B., Brody, A. W., Lewis, D. H., and Burgess, B. F., Jr.: Oscillation mechanics of lungs and chest in man. J. Appl. Physiol., *8*:587–594, 1956.

21. Ferris, B. G., Jr., Mead, J., and Opie, L. H.: Partitioning of respiratory flow resistance in man. J. Appl. Physiol., *19*:653–658, 1964.
22. Marshall, R., and DuBois, A. B.: The measurement of the viscous resistance of the lung tissues in normal man. Clin. Sci., *15*:161–170, 1956.
23. Macklem, P. T., and Mead, J.: Resistance of central and peripheral airways measured by a retrograde catheter. J. Appl. Physiol., *22*:395–401, 1967.
24. Hogg, J. C., Macklem, P. T., and Thurlbeck, W. M.: Site and nature of airway obstruction in chronic obstructive lung disease. New Engl. J. Med., *278*:1355–1360, 1968.
25. Hughes, J. M. B., Hoppin, F. G., Jr., and Mead, J.: Effect of lung inflation on bronchial length and diameter in excised lungs. J. Appl. Physiol., *32*:25–35, 1972.
26. Hahn, H. L., Graf, P. D., and Nadel, J. A.: Effect of vagal tone on airway diameters and on lung volume in anesthetized dogs. J. Appl. Physiol., *41*:581–589, 1976.
27. Klingele, T. G., and Staub, N. C.: Terminal bronchiole diameter changes with volume in isolated air-filled lobes of cat lung. J. Appl. Physiol., *30*:224–227, 1971.
28. Hoppin, F. G., Jr., Green, M., and Morgan, M. S.: Relationship of central and peripheral airway resistance to lung volume in dogs. J. Appl. Physiol., *44*:728–737, 1978.
29. Macklem, P. T.: Obstruction in small airways—a challenge to medicine. Am. J. Med., *52*:721–724, 1972.
30. Macklin, C. C.: X-ray studies on bronchial movements. Am. J. Anat., *35*:303–329, 1925.
31. Briscoe, W. A., and DuBois, A. B.: The relationship between airway resistance, airway conductance and lung volume in subjects of different age and body size. J. Clin. Invest., *37*:1279–1285, 1958.
32. Stubbs, S. E., and Hyatt, R. E.: Effect of increased lung recoil pressure on maximal expiratory flow in normal subjects. J. Appl. Physiol., *32*:325–331, 1972.
33. Mead, J., Takishima, T., and Leith, D.: Stress distribution in lungs: a model of pulmonary elasticity. J. Appl. Physiol., *28*:596–608, 1970.
34. Hyatt, R. E., and Flath, R. E.: Influence of lung parenchyma on pressure-diameter behavior of dog bronchi. J. Appl. Physiol., *21*:1448–1452, 1966.
35. Inoue, H., Inoue, C., and Hildebrandt, J.: Vascular and airway pressures, and interstitial edema, affect peribronchial fluid pressure. J. Appl. Physiol., *48*:177–185, 1980.
36. Wilson, A. G., Massarella, G. R., and Pride, N. B.: Elastic properties of airways in human lungs postmortem. Am. Rev. Respir. Dis., *110*:716–729, 1974.
37. Fry, D. L., Ebert, R. V., Stead, W. W., and Brown, C. C.: The mechanics of pulmonary ventilation in normal subjects and in patients with emphysema. Am. J. Med., *16*:80–97, 1954.
38. Fry, D. L., and Hyatt, R. E.: Pulmonary mechanics. A unified analysis of the relationship between pressure, volume and gasflow in the lungs of normal and diseased human subjects. Am. J. Med., *29*:672–689, 1960.
39. Hyatt, R. E.: Expiratory flow limitation. J. Appl. Physiol., *55*:1–8, 1983.
40. Green, M., Mead, J., and Turner, J. M.: Variability of maximal expiratory flow-volume. J. Appl. Physiol., *37*:67–74, 1974.

41. Mead, J.: Dysanapsis in normal lungs assessed by the relationship between maximal flow, static recoil, and vital capacity. Am. Rev. Respir. Dis., *121*:339–342, 1980.
42. Mead, J., Turner, J. M., Macklem, P. T., and Little, J. B.: Significance of the relationship between lung recoil and maximum expiratory flow. J. Appl. Physiol., *22*:95–108, 1967.
43. Pride, N. B., Permutt, S., Riley, R. L., and Bromberger-Barnea, B.: Determinants of maximal expiratory flow from the lungs. J. Appl. Physiol., *23*:646–662, 1967.
44. Dawson, S. V., and Elliott, E. A.: Wave-speed limitation on expiratory flow—a unifying concept. J. Appl. Physiol., *43*:498–515, 1977.
45. Elliott, E. A., and Dawson, S. V.: Test of wave-speed theory of flow limitation in elastic tubes. J. Appl. Physiol., *43*:516–522, 1977.
46. Mead, J.: Expiratory flow limitation: a physiologist's point of view. Fed. Proc., *39*:2771–2775, 1980.
47. Dosman, J., Bode, F., Urbanetti, J., Martin, R., and Macklem, P. T.: The use of helium-oxygen mixture during maximum expiratory flow to demonstrate obstruction in small airways in smokers. J. Clin. Invest., *55*:1090–1099, 1975.
48. Cosio, M. G., Ghezzo, H., Hogg, J. C., Corbin, R., Loveland, M., Dosman, J., and Macklem, P. T.: The relation between structural changes in small airways and pulmonary function tests. New Engl. J. Med., *198*:1277–1281, 1978.
49. Berend, N., Woolcock, A. J., and Marlin, G. E.: Correlation between the function and structure of the lung in smokers. Am. Rev. Respir. Dis., *119*:695–705, 1979.
50. Berend, N., and Thurlbeck, W. M.: Correlations of maximum expiratory flow with small airway dimensions and pathology. J. Appl. Physiol., *52*:346–351, 1982.
51. Woolcock, A. J., Vincent, N. J., and Macklem, P. T.: Frequency dependence of compliance as a test for obstruction in the small airways. J. Clin. Invest., *48*:1097–1106, 1969.
52. Otis, A. B., McKerrow, C. B., Bartlett, R. A., Mead, J., McIlroy, M. B., Selverstone, N. J., and Radford, E. P.: Mechanical factors in distribution of pulmonary ventilation. J. Appl. Physiol., *8*:427–443, 1956.
53. Macklem, P. T., and Mead, J.: Factors determining maximum expiratory flow in dogs. J. Appl. Physiol., *25*:159–169, 1968.
54. Macklem, P. T.: Airway obstruction and collateral ventilation. Physiol. Rev., *51*:368–436, 1971.
55. Hoffman, E. A., Behrenbeck, T., Chevalier, P. A., and Wood, E. H.: Estimation of regional pleural surface expansile forces in intact dogs. J. Appl. Physiol., *55*:935–948, 1983.
56. Gropper, M. A., Wiener-Kronish, J. P., and Lai-Fook, S. J.: Pleural liquid pressure (Ppl) in upright dogs measured through implanted rib capsules. Fed. Proc., *42*:1270 (abstract), 1983.
57. Hoffman, E. A., Lai-Fook, S. J., Wei, J., and Wood, E. H.: Regional pleural surface expansile forces in intact dogs by wick catheters. J. Appl. Physiol., *55*:1523–1529, 1983.
58. West, J. B., and Matthews, F. L.: Stresses, strains, and surface pressures in the lungs caused by its weight. J. Appl. Physiol., *32*:332–345, 1972.
59. Macklem, P. T.: Respiratory mechanics. Annu. Rev. Physiol., *40*:157–184, 1978.

60. Michels, D. B., and West, J. B.: Distribution of ventilation and perfusion during short periods of weightlessness. J. Appl. Physiol., 45:987–998, 1978.
61. Hubmayr, R. D., Walters, B. J., Chevalier, P. A., Rodarte, J. R., and Olson, L. E.: Topographical distribution of regional lung volume in anaesthetized dogs. J. Appl. Physiol., 54:1048–1056, 1983.
62. Milic-Emili, J., Henderson, J. A. M., Dolovich, M. B., Trop, D., and Kaneko, K.: Regional distribution of inspired gas in the lung. J. Appl. Physiol., 21:749–759, 1966.
63. Glazier, J. B., Hughes, J. M. B., Maloney, J. E., and West, J. B.: Vertical gradient of alveolar size in lungs of dogs frozen intact. J. Appl. Physiol., 23:694–795, 1967.
64. Engel, L. A., Grassino, A., and Anthonisen, N. R.: Demonstration of airway closure in man. J. Appl. Physiol., 38:1117–1125, 1975.
65. Leblanc, P., Ruff, F., and Milic-Emili, J.: Effects of age and body position on "airway closure" in man. J. Appl. Physiol., 28:448–451, 1970.
66. Mansell, A., Bryan, A., and Levison, H.: Airway closure in children. J. Appl. Physiol., 33:711–714, 1972.
67. Comroe, J. H., Jr., and Fowler, W. S.: Lung function studies. VI. Detection of uneven alveolar ventilation during a single breath of oxygen. Am. J. Med., 10:408–413, 1951.
68. Macklem, P. T.: Relationship between lung mechanics and ventilation distribution. Physiologist, 16:580–588, 1973.
69. Menkes, H. A., and Traystman, R. J.: Collateral ventilation. Am. Rev. Respir. Dis., 116:287–309, 1977.
70. Terry, P. B., Traystman, R. J., Newball, H. H., Batra, G., and Menkes, H. A.: Collateral ventilation in man. New Engl. J. Med., 298:10–15, 1978.
71. Robertson, P. C., Anthonisen, N. R., and Ross, D.: Effect of inspiratory flow rate on regional distribution of inspired gas. J. Appl. Physiol., 26:438–443, 1969.
72. Roussos, C. S., Fixley, M., Genest, J., Cosio, M., Kelley, S., Martin, R. R., and Engel, L. A.: Voluntary factors affecting the distribution of inspired gas. Am. Rev. Respir. Dis., 116:457–467, 1977.
73. Bake, B., Wood, L., Murphy, B., Macklem, P. T., and Milic-Emili, J.: Effect of inspiratory flow rate on regional distribution of inspired gas. J. Appl. Physiol., 37:8–17, 1974.
74. Cumming, G.: Gas mixing efficiency in the human lung. Respir. Physiol., 2:213–224, 1967.
75. Anthonisen, N. R., Robertson, P. C., and Ross, W. R. D.: Gravity-dependent sequential emptying of lung regions. J. Appl. Physiol., 28:589–595, 1970.
76. Piiper, J.: Series ventilation, diffusion in airways, and stratified inhomogeneity. Fed. Proc., 38:17–21, 1979.

5

Respiratory Muscles

INTRODUCTION

Spontaneous breathing, which must take place for a lifetime, requires the repetitive contraction of the muscles of respiration. The respiratory muscles also contribute to many specialized functions, such as sneezing, coughing, defecation, vomiting, and parturition. When viewed in this context, it is remarkable that, until recently, so little was known about these essential organs. Since publication of the first edition of this book, however, sufficient amounts of new and important information have been obtained to warrant inclusion of a separate chapter on the subject. Although an appreciation of how this knowledge contributes to the diagnosis and treatment of patients with respiratory diseases is just beginning, it is clear from the results of the studies that have been completed and from those that are underway that an exciting period of clinical application lies ahead. This chapter will summarize the present state of knowledge of respiratory muscle structure and function. Several excellent reviews are available to assist the interested reader who wishes to acquire more detailed knowledge about this rapidly expanding field.[1-4]

ANATOMY

During spontaneous breathing, the lungs inflate because contraction of the respira-

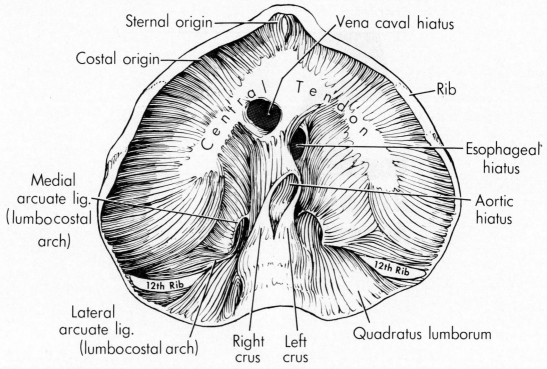

Figure 5–1. Schematic drawing of the human diaphragm showing fibers of costal and sternal origin, the location of the medial and lateral arcuate ligaments, the right and left crus, the central tendon, and other neighboring landmarks.

tory muscles generates sufficient force to enlarge the thoracic cavity. The thorax, which is that part of the body between the neck and abdomen, is encased by a bony framework of ribs that is shaped like a truncated cone. All 12 ribs articulate with the thoracic spine posteriorly and, except for ribs 11 and 12, connect to the sterum anteriorly. Ribs one to six are attached directly to the sternum by short extensions of cartilage; ribs seven to ten are connected to each other and to the sternum by a common segment of cartilage. Expansion and contraction of the thoracic cavity are accomplished by the three groups of respiratory muscles: (1) the diaphragm, (2) the intercostal and accessory muscles, and (3) the abdominal muscles.

Diaphragm

The diaphragm is a musculotendinous sheet that separates the thoracic cavity from the abdominal cavity and is the main source of inspiratory muscle force. The diaphragm consists of two distinct muscular components, the (sterno)costal portion and the crural portion, both of which insert into a central tendon (Fig. 5–1). It has long been known that the costal and crural portions of the diaphragm have distinct embryologic origins and segmental innervations and different fiber compositions, but only recently has it been established in experimental animals that the two parts have different mechanical actions when made to contract separately (see Decramer et al.[5] for review and additional references).

The costal portion of the diaphragm arises anteriorly from the xiphoid process and around the chest wall from the seventh to the twelfth ribs. The crural portion arises posteriorly, from the aponeurotic arches on both sides, and from the first to the third lumbar vertebral bodies on the right side, and from the first and second on the left side. The muscle fibers vary in length; they are longest in the posterolateral portion, where the greatest muscular excursion takes place. The normal diaphragm is perforated near its center by three separate openings, each called a hiatus, for the aorta, inferior vena cava, and esophagus. Branches of the vagus nerves pass through the esophageal hiatus, and the azygous vein and thoracic duct pass through the aortic hiatus. There are also tiny paravertebral perforations for entry of the splanchnic nerves. Because of the way the fibers originate from the bones and travel to the central tendon, triangular areas occur, in which spaces or clefts may exist. Anteriorly these are called Morgagni's foramina, and posteriorly they are known as the foramina of Bochdalek. Each of these areas of potential weakness can be the site of a hernia of abdominal contents into the thorax.

The diaphragm, like other skeletal muscles of the body, is comprised of muscle fibers that differ from each other in many morphologic, physiologic, and cytochemical characteristics; there is also considerable interspecies variation.[6] In humans, the myofibers are classified as intermediate in size, but they are extremely heterogeneous in diameter (Fig. 5–2). In keeping with their need to continuously contract and relax, the myofibrils of the diaphragm are richly supplied with blood vessels (Fig. 5–3). The close approximation between blood capillaries and myofibrils facilitates transfer by diffusion of O_2, CO_2, nutrients, and metabolites along the entire surface of the sarcolemma (external membrane).

The *phrenic nerve* appears to be the sole motor nerve to the diaphragm. Evidence in favor of extraphrenic innervation is inconclusive and controversial. The phrenic nerve arises in the neck from the fourth cervical nerve and is joined by branches from the third and fifth cervical segments. The branch from the fifth nerve is not invariably present and is called the accessory phrenic nerve. Innervation of the diaphragm in the dog is from the fourth to the sixth cervical nerves, and in the cat is mainly from the fifth and sixth segments, with inconsistent contributions from the fourth and seventh segments. In humans, as the phrenic nerves descend from the neck to the diaphragm, they pass anteriorly to the medial border of the anterior scalene muscle in the neck. On the right side the course of the nerve through the mediastinum is first in close association with the superior vena cava,

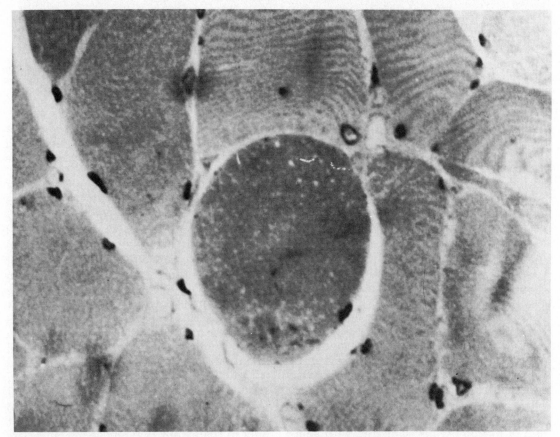

Figure 5–2. Light micrograph of the human diaphragm as seen in thick (1 μm) Epon section. Note the variation in fiber diameter. (Original magnification × 220.) (Reprinted by permission from Leak, L. V.: Gross and ultrastructural morphologic features of the diaphragm. Am. Rev. Respir. Dis., *119*(suppl.):3–21, 1979.)

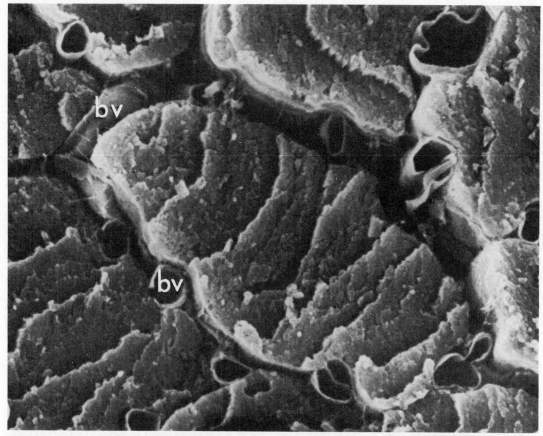

Figure 5–3. Low-power scanning electron micrograph showing myofibers in cross section surrounded by numerous blood vessels (bv). (Original magnification × 3000.) (Reprinted by permission from Leak, L. V.: Gross and ultrastructural morphologic features of the diaphragm. Am. Rev. Respir. Dis., *119*(suppl.):3–21, 1979.)

then anterior to the hilus of the right lung, and finally between the parietal pericardium and the mediastinal pleura to the diaphragm. The nerve pierces the diaphragm and sends the terminal branches to its inferior surface. On the left side the nerve passes between the left common carotid artery and the subclavian artery and in front of the aortic arch, after which its course is similar to that on the right.

The sensory innervation of the diaphragm is chiefly by the two phrenic nerves, except for the outermost perimeter, which is supplied by branches from the sixth to twelfth thoracic segmental nerves. Free sensory endings and pacinian corpuscles have been identified throughout the diaphragm. In contrast to the intercostal muscles, however, the concentration of muscle spindles and Golgi tendon organs in the diaphragm is very low, and there is a relative preponderance of tendon organs compared with spindles.[7] The difference in proprioceptive innervation between the two groups of respiratory

muscles is believed to reflect the greater involvement of the intercostal muscles in controlling movement and posture of the trunk.[8]

Action. The mechanical action of the diaphragm has been a subject of considerable interest to physicians and physiologists for centuries (see reference 2 for a historical review). After a multitude of studies in humans, there is now uniform agreement that during normal quiet breathing, inspiration depends mainly on contraction of the diaphragm. Furthermore, the mechanics of how the contractile force developed by the diaphragm expands the thorax have now been carefully analyzed, particularly by Mead and Goldman.[9, 10] When the diaphragm contracts, it pushes down on the abdominal contents and displaces the abdominal wall outward. The contracting diaphragm also tends to lift and to expand the rib cage but only to the extent that the abdomen resists being displaced and that the intraabdominal pressure rises. In other words, the diaphragm displaces the rib cage in part because the viscera serve as a fulcrum for its action, and in part because intraabdominal pressure increases. The latter effect is facilitated by what Mead[11] has called the area of apposition between the diaphragm and the rib cage. Over the area of apposition there is no lung interposed between the cephalad surface of the diaphragm and the inner surface of the chest wall. This arrangement enhances transmission of abdominal pressure across the diaphragm directly to the rib cage. Moreover, because the diaphragm behaves like a piston during much of inspiration (i.e., does not change its radius of curvature as it descends), the area of apposition tends to be maintained, thus promoting mechanical coupling between the abdomen and the thorax.

During inflation as total lung capacity (TLC) is approached, the diaphragm assumes its flattest configuration. Further muscle fiber shortening of a flattened diaphragm has an expiratory action by pulling the rib cage inward; this probably does not occur in normal subjects but is important in certain diseases (see subsequent discussion of hyperinflation).

In dogs, in which the action of the costal and crural parts of the diaphragm can be studied separately, the costal diaphragm, through its attachments to the ribs, expands the lower rib cage by contracting against the abdominal contents (fulcrum effect) and by raising intraabdominal pressure as just described. In contrast, the crural diaphragm, which has no rib attachments, has an expiratory action when abdominal pressure is prevented from increasing.[12] Based on these observations, Macklem and coworkers[13] proposed a model of diaphragmatic activity in which the two muscles were mechanically arranged in parallel at functional residual capacity (FRC), but as lung volume increased they functioned more and more as muscles arranged in series. Several predictions from this model about the mechanical behavior of the diaphragm have recently been confirmed in experiments in dogs.[5] However, the benefits, if any, of separate innervations and mechanical actions of the two parts of the diaphragm are poorly understood. A dissociation in the electrical activity between different parts of the diaphragm has been demonstrated in the dog during vomiting and eructation;[14] under these conditions the crural portion was silent, perhaps preventing its contrac-

tion from pinching off the esophagus, whereas the costal portion was active, contributing to the increase in abdominal pressure. Whether or not these effects, so far observed only in dogs, occur in humans remains to be seen. But the many similarities in diaphragmatic structure and function between the two species make this a good possibility.

Intercostal and Accessory Muscles

Between the ribs lie two bands of muscles, the external and internal intercostal muscles. The *external intercostal muscles* extend from the articulations between the ribs and vertebral bodies to the origin of the costal cartilages. In contrast, the *internal intercostal muscles* extend from the sternum only to the angles of the ribs. The internal intercostals are subdivided into interchondral (parasternal) and interosseous portions (Fig. 5–4).

Both internal and external intercostal muscles receive their motor and sensory innervation from the intercostal nerves, which arise from the first to twelfth thoracic segmental nerves. The lower intercostal nerves, which contribute a few sensory branches to the diaphragm, also supply the abdominal muscles. The intercostal muscles are richly supplied with proprioceptors such as muscle spindles and Golgi tendon organs. The contribution of these receptors to the control of breathing is considered in Chapter 10.

In contrast to previous beliefs that several muscles might serve as accessory muscles of inspiration, only the *scalene* (anterior, medial, and posterior) and *sternomastoid muscles* have important inspiratory functions in humans. However, because these muscles, especially the scalenes, are often used at rest and during relatively quiet breathing, it has been questioned whether or not they should be regarded as "accessory."[15]

Action. The mechanical action of the intercostal muscles on the rib cage has been a source of debate and controversy. The most widely held view is that the external intercostals and the interchondral (parasternal) portion of the internal intercostals are inspiratory, because they elevate the ribs to which they are attached; in contrast, the interosseous portions of the internal intercostals are expiratory because, when con-

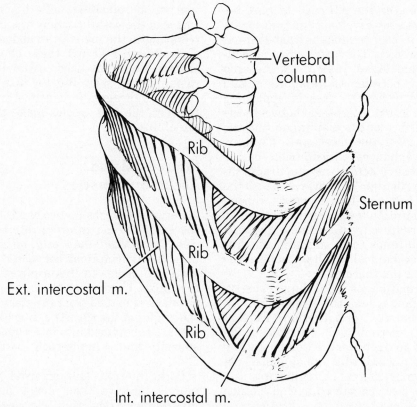

Vertebral column

Sternum

Rib

Rib

Ext. intercostal m.

Rib

Int. intercostal m.

Figure 5–4. Schematic drawing of part of the chest wall showing the location and orientation of the fibers in the external (Ext.) and internal (Int.) intercostal muscles (m).

tracting, they lower the ribs. This theory, which was inferred from the anatomic relations of the muscles (origins, insertions, and direction of fibers), has been supported by the results of electromyographic recordings in normal human subjects.[16]

Recently, however, this view has been challenged by De Troyer and coworkers[17, 18] on the basis of their experimental observations in dogs. In their first study, they found that while the animals were breathing with the inspiratory intercostal muscles alone, the ribs moved cephalad whereas the sternum moved caudad; barring species differences, they suggested that the cephalad motion of the sternum noted in humans is attributable to contraction of the scalene muscles.[17] In a more recent study, De Troyer and coworkers[18] separately stimulated the external and internal interosseous intercostal muscles (the latter group should be expiratory according to theory). At normal resting lung volume, both groups of intercostal muscles were inspiratory; in contrast, as the lungs were progressively inflated to above approximately half their inspiratory

capacity, the action was reversed and both groups became expiratory. Obviously, these findings cannot be applied directly to humans, but they suggest that rib cage movements may be far more complicated than previously suspected.

The scalene muscles, which elevate or fix the first two ribs, are recruited at approximately the same time during inspiration as the intercostal muscles; thus, they may be used at rest and are active during relatively quiet breathing. In contrast, the sternomastoids, which elevate the sternum, are recruited after about three-quarters of the vital capacity has been inhaled and are utilized only during strenuous breathing.[15]

Abdominal Muscles

Several muscles of the abdominal wall contribute to respiratory movements. Of these, the rectus, external and internal obliques, and transverse abdominal muscles are considered to function strictly during expiration. But, as will be pointed out, they may play an important role in quiet breathing by enhancing the inspiratory function of the diaphragm, particularly in the upright and sitting positions.

Action. It is generally believed that during exercise and other maneuvers that require vigorous breathing, the abdominal muscles are recruited and contribute to active (i.e., assisted) exhalation. Recently, De Troyer and coworkers[19] have performed experiments to determine how the various abdominal muscles act on the rib cage of a dog. By stimulating the muscles separately, the mechanical action of each could be examined. The *rectus abdominal muscles* were invariably expiratory (i.e., when stimulated, thoracic diameters decreased and sternal displacement was caudad), whereas the *external oblique muscles* had the opposite effect. The *internal oblique* and *transverse abdominal muscles* did not produce detectable displacement of the rib cage when stimulated.

These different actions are presumably related to the sites of rib cage attachment and fiber orientation of the various muscles. The net effect from the coordinated contraction of all the abdominal muscles should depend on the balance between the force related to muscle insertions, which deflates the rib cage and is expiratory, and the force causing an increase in abdominal pressure, which, as discussed previously, acts through the area of apposition to inflate the lower rib cage and thus is inspiratory.[19]

PHYSIOLOGY

The physiologic principles of skeletal muscle function are reasonably well known and can be used to differentiate clinical disorders associated with weakness and fatigue. The same general concepts are being applied to respiratory muscle function in health and disease with great benefit. But it must be remembered that the respiratory muscles differ from other skeletal muscles in several important respects. (1) They are the only skeletal muscles on which life depends; (2) they are under both voluntary and involuntary control; and (3) they deal chiefly with elastic and resistive loads, whereas most other skeletal muscles cope mainly with inertial loads. Furthermore, because they must contract repetitively for each person's lifetime, they are the skeletal muscles that are used the most.[2]

Force-Length Relationships

One of the intrinsic physiologic properties that respiratory muscles share with other skeletal muscles is that the active force developed is a function of the length of the muscle. In the respiratory system, as the lungs inflate the inspiratory muscles shorten and the expiratory muscles lengthen. Thus, one of the early ways of studying respiratory muscle mechanics was to use lung volume as an index of muscle length and to use the pressure developed at that volume as an index of force to approximate the force-length relationships of respiratory muscles.[20] The results of these studies showed that as lung volume increases, maximal inspiratory pressure decreases whereas maximal expiratory pressure increases, and vice versa during exhalation (Fig. 5–5). As might be expected, because of their greater muscle mass men generate higher maximal pressures than women, and there is some weakening of respiratory muscle strength with increasing age.

Because the various respiratory muscle groups can be made to lengthen differently to achieve the same lung volume and because the transformation from a force developed by respiratory muscles to a pressure acting on the system depends on the muscles' mechanical advantages and geometries, maximal inspiratory and expiratory volume-pressure curves are only an approximation of the force-length relationships of respiratory muscles. Moreover, such studies can only describe the characteristics of the entire system, and the approach provides no information about the contribution of the various separate muscle groups.

The relationships among diaphragmatic muscle length, contractile tension, and transdiaphragmatic pressure have been determined in the open-chest dog;[21] the force-length characteristics derived from this study are shown in Figure 5–6. Maximal active tension was observed at approximately 25 per cent beyond the *in situ* resting length, a finding that differs from other skeletal muscles in which maximal active tension occurs at approximately *in situ* resting length. Moreover, Figure 5–6 shows that the diaphragm still generates appreciable tension at lengths as short as 40 per cent of the *in situ* resting length; this condition also differs from that found in other skeletal muscles, in which tension becomes zero at 50 to 60 per cent of the *in situ* resting length.

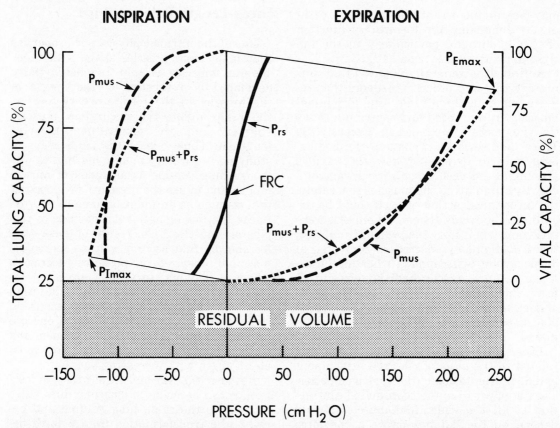

Figure 5–5. Volume-pressure diagram of the respiratory system (from Fig. 4–7), showing the pressures generated by the respiratory muscles (P_{mus}) and the muscles plus the recoil of the respiratory system ($P_{mus} + P_{rs}$) during inspiration and expiration. FRC = functional residual capacity; P_{Imax} = maximal inspiratory pressure; P_{Emax} = maximal expiratory pressure. (Reprinted by permission from Murray, J. F.: Respiration. *In* Smith, L. H., and Their, S. (eds.): Pathophysiology. Philadelphia, W. B. Saunders Company, 1985, pp. 753–854.)

Thus, the canine diaphragm appears to function effectively over a longer range of muscle fiber lengths than do other skeletal muscles. Similar findings were reported in studies of the hamster diaphragm by Farkas and Roussos.[22]

Investigators have noted that the diaphragm of the dog behaves much like a piston in that it descends into the abdomen without changing its radius of curvature very much; this means that the length-tension characteristics of the muscle are more important than Laplace relationships (see equation 10, Chapter 4), from changing geometry in explaining diaphragmatic mechanical function.[21] Moreover, as already pointed out, this behavior tends to preserve the area of apposition and to facilitate the action of abdominal pressure on the rib cage.

Recently, the force-length relationships of the human diaphragm have been inferred from pressure measurements and chest roentgenograms taken at different lung volumes.[23] The results differed from those obtained in directly studied muscles (see Fig. 5–6) in two important respects. First, no distinct peak of maximal active tension was observed near the resting muscle length. Second, the range of muscle length through which tension was developed was narrower in the human diaphragm than in the dog and hamster diaphragms. Whether these are methodological or species differences remains to be determined. Human diaphragmatic behavior was similar to that of the dog in that length was a far more important determinant of contractile force than the radius of curvature;[23] in neither species did the diaphragm change its geometry substantially through most of its range of contraction.

Force-Velocity Relationships

Another intrinsic mechanical property of skeletal muscle is the relationship between the force generated and the velocity of mus-

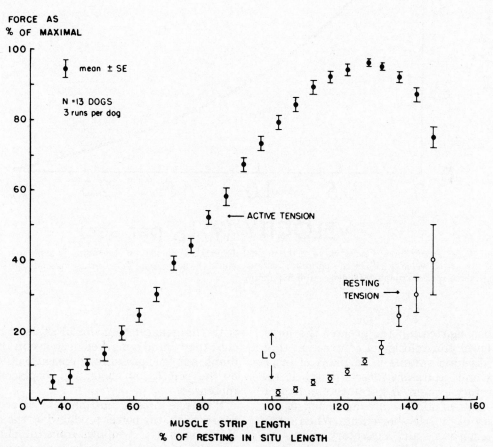

Figure 5–6. Active and passive length-tension diagrams obtained from a diaphragm strip preparation. Force was measured with a Grass force transducer. On the abscissa 100 per cent designates resting *in situ* length (Lo) as determined by the first appearance of passive tension. The ordinate is the active and passive force expressed as percentage of maximal active force. (Reprinted by permission from Kim, M. J., et al.: Mechanics of the canine diaphragm. J. Appl. Physiol., *41*:369–382, 1976.)

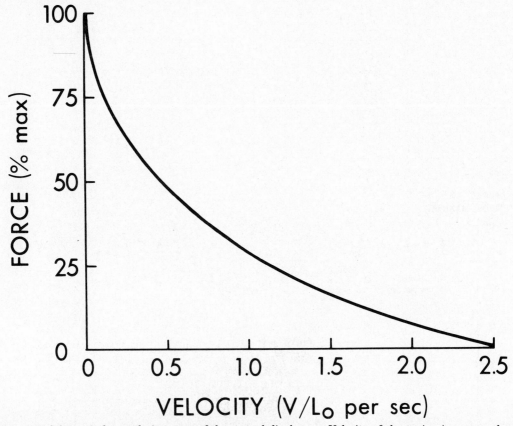

Figure 5–7. Schematic force-velocity curve of the normal diaphragm. Velocity of shortening is expressed as the ratio of the actual velocity (V) to the optimum resting length of the muscle (L_o). During vigorous breathing, developed force is approximately 50 per cent of maximum.

cle fiber shortening: the greater the force, the slower the velocity of contraction (Fig. 5–7). As lung volume is an index of inspiratory and expiratory muscle length in the respiratory system, inspiratory and expiratory rates of airflow are an index of the velocity of muscle shortening. When maximal inspiratory and expiratory efforts are made through different-sized orifices, to vary resistance to airflow, the maximal pressures exerted by the respiratory muscles decrease as the rate of airflow increases.[24, 25]

As pointed out in the previous section, the same lung volume can be attained by different respiratory muscle configurations. This limits the interpretation of not only pressure-volume data (see Fig. 5–5) but the results of pressure-flow studies as well. To avoid this pitfall and to obtain a direct assessment of the velocity of diaphragmatic fiber shortening, Goldman and coworkers[26] measured the rate of abdominal displacement with the rib cage fixed; in agreement

with the general behavior of skeletal muscles, they found a marked decrease in transdiaphragmatic pressure, a measure of force, as the velocity of abdominal displacement increased.

If muscle force is multiplied by velocity of contraction, the power produced by the muscle is obtained. It follows from the characteristics of the force-velocity curve (see Fig. 5–7) that power is zero at the two extremes: when force is maximal and velocity is zero and when force is zero and velocity is maximal. This means that there is a particular velocity of contraction at which power output is maximal. In a well-designed system (and the human body certainly is!), it is reasonable to expect the muscle to operate at that velocity. Disappointingly, inspiratory airflow rates and the velocities of muscle contraction are known to vary widely and to depend on the needs of the moment. Mechanical order could be restored, however, if it could be shown that the respiratory system is designed in such a way that as inspiratory demand increases, there is progressive recruitment of new inspiratory muscles rather than an increase in the force of contraction of all the muscles used in quiet breathing. When new muscles are recruited, there is a shift upward in the resulting force-velocity relationships and a corresponding shift to the right in velocity of maximum power output. By this means, muscle function may be coordinated in such a way that the muscles are always shortening at the velocity that will produce optimum power.[2] Evidence is becoming available to support this theory.[27, 28]

Energetics

All cells of the body require O_2 and nutrients to sustain their metabolic needs. Skeletal muscles differ from those organs whose metabolism remains relatively constant in that muscles must be able to increase their O_2 consumption more than twentyfold during the transition from rest to strenuous exercise. Increased O_2 requirements are satisfied through a combination of increased blood flow to and increased extraction of O_2 by the contracting muscles. Judging from the limited information available, respiratory muscles are similar to other skeletal muscles in their capacity to increase metabolism greatly. But the diaphragm, which has been the most extensively studied respiratory muscle, differs from other muscles in the mechanisms by which it meets increased O_2 demands and in several other important metabolic activities.

As the O_2 requirements of the diaphragm begin to increase, both blood flow and O_2 extraction increase; however, at high levels of contractile effort and O_2 consumption, extraction tends to plateau and blood flow continues to increase.[29] This dependency on perfusion is unlike that of other skeletal muscles and resembles that of the heart. Blood flow to limb skeletal muscles does not increase indefinitely and actually decreases or ceases during strenuous contractions. The results of most studies indicate that this phenomenon does not occur in the diaphragm.[29, 30] During sustained tetanic contractions, diaphragmatic blood flow is obstructed, but during intermittent contractions, even at maximal levels of trans-

diaphragmatic pressure, blood flow is not affected.[31] There is no doubt that when cardiac output is low and ventilatory demands are high, the diaphragm has to compete with other organs for its blood flow and that sometimes it does this unsuccessfully.[32] Under these extreme conditions mechanical ventilation may be life saving.

The efficiency of the contracting diaphragm in converting energy to work increases when ventilation is increased but decreases progressively in the presence of increased resistance to inspiratory airflow.[33] Approximately one-half of the energy utilized by the working diaphragm comes from carbohydrate metabolism, chiefly in the form of lactate utilization, and the remainder is presumably from lipids, chiefly in the form of fatty acids.[33] The canine diaphragm is known to be remarkably resistant to anaerobic metabolism, even while working hard in a hypoxic environment;[34] in this respect also the diaphragm differs from other skeletal muscles, which generate large quantities of lactate as they become hypoxic. Thus, the hemodynamic and metabolic attributes of the diaphragm, which more closely resemble the heart than other skeletal muscles, endow this key respiratory muscle with extraordinary endurance for high work loads.

Fatigue

The material in the previous section should not be misconstrued. The diaphragm is an exceptional muscle, beautifully designed for the task of breathing for a lifetime. But it is not capable of limitless feats of contractile effort. It can fatigue. Respiratory muscle fatigue, both of the diaphragm[35] and of the sternocleidomastoid muscle,[36] has been well demonstrated in carefully controlled experiments in normal human subjects. Moreover, as ways are being found to make the diagnosis, there is increasing evidence that respiratory muscle fatigue is important in a variety of clinical disorders associated with respiratory failure.

There are several types of muscle fibers that can be classified on the basis of their biochemical and electrophysiologic characteristics, including their resistance to fatigue. Respiratory muscles contain three types of fibers but are composed chiefly of two of them: type I, slow-twitch, high-oxi-

Table 5–1. PROPORTION OF TYPE I MUSCLE FIBERS IN HUMAN RESPIRATORY MUSCLES*

Age	Diaphragm	Internal Intercostal	External Intercostal
< 37 weeks gestation	9.7	21.8	24.7
Full-term infants	25.0	47.1	49.7†
2–10 years	55.4	62.3	69.4
Adults	54.6	59.7†	60.7†

*Data from Lieberman, D. A., et al.: Performance and histochemical composition of guinea pig and human diaphragm. J. Appl. Physiol., *34*:233–237, 1973; and Keens, T. G., et al.: Developmental pattern of muscle fiber types in human ventilatory muscles. J. Appl. Physiol., *44*:909–913, 1978.
†Only one value available.

dation fibers and type II, fast-twitch, low-oxidation fibers.[37] The developmental pattern of type I human respiratory muscle fibers is shown in Table 5–1. The increasing proportion of type I fibers during gestation and infancy is important because these fibers are approximately three times more efficient than type II fibers in sustaining an isometric contraction and thus are more resistant to fatigue. The corollary of this observation is that premature infants, who have only about 10 per cent type I fibers in their diaphragms, are ill-equipped to deal with the relatively high respiratory work loads of the newborn period.[38]

For practical purposes, fatigue has been defined as the inability of a muscle to continue to generate a required force.[3] When applied to the respiratory system, this term means that the respiratory muscles are unable to produce sufficient force to sustain adequate movement of air into and out of the lungs. There are two basic types of respiratory muscle fatigue: that resulting from lack of central neural drive ("central fatigue") and that resulting from failure in the performance of the muscle itself ("peripheral fatigue"). Thus, the site of fatigue may be at any level from the central nervous system to the contractile elements within the muscle fiber.

With few exceptions, most causes of respiratory muscle fatigue are peripheral and can be attributed to failure of metabolic regenerative processes in the muscle fiber. Usually, these can be related to an imbalance between increased demand for energy on the one hand and decreased supply of energy on the other. The factors that govern the energy demands of the respiratory muscles are the work that they need to perform, their strength, and their efficiency in converting energy to work. It follows that an increase in work or a decrease in strength or efficiency can lead to respiratory muscle fatigue.

The factors that determine energy supplies are more complex than those that regulate energy demand. The availability of energy supplies only becomes critical after local energy stores, particularly glycogen, are depleted. Thus, starvation or other catabolic states as well as prolonged submaximal breathing may deplete glycogen stores and contribute to respiratory muscle fatigue. Conditions in which energy supplies are reduced and which thereby predispose to respiratory muscle fatigue are a decrease in cardiac output, a low O_2 content of arterial blood from any cause, an inability to extract and use energy from the blood, and a low blood-substrate concentration.[3]

The presence of respiratory muscle fatigue can only be established in the laboratory and it can only be detected under conditions in which lung volume and chest wall geometry are carefully controlled and the patient's ability and motivation to cooperate are ensured. One of the best tests is to determine the relation between diaphragmatic contractility at different excitation frequencies and developed forces. The electromyogram is recorded as a measure of excitation, and transdiaphragmatic pressure is used as an index of force. (Transdiaphragmatic pressure is taken as the difference between pleural pressure, measured as described in Chapter 4 with an esophageal balloon, and gastric pressure, measured with a separate balloon placed in the stomach.) During this test, it is important to maintain isometric conditions by ensuring that the dimensions of the rib cage and abdomen remain constant. Diaphragmatic contractility has also been measured by transcutaneous stimulation of the phrenic nerve. A decrease in transdiaphragmatic pressure at a given stimulus frequency denotes fatigue (Fig. 5–8).

Recently, emphasis has been placed on using the electromyographic power spectrum in detecting inspiratory muscle fatigue.[39] A contracting muscle generates electromyographic signals of both high and low frequencies. As the muscle begins to fatigue, there is a shift in the electromyographic power spectrum, with a decrease in high-frequency components and an increase in low-frequency components. The validity of this technique has been reinforced by the observation that the shift in frequency spectrum coincided with a decrease in the rate of diaphragmatic relaxation, a well-established feature of incipient skeletal muscle fatigue.[40]

BREATHING

Breathing is achieved by changes in the size of the thoracic cavity, brought about by contraction of the respiratory muscles. Enlargement of the thorax can occur by displacement outward either of the rib cage or of the abdominal wall. For practical purposes, the sum of the volumes displaced by these two maneuvers equals the increase in volume of the thorax and this, in turn, equals the increase in volume of the lungs. The old notion that women breathe with their chests and men with their abdomens has been thoroughly discredited. Both sexes breathe in much the same way, using similar respiratory muscles. It has proved difficult, however, to analyze completely the contribution of each of the three groups of

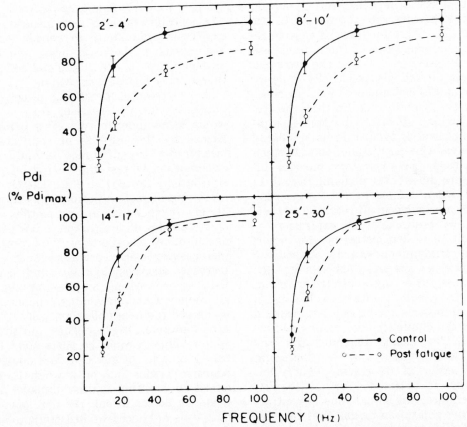

Figure 5–8. Pressure-frequency curves of the human diaphragm before and after fatigue. The curves represent results obtained in four subjects before fatigue and 2 to 4, 8 to 10, 14 to 17, and 25 to 30 minutes after fatigue. Solid curves represent the average of the three curves before diaphragmatic fatigue (control). Dotted curves represent the average of three curves at different times during recovery period. Transdiaphragmatic pressure (Pdi) is expressed as a percentage of the Pdi generated for a stimulation frequency of 100 Hz. Bars indicate ± 1 S.E. (From Roussos, C., and Macklem, P. T.: The respiratory muscles. By permission from New Eng. J. Med. 307:786–797, 1982.)

respiratory muscles to normal breathing in different body positions and under various conditions of stress. However, sufficient information is available to present a reasonably complete description of how breathing occurs in certain ordinary circumstances.

Rest

In humans breathing quietly at rest, the diaphragm is chiefly responsible for ventilation. However, it does not function alone. As already pointed out, both the inspiratory intercostal muscles[16] and (usually) the scalene muscles[15] are also active during quiet breathing. The abdominal respiratory muscles were generally considered to be inactive at rest, but recent evidence suggests that this is not the case, at least when healthy subjects are sitting or standing. In these body positions, Loring and Mead[41] demonstrated that at the end of expiration, normal (untrained) persons did not return to the FRC position determined by the passive relaxation characteristics of their lungs and chest wall (see Fig. 4–7 and the accompanying text for full discussion of the determinants of FRC). Values of FRC in these subjects were usually smaller than the "relaxed" FRC, an effect attributable to expiratory muscle activity; furthermore, judging from the relative positions of the abdomen and rib cage, the expiratory muscles involved were those of the abdominal wall. In contrast, when studied in the supine position, the same subjects all returned to their relaxed FRC positions at end-expiration.

In addition to demonstrating the importance of studying untrained instead of trained persons, the usual subjects for such experiments, these observations have important physiologic implications. The use of abdominal muscles during expiration would lengthen the diaphragm at the onset of inspiration. One should remember that the maximal force generated by the diaphragm does not occur at its resting length but occurs when it is stretched further (see Fig. 5–6); therefore, abdominal muscle contraction during expiration means that the efficiency of diaphragmatic contraction during inspiration will be increased because the muscle will be operating along a more favorable segment of its force-length curve. Apparently, in the supine position it is unnecessary to utilize this mechanical advantage, presumably because of other postural effects. Support for these considerations comes from the results of electromyographic studies of abdominal muscle activity during various breathing maneuvers in normal subjects.[42]

Exercise

There is less disagreement concerning the contribution of the various groups of respiratory muscles to breathing during exercise than during rest, but this may be because fewer detailed studies have been carried out in exercising subjects owing to the difficulties involved. As the demands for O_2 increase during exercise, more and more respiratory muscles are recruited to meet the body's needs for additional ventilation.[43] (The relationships among exercise, O_2 consumption, and ventilation are discussed in Chapter 11). At high exercise work loads, all respiratory muscles, both inspiratory and expiratory, contribute to ventilation, and movements of the arms, legs, and trunk, although they do not inflate and deflate the thorax, may facilitate breathing.

The O_2 cost of breathing progressively increases during exercise; this variable, which is an index of the work being performed by the muscles of respiration, is measured as the difference in total body O_2 consumption at rest and during increasing ventilatory efforts (Fig. 5–9). The O_2 cost of breathing at rest in normal subjects is relatively inexpensive, approximately 0.5 ml of O_2 per liter of ventilation, a low percentage of total O_2 consumption.[44] As ventilation increases however, respiratory muscle needs increase disproportionately and compete with other working muscles for available O_2. When ventilatory muscle demands for O_2 exceed the available supply of O_2, respiratory muscle fatigue ensues and the ventilatory effort cannot be sustained.[3] Respiratory muscle fatigue can develop even in healthy persons but only when they are forced to breathe against unusual loads. Under these conditions, the development of fatigue is enhanced by breathing gas mixtures low in O_2[45] or high in CO_2.[46] There are several reasons, therefore, why patients with lung disease are susceptible to respiratory muscle fatigue. Among the most important are that their muscles are often at a mechanical disadvantage (see below),

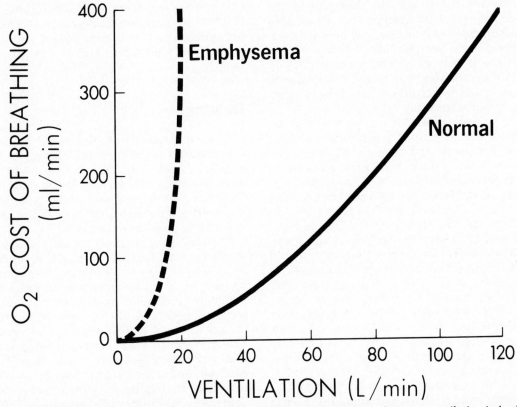

Figure 5–9. Respiratory muscle oxygen consumption (O_2 cost of breathing) in relation to ventilation in healthy persons (Normal) and in patients with increased work of breathing (Emphysema). (Data from Roussos, C., and Macklem, P. T.: The respiratory muscles. New Engl. J. Med., *307*:786–797, 1982 and Cherniack, R. M.: The oxygen consumption and efficiency of the respiratory muscles in health and emphysema. J. Clin. Invest. *38*:494–499, 1959.)

their O_2 cost of breathing is considerably greater than normal because of the extra work required to ventilate abnormal lungs and chest walls (see Fig. 5–9), [47] and they may be hypoxic or hypercapneic.

Disease

In general, respiratory diseases tend to increase the work of breathing or to place the respiratory muscles at a mechanical disadvantage, or both. A full discussion of the many abnormalities that may involve the respiratory muscles is beyond the intent of this book on normal structure and function; furthermore, some excellent reviews are available.[2–4] Two disorders will be analyzed because they enhance an understanding of normality.

Diaphragmatic Paralysis. The contribution of the intact diaphragm to normal breathing can be appreciated by studying patients with diaphragmatic disorders[48] or experimental animals after cutting both phrenic nerves.[17] When both halves of the diaphragm are unable to contract, no transdiaphragmatic pressure develops during inspiration and abdominal pressure remains equal to pleural pressure. Breathing can still occur because the chest cage becomes elevated and expanded owing to contraction of the remaining functional inspiratory intercostal and accessory muscles. But under these circumstances, as pleural pressure becomes more negative, the diaphragm and abdominal contents are sucked into the thorax, creating a paradoxical abdominal motion. Thus, inward displacement of the abdomen offsets much of the outward displacement of the rib cage, and breathing becomes very inefficient. To maintain a given level of ventilation despite total diaphragmatic paralysis, the intercostal and accessory muscles must do a great deal of extra external work, because they not only inflate the chest cage but they pull in the abdomen as well. Despite this formidable mechanical disadvantage, patients with paralysis of the two hemidiaphragms appear to have a reserve breathing capability in that they are able to increase ventilation to some extent by voluntary use of the remaining intact respiratory muscles.[48]

Hyperinflation. An increase in end-expiratory lung volume is a common clinical and physiologic finding that occurs in association with either bronchial obstruction from premature closure of the narrowed airways, or decreased elastic recoil of the lung from loss of tissue forces (see Chapter 4). In either case, the chest wall at FRC is more inflated than normal, and all of the inspiratory muscles are shorter than they should be at the onset of inspiration. These muscles, therefore, must operate on a less than optimum segment of their force-length curve, which means that to achieve a given level of ventilation the muscles require a greater than normal excitation and must generate a greater percentage of the maximum pressure available.[3] In addition, recent studies have revealed disturbances of contractility in the acutely shortened diaphragm that developed in addition to the decrease in tension that ordinarily accompanies muscle shortening.[49] These and other factors must contribute to diaphragmatic fatigability during acute hyperventilation such as may occur during an asthmatic attack. As discussed below, some adaptation may follow a chronic increase in FRC. When hyperinflation is extreme and the diaphragm is flattened, its function changes from that of an inspiratory to that of an expiratory muscle, because contraction now pulls the lower rib cage inward.

The mechanical consequences of hyperinflation tend to increase energy consumption for a given work load and to decrease efficiency.[3] These considerations demonstrate that the normal respiratory system is designed so that its muscles are operating at or near their positions of maximal mechanical utility. Deviations from this setting are usually associated with increased work of breathing and decreased efficiency. Some adaptation to chronic hyperinflation and shortening of inspiratory muscle length seems possible; Farkas and Roussos[50] recently showed that hamsters adapted to chronic hyperinflation from enzyme-induced emphysema by decreasing the number of functioning units (sarcomeres) in their diaphragms, which restored normal maximal tension at the new shorter operational length.

Training

One can predict from the many similarities between respiratory muscles and other skeletal muscles that the former might behave like the latter in response to training. This has now been shown to be true, both in healthy subjects[51] and in patients with various respiratory diseases.[52, 53]

Training programs are usually designed specifically to increase strength or endurance, sometimes both. Strength is improved by increasing the number of contractile elements or myofibrils; this is what happens in weight lifters and, by analogy, respiratory muscle strength can be improved by repeatedly performing maximal static inspiratory and expiratory pressure maneuvers.[51] In contrast, endurance is improved by increasing muscle capillary and mitochondrial densities and the muscles' overall oxidative enzyme capacity; this occurs in marathon runners and, again by analogy, takes place in respiratory muscles in response to repeated hyperventilation maneuvers.[51] Breathing through inspiratory resistances has been shown to improve both strength and endurance[54] and can easily be performed at home by using a simple pocket-sized device.

Diaphragmatic contractility is augmented during an infusion of aminophylline, an effect that can be abolished by verapamil, a calcium channel blocking drug.[55] Similar effects on contractility with resulting improved resistance to fatigue can be produced by aminophylline in healthy subjects and in patients with chronic airflow limitation.[56] But what matters to the patient and to the clinician is the effect of aminophylline at therapeutic concentrations. When this constraint is evaluated, the benefits of the drug on respiratory muscle function are less impressive.[57] Further research is clearly required and should be directed toward evaluating the effects of aminophylline in humans with lung disease. Nevertheless, training and use of pharmacologic agents offer interesting future prospects for improving respiratory muscle function in patients whose work of breathing is increased.

REFERENCES

1. Campbell, E. J. M., Agostoni, E., and Newsom Davis, J.: The Respiratory Muscles: Mechanics and Neural Control. Philadelphia, W. B. Saunders Co., 1970.
2. Derenne, J. P., Macklem, P. T., and Roussos, C.: The respiratory muscles: mechanics, control and pathophysiology. Parts I, II and III. Am. Rev. Respir. Dis., *118*:119–133, 373–390, 581–601, 1978.
3. Roussos, C., and Macklem, P. T.: The respiratory muscles. New Engl. J. Med., *307*:786–797, 1982.
4. Green, M., and Morham, J.: Respiratory muscles. *In* Flenley, D. L. (ed.): Recent Advances in Respiratory Medicine No 3. Edinburgh, Churchill Livingstone, 1983, pp. 1–20.
5. Decramer, M., De Troyer, A., Kelly, S., and Macklem, P. T.: Mechanical arrangement of costal and crural diaphragms in dogs. J. Appl. Physiol., *56*:1484–1490, 1984.
6. Leak, L. V.: Gross and ultrastructural morphologic features of the diaphragm. Am. Rev. Respir. Dis., *119*(Suppl.):3–21, 1979.
7. Corda, M., von Euler, C., and Lennerstrand, G.: Proprioceptive innervation of the diaphragm. J. Physiol. (Lond.), *178*:161–177, 1965.
8. von Euler, C.: On the neural organization of the motor control of the diaphragm. Am. Rev. Respir. Dis., *119*(Suppl.):45–49, 1979.
9. Konno, K., and Mead, J.: Measurement of the separate volume changes of rib cage and abdomen during breathing. J. Appl. Physiol., *22*:407–422, 1967.
10. Goldman, M. D.: Mechanical interaction between diaphragm and rib cage. Boston view. Am. Rev. Respir. Dis., *119*(Suppl.):23–26, 1979.
11. Mead, J.: Functional significance of the area of apposition of diaphragm to rib cage. Am. Rev. Respir. Dis., *119*(Suppl.):31–32, 1979.
12. De Troyer, A., Sampson, M., Sigrist, S., and Macklem, P. T.: Action of the costal and crural parts of the diaphragm on the rib cage in dog. J. Appl. Physiol., *53*:30–39, 1982.
13. Macklem, P. T., Macklem, D. M., and De Troyer, A.: A model of inspiratory muscle mechanics. J. Appl. Physiol., *55*:547–557, 1983.
14. Monges, H., Salducci, J., and Naudy, B.: Dissociation between the electrical activity of the diaphragmatic dome and crural muscular fibers during esophageal distention, vomiting, and eructation. A electromyographic study in the dog. J. Physiol. (Paris), *74*:541–554, 1978.
15. Raper, A. J., Thompson, W. T., Jr., Shapiro, W., and Patterson, J. L., Jr.: Scalene and sternomastoid muscle function. J. Appl. Physiol., *21*:497–502, 1966.
16. Taylor, A.: The contribution of the intercostal muscles to the effort of respiration in man. J. Physiol. (Lond.), *151*:390–402, 1960.
17. De Troyer, A., and Kelly, S.: Chest wall mechanics in dogs with acute diaphragm paralysis. J. Appl. Physiol., *53*:373–378, 1982.
18. De Troyer, A., Kelly, S., and Zin, W. A.: Mechanical action of the intercostal muscles on the ribs. Science, *220*:87–88, 1983.
19. De Troyer, A., Sampson, M., Sigrist, S., and Kelly, S.: How the abdominal muscles act on the rib cage. J. Appl. Physiol., *54*:465–469, 1983.
20. Rahn, H., Otis, A. B., Chadwick, L. E., and Fenn, W. O.: The pressure-volume diagram of the thorax and lung. Am. J. Physiol., *146*:161–178, 1946.
21. Kim, M. J., Druz, W. S., Danon, J., Macnach, W., and Sharp, J. T.: Mechanics of the canine diaphragm. J. Appl. Physiol., *41*:369–382, 1976.
22. Farkas, G. A., and Roussos, C.: Adaptability of the hamster diaphragm to exercise and/or emphysema. J. Appl. Physiol., *53*:1263–1272, 1982.
23. Braun, N. M. T., Arora, N. S., and Rochester, D. F.: Force-length relationship of the normal human diaphragm. J. Appl. Physiol., *53*:405–412, 1982.
24. Agostoni, E., and Fenn, W. O.: Velocity of muscle shortening as a limiting factor in respiratory airflow. J. Appl. Physiol., *15*:349–353, 1960.
25. Hyatt, R. E., and Flath, R. E.: Relationship of airflow to pressure during maximal respiratory effort in man. J. Appl. Physiol., *21*:477–482, 1966.
26. Goldman, M. D., Grassino, A., Mead, J., and Sears, J. A.: Mechanics of the human diaphragm during voluntary contraction. Dynamics. J. Appl. Physiol., *44*:840–848, 1978.
27. Pengally, L. D., Alderson, A. M., and Milic-Emili, J.: Mechanics of the diaphragm. J. Appl. Physiol., *30*:797–805, 1971.
28. Macklem, P. T., Gross, D., Grassino, A., and Roussos, C.: Partitioning of inspiratory pressure swings between diaphragm and intercostal/accessory muscles. J. Appl. Physiol., *44*:200–208, 1978.
29. Rochester, D. F., and Bettini, G.: Diaphragmatic blood flow and energy expenditure in the dog. Effects of inspiratory airflow resistance and hypercapnia. J. Clin. Invest., *57*:661–672, 1976.
30. Johnson, R. L., Jr., and Reid, M.: Limits of oxygen transport to the diaphragm. Am. Rev. Respir. Dis., *119*(Suppl.):113–114, 1979.
31. Buchler, B., Magder, S., Katsardis, H., Jammes, Y., and Roussos, C.: Effects of pleural pressure and abdominal pressure on diaphragmatic blood flow. J. Appl. Physiol., *58*:691–697, 1985.
32. Aubier, M., Trippenbach, T., and Roussos, C.: Respiratory muscle fatigue during cardiogenic shock. J. Appl. Physiol., *51*:499–508, 1981.
33. Rochester, D. F., and Briscoe, A. M.: Metabolism of the working diaphragm. Am. Rev. Respir. Dis., *119*(Suppl.):101–106, 1978.
34. Robertson, C. H., Jr., Foster, G. H., and Johnson, R. L., Jr.: The relationship of respiratory failure to the oxygen consumption of, lactate production by, and distribution of blood flow among respiratory muscles during increasing respiratory resistance. J. Clin. Invest., *59*:31–42, 1977.
35. Roussos, C. S., and Macklem, P. T.: Diaphragmatic fatigue in man. J. Appl. Physiol., *43*:189–197, 1977.
36. Moxham, J., Wiles, C. M., Newham, D., and Edwards, R. H. T.: Sternomastoid muscle function and fatigue in man. Clin. Sci., *59*:463–468, 1980.
37. Lieberman, D. A., Faulkner, J. A., Craig, A. B., Jr., and Maxwell, L. C.: Performance and histochemical composition of guinea pig and human diaphragm. J. Appl. Physiol., *34*:233–237, 1973.
38. Keens, T. G., Bryan, A. C., Levison, H., and Ianuzzo, C. D.: Developmental pattern of muscle fiber

types in human ventilatory muscles. J. Appl. Physiol., *44*:909–913, 1978.

39. Gross, D., Grassino, A., Ross, W. R. D., and Macklem, P. T.: Electromyogram pattern of diaphragmatic fatigue. J. Appl. Physiol., *46*:1–7, 1979.

40. Esan, S., Bellemare, F., Grassino, A., Permutt, S., Roussos, C., and Pardy, R. L.: Changes in relaxation rate with diaphragmatic fatigue in humans. J. Appl. Physiol., *54*:1353–1360, 1983.

41. Loring, S. H., and Mead, J.: Abdominal muscle use during quiet breathing and hyperpnea in uninformed subjects. J. Appl. Physiol., *52*:700–704, 1982.

42. Strohl, K. P., Mead, J., Banzett, R. B., Loring, S. H., and Kosch, P. C.: Regional differences in abdominal muscle activity during various maneuvers in humans. J. Appl. Physiol., *51*:1471–1476, 1981.

43. Grimby, G., Bunn, J., and Mead, J.: Relative contribution of rib cage and abdomen to ventilation during exercise. J. Appl. Physiol., *24*:159–166, 1968.

44. Otis, A. B.: The work of breathing. Physiol. Rev., *34*:449–458, 1954.

45. Lardin, J., Farkas, G., Prefant, C., Thomas, D., Macklem, P. T., and Roussos, C.: The failing inspiratory muscles under normoxic and hypoxic conditions. Am. Rev. Respir. Dis., *124*:274–279, 1981.

46. Juan, G., Calverley, P., Talamo, C., Schnader, J., and Roussos, C.: Effect of carbon dioxide on diaphragmatic function in human beings. New Engl. J. Med., *310*:874–879, 1984.

47. Cherniack, R. M.: The oxygen consumption and efficiency of the respiratory muscles in health and emphysema. J. Clin. Invest., *38*:494–499, 1959.

48. Newsom Davis, J., Goldman, M., Loh, L., and Casson, M.: Diaphragm function and alveolar hypoventilation. Quart. J. Med., *45*:87–100, 1976.

49. Farkas, G. A., and Roussos, C.: Acute diaphragmatic shortening: *in vitro* mechanics and fatigue. Am. Rev. Respir. Dis., *130*:434–438, 1984.

50. Farkas, G. A., and Roussos, C.: Diaphragm in emphysematous hamsters: diaphragm adaptability. J. Appl. Physiol., *54*:1635–1640, 1983.

51. Leith, D. E., and Bradley, M.: Ventilatory muscle strength and endurance training. J. Appl. Physiol., *41*:508–516, 1976.

52. Keens, T. G., Krastius, I. R. B., Wannamaker, E. M., Levison, H., Crozier, D. N., and Bryan, C.: Ventilatory muscle endurance training in normal subjects and patients with cystic fibrosis. Am. Rev. Respir. Dis., *116*:853–860, 1977.

53. Belman, M. J., and Mittman, C.: Ventilatory muscle training improves exercise capacity in chronic obstructive pulmonary disease patients. Am. Rev. Respir. Dis., *121*:273–280, 1980.

54. Pardy, R. L., Rivington, R. N., Despos, P. J., and Macklem, P. T.: The effects of inspiratory muscle training on exercise performance in chronic airflow limitation. Am. Rev. Respir. Dis., *123*:426–433, 1981.

55. Aubier, M., Murcino, D., Viires, N., Lecocguic, Y., and Pariente, R.: Diaphragmatic contractility enhanced by aminophylline: role of extracellular calcium. J. Appl. Physiol., *54*:460–467, 1983.

56. Murciano, D., Aubier, M., Lecocguic, Y., and Pariente, R.: Effects of theophylline on diaphragmatic strength and fatigue in patients with chronic obstructive pulmonary disease. New Engl. J. Med., *311*:349–353, 1984.

57. Moxham, J., and Green, M.: Aminophylline and the respiratory muscles. Bull. Eur. Physiopathol. Respir., *21*:1–6, 1985.

Chapter

6

Circulation

INTRODUCTION

The chief function of the pulmonary circulation is to deliver blood in a thin film to the terminal respiratory units so that gas exchange can take place. The anatomy of the pulmonary circulation is well suited for this purpose because it consists of inflow and outflow vessels that supply and drain an extensive capillary bed that occupies 85 to 95 per cent of the total alveolar surface and that provides an interface for the uptake of O_2 and elimination of CO_2 of potentially 126 ± 12 (standard error) m^2 in a normal human adult.[1] Although the lung is designed as an efficient gas exchanger, numerous factors operate continuously to influence gas transfer between air and blood by affecting whether or not incoming blood and inspired air are apposed in proportionate amounts. Chapter 4 considered the mechanisms that regulate the volume and distribution of inspired air to the terminal respiratory units; this chapter deals similarly with the volume and distribution of pulmonary blood flow.

The pulmonary circulation has additional functions besides gas exchange.[2] Some of these have been alluded to briefly elsewhere but are summarized as follows: (1) it acts as a filter of the venous drainage from virtually the entire body; (2) it provides substrates for the nutritional and metabolic needs of the lung parenchyma, including the synthesis of surfactant; (3) it serves as a reservoir of blood for the left ventricle; (4) it modifies the pharmacologic properties of a variety of circulating substances by biochemical transformation; and (5) it provides a large surface for the absorption of lung liquid that must occur immediately after birth or may take place in unusual circumstances (instillation of liquids therapeutically, drowning).

This chapter will consider the transport of blood through the lungs, particularly the factors that regulate the distribution of blood flow and vascular resistance within the lungs. The important roles of the pulmonary circulation in movement of liquid and solute into and out of the lungs and pleural space and in the processing of a variety of biochemical substances are considered further in Chapter 12.

PULMONARY BLOOD FLOW

After fetal shunt pathways have closed, the pulmonary circulation of a normal infant accommodates the entire output of the right ventricle, regardless of the amount ejected. Total pulmonary blood flow, as described earlier, is considerably different during fetal life from what it is after the newborn period; it may also differ from normal in persons with cardiovascular diseases, especially congenital heart abnormalities with shunts of blood from left to right or right to left. The output of the right ventricle is normally a little less than that of the left ventricle—the difference being due to drainage through bronchial veins and thebesian

veins that bypass the right ventricle. Cardiac output averages about 5 to 8 L/min in an adult at rest and may rise to 20 to 30 L/min during heavy exercise in a well-trained athlete.

Intravascular Pressures

Although blood flow to the lungs is higher than that to any other organ of the body, the pressure within pulmonary arteries is low, being about one-fifth of that within systemic arteries. A comparison of intravascular pressures in the pulmonary and systemic circulations is presented in Table 6–1. Not only is the pulmonary circulation a high flow–low pressure system in a subject at rest but it can also accommodate increases in cardiac output of up to three or four times resting values with only a small rise in inflow pressure. This means that pulmonary vascular resistance is low to begin with in a resting subject and is capable of substantial further reductions when pulmonary blood flow increases. The physiologic and clinical importance of changes in pulmonary vascular resistance has been recognized for many years and will be considered in greater detail in subsequent sections of this chapter.

Pulmonary venous pressure must be sightly higher than, but for practical purposes can be regarded as equal to, left atrial pressure. Left atrial pressure is normally higher than right atrial pressure, a condition that accompanies the increase in pul-

Table 6–1. COMPARISON OF PULMONARY AND SYSTEMIC HEMODYNAMIC VARIABLES DURING REST AND EXERCISE OF MODERATE SEVERITY IN NORMAL ADULT MAN

Condition	Rest (sitting)	Exercise
Oxygen consumption	300	2000 ml/min
Blood flow		
Cardiac output	6.3	16.2 L/min
Heart rate	70	135 beats/min
Stroke volume	90	120 ml/beat
Intravascular pressures		
Pulmonary arterial pressure	20/10	30/11 mm Hg
Mean	14	20 mm Hg
Left atrial pressure, mean	5	10 mm Hg
Brachial arterial pressure	120/70	155/78 mm Hg
Mean	88	112 mm Hg
Right atrial pressure, mean	3	1 mm Hg
Resistances		
Pulmonary vascular resistance	1.43	0.62 units*
Systemic vascular resistance	13.5	6.9 units*

*Units = mm Hg/L/min.

monary blood flow at birth and serves to close the foramen ovale. Knowledge of pulmonary venous and left atrial pressure values is essential to an assessment of the pulmonary circulation, but it is technically more difficult to measure pressures within the left atrium than pressures within the right heart chambers and pulmonary arterial circulation during cardiac catheterization. This presented a serious practical limitation to studies of the pulmonary circulation until it was learned that "wedge" pressures from an accessible pulmonary artery were almost identical with simultaneously measured pressures from the left atrium.[3]

A wedge pressure is obtained by occluding blood flow through a branch of the pulmonary artery by either wedging the end of a cardiac catheter or inflating a balloon surrounding the catheter in the vessel. Pressures recorded from the tip of the catheter under conditions of "no flow" reflect the pressure downstream within the vascular network at the site of the next freely communicating channels, i.e., pulmonary capillaries or small pulmonary veins.

The fact that wedge pressures from the pulmonary artery and left atrial pressures are nearly the same means that the decrease in pressure along the entire pulmonary venous system is very small. It is also recognized that pulmonary arterial end-diastolic pressure in normal subjects and in patients without lung disease provides a close approximation of their wedge pressure. This correspondence occurs because the total pressure difference across the lungs is normally small and because the pressure difference will be least at the end of diastole, when blood flow through the pulmonary circulation is lower than at any other instant during the cardiac cycle. This relationship, however, is *not* maintained in the presence of disorders of the pulmonary circulation, and, therefore, this method should not be used as a substitute for more accurate techniques of wedge pressure recording in patients with any form of lung disease.[4]

Pulmonary arterial and wedge pressures can now easily be measured outside the cardiac catheterization laboratory through the use of specially designed flexible catheters that can be "floated" through the venous system and right heart into the pulmonary circulation.[5] This technique is being widely and routinely applied to studies of the pulmonary circulation in both healthy subjects and seriously ill patients.

Distribution of Pulmonary Blood Flow

Soon after the technique of cardiac catheterization was introduced and direct measurements of pulmonary arterial pressures became available, Dock[6] suggested that the distribution of blood flow within the lungs must be uneven because the pulmonary circulation is a low-pressure system that is operating in a gravitational field. He also speculated that the presence of uneven blood flow would create important differences between regions of the lung in their local defense capabilities and adequacy of gas exchange. Fifteen years later, the development of radioactive gas techniques for assessing the distribution of pulmonary blood flow provided convincing confirmation of Dock's theory.

Regional pulmonary blood flow can be measured using radioactive tracers, whose uptake, release, or retention is a reflection of blood flow and whose presence can be detected by external counting. (1) Radiolabeled CO_2 ($C^{15}O_2$) was the first substance to be used to study the distribution of blood flow in the pulmonary circulation.[7] Its suitability depends upon monitoring the disappearance of an inhaled gas whose uptake from alveoli is determined by the blood flow to them. Because the indicator gas is breathed into the lungs, a region must be ventilated before perfusion to the region can be detected by diffusion of $C^{15}O_2$ into the bloodstream. (2) Radioactive, insoluble gases (such as ^{133}Xe) can be used to identify gas-filled alveoli that are perfused by pulmonary capillary blood.[8] A small amount of tracer gas dissolved in saline is injected intravenously, and as the blood containing the injectate flows through the lungs, the gas, because of its low solubility, diffuses from the blood into neighboring air-containing spaces; hence, the presence of radioactivity signifies perfusion of gas-filled alveoli in a given region. (3) Radiolabeled particles (such as ^{99m}Tc-labeled macroaggregated albumin), prepared at an appropriate size to be trapped within small pulmonary blood vessels during an attempted passage through the pulmonary circulation after intravenous injection, will be retained in and can be detected over perfused regions of the lungs.[9]

Thus each of these techniques differs from the others in how regional blood flow is detected: $C^{15}O_2$ depends on a ventilated pathway to reach the pulmonary circulation, ^{133}Xe depends on perfusion of gas-filled alveoli into which it can escape, and ^{99m}Tc-macroaggregates depend solely on patent vascular channels in which the tiny emboli finally impact.

Each of the procedures described has its advantages and disadvantages, but all have yielded similar evidence concerning the presence of a vertical gradient of blood flow from the top to the bottom of the lung. The topographic gradient of blood flow is determined by hydrostatic pressure differences in the pulmonary circulation caused by gravity and not, as is the case within the regional distribution of ventilation, by the vertical gradient of intrapleural pressure.* The difference between the factors affecting the distribution of ventilation on the one hand and the distribution of blood flow on the other can easily be demonstrated by studies performed with isolated lungs or open-chest animals; in these preparations, the vertical gradient of intrapleural pressure is abolished, but that due to hydrostatic pressure remains.

The importance of hydrostatic pressure differences is shown schematically in Figure 6–1. In the diagram, alveolar pressure is set realistically and for convenience at 0 cm H_2O; the importance of changes in alveolar pressure is considered below. It can be seen in Figure 6–1 that pulmonary arterial pressure, reflected by the height of the black column in the manometer, is insufficient to cause blood to rise all the way to the apex of the (schematic) lung in the upright position. The column of blood will rise in the lung as well as in the manometer to the level at which the pressure at the top of the column equals alveolar pressure; in other words, to a pressure of 0 cm H_2O in this model. At 5 cm below the top of the column the perfusion pressure is 5 cm H_2O, and at

15 cm below the top of the column, the perfusion pressure is 15 cm H_2O. Because the effect of hydrostatic pressure increases in a downward direction, more blood will perfuse a region 15 cm below the "top" of pulmonary arterial pressure than a region 5 cm below the top. Therefore, inflow pressure to any region of the lung is determined by the maximum pressure within the pulmonary artery, which determines the height to which blood will rise in the lungs (or in the manometer, as illustrated) and by how far the given region is below this level.

On the basis of these considerations, Dock[6] predicted and West and coworkers[7, 11] demonstrated that the topographic distribution of perfusion must be affected by the level of pulmonary artery pressure in relation to the total vertical dimensions of the lung. This explains why the apex of the lung receives less blood flow than the base in the upright position and why, at a constant pulmonary arterial pressure, the lung is more evenly perfused in the recumbent than in the upright position.

Figure 6–1 also demonstrates an important relationship between the pulmonary venous (or outflow) pressure and the distribution of blood within the lung. Pulmonary venous pressure is customarily low (see Table 6–1), and its hydrostatic effect, therefore, is to support a column of venous blood that reaches only part of the way up the total vertical height of the lung. As illustrated, the black column, like that on the inflow side, will also rise to the level within the lung and manometer, at which the pressure at the top of the column equals alveolar pressure. Below this level, the hydrostatic effect of venous pressure becomes increasingly great and will cause those vessels exposed to its influence either to open or to dilate, or both. Conversely, the amount of blood flow to the lung above the level at which venous pressure equals alveolar pressure is not influenced by (i.e., is out of "reach" of) venous pressure.

Alveolar pressure was deliberately assigned a value of zero in Figure 6–1, but it can be visualized that if alveolar pressure were changed, it would displace the column of blood a corresponding amount in the lung but not in the two manometers. For example, if alveolar pressure were plus 10 cm H_2O and inflow and outflow pressures were unchanged, as might occur through the application of positive end-expiratory pressure

*Gravity, in fact, contributes to the vertical gradient of pleural pressure by affecting the weight of the lungs (large animals) or the shape of the chest wall (small animals). However, in the intact thorax, the magnitude of the difference in pleural surface pressure from top to bottom of the lungs is much less than the difference in hydrostatic pressure.

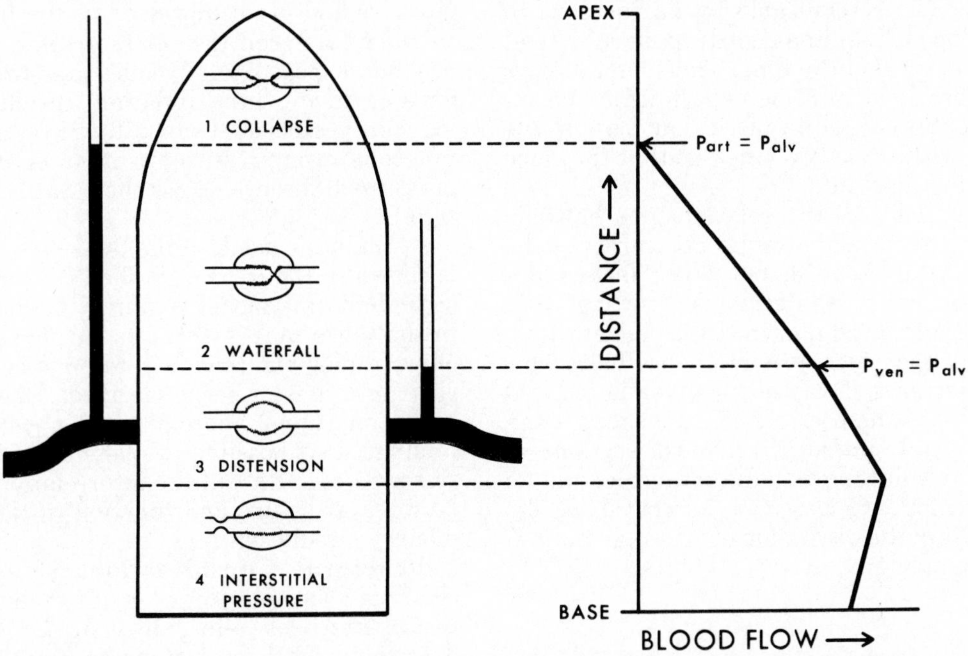

Figure 6–1. Schematic representation of the four zones of the lung in which different hemodynamic conditions govern blood flow. Alveolar pressure (Palv) is assumed to be 0; the heights of the black columns on the left and right of the lung represent the magnitude of pulmonary arterial (Part) and pulmonary venous (Pven) pressures, respectively. For discussion, see text (Adapted and reprinted by permission from Hughes, J. M. et al.: Effect of lung volume on the distribution of pulmonary blood flow in man. Respir. Physol., *4*:58–72, 1968.)

(PEEP), the profile of blood flow shown in the right-hand panel of Figure 6–1 would be displaced downward 10 cm, and the lungs accordingly would be perfused less completely.

These descriptions should suffice to show that all three pressures, pulmonary arterial, pulmonary venous, and alveolar, govern the distribution of blood in the lungs. The relationships among these pressures have been employed to subdivide the lung, as shown in Figure 6–1, into four zones with differing conditions of blood flow.

1. In *Zone 1,* alveolar pressure (P_{alv}) exceeds both pulmonary arterial (P_{PA}) and venous (P_{PV}) pressures ($P_{alv} > P_{PA} > P_{PV}$). There is no blood flow to this region because inflow pressure is everywhere lower than alveolar pressure.

2. In *Zone 2,* pulmonary arterial pressure exceeds alveolar pressure, but alveolar pressure exceeds pulmonary venous pressure ($P_{PA} > P_{alv} > P_{PV}$). In this region, blood flow increases progressively down the lung from the level of no flow ($P_{PA} = P_{alv}$) to the level at which alveolar and pulmonary venous pressures are equal ($P_{alv} = P_{PV}$). Because the effect of venous pressure is not transmitted to Zone 2, the resistance to blood flow through the zone is determined by the pressure difference from pulmonary artery to alveolus. This condition has been likened to a "sluice" or "waterfall" and can be simulated by a Starling resistor.[12, 13]

3. In *Zone 3,* pulmonary arterial pressure exceeds pulmonary venous pressure and pulmonary venous pressure exceeds alveolar pressure ($P_{PA} > P_{PV} > P_{alv}$). Resistance to blood flow in this region is determined by the pressure difference from pulmonary artery to pulmonary vein. Because this difference remains constant throughout Zone 3, at first glance there seems to be no reason for blood flow to increase below the level at which pulmonary venous and alveolar pressures are equal ($P_{PV} = P_{alv}$). However, the transmural distending pressure across the vessel wall increases with distance down the zone because pulmonary arterial and venous pressures both increase while alveolar pressure remains constant. The progressively increasing distending force alters the geometry of the intervening vascular pathways and lowers the resistance to blood flow through them.

In Figure 6–1, the junction between Zones

2 and 3 is recognizable by an increase in the slope of the line depicting blood flow at a given level of the lung. This is not always the case, and in some experiments the incremental change in blood flow may be the same within the two zones, so that the slope remains constant.

4. In *Zone 4,* the relationships between intravascular and alveolar pressures are the same as in Zone 3, but other factors are present that cause vascular narrowing.[10] Resistance to blood flow in the dependent lung regions may increase, and hence blood flow will decrease if vascular caliber is reduced because of the possible effects of increasing interstitial pressure (see next section) or local alveolar hypoxia (if airways leading to the region are closed or narrowed, as described in the discussion of "closing volume" in Chapter 4).

"Alveolar" and "Extraalveolar" Vessels

The model shown in Figure 6–1 certainly provides the best explanation that is currently available for the varying patterns of pulmonary blood flow observed in humans and experimental animals under physiologic and pathologic conditions. However, the applicability of the model depends upon the behavior of two distinct sets of blood vessels within the pulmonary circulation, which are differentiated by their perivascular pressures and their responses to lung inflation. (1) *Alveolar vessels* are exposed to alveolar

pressure and are compressed as the lung is inflated; (2) in contrast, *extraalveolar vessels* are not exposed to alveolar pressure and expand during lung inflation. In addition, alveolar vessels offer virtually no resistance to a collapsing pressure; in other words, the pressure difference across their walls is negligible.

A schematic model of the two set of vessels is shown in Figure 6–2. It should be emphasized that this model is purely operational in the sense that it accounts for physiologic observations but that its anatomic boundaries have never been specified. However, based on recent anatomic and physiologic findings, it is possible to make some tentative predictions about the interrelationships between structure and function in the pulmonary circulation.

Structural Considerations. It seems clear that extraalveolar vessels include arteries, arterioles, veins, and venules.[14] These diverse anatomic structures have one thing in common: a perivascular interstitial space surrounded by a connective tissue sheath that, as already pointed out (Chapter 2), accompanies the vessels deep into the terminal respiratory unit(s) they supply or drain. Moreover, recent measurements with micropipettes inserted into the perivascular interstitial spaces near the hilus have revealed pressures that are slightly more negative than pleural pressure and become even more so as the lungs are inflated.[15] Thus by definition, these vessels are extraalveolar because they are exposed to a pressure that differs from alveolar pressure and because the vessels expand during inflation owing to

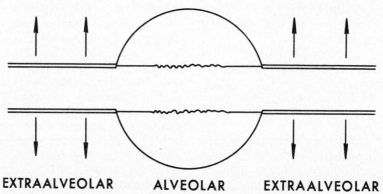

EXTRAALVEOLAR   ALVEOLAR   EXTRAALVEOLAR

Figure 6–2. Schematic representation of extraalveolar and alveolar vessels. The pressure surrounding extraalveolar vessels (arrows) is approximately the same as pleural pressure. In contrast, the pressure surrounding alveolar vessels is approximately the same as alveolar pressure. In addition, extraalveolar vessels are thick walled and resist collapse, whereas alveolar vessels are thin walled and readily collapsible. (Adapted and reprinted by permission from Hughes, J. M. et al.: Effect of lung volume on the distribution of pulmonary blood flow in man. Respir. Physiol., 4:58–72, 1968.)

the negative perivascular distending pressure (with respect to pleural pressure).

Of all the vessels that are exposed to alveolar pressure and that are compressed as the lungs inflate, the pulmonary capillaries seem the most obvious. But the transition from extraalveolar vessels to alveolar vessels is not clear-cut, and the results of morphometric studies have led to a somewhat confusing picture. Part of the confusion is related to methods of fixation in that the microcirculation looks completely different in lungs that are fixed through the airways compared with those that are fixed through the vasculature; also, the extent of lung inflation is extremely important (see Fig. 2–28). The careful morphometric studies by Gil and coworkers[16, 17] of the lungs of rodents fixed by vascular perfusion revealed pleats in the interalveolar septa near alveolar corners (i.e., where the walls of adjacent alveoli meet), which were formed by various degrees of infolding of the alveolar walls. Folds may also occur in the walls of the septa away from the corners. The pattern of folding is such that the cell nuclei and connective tissue elements are displaced inward away from the surface facing the alveolus, which is thereby composed almost exclusively of the thin portions of the septum.[18] In this manner, gas exchange capabilities are maintained even if the septum becomes folded. The pleats are a variable feature; they are more numerous at low lung volumes and seem to unfold as lung volume is increased. The extent of pleating may also be affected by the arteriovenous pressure difference across the local capillary network.

Folding of the interalveolar septa helps to explain the elusive *corner vessels,* a term that applies to those vessels in which red blood cells can be seen and through which blood presumably flows in regions of lung under Zone 1 conditions. These vessels were first described in the corners formed by the junctions of three alveolar septa, a location where the vessels are protected from (i.e., their perivascular pressure is less than) the prevailing alveolar pressure because of the small radius of curvature and the strong inward recoil of the overlying film of surfactant.[19] Recent morphologic evidence suggests that the corner vessels are located within the pleats that may occur in the interalveolar septa. Thus, when the septa are pleated to form corner vessels, the en-

folded capillaries are extraalveolar vessels in the sense that they are not exposed to alveolar pressure. However, when the septa unfold, the same capillaries become alveolar vessels because their surrounding pressure must now be much closer to the pressure in the neighboring alveoli.

Functional Considerations. When lungs of experimental animals are frozen and fixed under varying conditions of pulmonary arterial, venous, and alveolar pressures, the resultant histologic appearance reveals how perfusion probably takes place during life. Examination of the lungs prepared under Zone 1 conditions revealed that, except for corner vessels, few vessels with a diameter less than 30 μm contained red blood cells, few capillaries were open, and the interalveolar septa were thin. More red blood cells were evident in the capillaries of lungs studied under Zone 2 conditions; filling of the septum was patchy near the top but became more complete near the bottom of the zone. Even more red blood cells were evident in Zone 3, and the width of the capillaries increased substantially. These findings were interpreted as showing that when inflow and outflow hydrostatic pressures progressively increase, there is at first recruitment and then distention of pulmonary capillaries.[19] Somewhat different conclusions were reached from the results of other studies, which indicated that recruitment was the predominant mechanism throughout the lungs.[20]

In either case, the phenomenon of recruitment has led to a model of the pulmonary capillary circulation as a network of branching vessels, some of which may be perfused and others not, depending on the prevailing conditions. This model contrasts sharply with the concept of sheet-flow proposed by Fung and Sobin,[21] in which recruitment is impossible. In the model of sheet-flow, the microcirculation is depicted as a broad sheet lined on both sides by endothelium and bridged by regularly arranged endothelium-lined posts.

According to Gil,[14] it is now possible to reconcile some of the apparent structure-function inconsistencies. Based on morphometric observations, the limited number of probable capillary configurations is illustrated in Figure 6–3. Type A depicts the original histologic findings described by Glazier and coworkers[19] in Zone 1 and also

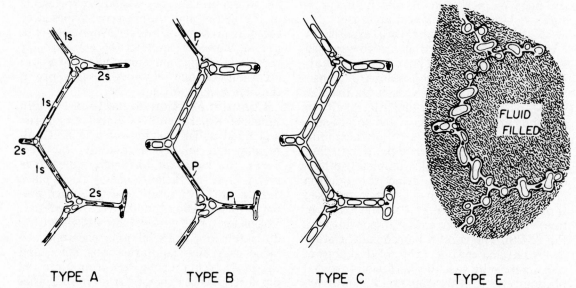

TYPE A   TYPE B   TYPE C   TYPE E

Figure 6–3. Simplified schematic representations of four types of capillary configurations described in the literature. As shown in type A, 1s are primary septa placed between different ducts; 2s are secondary septa placed between alveoli open to the same duct. On type B, P points at patches of closed septal capillaries. Corner pleats in real histologic specimens are usually larger. At this magnification level, the smoothness of the alveolar surface (particularly on type C) is exaggerated. Air-filled surfaces show no bumps except under connective tissue condensations, but gentle changes of curvature can occur. Type E is the configuration seen in flooded alveoli without a normal surfactant lining. (From Gil, J.: Organization of microcirculation of the lung. Ann. Rev. Physiol., 42:177–186, 1980. Reproduced, with permission, from the Annual Reviews Inc.)

includes the more recent notion that the corner vessels, the only obviously open parts of the capillary network, are inside septal pleats. Type B represents Zone 2, in which there is patchy capillary filling; some pleats are present but others have gone, and where there are pleats the corner vessels persist. Type C illustrates Zone 3, in which all the capillaries are filled; the septa have thickened, and corner vessels are rare; this configuration also conforms to the sheet-flow model.[21] For contrast, Type E displays the appearance of the capillary network in a lung fixed through the airways, and shows that the luminal surface is corrugated because the capillaries, no longer constrained by the interfacial forces of surfactant, are free to bulge into the alveolar spaces; it is easy to visualize how misleading notions about the geometry of the microcirculation could come from lungs fixed in such a manner.

Another point deserves reemphasis. Most of the information just discussed came from experiments in animals other than humans. Many more studies need to be carried out in humans to provide a clearer picture of the structure-function relationships of the human pulmonary microcirculation.

Total Interstitial Pressures

Both alveolar and extraalveolar vessels are surrounded by a perivascular space, but, as indicated, the pressures in the two interstitial compartments are different. The customary practice of referring to "tissue pressure" or to "interstitial pressure" is no longer tenable. Guyton and associates[22] have emphasized that the total pressure applied to a tissue surface is the sum of the liquid pressure (from the force of kinetic bombardment of the surface by molecules of the liquid) and the solid pressure (from the force attributable to actual points of contact between the surface and neighboring solid structures), so that

Total interstitial pressure =
    interstitial liquid pressure +
        interstitial solid pressure.   (1)

These concepts have been applied to the local factors that contribute to total interstitial pressures surrounding alveolar and extraalveolar vessels and are shown schematically in Figures 6–4 and 6–5.[23] In both examples, a force exists that favors liquid absorption from within the perivascular

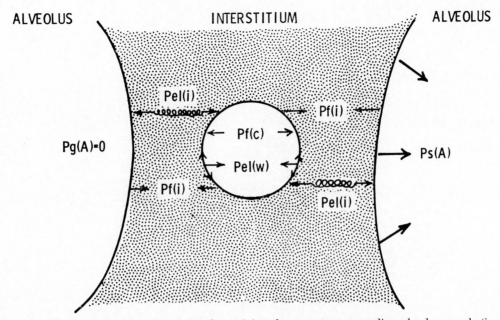

Figure 6–4. Schematic diagram of the forces determining the pressure surrounding *alveolar* vessels (i.e., total pericapillary pressure in the interstitium of the interalveolar septum). The arrows indicate the direction of action but not the magnitude of the pressures acting on the alveolar and capillary membranes. Pg(A) = alveolar gas pressure; Ps(A) = pressure arising from tension in the alveolar membrane (mainly surface tension); Pel (i) = solid elastic pressure arising from packing together of the solid elements in the interstitium; Pf(i) = fluid pressure in interstitial liquid; Pf(c) = fluid pressure in pulmonary capillaries; Pel(w) = pressure arising from elastic tension due to stretching of the capillary wall (assumes no active tension). The net balance of these forces is believed to result in a pericapillary pressure slightly less than alveolar pressure. For discussion, see text. (Reprinted by permission from Hughes, J. M.: Pulmonary interstitial pressure. Bull. Eur. Physiopathol. Respir., 7:1095–1123, 1971.)

space into the bloodstream; the absorptive force is due to the fact that colloid osmotic (oncotic) pressure exceeds the hydrostatic pressure within the blood vessel. Accordingly, liquid is absorbed from the interstitial space until the pressure generated by packing the solid tissue elements is sufficient to resist further absorption, and equilibrium is attained.

The difference between total interstitial pressures around alveolar and extraalveolar vessels is accounted for by the different lung structures that determine the point of equilibrium. For alveolar vessels (see Fig. 6–4), the balance occurs across the alveolar membrane (including the surfactant layer) and the capillary membrane. It is believed that pericapillary total interstitial pressure is less than alveolar pressure by an amount determined by alveolar surface forces. Calculations, both from presumed values of geometry and surface tension and from data from animal experiments, suggest that pericapillary total interstitial pressure ranges from 0 to minus 3 to 5 cm H_2O.[24, 25]

For extraalveolar vessels (see Fig. 6–5), the balance of forces that affect perivascular total interstitial pressure operates across the perivascular sheath that is attached to the lung parenchyma; consequently, the pressure on the alveolar side of the membrane (i.e., opposite the blood vessel lumen) is determined by the elastic recoil of the lung. Because elastic recoil pressure is equal and opposite to pleural pressure, it can be appreciated why extraalveolar perivascular total interstitial pressure is nearly the same as pleural pressure. Moreover, as mentioned in the case of conducting airways, the pressure surrounding extraalveolar vessels is believed to be at least as negative as and probably slightly more negative than pleural pressure; the increment of additional negativity is related to the extent to which the vessels do not follow the expansion of the remainder of the lung.[26] This phenomenon can also be visualized from Figure 6–5. During lung inflation, elastic recoil and the outward "pull" on the perivascular sheath increase; if the blood vessel

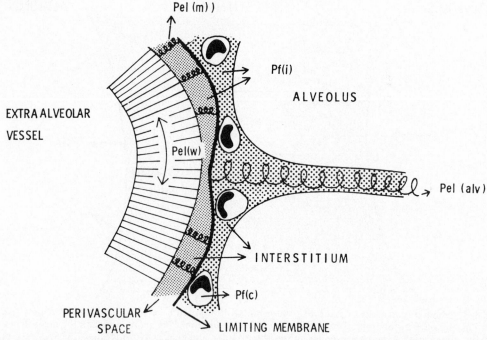

Figure 6–5. Schematic diagram of the forces determining the pressure surrounding *extraalveolar* vessels (i.e., perivascular interstitial pressure). Abbreviations as in Figure 6–4. Absorption of interstitial liquid from the perivascular space proceeds until deformation of the solid elements creates an elastic recoil pressure of the limiting membrane (i.e., the perivascular connective tissue sheath) itself [Pel(m)]. The limiting membrane is also exposed to the elastic recoil pressure of the alveolar parenchyma [Pel(alv)] generated by expansion of the lung. The net balance of these forces is believed to result in a pressure in the perivascular space slightly less than pleural pressure. (See Chapter 4 for discussion of the relationship between pleural pressure and elastic recoil pressure of the lung parenchyma.) (Reprinted by permission from Hughes, J. M.: Pulmonary interstitial pressure. Bull. Eur. Physiopathol. Respir., 7:1095–1123, 1971.)

wall resists this pull, the total interstitial pressure becomes more negative than if the vessel enlarged in proportion to the increase in lung volume. These predictions have been validated through direct measurements with micropipettes of perivenous interstitial fluid pressures near the hilus. This pressure is only slightly more negative than pleural surface pressure at low lung volumes, but the difference between the two pressures widens as lung volume is increased.[15] When intravascular pressure is high to begin with, the vessels are more rigid, so that lung volume has less influence on vascular caliber and perivascular pressure.[27]

Because the interstitial spaces throughout the lung are continuous, it follows that there must be a hydrostatic gradient of interstitial liquid pressure of 1 cm H_2O for every 1 cm of vertical distance in the lung. However, it is generally assumed that total interstitial pressure at any level within the lung is not affected by gravity, because any change in interstitial liquid pressure is offset by an

equal and opposite change in interstitial solid pressure. However, in pathologic disorders associated with pulmonary edema, the separation of tissue elements by the excess liquid accumulation nullifies the effect of solid pressures; under these conditions, a vertical hydrostatic gradient of total interstitial pressure can be demonstrated.[23]

Effects of Lung Inflation

Figure 6–6 shows the results of mean regional blood flow measurements at different lung volumes in seated normal subjects. It can be seen that the vertical gradient of blood flow is most evident when measured at TLC and that the gradient is reversed when measurements are made at RV. These variations cannot be explained by changes in the relationships among pulmonary arterial, pulmonary venous, and left atrial pressures, which presumably remained relatively constant during the study, but are

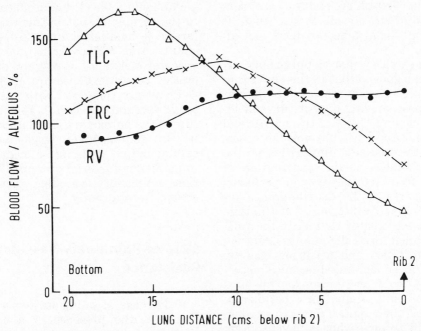

Figure 6–6. Blood flow per alveolus as a percentage of that expected if all alveoli were perfused equally, plotted against vertical distance from the bottom of the lung to the second rib. Points represent the mean values of both right and left lungs of subjects studied at total lung capacity (TLC), functional residual capacity (FRC), and residual volume (RV). Note the reduction in blood flow to the bottom of the lung that is more marked at FRC and RV than TLC. (Reprinted by permission from Hughes, J. M. et al.: Effect of lung volume on the distribution of pulmonary blood flow in man. Respir. Physiol., 4:58–72, 1968.)

believed to result from the influence of lung expansion on total interstitial pressure and on the caliber of extraalveolar vessels.[10] In addition, as stated previously, closure of airways in dependent regions, especially at low lung volumes, creates local alveolar hypoxia; this may cause, in turn, regional arterial vasoconstriction that also contributes to the redistribution of blood flow away from the involved areas.

At RV, the entire parenchyma is compressed, and total interstitial pressure is increased sufficiently to influence the topographic distribution of blood flow throughout the entire lung. At FRC, the upper half of the lung is expanded more than the lower half, which still demonstrates the effect of raised total interstitial pressure. When the lung is fully expanded to TLC, the only region where total interstitial pressure is still high enough to affect the caliber of extraalveolar vessels and to reduce blood flow is a small area at the bottom of the lung.

Stratification of Blood Flow

Although the distribution of pulmonary blood flow is governed chiefly by the transmural distending pressure and the distensibility of the vessel wall, other mechanisms can be detected as well. Morphometric studies of the pulmonary circulation leave no doubt that there is considerable variation in the length of available pathways from the main pulmonary artery to the terminal respiratory units; this must lead to different transit times for red blood cells traveling between the pulmonary valve and gas exchange units in various locations throughout the lung. In one carefully studied human lung specimen, it was found that the length of the pulmonary arteries from pulmonary valve to branches on the order of 50 μm in diameter averaged about 14 cm, with a range of 7 to 23 cm.[28] Thus, variation occurs between one distal unit and another. There is, moreover, variation within a single terminal respiratory unit; incoming blood

reaches the first-order respiratory bronchioles and their alveoli sooner than it
reaches more distal alveolar ducts and alveolar sacs.

The branching system of pulmonary arteries is analogous to that in the airways in
which the presence of pathways of different
lengths causes varying transit times of inhaled gas moving between the mouth and
the alveoli. And the physiologic consequences of the anatomic similarities are the
same: unevenness of the distribution of
blood flow from stratification of perfusion
and unevenness of the distribution of inspired air from stratification of ventilation.
It might be anticipated that since the variations in transit times affect the distribution
of both ventilation and perfusion, gas exchange might be facilitated because matching of the two is maintained. This is a
difficult problem to study, but experimental
data suggest that, contrary to expectation,
gas exchange is worse when both ventilation
and perfusion are stratified than when only
blood flow is unevenly distributed.[29]

PULMONARY VASCULAR RESISTANCE

Resistance to blood flow through the pulmonary circulation is calculated using the
same general equation for frictional resistance described on page 94. As before, the
flow resistance offered by a system is computed from the pressure difference "across"
the system and the flow through it. Pulmonary vascular resistance (PVR) is traditionally determined by the inflow pressure in
the pulmonary artery, the outflow pressure
in the pulmonary veins or left atrium (P_{LA}),
and the blood flow through the lungs (pulmonary blood flow), according to the equation:

$$\text{PVR, units} = \frac{P_{PA} - P_{LA}, \text{mmHg}}{\text{pulmonary blood flow, L/min}}. \quad (2)$$

However, as might be anticipated, because of the zonal distribution of inflow and
outflow pressures, this equation provides
only a global expression of numerous dis-
parate events. The effect of height has already been alluded to, and its effect on
pulmonary vascular resistances is considered subsequently.

Pulmonary blood flow is normally equal
to the cardiac output but at times may be
larger or smaller if intracardiac or other
shunts exist. Values for normal pulmonary
vascular resistance at rest and during moderately severe exercise are given in Table
6–1 and are compared with values of systemic vascular resistance. The striking feature of the pulmonary circulation is its ability to accommodate large increases in
cardiac output with only a modest increase
in pulmonary arterial pressure. This means
that pulmonary vascular resistance decreases substantially.

Sites of Pulmonary Vascular Resistance

A decrease of pulmonary vascular resistance, in the presence of a constant or
slightly increased pulmonary arteriovenous
pressure difference, indicates that the cross-
sectional area of those vessels that are the
principal sites of resistance to blood flow
must increase. Recent findings have helped
to localize these sites, at least in one experimental model. Furthermore, the new observations have reinforced the long-standing
belief that, in contrast with the systemic
circulation in which resistance to blood flow
through capillaries is a small fraction of the
total systemic vascular resistance, a substantial portion of the total pulmonary vascular resistance in dogs resides in capillaries—34 per cent in one study[30] and 53 per
cent in another.[31]

An important advance in our knowledge
concerning the distributions of pressures
and vascular resistances in the pulmonary
circulation was recently made by Bhattacharya and Staub,[32] who measured microvascular pressures with micropipettes in an
isolated perfused dog lung. The profile of
the distribution of vascular resistance under
Zone 3 conditions is shown in Figure 6–7.
Note that the large resistance (46 per cent)
lies in the capillaries of the alveolar septum,
most of the remainder is in arterioles (20 to
50 μm in diameter), and there is negligible
resistance from venules (20 μm in diameter)
to pulmonary veins. Further analysis of
these data suggests that they apply to the
lungs as a whole and could be compatible
with either network or sheet-flow models of
the microcirculation.[33]

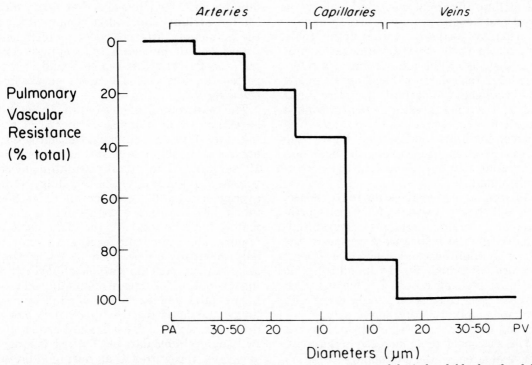

Figure 6–7. Profile of vascular resistance (pressure drop) in various segments of the isolated, blood-perfused dog lung under zone III conditions. The ordinate represents per cent resistance from zero in the pulmonary artery (PA) to 100 per cent in the pulmonary vein (PV). Most of the resistance lies within the microcirculation, as expected. The largest single resistance is in the alveolar wall capillaries (46 per cent of total). (Reprinted by permission from Bhattacharya, J., and Staub, N. C.: Direct measurements of microvascular pressures in the isolated perfused dog lung. Science, *210:*327–328, 1980. Copyright 1980 by the American Association for the Advancement of Science.)

Because the major pressure drop of blood flowing through the pulmonary circulation occurs across the pulmonary capillaries, it is prudent to examine how the vessels behave under dynamic conditions. The pattern of filling in the pulmonary capillary bed has been examined because it was reasoned that if recruitment were determined by the opening of a previously closed small artery, all capillaries in the region supplied by that artery would be filled with blood. This would lead to a "patchwork" pattern of filling in Zone 2 because all arteries would not open simultaneously, but owing to variations in their critical opening pressures, some would be open and some would remain closed at a given level of pressure in the lung.[34] It was discovered, however, that capillary recruitment did not vary from one arteriolar "domain" to another but that changes occurred within the network supplied by a single arteriole; this was revealed by finding red blood cells in some capillaries of an interalveolar septum while adjacent capillaries were empty. Under Zone 3 conditions, all capillaries in a given septum were filled. The random filling of capillaries in a net-

work under Zone 2 conditions suggests that the pressure drop across a single channel of the network must be small and that hemodynamic changes occurring in one part of the segment probably affect those in neighboring segments. Thus, unstable flow conditions, which help to account for the intermittency of pulmonary capillary flow that has been observed directly in many experimental preparations, are created. From these studies, it is apparent that no simple relationship exists between the pressure acting from one end of the capillary network to the other and the morphometric appearance of the capillaries. Gil[14] has postulated the existence of low-resistance channels ("preferential paths") in the septa separating adjacent alveolar ducts, with the capillaries of the interalveolar septa serving as collateral vessels.

Effects of Lung Height

The normal adult human lung has a height of about 25 cm in the vertical position at FRC, of which about 15 cm lies above the left atrium. If normal mean pulmonary arterial and venous pressures are 19 and 11 cm H_2O, respectively (values from Table 6–1, converted to cm H_2O), one can appreciate that, using the left atrium as a reference level, the column of blood on the inflow side is sufficient to perfuse the entire lungs and that outflow pressure creates Zone 3 conditions up to about two-thirds of the way between the hilus and the apex. Most of the lungs, therefore, are in Zone 3; there is a small Zone 2 and no Zone 1 in the normal adult human.

As cardiac output rises during exercise, both pulmonary arterial and venous pressures also rise (see Table 6–1). Overall pulmonary vascular resistance decreases as the relatively high vascular resistance Zone 2 becomes converted, finally in entirety, to the lower resistance Zone 3.[35] For practical purposes this conversion should recruit all available capillaries and apply a high distending pressure to most of them. The net result is a considerable increase in the cross-sectional area of the pulmonary capillary bed and a consequent lowering of local vascular resistance, because, as stated, the capillaries offer most of the resistance to blood flow through the pulmonary circulation.

Pulmonary Blood Volume

It is not widely appreciated that the pulmonary arteries and arterioles differ from the bronchi and bronchioles, with which they travel in close relationship, in that the cross-sectional area of the vessels *decreases* rather than increases moving from the hilus toward the periphery of the lung. This fact is implicit in the data of Bhattacharya and Staub,[32] which shows that an appreciable proportion of total pulmonary vascular resistance resides in arteries 20 to 50 μm in diameter (see Fig. 6–7). The difference between vessels and airways is explained by the branching pattern of arteries in which the two daughter branches each have a smaller diameter than the corresponding bronchial branches. A corollary of this observation is that most of the intraarterial blood volume is contained in the large central elastic arteries and not in the small peripheral muscular branches.[36] Veins behave similarly but contain, surprisingly, even less blood than the arteries; this is because the pulmonary venous system ter-

minates with the four veins that empty into the left atrium. Thus, when compared with the pulmonary arterial system, which continues to a single vessel, the two most central venous branches, which would be expected to contain the most blood, are "missing."[37]

The total volume of blood in the lungs can be estimated in humans by means of the indicator dilution technique. Normal values are about 295 ml/m^2 body surface, or roughly 10 per cent of the total circulating blood volume.[38] Accordingly, the two lungs of an average-sized adult man contain about 500 ml of blood, which accounts for approximately half the total weight of the excised organs. The pulmonary capillaries contain only about 75 ml of blood in the resting state but can accommodate much more during exercise. The mean maximum pulmonary capillary blood volume of adult human lungs calculated from morphometric measurements is 213 ± 31 (standard error) ml.[1] Although reliable data are limited, it is now generally recognized that during exercise total pulmonary blood volume tends to remain constant, and increases of more than 20 per cent seldom occur despite marked increases in cardiac output. These findings, taken in concert with the observation that pulmonary vascular resistance decreases during exercise, mean either that there is a redistribution of intrapulmonary blood volume from large vessels into the capillaries, or that the small increase in total vascular volume that does occur is entirely taken up by the capillaries, or both. The constancy of pulmonary blood volume was also shown in other experiments in which total circulating blood volume was expanded and cardiac output increased.[38]

Pulmonary Vascular Distensibility

The observations just cited, which emphasize the stability of pulmonary blood volume, may seem at first glance to conflict with reports that emphasize the distensibility of the pulmonary vascular bed. It is known, for example, that nearly 70 per cent of the right ventricular stroke volume is retained in pulmonary arteries during systole for distribution to the pulmonary capillaries during the ensuing diastole.[39] Although the "storage capacity" is affected by changes in heart rate and pulmonary arterial pressure, its presence appears to belie statements about the constancy of pulmonary blood volume.

This apparent paradox can be explained by the fact that measurements of pulmonary blood volume by the conventional method, the indicator dilution technique (multiplying mean transit time by the blood flow through the pulmonary circulation), eliminate variations in volume during a single heartbeat. Thus, in any given segment of the pulmonary circulation the volume varies from moment to moment during the cardiac cycle, but when averaged over several beats, the volume in the entire pulmonary vascular bed tends to remain constant despite changing cardiac output.

Accommodation of blood during systole and its release during the subsequent diastole means that the pulmonary arterial system is pulsatile, a feature that has been recognized for decades through the use of fluoroscopy. It is now known from studies performed with the body plethysmograph that blood flow through the pulmonary capillaries is also pulsatile,[40] and other experimental data demonstrated that venous blood flow is pulsatile as well, reflecting the trans-

mission of pulsations through "open" arteries and capillaries into the veins.[41] Figure 6–8 shows examples of the pulse wave characteristics of pulmonary capillaries and pulmonary veins. The transmission of pulse waves through the pulmonary circulation depends on the characteristics of the blood vessel walls and on the frequency of the impulses (determined by heart rate).[42] Pulmonary vasoconstriction induced by drugs (e.g., serotonin) or hypoxia in experimental animals has been shown to produce a decrease in arterial distensibility and, as expected, an increase in pulse wave velocity.[39]

In humans, pulmonary blood volume does not change in proportion to total circulating blood volume when total volume is increased or decreased;[37] this constancy indicates that changes in pulmonary vasomotor tone must occur. In addition, similar experiments in which autonomic blocking drugs were used provide convincing evidence that the distensibility of the pulmonary circulation is regulated by neurogenic stimuli that operate to keep blood volume in the lungs constant, within fairly narrow limits.[43] Thus, factors seem to be acting to prevent "overloading" of the pulmonary circulation; if this assump-

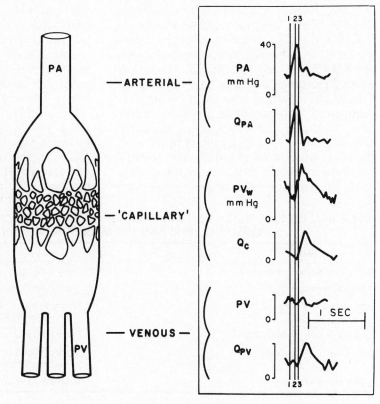

Figure 6–8. Schematic diagram showing the transformation of the pressure and flow pulses from the pulmonary artery to the pulmonary vein. PA = pulmonary arterial pressure; Q_{PA} = pulmonary arterial flow; PV_w = pulmonary venous wedge pressure; Q_c = pulmonary capillary flow; PV = pulmonary venous pressure; Q_{PV} = pulmonary venous flow. The interval 1–2 is the transmission time (0.09 sec) for the pulse from the pulmonary artery to capillaries; the interval 2–3 is the transmission time (0.03 sec) from the capillaries to pulmonary veins. (Reprinted by permission from Morkin, E. et al.: Pattern of blood flow in the pulmonary veins of the dog. J. Appl. Physiol., 20:1118–1128, 1965.)

tion is correct, these mechanisms can be considered "protective," and if they are deficient or overwhelmed, pulmonary vascular congestion may develop.

Factors Affecting Vascular Resistance

A logical extension of the considerations analyzed in previous sections is that total pulmonary vascular resistance is determined by the interaction of several different mechanisms. These can be conveniently divided into *passive* (Table 6–2) and *active* (Table 6–3) influences. Alterations in resistance from a "passive" process indicate that changes in the caliber of pulmonary blood vessels are secondary responses to changing mechanical conditions within the lungs or to hemodynamic events in the systemic circulation. In contrast, alterations in pulmonary vascular resistance from an "active" process imply that contraction or relaxation of the smooth muscles of blood vessel walls has occurred in response to neural, humoral, or chemical stimuli.

Two points should be stressed about interpretation of studies that have attempted to discover the mechanisms underlying any induced changes in pulmonary vascular resistance. First, the investigation must have included measurements of left atrial pressure, or a suitable substitute, such as wedge pressure, before any meaningful conclusions about resistance changes can be reached. This is an important constraint because the pulmonary arteriovenous pressure difference is small, and changes in left atrial pressure have a considerable influence on the calculated value of pulmonary vascular resistance. Second, it is impossible to demonstrate conclusively active pulmonary

vasoconstriction or vasodilatation in the presence of changing conditions that also cause passive alterations in the caliber of the vessels. (An exception to this occurs if the vasomotor responses are opposite to and prevail over those from associated passive variations.)

Passive Changes in Vascular Resistance

Included in Table 6–2 are six factors that, when changed, cause secondary changes in pulmonary vascular resistance by imposing a passive increase or decrease in the caliber of blood vessels. Changing one mechanical variable in the respiratory system frequently causes changes in another variable; for example, increasing left atrial pressure or alveolar pressure causes an increase in pulmonary arterial pressure and pleural pressure, respectively. For this reason, in order to study the effects of variations of a single factor, it is necessary (although difficult experimentally) to hold all other factors constant. It is obvious that these rigorous requirements cannot be met in a study of human pulmonary circulation, so most of the available evidence has been derived from studies of isolated lungs from experimental animals. Despite this limitation, there is good reason to believe that the general conclusions from these studies describe the behavior of pulmonary blood vessels in humans.

Pulmonary Arterial Pressure. As pulmonary arterial pressure is raised (either by raising the height of a perfusion reservoir or by increasing flow), with lung volume and left atrial pressure held constant, pulmonary vascular resistance decreases.[44] The

Table 6–2. FACTORS THAT WHEN VARIED CAUSE "PASSIVE" CHANGES IN PULMONARY VASCULAR RESISTANCE (PVR) AND THE DIRECTION OF THE RESPONSES

Factor	Response
Pulmonary arterial pressure (P_{PA})	Increased P_{PA} causes decreased PVR
Left atrial pressure (P_{LA})	Increased P_{LA} causes decreased PVR
Transpulmonary pressure (P_l)	Increase and decrease of P_l from value at FRC cause increased PVR
Total interstitial pressure (P_{Is})	Increased P_{Is} causes increased PVR
Pulmonary blood volume	Shift of blood from systemic vessels into lung vessels causes decreased PVR
Whole blood viscosity	Increase in viscosity causes increased PVR

Table 6–3. IMPORTANT CAUSES OF "ACTIVE" CHANGES IN PULMONARY VASCULAR RESISTANCE (PVR) AND THE DIRECTION OF THE RESPONSES

Factor	Response
Neurogenic Stimuli	
Sympathetic stimulation	Increases PVR in experimental animals; no effect in humans
Parasympathetic stimulation	Decreases PVR in experimental animals with preexisting vasoconstriction; no effect in humans
Humoral Substances	
Norepinephrine, serotonin, histamine, angiotensin, fibrinopeptides, prostaglandin $F_{2\alpha}$	Vasoconstriction; serotonin has no effect in humans
Acetylcholine, bradykinin, prostaglandin E_1, prostacyclin (prostaglandin I_2)	Vasodilatation; bradykinin affects humans with pulmonary hypertension
Chemical Stimuli	
Alveolar hypoxia	Increases PVR
Alveolar hypercarbia	Increases PVR in experimental animals; no effect in humans
Acidemia (decreased pH)	Increases PVR

increase in inflow pressure causes an increase in transmural distending pressure, which, by increasing the cross-sectional areas of the pulmonary arterial system and capillary network through dilatation and recruitment, decreases resistance to blood flow. As shown in Figure 6–9, the effect of changing pulmonary arterial pressure on pulmonary vascular resistance is lessened when left atrial pressure is high to begin with, because this maneuver separately dilates and recruits pulmonary blood vessels.[45]

Left Atrial Pressure. When left atrial pressure is raised, and pulmonary arterial pressure and lung volume are kept constant, pulmonary vascular resistance decreases, as shown in Figure 6–10. As might be expected from the relationships between pulmonary arterial and left atrial pressures, the effect of changing left atrial pressure on pulmonary vascular resistance diminishes if pulmonary arterial pressure is high at the outset.[44] Similarly, the effect on vascular resistance is augmented if pulmonary arterial pressure is allowed to increase as left atrial pressure is raised, a circumstance more closely resembling normal relationships then a change in left atrial pressure alone.

Transpulmonary Pressure. A distinction has already been made between alveolar vessels and extraalveolar vessels on the basis of the different pressures surrounding the two "types" of vascular channels and how they respond to inflation of the lungs.

In fact, the reason alveolar and extraalveolar vessels behave oppositely during inflation is linked to the differences in prevailing perivascular pressures (see earlier section on Total Interstitial Pressures). As the lungs are inflated, the interstitial pressure around extraalveolar vessels becomes more negative relative to pleural pressure and exerts a force that serves to distend the vessels.[46] In contrast, alveolar vessels are exposed to external mechanical forces during inflation that cause them to lengthen and to flatten. Accordingly, as shown schematically in Figure 6–11, the resistance offered by alveolar and extraalveolar vessels changes in opposite directions during inflation of the lung from RV to TLC.[47]

At low lung volumes, the relatively weak perivascular distending pressure and the kinking that occurs as extraalveolar vessels shorten increase resistance to flow through them; as lung volume increases, kinking disappears and distending pressure increases. At high lung volumes, although extraalveolar vessels are maximally dilated but lengthened, alveolar vessels are stretched and flattened and thus offer increased resistance to blood flow. The curves shown in Figure 6–11 must be regarded as speculative, because it appears as though there are considerable differences among species in the behavior of the pulmonary circulation during lung inflation. In contrast to the lungs of dogs, in which arteries distend as excised lobes are inflated,[46] intact

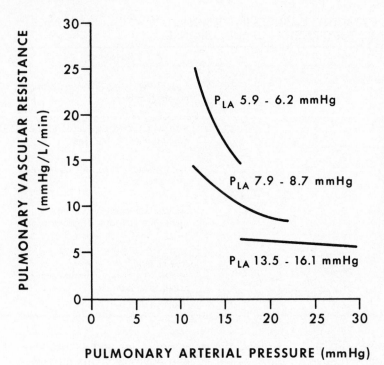

Figure 6–9. Diagrammatic representation of the results of perfusion experiments showing the effects of changes in pulmonary arterial pressure on pulmonary vascular resistance at three different ranges of left atrial pressure (P_{LA}). As pulmonary arterial pressure is increased, pulmonary vascular resistance decreases; but the effect progressively lessens as left atrial pressure is raised. (Adapted from Borst, H. G. et al.: Influence of pulmonary arterial and left atrial pressures on pulmonary vascular resistance. Circ. Res., 4:393–399, 1956 by permission of the American Heart Association, Inc.)

Figure 6–10. Diagrammatic representation of the results of perfusion experiments showing the effects of changes in left atrial pressure on pulmonary vascular resistance at two different values of transpulmonary pressure (P_1); pulmonary arterial pressure (P_{PA}) was held constant at 26 mm Hg throughout. As left atrial pressure is increased, pulmonary vascular resistance decreases. The influence of transpulmonary pressure is explained by the effects of lung inflation on pulmonary vascular resistance (see text and Fig. 6–11). (Adapted and reprinted by permission from Roos, A. et al.: Pulmonary vascular resistance as determined by lung inflation and vascular pressures. J. Appl. Physiol., 16:77–84, 1961.)

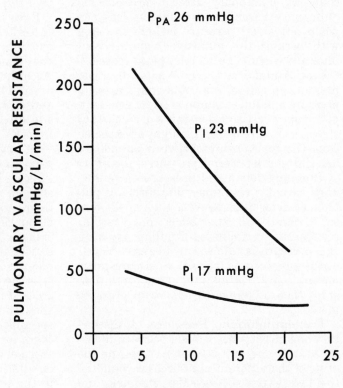

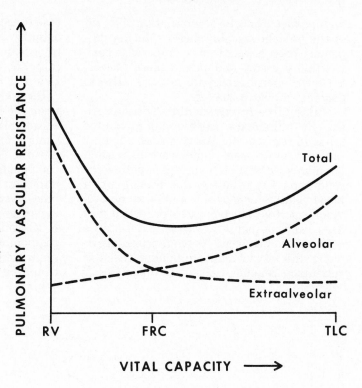

Figure 6–11. Schematic representation of the effects of changes in vital capacity on total pulmonary vascular resistance and the contributions to the total afforded by alveolar and extraaveolar vessels. During inflation from residual volume (RV) to total lung capacity (TLC), resistance to blood flow through alveolar vessels increases, whereas resistance through extraalveolar vessels decreases. Thus changes in total pulmonary vascular resistance form a U-shaped curve during lung inflation, with the nadir at functional residual capacity (FRC).

sheep lungs and excised human lungs (at high intravascular pressure) demonstrate vascular narrowing during inflation.[48, 49] The diagram accurately reflects, however, the belief that total pulmonary vascular resistance is minimal at FRC and that both increases and decreases in lung volume from the resting position are associated with increased resistance to blood flow. The magnitude of the changes depicted is arguable.

Much of the uncertainty about the actual *in vivo* effects of inflation on pulmonary vascular resistance comes from studies of isolated perfused lungs or lobes inflated either by positive pressure applied to the airways or by negative pressure applied around the lung. As Permutt[50] rightly emphasized, neither experimental model accurately simulates the events that occur with normal breathing. During an ordinary inspiration, pulmonary arterial pressure increases relative to pleural pressure and maintains its relationship to alveolar pressure; this behavior is simulated in negative pressure experiments. In contrast, during a natural breath, left atrial pressure decreases in concert with pleural pressure, conditions that occur during positive pressure experiments.[35] Analysis in humans of

the effects of breathing on pulmonary vascular resistance is further complicated by changes in cardiac output.

Perivascular Pressure. All vessels have pressure applied to their outside walls, and as indicated earlier, the perivascular (total interstitial) pressure differs between the two "types" of pulmonary blood vessels. Perivascular pressure surrounding alveolar vessels is normally the same or slightly lower than alveolar pressure, owing to the retractive force created by the film of surfactant that lines alveolar walls and the radius of curvature of the surface. Where the septa are flat, the effect on underlying capillaries is negligible. If surface tension rises, so does the inward "pull" of the film, and the pericapillary pressure will become more negative. This phenomenon lowers resistance to blood flow through alveolar vessels, but it also has important implications for the movement of liquid and solute (see Chapter 12). The total interstitial pressure surrounding extraalveolar vessels is normally a little less than pleural pressure, and it becomes even lower as lung volumes are increased. Total interstitial pressure around extraalveolar vessels is increased at low lung volumes for reasons already discussed. One might expect that the accumulation of liquid in the bronchovascular sheaths during pulmonary edema would serve to increase perivascular pressure and narrow blood vessels. However, morphometric data have failed to demonstrate such changes.[51]

Pulmonary Intravascular Volume. Although pulmonary intravascular volume tends to remain relatively constant, it may increase or decrease under certain normal circumstances and in a variety of pathologic conditions. Regardless of the mechanism, if blood volume increases, it must distend previously perfused blood vessels or recruit new ones, and pulmonary vascular resistance will tend to decrease. As emphasized previously, the fall in total pulmonary vascular resistance depends upon how much (local) resistance decreases in those vessels that actually increase their cross-sectional area to accommodate the extra volume; changes in pulmonary capillary dimensions are particularly important.

Blood Viscosity. Blood viscosity depends upon the intravascular hematocrit ratio, the characteristics of red blood cells (especially their deformability), and the composition of plasma. Although measurement of these components presents difficulty and the contribution of blood viscosity to total pulmonary vascular resistance is hard to assess, experimental evidence is now available (Fig. 6–12) that demonstrates that an increase in pulmonary vascular resistance accompanies an increase in blood viscosity induced by changing hematocrit ratio.[52, 53]

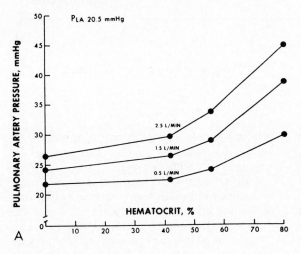

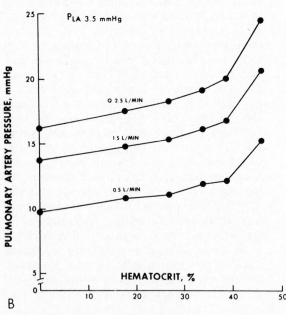

Figure 6–12. Experimental results showing the effect of changes in hematocrit on the pulmonary arterial pressure required to produce a given blood flow. Left atrial pressure (P_{LA}) was constant at 20.5 mm Hg in *A* and 3.5 mm Hg in *B*. As hematocrit increases, progressively more pressure is required to overcome the contribution of increasing blood viscosity to resistance to blood flow. (Reprinted by permission from Murray, J. F. et al.: Viscosity effects on pressure-flow relations and vascular resistance in dogs' lungs. J. Appl. Physiol., *27*:336–341, 1969.)

Active Changes
in Vascular Resistance

Table 6–3 lists the chief neurogenic, humoral, and chemical causes of active pulmonary vasomotor reactions. But in view of the difficulties inherent in designing suitable experiments, it is not surprising that considerable doubt still exists about the mechanism of action of numerous common physiologic or pharmacologic stimuli.

Neurogenic Stimuli. Pulmonary arteries and, to a lesser extent, veins are innervated with nerve fibers from the sympathetic trunks and the vagus nerves. Despite the presence of a definite vascular nervous plexus, which (as a first assumption) must have functional significance, it has been extremely difficult to document vasomotor response to electrical stimulation of either sympathetic or parasympathetic pathways in experimental animals. Furthermore, inferences from this approach do not necessarily apply to neuromotor control under more natural conditons. Studies in dogs have demonstrated that sympathetic nerve stimulation increased pulmonary arterial tone and pulse wave transmission through the circulation;[54] although no vasoconstriction was evident in these experiments, recent investigations, using different methods, revealed a vasoconstrictor response.[55] The consensus concerning stellate ganglion (sympathetic) stimulation is that it increases both pulmonary arterial wall stiffness and calculated vascular resistance, although the latter effect is smaller and less consistent.[56]

More recent studies of the effects of vagal nerve stimulation in the cat indicate that the nerve contains both sympathetic and parasympathetic efferent fibers that innervate the pulmonary vascular bed.[57] Through the use of appropriate blocking drugs, it has been shown that stimulation of the sympathetic fibers in the vagus caused vasoconstriction, whereas stimulation of the parasympathetic fibers caused vasodilation; a vasodilator response could only be elicited when some degree of vasocontriction was already present. Intrathoracic nerve stimulation experiments are obviously impossible to carry out in humans. However, studies with neurogenic blocking drugs have been performed and have led to the conclusion that the autonomic nervous system exerts little or no control over the pulmonary circulation in the normal human adult.[58]

Humoral Agents. Several naturally occurring humoral agents are thought to initiate either vasoconstrictor or vasodilator responses from different segments of the pulmonary vascular bed. Most of this information was derived from studies of animals that were given large doses of the test substance. Because it is well known that drugs have different effects in different species and that the action may be dose dependent, some reservation is always necessary in translating the results from animal studies into inferences about the regulation of the human pulmonary circulation. Within these limitations, it is believed that several humoral substances exert vasomotor control over the pulmonary circulation.[59] Among the vasoconstrictors are catecholamines, angiotensin, histamine, prostaglandin $F_{2\alpha}$, and fibrinopeptides; among the vasodilators are isoproterenol, prostacyclin, and acetylcholine (only in an already constricted vascular bed). Serotonin produces unequivocal vasoconstriction in experimental animals but not in humans.

The results of studies with various pharmacologic agents indicate that pulmonary blood vessels have receptors for neurotransmitters (alpha and beta agonists, acetylcholine) that appear to have functions independent of autonomic nervous system activity.[59] But the roles of these receptors, as well as those of a variety of other vasoactive substances in the control of the pulmonary circulation in health and disease, are totally speculative.

Chemical Substances. Of all the ways in which the pulmonary circulation can be made to dilate or constrict, the arterial vasoconstriction that follows exposure to alveolar hypoxia is the most physiologically relevant and convincing. Yet we still do not know how the reaction is mediated. Because the response occurs in the isolated lung, functional neurohumoral mechanisms are not required, and the vasoconstriction appears to be produced locally.[60] However, recent evidence suggests that the sympathetic nervous system may also contribute to the total response in intact animals.[61] The reaction depends upon the P_{O_2} in the alveolus and, to a much lesser extent, on that in the bloodstream.[62] These observations have led to extensive investigation of the mechanisms that cause pulmonary arteries to constrict in response to alveolar hypoxia. There is suggestive but inconclusive evidence in favor of a locally generated chemical media-

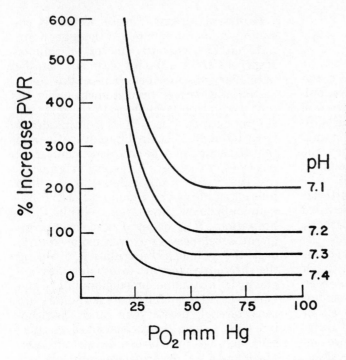

Figure 6–13. Diagram of the average results from experiments in newborn calves showing the effect of changes in inspired P_{O_2} on pulmonary vascular resistance (PVR) under conditions of different arterial blood pH. As inspired P_{O_2} is decreased, pulmonary vascular resistance increases; this effect becomes exaggerated and occurs at progressively higher P_{O_2} values as pH is decreased. (Reprinted by permission from Rudolph, A. M., and Yuan, S.: Response of the pulmonary vasculature to hypoxia and H⁺ ion concentration changes. J. Clin. Invest., *45*:399–411, 1966.)

tor, histamine being the leading candidate, or a direct action of hypoxia on pulmonary vascular smooth muscle.[63]

Several studies in humans[64] and experimental animals[65] have documented the synergistic interrelationship between the effects of alveolar hypoxia and acidosis on pulmonary vascular resistance. As shown in Figure 6–13, the influence of hypoxia becomes progressively greater as arterial pH is lowered. At the present time it is impossible to say what, if any, direct effect CO_2 has on the pulmonary circulation. In studies in humans its influence was trivial.[66] Because an increase or decrease in [H⁺] causes a respective increase or decrease in pulmonary vascular resistance, it is likely that any effects of changes in alveolar or blood P_{CO_2} will be mediated in large part by the corresponding changes in pH.

Many endogenous vasoactive hormones have been synthesized and are available as drugs. Most of the naturally occurring agents identified previously have been given to humans and have elicited the responses indicated. Other pulmonary vasoconstrictors are metaraminol, phenylephrine, and bretylium tosylate. Among the vasodilators are isoproterenol, dopamine, hydralazine, diazoxide, phentolamine, and tolazoline (for reference, see the review by Bergofsky[59]). These drugs are being increasingly used in the treatment of patients with pulmonary

vascular disorders, but they should only be given under carefully controlled conditions because the hemodynamic consequences are unpredictable and dangerous; in most instances, vasodilation of systemic blood vessels precedes and outweighs any effect on the pulmonary circulation.

REFERENCES

1. Gehr, P., Bachofen, M., Weibel, E. R.: The normal human lung: ultrastructure and morphometric estimation of diffusing capacity. Respir. Physiol., *32*:121–140, 1978.
2. Heinemann, H. O., and Fishman, A. P.: Nonrespiratory functions of mammalian lung. Physiol. Rev., *49*:1–47, 1969.
3. Hellems, H. K., Haynes, F. W., and Dexter, L.: Pulmonary "capillary" pressure in man. J. Appl. Physiol., *2*:24–29, 1949.
4. Jenkins, B. S., Bradley, R. D., and Branthwaite, M. A.: Evaluation of pulmonary arterial end-diastolic pressure as an indirect estimate of left atrial mean pressure. Circulation, *42*:75–78, 1970.
5. Swan, H. J. C., Ganz, W., Forrester, J., Marcus, H., Diamond, G., and Chonette, D.: Catheterization of the heart in man with use of a flow-directed balloon-tipped catheter. New Engl. J. Med., *283*:447–451, 1970.
6. Dock, W.: Apical localization of phthisis. Its significance in treatment by prolonged rest in bed. Am. Rev. Tuberc., *53*:297–305, 1946.
7. West, J. B., and Dollery, C. T.: Distribution of blood flow and ventilation-perfusion ratio in the lung, measured with radioactive CO_2. J. Appl. Physiol., *15*:405–410, 1969.

8. Ball, W. C., Jr., Stewart, P. B., Newsham, L. G. S., and Bates, D. V.: Regional pulmonary function studied with xenon. J. Clin. Invest., *41*:519–531, 1962.

9. Wagner, H. N., Jr., Sabiston, D. C., Jr., Iio, M., McAfee, J. G., Meyer, J. K., and Langan, J. K.: Regional pulmonary blood flow in man by radiois-otope scanning. JAMA, *187*:601–603, 1964.

10. Hughes, J. M. B., Glazier, J. B., Maloney, J. E., and West, J. B.: Effect of lung volume on the distribution of pulmonary blood flow in man. Respir. Physiol., *4*:58–72, 1968.

11. West, J. B., Dollery, C. T., and Naimark, A.: Distribution of blood flow in isolated lung; relation to vascular and alveolar pressures. J. Appl. Physiol., *19*:713–724, 1964.

12. Banister, J., and Torrance, R. W.: The effects of the tracheal pressure upon flow: pressure relations in the vascular bed of isolated lungs. Quart. J. Exp. Physiol., *45*:352–367, 1960.

13. Permutt, S., Bromberger-Barnea, B., and Bane, H. N.: Alveolar pressure, pulmonary venous pressure, and the vascular waterfall. Med. Thorac., *19*:239–260, 1962.

14. Gil, J.: Organization of microcirculation of the lung. Annu. Rev. Physiol., *42*:177–186, 1980.

15. Lai-Fook, S. J.: Perivascular interstitial fluid pressure measured by miropipettes in isolated dog lung. J. Appl. Physiol., *52*:9–15, 1982.

16. Gil, J.: Morphologic aspects of alveolar microcir-culation. Fed. Proc., *37*:2462–2465, 1978.

17. Gil, J., Bachofen, H., Gehr, P., and Weibel, E. R.: The alveolar volume to surface area relationship in air- and saline-filled lungs by vascular perfusion. J. Appl. Physiol., *47*:990–1001, 1979.

18. Weibel, E. R., Untersee, P., Gil, J., and Zulauf, M.: Morphometric estimation of pulmonary diffusing capacity. IV. Effect of varying positive pressure inflation of air spaces. Respir. Physiol., *18*:285–308, 1973.

19. Glazier, J. B., Hughes, J. M. B., Maloney, J. E., and West, J. B.: Measurements of capillary dimen-sions and blood volume in rapidly frozen lungs. J. Appl. Physiol., *26*:65–76, 1969.

20. Maseri, A., Caldini, P., Harward, P., Joshi, R. C., Permutt, S., and Zierler, K. L.: Determinants of pulmonary vascular volume. Recruitment versus distensibility. Circ. Res., *31*:218–228, 1972.

21. Fung, Y. C., and Sobin, S. S.: Pulmonary alveolar blood flow. Circ. Res., *30*:470–490, 1972.

22 Guyton, A. C., Granger, H. J., and Taylor, A. E.: Interstitial fluid pressure. Physiol. Rev., *51*:527–563, 1971.

23. Hughes, J. M.: Pulmonary interstitial pressure. Bull. Eur. Physiopathol. Respir., 7:1095–1123, 1971.

24. Bruderman, I., Somers, K., Hamilton, W. K., Tooley, W. H., and Butler, J.: Effect of surface tension in circulation in the excised lungs of dogs. J. Appl. Physiol., *19*:707–712, 1964.

25. Staub, N. C.: Pulmonary edema. Physiol. Rev., *54*:678–811, 1974.

26. Mead, J., Takishima, T., and Leith, D.: Stress distribution in lungs: a model of pulmonary elas-ticity. J. Appl. Physiol., *28*:596–608, 1970.

27. Lai-Fook, S. J.: A continuum mechanics analysis of pulmonary vascular interdependence in isolated dog lobes. J. Appl. Physiol., *46*:419–429, 1979.

28. Cumming, G., Henderson, R., Horsfield, K., and Singhal, S. S.: The functional morphology of the pulmonary circulation. *In* Fishman, A. P., and Hecht, H. H. (eds.): The Pulmonary Circulation and Interstitial Space. Chicago, University of Chi-cago Press, 1969, pp. 327–340.

29. West, J. B., Maloney, J. E., and Castle, B. L.: Effect of stratified inequality of blood flow on gas ex-change in liquid-filled lungs. J. Appl. Physiol., *32*:357–361, 1972.

30. Brody, J. S., Stemmeler, E. J., and DuBois, A. B.: Longitudinal distribution of vascular resistance in the pulmonary arteries, capillaries, and veins. J. Clin. Invest., *47*:783–799, 1968.

31. Schleier, J.: Der Energieverbrauch in der Blut-bahn. Pflügers Arch. Gesamte Physiol., *173*:172–204, 1919.

32. Bhattacharya, J., and Staub, N. C.: Direct meas-urements of microvascular pressures in the isolated perfused dog lung. Science, *210*:327–328, 1980.

33. Overholser, K. A., Bhattacharya, J., and Staub, N. C.: Microvascular pressure in the isolated, perfused dog lung: comparison between theory and meas-urement. Microvasc. Res., *23*:67–76, 1982.

34. Warrell, D. A., Evans, J. W., Clarke, R. O., Kin-gaby, G. P., and West, J. B.: Pattern of filling in the pulmonary capillary bed. J. Appl. Physiol., *32*:346–356, 1972.

35. Culver, B. H., and Butler, J.: Mechanical influences on the pulmonary circulation. Annu. Rev. Physiol., *42*:187–198, 1980.

36. Singhal, S., Henderson, R., Horsfield, K., Harding, K., and Cumming, G.: Morphometry of the human pulmonary arterial tree. Circ. Res., *33*:190–194, 1973.

37. Horsfield, K., and Gordon, W. I.: Morphometry of pulmonary veins in man. Lung, *159*:211–218, 1981.

38. De Freitas, F. M., Faraco, E. Z., deAzevedo, D. F., Zaduchliver, J., and Lewin, T.: Behavior of normal pulmonary circulation during changes of total blood volume in man. J. Clin. Invest., *44*:366–378, 1965.

39. Lee, G. de J.: Regulation of the pulmonary circu-lation. Br. Heart J., *33*(Suppl.):15–26, 1971.

40. Lee, G. de J., and DuBois, A. B.: Pulmonary cap-illary blood flow in man. J. Clin. Invest., *34*:1380–1390, 1955.

41. Morkin, E., Collins, J. A., Goldman, H. S., and Fishman, A. P.: Pattern of blood flow in the pul-monary veins of the dog. J. Appl. Physiol., *20*:1118–1128, 1965.

42. Maloney, J. E., Bergel, D. H., Glazier, J. B., Hughes, J. M. B., and West, J. B.: Transmission of pulsatile blood pressure and flow through the iso-lated lung. Circ. Res., *23*:11–24, 1968.

43. Guintini, C., Maseri, A., and Bianchi, R.: Pulmo-nary vascular distensibility and lung compliance as modified by dextran infusion and subsequent atropine injection in normal subjects. J. Clin. In-vest., *45*:1770–1789, 1966.

44. Roos, A., Thomas, L. J., Jr., Nagel, E. L., and Prommas, D. C.: Pulmonary vascular resistance as determined by lung inflation and vascular pres-sures. J. Appl. Physiol., *16*:77–84, 1961.

45. Borst, H. G., McGregor, M., Whittenberger, J. L., and Berglund, E.: Influence of pulmonary arterial and left atrial pressures on pulmonary vascular resistance. Circ. Res., *4*:393–399, 1956.

46. Benjamin, J. J., Murtagh, P. S., Proctor, D. F., Menkes, H. A., and Permutt, S.: Pulmonary vas-cular interdependence in excised dog lobes. J. Appl. Physiol., *37*:887–894, 1974.

47. Howell, J. B. L., Permutt, S., Proctor, D. F., and Riley, R. L.: Effect of inflation of the lung on different parts of pulmonary vascular bed. J. Appl. Physiol., 16:71–76, 1961.

48. Maloney, J. E., Cannata, J., and Ritchie, B. C.: The influence of transpulmonary pressure on the diameter of small arterial blood vessels in the lung. Microvasc. Res., 11:57–66, 1976.

49. Kalk, J., Benjamin, J. J., Comite, H., Hutchins, G., Traystman, R., and Menkes, H. A.: Vascular interdependence in postmortem human lungs. Am. Rev. Respir. Dis., 112:505–511, 1975.

50. Permutt, S.: Mechanical influences on water accumulation in the lungs. In Fishman, A. P., and Renkin, E. M. (eds.): Pulmonary Edema. Bethesda, MD, American Physiological Society, 1979, pp. 174–194.

51. Ritchie, B. C., Shauberger, G., and Staub, N. C.: Inadequacy of perivascular edema hypothesis to account for the distribution of pulmonary blood flow in lung edema. Circ. Res., 24:807–814, 1969.

52. Murray, J. F., Karp, R. B., and Nadel, J. A.: Viscosity effects on pressure-flow relations and vascular resistance in dogs' lungs. J. Appl. Physiol., 27:336–341, 1969.

53. Buceus, D., and Pain, M. C. F.: Influence of hematocrit, blood gas tensions, and pH on pressure-flow relations in the isolated canine lung. Circ. Res., 37:588–596, 1975.

54. Ingram, R. H., Szidon, J. P., Skalak, R., and Fishman, A. P.: Effects of sympathetic nerve stimulation on the pulmonary arterial tree of the isolated lobe perfused in situ. Circ. Res., 22:801–815, 1968.

55. Kadowitz, P. J., and Hyman, A. L.: Effect of sympathetic nerve stimulation on pulmonary vascular resistance in the dog. Circ. Res., 32:221–227, 1973.

56. Dowing, S. E., and Lee, J. C.: Nervous control of the pulmonary circulation. Annu. Rev. Physiol., 42:199–210, 1980.

57. Nandiwada, P. A., Hyman, A. L., and Kadowitz, P. J.: Pulmonary vasodilator response to vagal stimulation and acetylcholine in the cat. Circ. Res., 53:86–95, 1983.

58. Widdicombe, J. G., and Sterling, G. M.: The autonomic nervous system and breathing. Arch. Intern. Med., 126:311–329, 1970.

59. Bergofsky, E. H.: Humoral control of the pulmonary circulation. Annu. Rev. Physiol., 42:221–223, 1980.

60. Glazier, J. B., and Murray, J. F.: Sites of pulmonary vasomotor reactivity in the dog during alveolar hypoxia and histamine infusion. J. Clin. Invest., 50:2550–2558, 1971.

61. Porcelli, R. J., Vian, A. T., Naftchi, N. E., and Bergofsky, E. H.: β-Receptor influence on lung vasoconstrictor responses to hypoxia and humoral agents. J. Appl. Physiol., 43:612–616, 1977.

62. Marshall, C., and Marshall, B.: Site and sensitivity for stimulation of hypoxic pulmonary vasoconstriction. J. Appl. Physiol., 55:711–716, 1983.

63. Fishman, A. P.: Vasomotor regulation of the pulmonary circulation. Annu. Rev. Physiol., 42:211–220, 1980.

64. Harvey, R. M., Enson, Y., Betti, R., Lewis, M. L., Rochester, D. F., and Ferrer, M. I.: Further observations on the effect of hydrogen ion on the pulmonary circulation. Circulation, 35:1019–1027, 1967.

65. Rudolph, A. M., and Yuan, S.: Response of the pulmonary vasculature to hypoxia and H^+ ion concentration changes. J. Clin. Invest., 45:399–411, 1966.

66. Fishman, A. P., Fritts, H. W., Jr., and Cournand, A.: Effects of breathing carbon dioxide upon the pulmonary circulation. Circulation, 22:220–225, 1960.

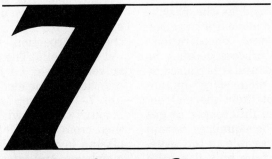

Chapter

Diffusion of Gases, Oxyhemoglobin Equilibrium, and Carbon Dioxide Equilibrium

INTRODUCTION

Diffusion causes O_2 molecules to move from alveolar gas into pulmonary capillary blood and also from peripheral tissue capillary blood into contiguous cells. Movement of CO_2 molecules is also governed by diffusion but is normally in the opposite direction to that of O_2. Both gases undergo chemical reactions in the bloodstream at the start and finish of their journeys between the lungs and the peripheral tissues: O_2 reacts solely with hemoglobin, and CO_2 reacts in part with hemoglobin and in part with water to form HCO_3^-. The reversible chemical reactions between hemoglobin and O_2 and CO_2 are complementary and add considerably to the transport capacity of the blood. This chapter will consider these essential first steps in the process of gas exchange between the inspired air brought into the lungs and distributed through them by ventilation (Chapter 4) and the blood delivered to and removed from the pulmonary capillaries by the circulation (Chapter 6).

163

DIFFUSION

Diffusion can be defined as the passive tendency of molecules to move from a region of higher to one of lower concentration.[1] Diffusion is a passive process because no extra energy is required, and it is caused by molecules moving "by themselves" in random fashion because of their thermal energy; as a consequence, differences in gas concentration tend to be equalized within the various regions accessible to the molecules. Diffusion differs from bulk flow, also known as *convection,* in that there is no net transport of matter but merely a rearranging of those molecules already present that acts to even out differences in gas concentration.

Exchange of O_2 and CO_2 in the lung takes place in three separate steps, each involving diffusion: (1) diffusion of molecules within the gas spaces of the terminal respiratory units, (2) diffusion of O_2 and CO_2 across the air-blood barrier, and (3) diffusion and chemical reaction within the plasma and red blood cells. The anatomic structures involved and the barriers to these steps are indicated in the electron micrograph in Figure 7–1. Oxygen molecules must diffuse through the gas within the alveolar spaces, then cross the air-blood barrier, traverse a plasma layer of variable thickness and the membrane and interior of the red blood cell, and finally combine with hemoglobin.

Gas Phase Diffusion

As indicated in Chapter 4, bulk movement of inspired fresh air proceeds outward in the

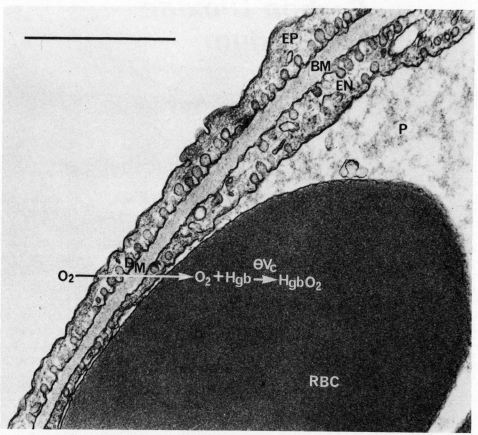

Figure 7–1. Electron micrograph showing the pathway for O_2 diffusion across the air-blood barrier in a human lung. An O_2 molecule must cross the epithelium (EP), basement membrane (BM), endothelium (EN), plasma layer (P), and red blood cell (RBC) membrane; resistance to movement through these barriers comprises the membrane component (D_M) of the total resistance to diffusion. After entering the red blood cell, O_2 must combine chemically with hemoglobin (Hgb); this reaction comprises the resistance imposed by the capillary blood volume (Vc) and rate of chemical combination (Θ). For discussion, see text. Horizontal bar = 1 μm. ($\times$ 41,500. Courtesy of Dr. Ewald R. Weibel.)

tracheobronchial tree to about as far as the alveolar ducts. The rate of movement of the inspirate slows progressively until finally it is so slow that it becomes superseded by movement of individual gas molecules, because of their own kinetic energy. The locations at which convection gives way to diffusion are also those at which large changes in gas composition occur and, accordingly, set the limits for the anatomic dead space of the conducting air passages as originally defined by Fowler[2] (see next Chapter for further details). This transition zone can be shifted proximally or distally by variations in respiratory frequency, lung volume, or gas density. But in all instances, final mixing between newly inspired fresh air and residual gas within the terminal respiratory units takes place by diffusion.

The importance of gas phase diffusion can be illustrated by studying the elimination from the lungs of an inspirate containing both an inert gas, which diffuses rapidly, and a suspension of aerosol particles, 0.5 μm in diameter, which because of their size diffuse much more slowly than the gas.[3] A plot of the concentration at the mouth of two such tracers following a 600 ml inspiration followed by exhalation to RV is shown in Figure 7–2. After the dead space is cleared, the concentration of the diffusible

gas reaches a near plateau throughout all of expiration, whereas the aerosol is completely washed out after 1500 ml have been exhaled. The plateau indicates that gas mixing was virtually complete, and the difference between the two tracers demonstrates that molecular diffusion accounted for the mixing of the gas.

The extent to which equilibration of gas occurs both within and among neighboring terminal respiratory units is a matter of considerable controversy. Proponents of the concept of *stratified inhomogeneity* contend that there is sufficient diffusion limitation within the gas phase to restrict the exchange of respiratory gases.[4] Others believe that sequential filling or emptying is important, whereas still others hold that interaction between convection and diffusion in asymmetrical terminal respiratory units accounts for nonuniformity of alveolar gas concentrations.[5] But regardless of the mechanism, the consensus is clear that during inspiration, concentration gradients of inspired gas extend from the central to the peripheral regions of the terminal respiratory units. How much resistance to uniform mixing contributes to the total resistance to O_2 uptake is arguable, but it may be appreciable. It is also clear that to whatever extent gas phase diffusion is imperfect in

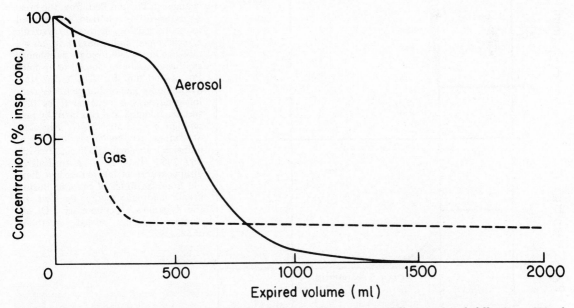

Figure 7–2. Concentration at the mouth of an insoluble gas (He) and a nondiffusing aerosol, following a 600 ml inspiration of each, plotted against expired volume. The 0.5 μm aerosol particles, which trace out convective flow, are absent after 1500 ml of exhalation. In contrast, gas concentration is almost constant until end of expiration. The difference between the two curves shows influence of molecular diffusion. (Reprinted by permission from Muir, D. C. F.: Bulk flow and diffusion in the airways of the lung. Brit. J. Dis. Chest, *60*:169–176, 1966.)

normal lungs, the disturbance is likely to be amplified in the presence of disease.[6]

Membrane Diffusion

As mixed venous blood begins to flow through pulmonary capillaries, the blood becomes exposed to alveolar gas that contains O_2 at a higher concentration and CO_2 at a lower concentration than that which exists within the blood at that moment. Because of the prevailing differences in concentrations, O_2 diffuses from the alveolus into the pulmonary capillary blood and CO_2 diffuses in the opposite direction, as depicted in Figure 7–3. Normally, this exchange takes place rapidly, and equilibrium between the pressures of O_2 and CO_2 within the gas phase and the plasma is achieved in about 0.25 sec. If cardiac output is 6 L/min (100 ml/sec) and pulmonary-capillary blood

volume is 75 ml (see next section), the average transit time for blood to traverse the total capillary network is 0.75 sec. Thus, diffusion equilibrium occurs in about one-third of the time available under resting conditions, and there is substantial reserve to accommodate increases in cardiac output and velocity of blood flow.

Blood Phase Diffusion

The instant that O_2 molecules cross the air-blood barrier and enter the plasma a new concentration difference for O_2 is established between the plasma and the hemoglobin-combining sites within red blood cells. This difference causes O_2 to move through the plasma and across the cell's membrane and within its interior to the sites of chemical reaction with hemoglobin. It was originally believed that the combination between

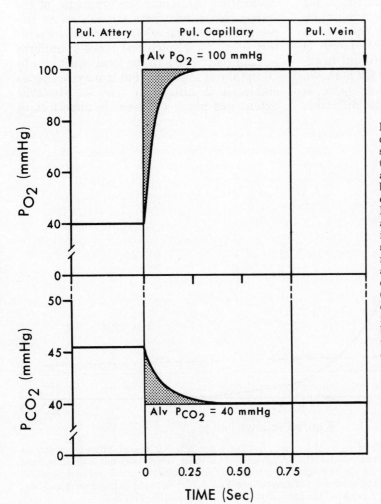

Figure 7–3. Schematic diagram of the changes in Po_2 and Pco_2 from the pressures prevailing in mixed venous blood (pulmonary artery) to those in systemic arterial blood (pulmonary vein) as red blood cells travel through pulmonary capillaries and are exposed to alveolar Po_2 of 100 mm Hg. The mean time available for gas exchange under resting conditions is believed to be 0.75 second. Adapted and reprinted by permission from Staub, N. C.: Alveolar-arterial oxygen tension gradient due to diffusion. J. Appl. Physiol., *18*:673–680, 1963; Hyde, R. W. et al.: Rate of disappearance of labeled carbon dioxide from the lungs of humans during breath holding: a method for studying the dynamics of pulmonary CO_2 exchange. J. Clin. Invest., *47*:1535–1552, 1968.)

O_2 and hemoglobin occurred virtually instantaneously; however, because of the work of Roughton and Forster,[9] it is now known that the reaction rate is finite and imposes a measurable delay on the diffusion process. This knowledge provided the basis for the development of techniques to subdivide the total resistance to diffusion imposed by the structures within the lung into the resistance to the movement of gases afforded by (1) the air-blood barrier, plasma layer, and red blood cell membrane, and (2) the time required for the chemical combination with hemoglobin in the interior of the red blood cell (see later section).

Measurement of Diffusing Capacity

The diffusing capacity of the lung for any gas (DL_G) indicates the quantity of that gas that diffuses across the air-blood barrier per unit time ($\dot{V}_G$) in response to the difference existing between the mean pressure of the gas in alveolar air ($P\bar{A}_G$)and the mean pressure of gas in capillary blood ($P\bar{C}_G$):

$$DL_G = \frac{\dot{V}_G}{P\bar{A}_G - P\bar{C}_G}, ml/min \times mm\ Hg. \quad (1)$$

The quantity of an individual gas that will diffuse in response to a given pressure difference is determined by the solubility and diffusivity of the gas in the alveolar-capillary membrane, the surface area and thickness of the membrane, and in some cases the rate of chemical reaction within the bloodstream. Most inert gases diffuse readily between gas and blood phases, and equilibrium between the concentrations in the alveolar gas and blood is reached rapidly; for example, N_2 achieves 90 per cent equilibration across the air-blood barrier in about 0.005 sec. Therefore, the amount of inert gas that can be taken up or given off by the pulmonary circulation is not detectably limited by the diffusion properties of the lung and its contents but is determined solely by the solubility of the gas and the volume of blood and tissue into which it can dissolve. These phenomena preclude the use of all inert gases for the measurement of pulmonary diffusing capacity but have been used to advantage by employing certain highly soluble gases, such as acetylene or N_2O, to measure effective pulmonary blood flow and

lung tissue volume in experimental animals and humans.[10]

The only two gases that can be used to measure the diffusing capacity of the lung are O_2 and CO. These two gases are suitable test substances because of their unique ability to combine with hemoglobin. Thus, both have to diffuse across the alveolar-capillary membrane in such large quantities to saturate the available hemoglobin at the gas pressure prevailing in the alveoli that it may not be possible for them to reach complete equilibrium before the hemoglobin-containing red blood cells reach the end of their journeys through pulmonary capillaries. A detectable alveolar end-capillary pressure difference for O_2 only exists in normal subjects when they exercise heavily or breathe low O_2 mixtures. However, a difference between gas and blood phases always exists for CO under ordinary testing conditions because the capacity of hemoglobin for CO is so high at very low PCO (100 per cent saturation occurs at about 0.5 mm Hg); also, the pressure difference under ordinary testing conditions and the tissue solubility of CO are very low.

Measurement of pulmonary diffusing capacity for O_2 (DL_{O_2}) is complicated and subject to technical difficulties (especially in patients with lung disease) because, as can be seen from Equation 1, it requires simultaneous assessment of mean alveolar and mean pulmonary capillary PO_2 values. The former can be approximated by direct measurement, but the latter must be derived mathematically using the technique of Bohr integration.[1] In contrast, CO is ideally suited for the measurement of pulmonary diffusing capacity (DL_{CO}) because its affinity for hemoglobin is 200 times that of O_2. When CO is inhaled in low concentrations, all the molecules that enter the red blood cell are bound by hemoglobin, so that for practical purposes the mean capillary PCO is zero. Accordingly, Equation 1 reduces to

$$DL_{CO} = \frac{\dot{V}_{CO}}{P\bar{A}_{CO}}, ml/min \times mm\ Hg. \quad (2)$$

Several methods using CO are available and widely employed to measure pulmonary diffusing capacity; discussions about the advantages and disadvantages of the different techniques are provided in several sources[1, 11, 12] and will not be reviewed here. Although CO and O_2 are used to measure the same process, it should be remembered that there is a considerable reserve available for O_2 diffusion before limitation (i.e., an alveolar end-capillary difference) occurs but that CO diffusion is limited normally and may be even further limited by disease before O_2 uptake becomes impaired. The difference in behavior between O_2 and CO accounts for the fact that DL_{CO} must usually be reduced to less than 45 per cent and less than 65 per cent of predicted values in patients at rest and during exercise, respectively, before diffusion impairment for O_2 causes arterial PO_2 to decrease.[13] (See Chapter 8 for further explanation.) However, tests of DL_{CO} are widely employed and are quite useful in the diagnosis and management of various forms of chronic obstructive pulmonary disease, interstitial pulmonary diseases, and disorders of the pulmonary circulation.[12, 14, 15]

It is theoretically possible to predict DL_{O2} from DL_{CO}, but simultaneous measurements of DL using the two gases reveal that observed DL_{O2} is always considerably less than the value predicted from DL_{CO}.[7] Part of the discrepancy undoubtedly relates to uncertainties about the assumptions that underlie the conversion of DL_{CO} to DL_{O2}. Another part is believed to originate from the random differences in the times individual red blood cells spend traversing pulmonary capillaries; a wide spectrum of exposure times to alveolar gas, and hence regional variations in DL, is implicit in the structure-function models of the alveolar-capillary network that have been developed by several investigators.[16, 17] Although regional differences in diffusing capacity based on variations in blood flow can be inferred from studies such as those cited, it is doubtful whether the changes are of sufficient magnitude to result in an alveolar-arterial PO_2 difference in healthy persons breathing ambient air at sea level. This mechanism becomes greatly exaggerated at high altitudes, where it may have considerable functional importance. The remarkable ascent of Mount Everest (altitude 8848 m) by Messner and Habeler without supplementary O_2 in May 1978 renewed interest in the problem of altitude-induced diffusion limitation across the air-blood barrier of the lungs and led to a computer analysis of the conditions assumed to prevail at the summit.[18] In 1981, to culminate an extraordinary scientific expedition, direct measurements of gas exchange were made on the summit of Mount Everest.

At the highest point on earth, where alveolar PO_2 was 35 mm Hg, diffusion limitation caused a calculated alveolar-end-capillary PO_2 difference of 7 mm Hg.[19]

Components of Diffusing Capacity

Because the solubility and diffusivity of CO and O_2 in the body tissues and fluids are constant physicochemical properties, barring an extraordinary change in the chemical composition of the alveolar-capillary membrane, the major variables affecting the total diffusion resistance ($1/DL$) are (1) the resistance to diffusion of the test gas across the alveolar-capillary membrane, capillary plasma, and red blood cell membrane (the membrane component, $1/DM$) and (2) the resistance to diffusion within the red blood cells imposed by the chemical reaction of the test gas with hemoglobin (the intravascular component, $1/\theta VC$). The second factor derives from the volume of blood in the pulmonary capillary (VC) and the rate (θ) at which the available hemoglobin can combine chemically with the test gas.[9] The total resistance to diffusion can therefore be expressed as the sum of the component resistances:*

$$\frac{1}{DL} = \frac{1}{DM} + \frac{1}{\theta VC}. \quad (3)$$

Equation 3 not only is useful for conceptual purposes but also can be used in studies of patients to solve graphically for values of DM and VC (Fig. 7-4). The principle of the method for subdividing DL into its components depends upon the variations in θ that can be determined *in vitro* in a rapid reaction apparatus by changing the concentrations of O_2 and CO in the test mixture (due to competition between gases for positions in the hemoglobin molecule). Extensive data for θ are limited, especially in pathologic conditions in which the reaction rates may vary. Measurements of DL using gas mixtures similar to those from which θ was measured, and assuming that θ is the same *in vivo* as it is in the reaction chamber,

*If DL, DM, and θVC are viewed as analogues of conductance, a variable that expresses an enhancement of flow, the use of the reciprocal to express their resistances to gas exchange becomes more understandable.

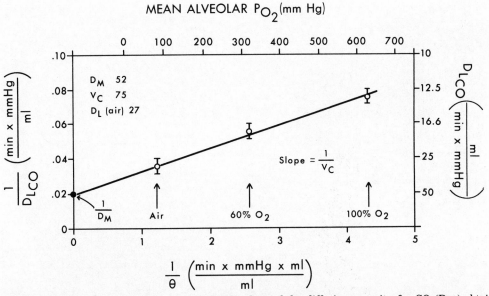

Figure 7–4. A plot demonstrating how experimental values of the diffusing capacity for CO (DL_{co}) obtained at different alveolar PO_2 values can be analyzed mathematically to obtain the subdivisions of total diffusing capacity: diffusing capacity of the membrane (DM) and pulmonary capillary blood volume (Vc). Changing alveolar PO_2 changes the reaction coefficient (θ) and allows $1/DL$ to be plotted against $1/\theta$. Under these conditions, DM is derived from the value of the Y-intercept and Vc from the slope of the line. For further discussion, see text.

permit derivation of the variables DM and Vc by plotting the results as shown in Figure 7–4. The results differ in normal subjects, mainly in DM, depending upon the method used to measure DL_{CO}.

Factors Affecting Diffusing Capacity

As indicated in Chapter 2, 85 to 95 per cent of the alveolar surface of the human lung is normally covered with pulmonary capillaries, and the air-blood interface, when fully expanded, exceeds 100 m². The extensive distribution of the alveolar-capillary network is vividly displayed in an inflated, injected frog lung (Fig. 7–5), and the thinness of the air-blood barrier in humans has been demonstrated (see Fig. 7–1). From the morphometric measurements of human lungs provided in Table 7–1 and estimates of the necessary physical coefficients, it is possible to compute values for the diffusing capacity of O_2 that vary from 125 to 263 ml/min × mm Hg, depending on the coefficients used, which is about twice the value found in exercising subjects.[21] Much of the discrepancy is accounted for by the fact that

the anatomic studies, because of the need to retain blood cells and plasma, were performed on lungs fixed via the airways; as already emphasized, this method of fixation causes the capillaries to protrude into the alveolar surface (see Fig. 2–27) and overestimates the actual surface of the air-blood barrier in an air-filled lung by some 25 to 50 per cent, depending on the degree of inflation. When this is taken into account and when the set of lowest physical coefficients is used for the calculation, values of "morphometric" diffusing capacity for O_2 (62 to 91 ml/min × mm Hg) correspond to those measured in humans during strenuous exercise.[21, 22]

It is known that DL varies from one mammalian species to another, according to body mass and not in proportion to O_2 needs.[24] Weibel[25] has attempted to explain this apparent paradox by the hypothesis that larger animals need a relatively larger DL_{O_2} because their alveolar end-capillary PO_2 difference (i.e., the driving force for diffusion) is lower than that of small animals. Among humans, DL varies from one person to another chiefly according to body build; consequently, DL will correlate with other indexes of physical dimensions, such as height, weight, and alveolar volume. The

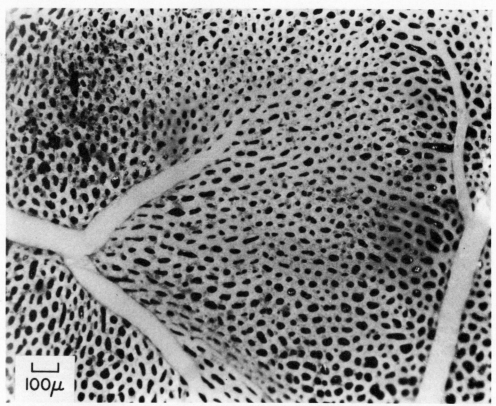

Figure 7–5. Micrograph of the capillaries of a frog lung following the injection of opaque material into the vasculature. The arteriole in the upper right supplies part of the capillary network; drainage occurs through the collecting venules on the left. Horizontal bar = 100 μm. (× 78. Reprinted by permission from Maloney, J. E., and Castle, B. L.: Pressure-diameter relations of capillaries and small blood vessels in frog lung. Respir. Physiol., 7:150–162, 1969.)

D_L increases during growth and then decreases gradually with age after maturity (see Chapter 14), presumably because of the loss of internal surface area, including pulmonary capillaries, during senescence.[26] The alveolar volume at which the measurements were made affects $D_{L_{CO}}$ values to some extent. It also is known that D_L may be influenced by changing metabolic needs and by the availability of O_2 (see Chapter 2, section on Adaptation). The most conspicuous example of this response in humans is the increased $D_{L_{CO}}$ of natives of high altitudes.[27]

Of the two component variables that affect values of D_L, the most important by far is V_C; this is true in normal subjects as well as in many patients with pulmonary diseases. Changes in D_M are much less common. The D_L was shown to vary markedly, as might be expected, when V_C was changed by regulating pulmonary arterial and left atrial pressures.[28] When left atrial pressure was low, raising pulmonary artery pressure increased D_L substantially (Fig. 7–6). The effect was diminished when left atrial pressure was high at the outset. These results can be explained by the effect of changing intravascular pressures on recruitment and distensibility of pulmonary capillaries and hence V_C. An increase in the number and volume of capillaries being perfused probably also accounts for the increase in $D_{L_{CO}}$ observed during exercise and with changes from the upright to the supine position. Similarly, the changes in D_L induced by certain drugs can be explained as a reflection of the effect of the drugs on V_C.

Because the quantity of O_2 or CO that can be taken up by the bloodstream depends upon the amount of hemoglobin present in the pulmonary capillaries, V_C and hence D_L vary proportionately with hemoglobin concentration. To avoid misinterpreting values of D_L in patients with anemia and polycythemia, the hemoglobin concentration should be known or determined at the time

Table 7–1. MORPHOMETRIC AND PHYSIOLOGIC VARIABLES RELATED
TO TOTAL PULMONARY DIFFUSING CAPACITY (DL) FOR O_2 AND CO,
MEMBRANE DIFFUSING CAPACITY (DM), AND PULMONARY CAPILLARY BLOOD
VOLUME (Vc) IN NORMAL ADULT HUMANS

	Mean	**± 1 S.E.**
Morphometric*		
Height, cm	177	3
Weight, kg	74	4
Body surface area, m²		
Total lung capacity	4341	285
Alveolar surface area (SA), m²	143	12
Capillary surface area (Sc), m²	126	12
Sc/SA		
Vc, ml	213	31
Mean thickness tissue barrier, μm	0.62	0.04
Mean thickness plasma barrier, μm	0.15	0.01
DL_{O_2} maximum, ml/min × mm Hg	263	34
DL_{O_2} minimum, ml/min × mm Hg	125	18
Physiologic†		
DL_{CO} (single breath, rest), ml/min × mm Hg	24	—
DL_{CO} (steady state, rest), ml/min × mm Hg	20	—
DL_{CO} (steady state, exercise), ml/min × mm Hg	53	—
DM_{CO} (single breath, rest), ml/min × mm Hg	52	—
Vc (single breath, rest), ml	75	—
DL_{O_2} (exercise), ml/min × mm Hg	85	—

*Data from Gehr, P., Bachofen, M., and Weibel, E. R.: The normal human lung: ultrastructural and morphometric estimation of diffusion capacity. Respir. Physiol., *32*:121–140, 1978.

†Data from Turino, G. M., Bergofsky, E. H., Goldring, R. M., and Fishman, A. P.: Effect of exercise on pulmonary diffusing capacity. J. Appl. Physiol., *18*:447–456, 1963 and Hamer, N. A.: The effect of age on the components of pulmonary diffusing capacity. Clin. Sci., *23*:85–93, 1962.

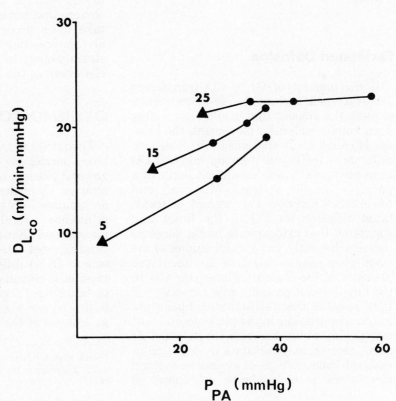

Figure 7–6. The effects of changes in pulmonary arterial pressure (PPA) on single breath diffusing capacity for CO (DL_{co}) at three different left atrial pressures (5, 15, and 25 mm Hg) in a blood-perfused dog lung. The value at the left of each line (▲) was obtained at zero blood flow; subsequent values (●) were obtained after PPA was raised by increasing flow. (Reprinted from Karp, R. B. et al.: Regulation of pulmonary capillary blood volume by pulmonary arterial and left atrial pressures. Circ. Res., *22*:1–10, 1968 by permission of the American Heart Association, Inc.)

DL is measured, and the observed value of DL should be corrected accordingly.

Owing to its solubility in water, CO_2 is approximately 20 times more diffusible than O_2. This has led to the generally accepted belief that in pulmonary disorders associated with impaired diffusion, O_2 exchange is affected considerably more than CO_2 exchange. This is not necessarily true because the *diffusivity* of a gas in the lungs, the rate of transfer across the air-blood barrier, is not always the same as the *rate of diffusion equilibration,* the rate at which the partial pressure of the gas in the capillary blood approaches that in the alveolar gas. Although the diffusivity of CO_2 is 20 times faster than that of O_2, the rate of diffusion equilibration of CO_2 is the same or even slower than that of O_2, chiefly because of the slope of the CO_2 equilibrium curve (see later section).[29] The slightly longer time course for CO_2 equilibration is reflected in Figure 7–3. However, the effects of the changes on O_2 and CO_2 are such that the alveolar end-capillary difference for P_{CO_2} is approximately one-twentieth that for P_{O_2} (see Fig. 8–3) and thus for practical purposes is negligible. Further discussion about CO_2 exchange is provided at the end of this chapter.

Facilitated Diffusion

If the amount of O_2 or CO transferred across a tissue such as the air-blood barrier exceeds the amount that would occur solely from kinetic molecular movement, the process is called facilitated diffusion. Based on differences in DL_{CO} at varying inspired CO concentrations, which should not occur in a purely passive system, Mendoza and coworkers[30] proposed the concept of facilitated diffusion for CO in the lungs and suggested that cytochromes might serve as carriers. Recently, two careful studies of the same phenomenon failed to document the presence of facilitated diffusion for CO in the lungs, and it probably does not exist.[31, 32] It is possible that facilitated diffusion enhances gas transfer in the placenta and that myoglobin, which has been established as an O_2 carrier, may facilitate O_2 diffusion in skeletal muscles.[33] But as matters stand now, there is no evidence in support of facilitated diffusion for either O_2 or CO in normal human lungs.

Site of Gas Exchange

Throughout the previous section it was implied that the pulmonary capillary is the sole site of gas exchange. This is not necessarily true, because investigators have shown that H_2 and O_2 will diffuse from alveoli into human pulmonary arteries with an internal diameter as large as 3.0 mm.[34] Similarly, Staub[35] noted a color change signifying oxygenation of blood in pulmonary arteries up to 200 μm in diameter in cats breathing 100 per cent O_2. Although in some of the experimental studies unphysiologic concentration differences between gas and blood phases were used, it is not surprising that some diffusion of gases into pulmonary arterioles occurs, because small blood vessels are often nearly completely surrounded by alveoli, and thus a relatively short diffusion pathway is created (see Fig. 2–15). Because the quantity of O_2 or CO_2 that diffuses across the air-blood barrier is inversely proportional to the length of the diffusion pathway and directly proportional to the surface area involved, it becomes obvious that virtually all gas exchange must take place across the thin portion of the alveolar-capillary membrane. Similar constraints apply to diffusion across capillaries elsewhere in the body.[36]

OXYHEMOGLOBIN EQUILIBRIUM

The initial movement of O_2 across the air-blood barrier takes place between alveolar gas and plasma, but as indicated earlier, as soon as O_2 molecules enter and begin to accumulate in plasma, a new concentration difference is established between O_2 in the plasma and that in the interior of the circulating red blood cell. This difference causes O_2 to diffuse into the cells, where most of it combines chemically with hemoglobin. Each 1.0 gm of hemoglobin can react with and serve as the carrier for as much as 1.34 ml of O_2.* Thus, the O_2 *capacity* of

---

*Some investigators use 1.38, which is the theoretical value based on a hemoglobin Fe content of 0.339 per cent.[37]

the blood is determined by the concentration of "active" hemoglobin (i.e., the hemoglobin that is chemically able to combine with O_2 [see later section]) in the blood and can be computed according to the following equation:

$$O_2 \text{ capacity, ml/100 ml} = \text{hemoglobin, gm/100 ml,} \times 1.34, \text{ml/gm.} \quad (4)$$

Not every O_2 molecule reacts with hemoglobin, and a small quantity of O_2 is present in physical solution in the bloodstream (O_2 dissolved), according to the solubility of O_2 (0.003 ml O_2/100 ml plasma/mm Hg P_{O_2}) and the partial pressure of O_2 in the plasma. The O_2 content of the blood is the actual amount of O_2 present in the blood, both chemically combined with hemoglobin and dissolved in plasma.

The relationship between the actual amount of O_2 combined with the hemoglobin contained in a given amount of blood and the O_2 capacity of that quantity of hemoglobin determines the per cent saturation of hemoglobin (S_{O_2}):

$$S_{O_2}, \% = \frac{O_2 \text{ content} - O_2 \text{ dissolved}}{O_2 \text{ capacity}} \times 100. \quad (5)$$

Instead of performing the laborious individual measurements necessary to compute per cent saturation of hemoglobin according to

Equation 5, values are usually obtained directly from spectrophotometric analysis of blood or derived indirectly from simple measurements of P_{O_2}, pH, and temperature.

Values for arterial and mixed venous blood composition in normal adults are given in Table 7–2. About 65 times more O_2 is carried in arterial blood combined with hemoglobin than is dissolved in plasma and cells, thus emphasizing the importance of hemoglobin as an O_2 carrier.

Oxyhemoglobin Equilibrium Curve

The reversible chemical reaction between O_2 and hemoglobin is defined by the oxyhemoglobin equilibrium curve (Fig. 7–7), which relates the per cent saturation of hemoglobin to the P_{O_2}. The characteristic feature of the O_2 equilibrium curves of most mammalian hemoglobin is their sigmoid shape, a configuration that indicates that the affinity for O_2 progressively increases as successive molecules of O_2 combine with hemoglobin. The sigmoid shape of the curve is physiologically advantageous because the flat upper portion allows arterial O_2 content to remain high and virtually constant despite fluctuations in arterial P_{O_2}, and the middle steep segment enables large quantities of O_2 to be released at the P_{O_2} pre-

Table 7–2. NORMAL VALUES FOR ARTERIAL AND MIXED VENOUS BLOOD COMPOSITION IN A 25 YEAR OLD PERSON AT REST*

Variable	Arterial Blood	Mixed Venous Blood
P_{O_2}, mm Hg	100	40
P_{CO_2} mm Hg	40	46
pH, units	7.40	7.36
Temperature, °C	37.0	37.0
Hemoglobin, gm/100 ml	14.9	14.9
O_2 capacity, ml/100 ml	20.0	20.0
O_2 content, ml/100 ml	19.80	14.62
Combined with hemoglobin	19.50	14.50
Dissolved O_2	0.30	0.12
Hemoglobin saturation, %	97.5	72.5
CO_2 content, ml/100 ml	49.0	53.1
Carbamino CO_2	2.2	3.1
Bicarbonate CO_2	44.2	47.0
Dissolved CO_2	2.6	3.0

*Data in part from Severinghaus, J. W.: Blood oxygen dissociation line charts: man. In Altman, P. C., and Dittmer, D. S. (eds.): Respiration and Circulation. Bethesda, Maryland, Federation of Experimental Biology, 1971, pp. 204–206; Singer, R. B.: Blood gas variables, factors, and constants: man. In Altman, P. C., and Dittmer, D. S. (eds.): Respiration and circulation. Bethesda, Maryland, Federation of Experimental Biology, 1971, p. 140.

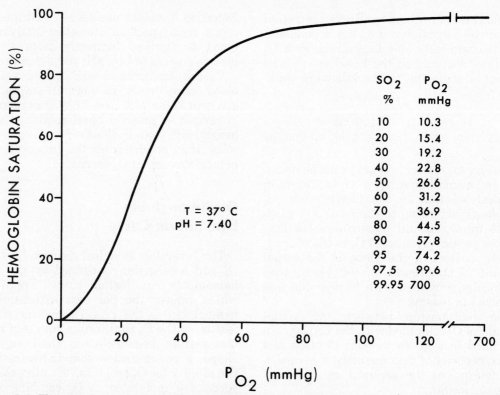

SO_2 %	PO_2 mmHg
10	10.3
20	15.4
30	19.2
40	22.8
50	26.6
60	31.2
70	36.9
80	44.5
90	57.8
95	74.2
97.5	99.6
99.95	700

Figure 7–7. The normal oxyhemoglobin dissociation curve for humans. Values for hemoglobin saturation (SO_2) at different PO_2 values, under standard conditions of temperature and pH, are indicated. (Data from Severinghaus, J. W.: Blood oxygen dissociation line charts: man. *In* Altman, P. C., and Dittmer, D. S. (eds.): Respiration and Circulation. Bethesda, Maryland, Federation of Experimental Biology, 1971, pp. 204–206.)

vailing in the peripheral capillaries. The affinity between O_2 and hemoglobin is conventionally expressed as the PO_2 at which the available hemoglobin is half saturated (P_{50}) under standard conditions of temperature (37°C) and pH (7.40).

The P_{50} of human blood is normally 26.6 mm Hg, but this value is known to vary considerably both in normal subjects under certain conditions and in patients with a variety of diseases. The effects of shifts in the position of the oxyhemoglobin equilibrium curve are depicted schematically in Figure 7–8; note that hemoglobin concentration has been arbitrarily set at 14.9 gm/100 ml so that O_2 capacity (i.e., 100 per cent saturation) is 20.0 ml/100 ml and arteriovenous (or tissue) O_2 differences can be easily derived. When the affinity of hemoglobin for O_2 increases, O_2 is taken up more readily and released less readily at any given PO_2; under these circumstances, the equilibrium curve is shifted to the left (curve B) of the normal curve (curve A), and the P_{50} is lower than usual (Fig. 7–8). When the affinity of hemoglobin for O_2 decreases, the new curve

is shifted to the right (curve C) of the normal one and the P_{50} increases. When arterial PO_2 is normal, shifts in the curves in either direction influence the *release* of O_2 in the tissues considerably more than the *uptake* of O_2 in the lungs. This phenomenon is also depicted in Figure 7–8 by the convergence of the flat portions (exaggerated for schematic effect) and the separation of the steep segments of the three curves. A decrease in O_2 affinity (curve C, $P_{50} = 30.6$ mm Hg) is physiologically useful because it increases the amount of O_2 released at the tissues, where PO_2 is 40 mm Hg, by 1.6 ml/100 ml. In other words, the shift from curve A to curve C increases O_2 release from 4.5 to 6.1 ml/100 ml. In contrast, an increased O_2 affinity (curve B, $P_{50} = 22.6$ mm Hg) is disadvantageous because it reduces the amount of O_2 normally available to the tissues by 1.6 ml/100 ml, or from 4.5 to 2.9 ml/100 ml. When arterial PO_2 is low, as in the hypoxia of high altitude and of severe pulmonary diseases, an increase in P_{50} may not be physiologically useful because it impairs O_2 uptake by arterial blood as much as or even

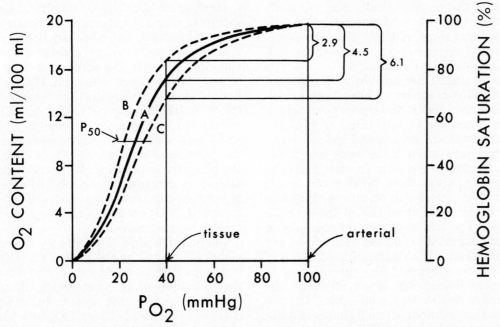

Figure 7–8. Schematic diagram showing the effects of increases and decreases in O_2 affinity on the amount of O_2 available at the P_{O_2} values prevailing in arterial blood and at the tissues. P_{50} = P_{O_2} at which hemoglobin saturation is 50 per cent. Hemoglobin concentration is assumed for convenience to be 14.9 gm/100 ml; therefore, O_2 content at 100 per cent saturation is 20 ml/100 ml. Curve A = normal blood; curve B = blood with increased affinity (decreased P_{50}); curve C = blood with decreased affinity (increased P_{50}). For further discussion, see text.

more than it facilitates O_2 release by capillary blood.

The results of computer modeling studies support the concept that there is no unique value of P_{50} at which gas exchange in humans is optimal.[40] When arterial P_{O_2} is normal or only moderately reduced, a high P_{50} is advantageous because it favors O_2 unloading in peripheral capillaries and serves to increase venous P_{O_2}. In contrast, when arterial P_{O_2} is decreased, a low P_{50} is better able to maintain satisfactory values of venous P_{O_2}, especially in organs like the heart, in which the arteriovenous O_2 difference is high. These findings probably explain why P_{50} is not fixed and why it can adapt remarkably well to changing physiologic conditions.

Factors Affecting Oxyhemoglobin Equilibrium

Hemoglobin has probably been studied more thoroughly than any other protein, and a considerable amount of information is now available concerning the relationships between the structure of hemoglobin and its chemical properties.[41] A single molecule of adult hemoglobin consists of two pairs of polypeptide chains: the α-chains containing 141 amino acid residues and the β-chains containing 146. Each chain is twisted into several folds that form a kind of basket into which the Fe-containing heme group fits neatly. The four chains are symmetrically arranged in a tetramer that is held together by chemical contacts, primarily between unlike units ($\alpha_1\beta_1$ and $\alpha_1\beta_2$). Of great importance is the evidence that hemoglobin undergoes conformational changes when it reacts with O_2; thus the hemoglobin molecule can be said to breathe, because it expands when bereft of O_2 and contracts when combined with O_2. Shifts in the molecular structure of hemoglobin are also caused by reactions with CO_2, H^+, and certain organic phosphates (particularly 2,3-diphosphoglycerate [DPG]). All the substances that exert an interdependent effect on the chemical bonding properties of hemoglobin are known collectively as *ligands*. This means that the concentration within red blood cells of any one of the ligands affects the ability of hemoglobin to combine with any of the others. Moreover, this mechanism accounts for many of the physiologically and clinically significant shifts in oxyhemoglobin dissociation relationships. (Details about hemoglobin-ligand chemistry are reviewed by Kilmartin and Rossi-Bernardi.[42])

Two states of hemoglobin with different structural conformations have been distinguished chemically: the *deoxy* form, which occurs when the O_2-combining sites at the heme groups are empty, and the *oxy* form, which occurs when these sites are filled. Exactly when the change in state from the deoxy to the oxy form takes place is not known, but it seems to require combination with O_2 by more than two of the four Fe atoms.[43] The two structures of hemoglobin and the sigmoid O_2 dissociation curve are characteristic for substrate-ligand binding of allosteric enzymes.* The current view is to regard hemoglobin as an allosteric enzyme that reacts with a substrate, O_2; the interactions between α and β chains and the conformational changes of the molecule that result from reactions with other ligands affect the affinity for O_2.[45] A summary of the effects of different ligands and other alterations in the hemoglobin molecule is presented in Table 7-3.

---

*"An enzyme may possess two separate sites which can bind ligands—the active site, where catalysis occurs, and the allosteric ('other') site where a modifier may bind."[44]

Hydrogen Ion. The O_2 affinity of hemoglobin is strongly influenced by changes in intracellular pH, the so-called Bohr effect. As will be explained in greater detail in Chapters 8 and 9, the addition or removal of CO_2 has a direct effect on H_2CO_3 and hence on H^+ concentration (symbolized $[H^+]$). In the lungs, $[H^+]$ falls as CO_2 is eliminated from pulmonary capillary blood and oxyhemoglobin affinity is increased; in the peripheral capillaries, CO_2 is added to the bloodstream, causing $[H^+]$ to rise and O_2 affinity to decrease. The combined effect is physiologically favorable because it enhances both O_2 uptake in the lungs and O_2 release to the tissues.

Carbon Dioxide. The affinity of hemoglobin is affected by the presence of CO_2 in two ways: first, as noted previously, through the formation of H^+ that reacts, in turn, with hemoglobin, and second, by a direct chemical reaction between CO_2 and hemoglobin, with the formation of carbamino compounds. Similar to a rise in $[H^+]$, a rise in carbamino compounds decreases O_2 affinity. Thus, the methods by which hemoglobin handles O_2 and CO_2 reciprocally augment the uptake and release of both gases in the lungs and tissues.

Organic Phosphates. The oxyhemoglobin equilibrium curve of hemoglobin stripped from its red blood cells lies far to

Table 7–3. THE EFFECT OF VARIOUS INFLUENCES ON OXYHEMOGLOBIN AFFINITY AND P_{50}*

Influence	O_2 Affinity	P_{50}
CO₂ concentration		
Increased	Decreased	Increased
Decreased	Increased	Decreased
pH		
Increased (alkalemia)	Increased	Decreased
Decreased (acidemia)	Decreased	Increased
2,3-Diphosphoglycerate		
Increased	Decreased	Increased
Decreased	Increased	Decreased
CO-hemoglobin, methemoglobin		
Increased	Increased	Decreased
Abnormal hemoglobins		
Chesapeake	Increased	Decreased
Yakima	Increased	Decreased
Rainier	Increased	Decreased
E	Decreased	Increased
Seattle	Decreased	Increased
Kansas	Decreased	Increased

*Data in part from Stamatoyannopoulos, G. et al.: Abnormal hemoglobins with high and low oxygen affinity. Annu. Rev. Med., *22:*221–234, 1971.

the left of the normal curve, even though pH and temperature are normal; furthermore, the position of the displaced curve can be moved to the right by the addition of certain organic phosphates, notably adenosine triphosphate (ATP) and DPG. The DPG is present in only trace amounts in most mammalian cells as an intermediate of glycolysis, but in red blood cells DPG is four times more plentiful than ATP and has a molar concentration equivalent to hemoglobin.[46] Because the synthesis of DPG increases during anaerobic conditions, red blood cells are equipped with their own inbuilt mechanism for responding to hypoxia in a manner that facilitates O_2 release to the tissues. Figure 7–9 shows the relationship between changes in DPG concentration and P_{50} in patients with cardiac disease.[47] The time course of the appearance of changes in intracellular DPG varies with different kinds of anaerobic stress; increased concentrations of DPG have been observed after only ten minutes of vigorous exercise[48] but as long as one to two days after ascent to high altitude.[49]

Increased synthesis of DPG appears to be an important component of the adaptive responses in normal persons to an acute need for more tissue O_2; increased DPG concentrations in red blood cells with corresponding increases in P_{50} and decreases in O_2 affinity occur in numerous diseases characterized by reduction in available O_2 (e.g., anemia, right-to-left shunts, congestive heart failure). In contrast, low levels of erythrocyte DPG and increased O_2 affinity have been observed in stored blood and in blood of patients with hypophosphatemia, hexokinase deficiency, and septic shock.

Hemoglobin Concentration. Oxygen affinity has been shown to be dependent upon the concentration of hemoglobin in hemolysates. Because a similar effect has been demonstrated in intact cells, the mean corpuscular hemoglobin concentration should be taken into account when evaluating the position of the oxyhemoglobin equilibrium curve.[50]

Carbon Monoxide Hemoglobin. Carbon monoxide and O_2 compete with each other for combination sites on the hemoglobin molecule, but CO has 200 times greater affinity than O_2. The result of the formation

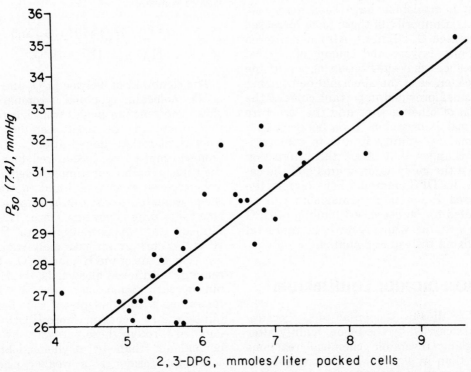

Figure 7–9. Relation between hemoglobin affinity for O_2, expressed as P_{50} measured at pH 7.4, and 2,3-diphosphoglycerate (2,3-DPG) in 39 patients with clinical evidence of cardiac disease. (Reprinted by permission from Woodson, R. D. et al.: The effect of cardiac disease on hemoglobin-oxygen binding. J. Clin. Invest., *49*:1349–1356, 1970.)

of carboxyhemoglobin is to increase the affinity of the remaining Fe atoms for O_2. Exposure to CO has two dire consequences: it lowers the O_2 capacity of the blood by reducing the amount of hemoglobin that can combine with O_2, and it causes a progressive leftward shift of the oxyhemoglobin equilibrium curve that increasingly impairs the unloading of those O_2 molecules that are able to combine with hemoglobin.[37] Both mechanisms contribute to the production of severe tissue hypoxia and explain why the formation of 50 per cent CO hemoglobin has much more serious clinical consequences than when hemoglobin concentration is reduced to half normal by various forms of anemia.

Methemoglobin. Methemoglobin is formed when the Fe atoms are oxidized from the ferrous to the ferric state. As this occurs successively among the four heme groups, the O_2 affinity of the remaining unoxidized Fe atoms increases. The effect of methemoglobin on peripheral capillary O_2 unloading and the production of tissue hypoxia is qualitatively the same but quantitatively less than that produced by equal amounts of CO hemoglobin.[51]

Abnormal Hemoglobins. Over 100 abnormal hemoglobins have been described, but only a minority of these have increased or decreased O_2 affinity.[45] Although altered O_2 affinity is rare and seldom of clinical significance, characterization of the amino acid sequences of the abnormal hemoglobin species has provided important clues to the location of binding sites and the structure of normal hemoglobin. It is believed that abnormal O_2 affinity is due to conformational changes that affect the interaction between the polypeptide chains and the capability for DPG binding.[30] For example, the decreased P_{50} of fetal hemoglobin can be attributed to the decreased binding of DPG by the γ-chains, which occur in normal fetal hemoglobin instead of β-chains.

CARBON DIOXIDE EQUILIBRIUM

Carbon dioxide is similar to O_2 because both are carried by the blood, mainly after undergoing reversible chemical reactions rather than in physical solution (see Table 7–2). In contrast to O_2, for which combination with hemoglobin is the only (single) process involved, several different chemical reactions play a role in the transport of CO_2 from the tissues to the lungs.[52] Perhaps the best way of describing the mechanisms by which CO_2 is carried in the blood is to examine the various pathways between the sources of CO_2 and its elimination from the body.

Chemical Reactions

Carbon dioxide is one of the end products of aerobic cellular metabolism, and thus is being continuously produced virtually everywhere in the body. After CO_2 is formed by cells, it diffuses into the blood plasma, owing to a concentration difference between the cell interior and the neighboring capillary blood. Most of the CO_2 that enters the blood passes into red blood cells, where it undergoes one of two possible chemical reactions. The remaining amount is carried in plasma in physical solution (i.e., dissolved), according to the solubility of CO_2 (0.065 ml CO_2/100 ml plasma/mm Hg P_{CO_2}).

1. Of the CO_2 that diffuses into red blood cells, the greater part enters into the reversible formation of HCO_3^- through a series of reactions:

$$CO_2 + H_2O \rightleftharpoons H_2CO_3, \text{ and} \qquad (6)$$

$$H_2CO_3 \rightleftharpoons H^+ + HCO_3^-. \qquad (7)$$

The combination between CO_2 and H_2O is of the molecular type and is comparatively slow. The reaction moves from left to right (hydration) in the tissue capillaries and from right to left (dehydration) in the pulmonary capillaries. Inside red blood cells the rates of both hydration and dehydration are accelerated several hundred times by the presence of *carbonic anhydrase,* a potent zinc-containing enzyme. Once H_2CO_3 is formed, its transformation into H^+ and HCO_3^- occurs by an extremely rapid ionic reaction. Some of the H^+ and HCO_3^- formed remains within red blood cells, the H^+ combining with hemoglobin and the HCO_3^- combining with K^+ displaced from hemoglobin by the H^+ reaction. More H_2CO_3 can be handled through these pathways by deoxyhemoglobin than by oxyhemoglobin, because the former is a weaker acid and, therefore, a better buffer than the latter (see Chapter 9 for a more complete discussion of buffers).

Some of the HCO_3^- formed by the ionization of H_2CO_3 diffuses out of the red blood cell into the plasma because the membrane is much more permeable to negatively charged anions, such as HCO_3^- and Cl^-, than to positively charged cations, such as K^+ and Na^+. This movement tends to set up an electrostatic difference across the cell membrane that is neutralized by the movement of Cl^- from the plasma into the red blood cell (the "chloride shift").

2. The smaller fraction of CO_2 that enters red blood cells combines reversibly with hemoglobin to form carbamino compounds. As is the case with the capacity of hemoglobin to combine with the H^+ formed from H_2CO_3, more CO_2 is bound in the form of carbamino compounds by deoxyhemoglobin than by oxyhemoglobin.

Although carbonic anhydrase accelerates the equilibration between PCO_2 and H^+ and HCO_3^- within red blood cells, it should have no effect on the speed of the reactions in plasma. The uncatalyzed alkalinization of plasma (pH increases from 7.36 to 7.40; see Table 7–2) requires much more time than blood actually spends flowing through the pulmonary capillaries, and thus would be expected to proceed to completion in the pulmonary veins and systemic circulation. But when this expected delay in pH adjustment was looked for experimentally, it could not be found; effluent blood from pulmonary capillaries changed its pH very little (approximately 0.01 unit) or not at all.[52] It was subsequently shown that a source of carbonic anhydrase was available to plasma in pulmonary capillaries, even though it was not in the plasma itself, and this observation led to the discovery of the enzyme first in lung tissue homogenates and, more recently, in pulmonary endothelial cells.[53] Finding carbonic anhydrase in the endothelium explains why plasma pH changes can keep up with those in red blood cells. Enns and Hill[54] have made the interesting suggestion that the presence of the enzyme in the air-blood barrier may facilitate CO_2 diffusion by enabling some of the total CO_2 flux through tissue to occur in the form of HCO_3^-; but if this were the case, it would be more appropriate for the enzyme to be located throughout the alveolar-capillary membrane and not just on the endothelial side.[55] Furthermore, other investigators have concluded that the main effect of pulmonary vascular carbonic anhydrase is on the rate of equili-

bration of plasma pH and not on CO_2 elimination.[56]

Another unsolved problem concerning CO_2 exchange is whether or not, under steady state conditions, alveolar-to-arterial PCO_2 differences ever occur. Several groups of investigators have reported that alveolar PCO_2 may exceed arterial PCO_2, sometimes by a substantial amount (see Hlastala and Robertson[57] for a review and additional references). In contrast, Scheid and Piiper[58] concluded that such differences were artifactual and attributable to technical errors. However, this conclusion needs to be reexamined in the light of the results of recent experiments using a clever new model, with which positive alveolar-arterial PCO_2 differences of 2 to 25 mm Hg were observed.[59] No clues to possible mechanisms have been provided, although the old notion of active transport of CO_2 now needs to be reconsidered.

Carbon Dioxide Equilibrium Curve

The CO_2 equilibrium curves of oxygenated and deoxygenated blood are shown in Figure 7–10. The curves are nearly linear in the physiologic range (PCO_2 40 to 50), and considerably more, about 6 ml/100 ml, CO_2 is bound at any given PCO_2 within that range by deoxyhemoglobin rather than by oxyhemoglobin. The shift from the lower to the upper curve in Figure 7–10 occurs during the deoxygenation of blood as it flows through tissue capillaries and adds, in turn, to the capacity of blood to take up CO_2; this enhancement of CO_2 transport is known as the Haldane effect and is believed by some to be physiologically of far greater importance than the converse influence of CO_2 (through formation of H^+) on O_2 transport ("Bohr effect," see preceding section). There are two components to the Haldane effect that depend upon chemical differences between deoxyhemoglobin and oxyhemoglobin: about 70 per cent is due to the augmented capacity of deoxyhemoglobin to form carbamino compounds, and the remainder is due to the enhanced ability of deoxyhemoglobin to absorb H^+ and release base (i.e., buffer the ionization products of H_2CO_3).

Because there are no suitable methods that allow in vivo studies of the physiologic usefulness of the Bohr and Haldane effects,

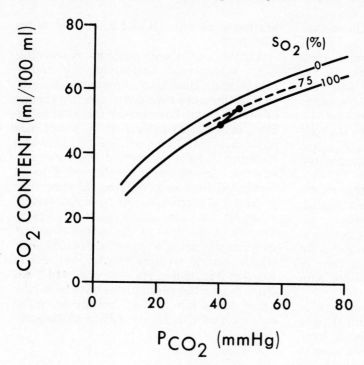

Figure 7–10. Normal CO_2 equilibration (dissociation) curves for whole blood at 0, 75, and 100 per cent oxyhemoglobin saturation (So_2). The heavy line connecting the two points shows the usual extent of the Haldane effect in arterial and venous blood.

which for practical purposes are mirror images of each other, estimations of their respective benefits have been based on the results of *in vitro* analyses or computer models. Using sophisticated computer programs, Grant[60] recently concluded that the Bohr and Haldane effects do not provide any major advantage for gas exchange in the lungs, even in the presence of certain simulated abnormalities; he did find, however, an appreciable influence on tissue gas exchange that tended to decrease mixed venous Pco_2 and tissue acidosis.

To summarize, CO_2 is carried in the bloodstream partly in red blood cells, both as HCO_3^- and bound to hemoglobin as carbamino compounds, and partly in plasma, as HCO_3^-; because of the relatively high solubility of CO_2 (compared with O_2), an appreciable portion is in physical solution. In the pulmonary capillaries, all of the chemical reactions that occur in tissue capillaries proceed in the reverse direction. The amounts of each form of CO_2 in arterial and venous blood are shown in Table 7–2. Intraerythrocyte carbonic anhydrase also plays an indispensable role in the lungs by catalyzing the dehydration of H_2CO_3 into CO_2 and H_2O; without the enzyme, or in the presence of carbonic acid inhibitors, the release of CO_2 does not proceed to equilibrium during the time that red blood cells spend traversing the pulmonary capillary, and a

difference develops between the CO_2 concentration in end-capillary blood and that in alveolar gas. The presence of carbonic anhydrase in endothelial cells allows pH changes in the plasma to keep pace with those in red blood cells.

Thus, the normal processes concerned with CO_2 elimination begin with diffusion from the sites of CO_2 production into the bloodstream, include chemical reactions within red blood cells and plasma that greatly increase the carrying capacity of the blood, and end, again, with diffusion of CO_2 out of the blood in pulmonary capillaries into the alveoli.

REFERENCES

1. Forster, R. E.: Exchange of gases between alveolar air and pulmonary capillary blood: pulmonary diffusing capacity. Physiol. Rev., 37:391–405, 1957.
2. Fowler, W. S.: Lung function studies. II. The respiratory dead space. J. Physiol. (Lond.), 107:405–416, 1948.
3. Muir, D. C. F.: Bulk flow and diffusion in the airways of the lung. Br. J. Dis. Chest, 60:169–176, 1966.
4. Hlastala, M. P.: Diffusion in lung gas and across alveolar membrane in mammalian lungs. Fed. Proc., 41:2122–2124, 1982.
5. Engel, L. A.: Gas mixing within the acinus of the lung. J. Appl. Physiol., 54:609–618, 1983.
6. Staub, N. C.: Time-dependent factors in pulmonary gas exchange. Med. Thorac., 22:132–145, 1965.
7. Staub, N. C.: Alveolar-arterial oxygen tension gra-

dient due to diffusion. J. Appl. Physiol., *18*: 673–680, 1963.

8. Hyde, R. W., Puy, R. J. M., Raub, W. F., and Forster, R. E.: Rate of disappearance of labeled carbon dioxide from the lungs of humans during breath holding: a method for studying the dynamics of pulmonary CO_2 exchange. J. Clin. Invest., 47:1535–1552, 1968.

9. Roughton, F. J. W., and Forster, R. E.: Relative importance of diffusion and chemical reaction rates in determining rate of exchange of gases in the human lung, with special reference to true diffusing capacity of pulmonary membrane and volume of blood in the lung capillaries. J. Appl. Physiol., 11:290–302, 1957.

10. Overland, E. S., Gupta, R. N., Huchon, G. J., and Murray, J. F.: Measurement of pulmonary tissue volume and blood flow in persons with normal and edematous lungs. J. Appl. Physiol., 51:1375–1383, 1981.

11. Forster, R. E.: Diffusion of gases. *In* Fenn, W. O., and Rahn, H. (eds.): Handbook of Physiology, Section 3. Respiration. Vol. I. Washington, D.C., American Physiological Society, 1964, pp. 839–872.

12. Bates, D. V., Macklem, P. T., and Christie, R. V.: Respiratory Function in Disease. An Introduction to the Integrated Study of the Lung. Philadelphia, W. B. Saunders Co., 1971, pp. 75–90.

13. Gold, W. M., Burgess, J. H., and Nadel, J. A.: Unpublished observations.

14. Thurlbeck, W. M., Henderson, J. A., Fraser, R. G., and Bates, D. V.: Chronic obstructive lung disease. A comparison between clinical, roentgenologic, functional and morphologic criteria in chronic bronchitis, emphysema, asthma and bronchiectasis. Medicine, 49:81–145, 1970.

15. Burgess, J. H.: Pulmonary diffusing capacity in disorders of the pulmonary circulation. Circulation, 49:541–550, 1974.

16. Hyde, R. W., Rynes, R., Power, G. G., and Nairn, J.: Determination of distribution of diffusing capacity in relation to blood flow in the human lung. J. Clin. Invest., 46:463–474, 1967.

17. Johnson, R. L., and Miller, J. M.: Distribution of ventilation, blood flow, and gas transfer coefficients in the lung. J. Appl Physiol., 25:1–15, 1968.

18. West, J. B., and Wagner, P. D.: Predicted gas exchange on the summit of Mt. Everest. Respir. Physiol., 42:1–16, 1980.

19. West, J. B., Hackett, P. H., Maret, K. H., Milledge, J. S., Peters, R. M., Pizzo, C. J., and Winslow, R. M.: Pulmonary gas exchange on the summit of Mt. Everest. J. Appl. Physiol., 55:678–687, 1983.

20. Maloney, J. E., and Castle, B. L.: Pressure-diameter relations of capillaries and small blood vessels in frog lung. Respir. Physiol., 7:150–162, 1969.

21. Gehr, P., Bachofen, M., and Weibel, E. R.: The normal human lung: ultrastructural and morphometric estimation of diffusion capacity. Respir. Physiol. 32:121–140, 1978.

22. Turino, G. M., Bergofsky, E. H., Goldring, R. M., and Fishman, A. P.: Effect of exercise on pulmonary diffusing capacity. J. Appl. Physiol., 18:447–456, 1963.

23. Hamer, N. A.: The effect of age on the components of the pulmonary diffusing capacity. Clin. Sci., 23:85–93, 1962.

24. Weibel, E. R., and Taylor, C. R. (eds.): Design of the mammalian respiratory system. Respir. Physiol., 44:1–164, 1981.

25. Weibel, E. R.: Is the lung built reasonably? Am. Rev. Respir. Dis., *128*:752–760, 1983.

26. Thurlbeck, W. M.: The internal surface area of nonemphysematous lungs. Am. Rev. Respir. Dis., *95*:765–773, 1967.

27. Guleria, J. S., Pande, J. N., Sethi, P. K., and Roy, S. B.: Pulmonary diffusing capacity at high altitude. J. Appl. Physiol., *31*:536–543, 1971.

28. Karp, R. B., Graf, P. D., and Nadel, J. A.: Regulation of pulmonary capillary blood volume by pulmonary arterial and left atrial pressures. Circ. Res., *22*:1–10, 1968.

29. Wagner, P. D.: Diffusion and chemical reaction in pulmonary gas exchange. Physiol. Rev., *57*: 257–312, 1977.

30. Mendoza, C., Peavy, H., Burns, B., and Gurtner, G.: Saturation kinetics for steady-state pulmonary CO transfer. J. Appl. Physiol., *43*:880–884, 1977.

31. Meyer, M., Lessner, W., Scheid, P., and Piiper, J.: Pulmonary diffusing capacity for CO independent of alveolar CO concentration. J. Appl. Physiol., *51*:571–576, 1981.

32. Jones, H. A., Clark, J. C., Davies, E. E., Forster, R. E., and Hughes, J. M. B.: Rate of uptake of carbon monoxide at different inspired concentrations in humans. J. Appl. Physiol., *52*:109–113, 1982.

33. Wittenberg, J. B.: Myoglobin-facilitated oxygen diffusion: role of myoglobin in oxygen entry into muscle. Physiol. Rev., *50*:559–636, 1970.

34. Sobel, B. J., Bottex, G., Emirgil, C., and Gissen, H.: Gaseous diffusion from alveoli to pulmonary vessels of considerable size. Circ. Res., *13*:71–79, 1963.

35. Staub, N. C.: Gas exchange vessels in the cat lung. Fed. Proc., *20*:107, 1961.

36. Krogh, A.: the Anatomy and Physiology of Capillaries. New York, Hafner, 1959, pp. 22–46, 267–274.

37. Roughton, F. J. W.: Transport of oxygen and carbon dioxide. *In* Fenn, W. O., and Rahn, H. (eds.): Handbook of Physiology, Section 3. Respiration. Vol. I. Washington, D.C., American Physiological Society, 1964, pp. 767–825.

38. Severinghaus, J. W.: Blood oxygen dissociation line charts: man. *In* Altman, P. C., and Dittmer, D. S. (eds.): Respiration and Circulation. Bethesda, Maryland, Federation of Experimental Biology, 1971, pp. 204–206.

39. Singer, R. B.: Blood gas variables, factors, and constants: man. *In* Altman, P. C., and Dittmer, D. S. (eds.): Respiration and Circulation. Bethesda, Maryland, Federation of Experimental Biology, 1971, p. 140.

40. Willford, D. C., Hill, E. P., and Moores, W. Y.: Theoretical analysis of optimal P_{50}. J. Appl. Physiol., *52*:1043–1048, 1982.

41. Perutz, M. F.: Structure and mechanism of haemoglobin. Br. Med. Bull., *32*:195–208, 1976.

42. Kilmartin, J. V., and Rossi-Bernardi, L.: Interaction of hemoglobin with hydrogen ions, carbon dioxide, and organic phosphates. Physiol. Rev., *53*:836–890, 1973.

43. Gibson, Q. H., and Parkhurst, L. J.: Kinetic evidence for a tetrameric functional unit in hemoglobin. J. Biol. Chem., *243*:5521–5524, 1968.

44. Harper, H. A.: Review of Physiological Chemistry. 13th Ed. Los Altos, California, Lange Medical Publications, 1971, p. 149.

45. Stamatoyannopoulos, G., Bellingham, A. J., Len-

fant, C., and Finch, C. A.: Abnormal hemoglobins with high and low oxygen affinity. Annu. Rev. Med., *22*:221–234, 1971.

46. Bunn, H. F., and Jandl, J. H.: Control of hemoglobin function within the red cell. New Engl. J. Med., *282*:1414–1420, 1970.

47. Woodson, R. D., Torrance, J. D., Shappell, S. D., and Lenfant, C.: The effect of cardiac disease on hemoglobin-oxygen binding. J. Clin. Invest., *49*: 1349–1356, 1970.

48. Faulkner, J. A., Brewer, G. J., and Eaton, J. W.: Adaptation of the red blood cell to muscular exercise. *In* Brewer, G. J. (ed.): Red Cell Metabolism and Function. New York, Plenum, 1970, pp. 213–227.

49. Lenfant, C., Torrance, J., English, E., Finch, C. A., Reynafarje, C., Ramos, J., and Faura, J.: Effect of altitude on oxygen binding by hemoglobin and on organic phosphate levels. J. Clin. Invest., *47*: 2652–2656, 1968.

50. Bellingham, A. J., Detter, J. C., and Lenfant, C.: Regulatory mechanisms of hemoglobin oxygen affinity in acidosis and alkalosis. J. Clin. Invest., *50*:700–706, 1971.

51. Darling, R. C., and Roughton, F. J. W.: The effect of methemoglobin on the equilibrium between oxygen and hemoglobin. Am. J. Physiol., *137*:56–68, 1942.

52. Forster, R. E.: Diffusion and chemical reaction as limiting factors in CO_2 equilibration in lungs. Fed. Proc., *41*:2125–2127, 1982.

53. Ryan, V. S., Whitney, P. L., and Ryan, J. W.: Localization of carbonic anhydrase on pulmonary artery endothelial cells in culture. J. Appl. Physiol., *53*:914–919, 1982.

54. Enns, T., and Hill, E. P.: CO_2 diffusing capacity in isolated dog lung lobes and the role of carbonic anhydrase. J. Appl. Physiol., *54*:483–490, 1983.

55. Effros, R. M., Mason, G., and Silverman, P.: Asymmetric distribution of carbonic anhydrase in the alveolar-capillary barrier. J. Appl. Physiol., *51*: 190–193, 1981.

56. Bidani, A., Mathew, S. J., and Crandall, E. D.: Pulmonary vascular carbonic anhydrase activity. J. Appl. Physiol., *55*:75–83, 1983.

57. Hlastala, M. P., and Robertson, H. T.: Evidence for active elimination of carbon dioxide from the lung. *In* West, J. B. (ed.): Pulmonary Gas Exchange. Vol II. New York, Academic Press, 1980, pp. 241–273.

58. Scheid, P., and Piiper, J.: Blood/gas equilibrium of carbon dioxide in lungs—a critical view. Respir. Physiol., *39*:1–31, 1980.

59. Green, J. F., Sheldon, M., Gurtner, G.: Alveolar-to-arterial P_{CO_2} differences. J. Appl. Physiol., *54*:349–354, 1983.

60. Grant, B. J. B.: Influence of Bohr-Haldane effect on steady-state gas exchange. J. Appl. Physiol., *52*:1330–1337, 1982.

Chapter

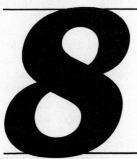

Gas Exchange and Oxygen Transport

INTRODUCTION

Movement of O_2 and CO_2 between gas and blood in the lungs and between cells and blood in the tissues of the body takes place by diffusion. As emphasized in the previous chapter, the transport capacity of blood for both O_2 and CO_2 is considerably increased by the chemical reactions that occur in the bloodstream, mainly with hemoglobin. But these essential features of gas exchange are only the first and the last mechanisms in the continuum of physiologic processes that ensures a steady flow of O_2 from the ambient air to the intracellular mitochondria and of CO_2 in the opposite direction. This chapter considers how O_2 uptake and CO_2 elimination take place in the lungs under idealized conditions and how deviations from the ideal occur in normal subjects and in patients with pulmonary disorders. Recent reviews of the subject are available.[1, 2]

Pulmonary gas exchange can be viewed as occurring solely under the control of and within the structures that comprise the respiratory system. In contrast, transport of O_2 and CO_2 is a multisystem process that involves not only the respiratory system but the circulatory and hemoglobin-regulating systems as well. This chapter also describes

183

the three components of O_2 transport and how they are interrelated under normal and stressful circumstances.

GAS EXCHANGE

The diffusion of O_2 and CO_2 between alveolar gas and blood in the pulmonary capillaries and their reversible reactions with hemoglobin take place continuously in the approximately 100,000 terminal respiratory units in the lungs; moreover, the adequacy of respiration in *each gas exchange unit* depends upon the apposition of a thin film of mixed venous blood with just the right amount of fresh air, so that the blood becomes fully oxygenated and part of its CO_2 is eliminated. The local matching of ventilation and perfusion is the critical determinant of gas exchange, and a deficiency or excess of ventilation relative to the amount of blood flow leads to either inadequate or wasteful respiration. It is impossible to evaluate the completeness of gas exchange within individual units, but the over-all effectiveness can be assessed through examination of the composition of arterial blood and alveolar gas. Other, much more complicated methods are available for analyzing the adequacy of gas exchange, but no technique allows an exact description of all the complex phenomena involved.

Normal values for the gas pressures prevailing at sea level (barometric pressure = 760 mm Hg) for the individual gases, P_{O_2}, P_{CO_2}, P_{N_2}, and P_{H_2O}, in ambient air, conducting airways, gas exchange units, and mixed venous and arterial blood are indicated in Table 8–1. Ambient air consists primarily of N_2 and O_2, all other gases being present in negligible amounts except water vapor, the pressure of which varies considerably depending upon local temperature and humidity. As air is inhaled, it is warmed

and fully saturated with water vapor at the subject's body temperature (P_{H_2O} at 37° C = 47 mm Hg). It was originally believed that the heating and humidification of inspired air were nearly completed by the time the inspirate reached the posterior pharynx or larynx and that the tracheobronchial system did not contribute to the process; now it is known that dry frigid air can penetrate to airways at least as small as 2 mm in diameter before conditioning is complete.[3] Regardless of where transfer of water vapor into the inspired airstream occurs, its addition has the effect of diluting the inspired mixture of N_2 and O_2, and it reduces their respective pressures within the conducting airways to the values indicated (see Table 8–1). After the inspirate reaches the terminal respiratory units, gas exchange takes place. More O_2 is removed than CO_2 is added, which causes the volume of each unit to diminish slightly and raises the concentration and pressure of N_2 within the gas phase slightly. This is known as the respiratory exchange effect. (Under steady-state conditions, the respiratory exchange ratio [R] is determined by metabolic events, the O_2 consumption [$\dot{V}_{O_2}$] and the CO_2 production [$\dot{V}_{CO_2}$]; $R = \dot{V}_{CO_2}/\dot{V}_{O_2}$ and is normally about 0.8.)

"Ideal" Relationships

Before considering the complexities of gas exchange in normal human lungs, it is useful to examine the behavior of the greatly simplified two-compartment lung model shown in Figure 8–1, which has been slightly modified from a diagram originally used by Comroe and associates.[4] In this and subsequent figures, the hemoglobin concentration is assumed to be 15.0 gm/100 ml and the arteriovenous difference in blood flowing through the lungs for O_2 is 4.6 ml/100 ml

Table 8–1. NORMAL GAS PRESSURES (in mm Hg) IN A YOUNG ADULT DURING INSPIRATION, IN AMBIENT AIR, CONDUCTING AIRWAYS, TERMINAL UNITS (ALVEOLI), AND ARTERIAL AND MIXED VENOUS BLOOD

	Ambient Air	Conducting Airways	Terminal Units	Arterial Blood	Mixed Venous Blood
P_{O_2}	156	149	101	95	40
P_{CO_2}	0	0	40	40	46
P_{H_2O}	15*	47	47	47	47
P_{N_2}	589	564	572	572	572
P_{TOTAL}	760	760	760	754	705

*P_{H_2O} varies according to humidity and has a proportionate effect on P_{O_2} and P_{N_2}.

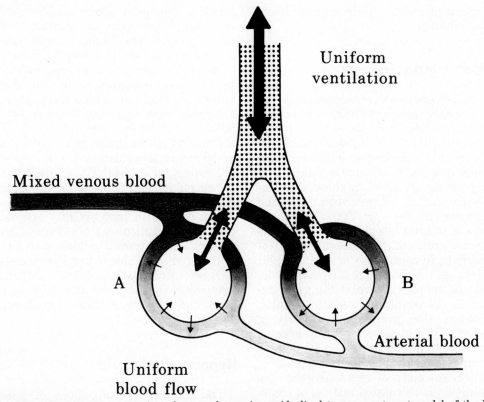

Uniform
ventilation

Mixed venous blood

A

B

Arterial blood

Uniform
blood flow

Figure 8–1. Schematic representation of gas exchange in an idealized two-compartment model of the lung in which there is uniform distribution of ventilation and blood flow. (Adapted from Comroe, J. H., Jr. et al.: The Lung. Clinical Physiology and Pulmonary Function Tests. 2nd Ed. Chicago, 1962, pp. 1–390. Reprinted by permission from the authors and Year Book Medical Publishers, Inc.)

	A	B	A + B	Units
Alveolar ventilation	2.4	2.4	4.8	L/min
Pulmonary blood flow	3.0	3.0	6.0	L/min
Ventilation-perfusion ratio	0.8	0.8	0.8	
Mixed venous P_{O_2}	40	40	40	mm Hg
Mixed venous S_{O_2}	70	75	75	per cent
Mixed venous P_{CO_2}	46	46	46	mm Hg
Alveolar P_{O_2}	101	101	101	mm Hg
Arterial P_{O_2}	101	101	101	mm Hg
Arterial S_{O_2}	97.5	97.5	97.5	per cent
Arterial P_{CO_2}	40	40	40	mm Hg
Alveolar-arterial P_{O_2} difference	0	0	0	mm Hg

and for CO_2 is 3.7 ml/100 ml. The large, double-pointed arrows indicate both the magnitude and the distribution of ventilation. The small arrows indicate diffusion of O_2 and CO_2 between alveolar gas and pulmonary capillary blood. The "arterialization" of blood is signified by the change in shading from black (mixed venous blood) to light gray (arterial blood).

In Figure 8–1, alveolar ventilation and blood flow are uniformly distributed to the gas exchange units; normally, there is less alveolar ventilation than pulmonary blood flow and the over-all *ventilation-perfusion*

ratio of the lung is 0.8. Because diffusion equilibrium is attained between the blood and gas phases, the values for both P_{O_2} and P_{CO_2} are the same in alveolar gas as in end-capillary and arterial blood. The essential feature of "ideal" gas exchange is that both ventilation and blood flow are distributed uniformly to the two gas exchange units; accordingly, there is no alveolar-arterial P_{O_2} difference. A small alveolar-arterial P_{O_2} difference occurs even in healthy persons (note that the values in Table 8–1 reveal an alveolar-arterial P_{O_2} difference of 6 mm Hg in a normal young adult), and an increased difference is one of the hallmarks of abnormal O_2 exchange.

Alveolar-Arterial Difference

The effectiveness of gas exchange by the lungs is usually assessed through measurements of Po_2 and Pco_2 in arterial blood. However, as will be shown, additional information about the mechanisms that underlie any abnormalities (if present) is obtained by relating values in blood to those simultaneously present in mean alveolar gas: the *alveolar-arterial* Po_2 *or* Pco_2 *difference.* Analysis of arterial blood gas composition is simple and accurate, but measurements of Po_2 and Pco_2 in continuous or spot samples of expired gas, although readily available, may not be representative of the gas composition in *all* terminal respiratory units; furthermore, the greater the underlying pathophysiologic abnormality, the greater the difficulty in obtaining a satisfactory specimen of alveolar gas. For these reasons, a practical estimate of mean alveolar gas concentration is calculated instead of measured by using the *alveolar air equation;* for mean alveolar Po_2 (PA_{O_2}):

$$PA_{O_2} = PI_{O_2} - PA_{CO_2}\left[FI_{O_2} + \frac{1 - FI_{O_2}}{R}\right], \quad (1)$$

where PI_{O_2} = Po_2 of inspired gas; PA_{CO_2} = alveolar Pco_2 (usually assumed to equal arterial Pco_2); FI_{O_2} = fractional concentration of O_2 in inspired gas; and R = respiratory exchange ratio (see above).

Disturbances of Gas Exchange

Measurements of arterial Po_2 and Pco_2 and calculations of alveolar-arterial Po_2 differences provide a handy clinical guide to the over-all adequacy of respiration. If abnormal values are obtained, further studies are often necessary to determine which one, or more, of the various processes that contribute to gas exchange are at fault. Normal values for Po_2, but not for Pco_2, vary considerably with age (see Chapter 14), and both Po_2 and Pco_2 are influenced by the altitude at which the subject is living when sampling is performed.

Finding an arterial Po_2 value below the range for normal subjects of the same age establishes the presence of *arterial hypoxia.* When defined in terms of Po_2, arterial hypoxia can result *only* from disturbances of respiration or from a reduction in the Po_2 of inspired air (Table 8–2).* *Hypercapnia,* or CO_2 retention, is defined as an elevation of arterial Pco_2 above the normal range; *hypocapnia* is a lower than normal arterial Pco_2.

Hypoventilation

The simplest derangement of gas exchange occurs when insufficient fresh air is breathed *(hypoventilation)* to provide enough new O_2 molecules to raise pulmonary capillary Po_2 to normal levels and to allow sufficient CO_2 to leave the bloodstream. When this situation develops, as shown in Figure 8–2, the quantity of O_2 in both arterial and venous blood must decrease, and the amount of CO_2 must increase. Although the blood gas abnormali-

---

*Some definitions exclude the presence of intracardiac right-to-left shunts of blood as a "respiratory" cause of arterial hypoxia. But as will be pointed out, right-to-left shunts are one of the major causes of a decreased arterial Po_2, and it does not matter where the shunt pathway exists.

Table 8–2. CAUSES OF ARTERIAL HYPOXIA (A REDUCTION IN Po_2) AND THEIR EFFECT ON ALVEOLAR-ARTERIAL Po_2 DIFFERENCES ([A-a]Po_2)

Cause	Effect on Arterial Po_2	Effect on (A-a)Po_2
Hypoventilation	Decreased	No change
Diffusion abnormality	No change or decreased*	No change or increased*
Ventilation-perfusion imbalance	Decreased	Increased
Right-to-left shunt	Decreased	Increased
Reduction in inspired Po_2	Decreased	No change

*Effects of diffusion abnormalities are infrequently encountered at rest but are more likely to be evident during exercise or at high altitude.

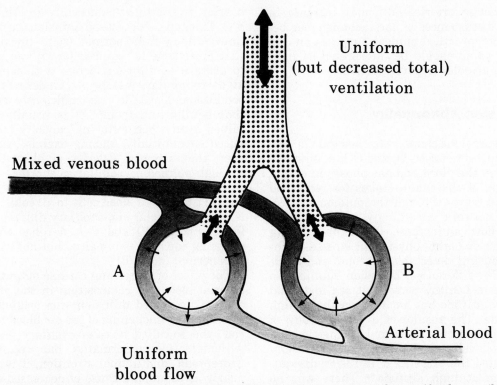

Figure 8–2. Schematic representation of the effects of hypoventilation on gas exchange. Alveolar ventilation is one-half that in Figure 8–1. (Adapted from Comroe, J. H., Jr. et al.: The Lung. Clinical Physiology and Pulmonary Function Tests. 2nd Ed. Chicago, 1962, pp. 1–390. Reprinted by permission from the authors and Year Book Medical Publishers, Inc.)

	A	B	A + B	Units
Alveolar ventilation	1.2	1.2	2.4	L/min
Pulmonary blood flow	3.0	3.0	6.0	L/min
Ventilation-perfusion ratio	0.4	0.4	0.4	
Mixed venous Po_2	34	34	34	mm Hg
Mixed venous So_2	64.3	64.3	64.3	per cent
Mixed venous Pco_2	90	90	90	mm Hg
Alveolar Po_2	53	53	53	mm Hg
Arterial Po_2	53	53	53	mm Hg
Arterial So_2	87.2	87.2	87.2	per cent
Arterial Pco_2	80	80	80	mm Hg
Alveolar-arterial Po_2 difference	0	0	0	mm Hg

ties that result from hypoventilation may be severe, it should be noted that if ventilation and blood flow remain uniformly distributed, as they are in Figure 8–2, no alveolar-arterial difference develops for either O_2 or CO_2.

Pure hypoventilation is a relatively uncommon clinical event; in most instances, hypoventilation coexists with one or more other causes of arterial hypoxia. When pure hypoventilation occurs, it is usually caused by depression of the central nervous system from anesthesia or sedative drugs, or by neuromuscular diseases that affect respiratory muscle function. In these disorders both the amount of air that is breathed in through the nose or the mouth *(minute ventilation)* and the amount that reaches the gas exchange units *(alveolar ventilation)* are reduced. The CO_2 pressure in alveolar gas (PA_{CO_2}) and arterial blood (Pa_{CO_2}) can be expressed by the relationship

$$PA_{CO_2} = Pa_{CO_2} = K \frac{\dot{V}_{CO_2}}{\dot{V}A}, \qquad (2)$$

where $\dot{V}_{CO_2}$ is the CO_2 output (or production), $\dot{V}A$ is the alveolar ventilation, and K is a constant. This equation indicates that if CO_2 production remains constant, halving alveolar ventilation doubles arterial Pco_2.

Although arterial P_{CO_2} may increase in other disturbances of gas exchange (see below), for practical clinical purposes an elevated value should be interpreted as indicating alveolar hypoventilation.

Diffusion Abnormality

The previous chapter stressed that in normal subjects at rest, O_2 and CO_2 equilibrate between the blood and gas phases in only a fraction of the time it takes for red blood cells to travel through the pulmonary capillary network; accordingly, the velocity of blood flow can increase considerably during exercise and other physiologic stresses without causing detectable alveolar end-capillary P_{O_2} differences. Diffusion equilibrium occurs in healthy persons at sea level and at low altitude but not necessarily at high altitude. The results of a recent study of normal subjects at rest and during exercise at sea level and simulated altitudes demonstrated the presence of diffusion disequilibrium at high altitude.[4a] There was no evidence of diffusion limitation at sea level or at 1524 m (5,000 ft.), even during moderately heavy exercise. However, an alveolar-arterial P_{O_2} difference attributable to incomplete diffusion was found during exercise (not at rest) at 3049 m (10,000 ft.), and the difference became even greater at 4573 m (15,000 ft.) These data provide the most direct evidence to date of the important contribution of diffusion disequilibrium to gas exchange in normal unacclimatized humans exercising at high altitude.

Many patients with lung disease have abnormal diffusing capacities, as measured in the pulmonary function laboratory with CO. But diffusion disequilibrium, manifested by an alveolar end-capillary P_{O_2} difference—in these patients while at rest—is unusual. In contrast, abnormalities of diffusion are much more likely to affect arterial blood gas composition during exercise and the effects are magnified at altitude. Exercise-induced desaturation occurs whether the abnormality of diffusion results from lengthening of the diffusion·pathway across the alveolar-capillary membrane or from a decrease in pulmonary capillary blood volume.

The explanation for the enhanced effect of exercise in producing arterial hypoxia in the presence of a given abnormality of diffusion caused by thickening of the air-blood barrier is shown schematically in Figure 8–3. This type of decreased diffusion (dashed lines) differs from normal (solid lines) in that more time is required for O_2 and CO_2 to achieve equilibrium across a thickened alveolar-capillary membrane. Under resting conditions, blood flow is sufficiently slow that equilibrium (point A) is usually attained even when diffusing capacity is reduced substantially. During exercise, however, the increased velocity of blood flow through pulmonary capillaries shortens the time available for diffusion; when the exposure time of red blood cells to alveolar gas is halved, alveolar end-capillary differences for O_2 (point B') and CO_2 develop when diffusing capacity is impaired but not when it is normal (point B).

The effect of increasing cardiac output on arterial blood gas composition in the presence of decreased diffusion was originally attributed to thickening of the air-blood barrier, the so-called *alveolar-capillary block*. Although this abnormality has received widespread (and undue) attention, it is not nearly as common a cause of decreased diffusing capacity measurements as is a reduction in pulmonary capillary blood volume. In this circumstance, the mechanism of arterial hypoxia is different from that which exists when the alveolar-capillary membrane is thickened; a reduction in pulmonary capillary blood volume is also displayed in Figure 8–3. As capillaries are progressively destroyed or obstructed, previously unperfused capillaries are successively recruited until finally the velocity of blood flow through the remaining vessels increases. When the disease process is severe, the time available for gas exchange in these patients at rest may be as short as it is in normal subjects during exercise (point B); consequently, during exercise the short pulmonary capillary transit times become even shorter, and failure of equilibration occurs (point C).

Ventilation-Perfusion Imbalance

In contrast to the ideal condition described previously, the distributions of inspired air and pulmonary capillary blood are neither uniform nor proportionate to each other. As emphasized in Chapters 4 and 6, the distributions of ventilation and blood flow can be shown to vary with such common events as changes in body position and changes in

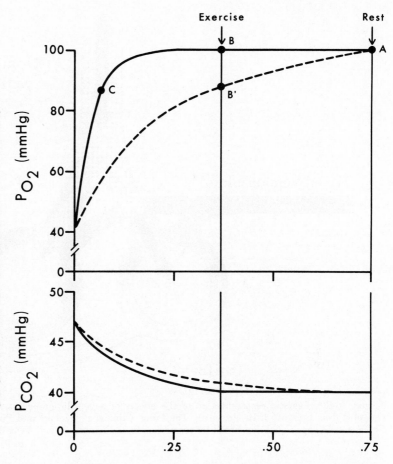

Figure 8–3. Schematic diagram showing the time course of changes in P_{O_2} and P_{CO_2} at rest and during exercise in normal subjects and in patients with decreased diffusing capacities from thickened alveolar-capillary membranes and decreased pulmonary capillary blood volumes. At rest, equilibration occurs between the pressures in the blood and gas phases (point A) in both normal subjects (solid line) and patients with decreased diffusing capacities from a thickened air-blood barrier (dashed line); during exercise, because the time available for gas exchange is shortened, equilibration occurs in normal subjects (point B) but not in patients (point B'). When the capillary bed is destroyed or obstructed, the velocity of blood flow increases in the remaining vessels under resting conditions (point B); during exercise, equilibration is no longer possible (point C).

TIME SPENT IN PULMONARY CAPILLARY
(Sec)

lung volume. Thus, there is always some variable degree of ventilation-perfusion imbalance present, even in normal subjects. Moreover, increased (above normal) mismatching of ventilation and perfusion is by far the most common cause of arterial hypoxia in patients with disorders affecting the respiratory system. It is worthwhile, therefore, to consider how ventilation-perfusion abnormalities occur, as well as their consequences.

The two-compartment model used to depict ideal gas exchange has been modified to that shown in Figure 8–4. The composition of mixed venous blood, total blood flow, and the distribution of blood are the same as in Figure 8–1. However, the same total alveolar ventilation is now distributed unevenly between the two gas exchange units, so that Unit A receives three times more inspired gas than Unit B. Because blood

flow is equally distributed to the two units, the ventilation-perfusion ratios ($\dot{V}A/\dot{Q}$) differ and cause the alveolar and end-capillary gas compositions to vary as shown. The O_2 and CO_2 contents of the end-capillary blood from each alveolus are determined by the gas pressures in the alveoli, which are in equilibrium with the end-capillary blood, and by the respective hemoglobin equilibration curves for the two gases. To derive the final composition of arterial blood after the two effluent vascular pathways mix, it is necessary first to sum algebraically* the contents (or saturations), *not the pressures*, and then to determine the resulting pressures from the oxyhemoglobin and CO_2 equi-

---

*In Figure 8–4, simple addition and division by two are all that are required, because blood flow is equally distributed; if blood flow to the two alveoli had been uneven, as in the case of ventilation, algebraic weighting would have been necessary.

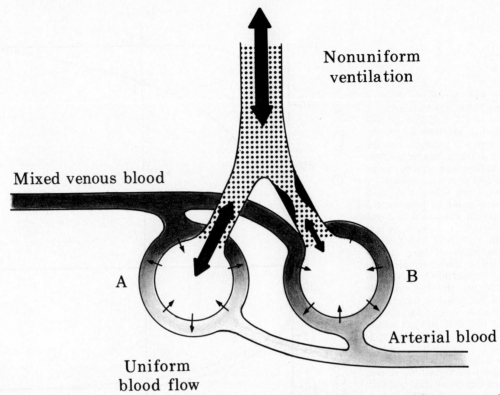

Nonuniform ventilation

Mixed venous blood

A

B

Arterial blood

Uniform blood flow

Figure 8–4. Schematic representation of the effects of a ventilation-perfusion abnormality on gas exchange. (Adapted from Comroe, J. H., Jr. et al.: The Lung. Clinical Physiology and Pulmonary Function Tests. 2nd Ed. Chicago, 1962, pp. 1–390. Reprinted by permission from the authors and Year Book Medical Publishers, Inc.)

	A	B	A + B	Units
Alveolar ventilation	3.6	1.2	4.8	L/min
Pulmonary blood flow	3.0	3.0	6.0	L/min
Ventilation-perfusion ratio	1.2	0.4	0.8	
Mixed venous P_{O_2}	40	40	40	mm Hg
Mixed venous S_{O_2}	75	75	75	per cent
Mixed venous P_{CO_2}	46	46	46	mm Hg
Alveolar P_{O_2}	114	77	105	mm Hg
Arterial P_{O_2}	114	77	89	mm Hg
Arterial S_{O_2}	98.2	95.4	96.8	per cent
Alveolar P_{CO_2}	36	45	38.3	mm Hg
Arterial P_{CO_2}	36	45	40.5	mm Hg
Alveolar-arterial P_{O_2} difference	0	0	16	mm Hg

librium curves (see Fig. 7–7 and 7–10); this procedure is required because of the alinear characteristics of both curves.

The final composition of mixed alveolar gas is derived by summing the gas tensions and algebraically allowing for the differences in ventilation to the two units. (In Fig. 8–4, [3(114) + 77]/4 = 105, for P_{O_2}.)

An important consequence of a ventilation-perfusion imbalance is evident even in this simplified diagram and analysis: *there must be a difference between the O_2 and CO_2 pressures in mixed alveolar gas and arterial blood.* The alveolar-arterial P_{O_2} difference

is 16 mm Hg, and the arterial-alveolar P_{CO_2} difference is 2.2 mm Hg in the example chosen. Alveolar-arterial differences occur because the relative overventilation of one unit does not fully compensate—by adding extra O_2 or by eliminating extra CO_2—for the disturbances created by underventilating the other unit. The failure to compensate is greater in the case of O_2 than in that of CO_2 owing to the flatness of the upper part of the oxyhemoglobin dissociation curve compared with the CO_2 dissociation curve. Increased ventilation raises alveolar P_{O_2} but adds little "extra" O_2 (content) to the bloodstream; in contrast, the steeper slope of the CO_2 curve allows more CO_2 to be eliminated when ventilation increases.

The calculations used to derive the values shown (see Fig. 8–4) are useful for illustrative purposes but are not completely accurate because mixed venous blood composition is held constant and is not affected, as it would be, by the circulation of arterial blood with reduced O_2 and increased CO_2 through the tissues of the body. A detailed and elegant computer analysis of a ten-compartment lung model, which takes these and other mathematical complexities into account, has been developed by West.[5] Figure 8–5 is reproduced from his work and shows the effect of increasing ventilation-perfusion inequality on gas exchange, the amount of venous admixture (see subsequent section), and the amount of wasted alveolar ventilation (see subsequent sec-

tion). As the inequality increases, arterial Po_2 falls continuously and precipitously, and arterial Pco_2 rises gradually at first and then more swiftly. This means, contrary to the usual teaching, that ventilation-perfusion imbalance can be a significant cause of CO_2 retention in patients with pulmonary disease.[6] This statement at first glance may appear to conflict with the common clinical observations that patients with many forms of pulmonary disease (e.g., emphysema and bronchial asthma) may have severe arterial hypoxia caused by ventilation-perfusion abnormalities but may also have arterial Pco_2 levels that are normal or, at times, even lower than normal. This apparent discrepancy is explained by the fact that these patients are ventilating more than is normal, and because of the respective shapes and positions of the equilibrium curves for O_2 and CO_2, hyperventilation of the ventil-

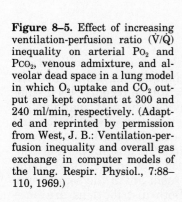

Figure 8–5. Effect of increasing ventilation-perfusion ratio ($\dot{V}/\dot{Q}$) inequality on arterial Po_2 and Pco_2, venous admixture, and alveolar dead space in a lung model in which O_2 uptake and CO_2 output are kept constant at 300 and 240 ml/min, respectively. (Adapted and reprinted by permission from West, J. B.: Ventilation-perfusion inequality and overall gas exchange in computer models of the lung. Respir. Physiol., 7:88–110, 1969.)

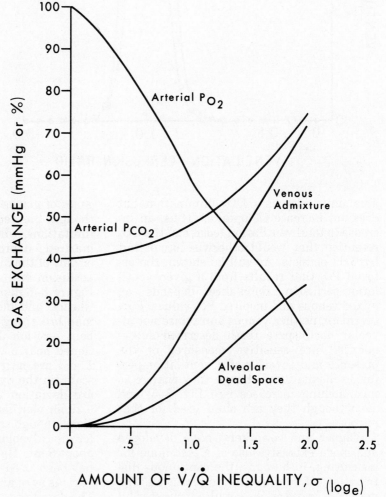

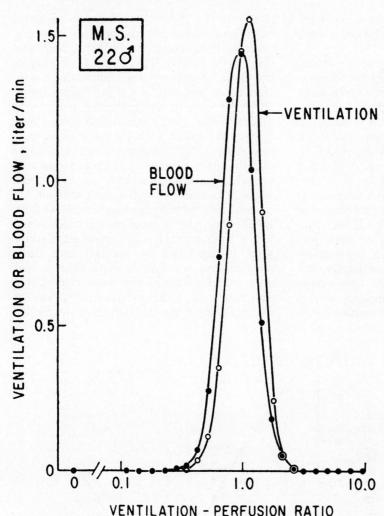

Figure 8–6. The distributions of ventilation and blood flow in a normal 22 year old man. Both distributions are positioned about a ventilation-perfusion ratio close to 1.0; the curves are symmetrical on a log scale with no areas of high or low ventilation-perfusion ratios, and there is no shunt (ventilation-perfusion ratio = zero). (Reprinted by permission from Wagner, P. D., et al.: Continuous distributions of ventilation-perfusion ratios in normal subjects breathing air and 100% O_2. J. Clin. Invest., *54*:54–68, 1974.)

able units increases CO_2 elimination but does not increase O_2 uptake.[6] Thus, an increase in total ventilation "corrects" the CO_2 retention that would otherwise occur, but hypoxia persists. As will be shown, the arterial Po_2 that results from a given ventilation-perfusion imbalance depends on mixed venous and inspired Po_2 values. Furthermore, neither venous admixture nor alveolar dead space (both described subsequently) are sensitive measures of the presence and severity of a ventilation-perfusion inequality, although they change as mismatching increases (see Fig. 8–5) and even though they are often used for that purpose.

Wagner and coworkers[8] have developed and made extensive use of a technique for measuring, in humans, the continuous distributions of ventilation and perfusion. The method is based on the simultaneous steady-state elimination by the lung of six inert gases of markedly different solubilities. Although the technique has some inherent limitations, which have recently been summarized,[9] it provides the best available overview of the distribution of ventilation and perfusion in humans in health and disease. Figure 8–6 depicts the distributions of ventilation and blood flow in a normal young man breathing room air in the semirecumbent position. Both distributions are positioned near a ventilation-perfusion ratio of 1 and are narrow and symmetric on a log scale (in the example shown, the log standard deviation was 0.32 for blood flow and 0.29 for ventilation). However, these dispersions, though small, are sufficient to account for an alveolar-arterial Po_2 difference of about 6 mm Hg (see Table 8–1). The method has been used to study healthy subjects of various ages and in different body positions. The results confirm the long-standing belief that the unevenness of the distribution of ventilation-perfusion ratios found in young adults worsens with increasing age and that regions of high ventilation-perfusion ratios develop with changes from the supine to the sitting position; the latter findings are consistent with the known effects of posture on the topographic distribution of ventilation, blood flow, and lung volumes discussed in Chapters 4 and 6.

Right-to-Left Shunts

Another departure from ideal gas exchange is caused by right-to-left shunts of blood in the lungs; these are found to a slight degree in normal subjects and may be of considerable magnitude in patients with pulmonary disease. A schematic representation of the effects of a right-to-left shunt upon gas exchange is shown in Figure 8–7. Alveolar ventilation, distribution of ventilation, and composition of mixed venous blood are the same as they were under ideal conditions, but distribution of cardiac output is different. The total blood flow remains the same (6 L/min), but only 2 L/min each, instead of 3 L/min each, reaches Units A and B; the remaining 2 L/min flows through the shunt pathway. In other words, there is

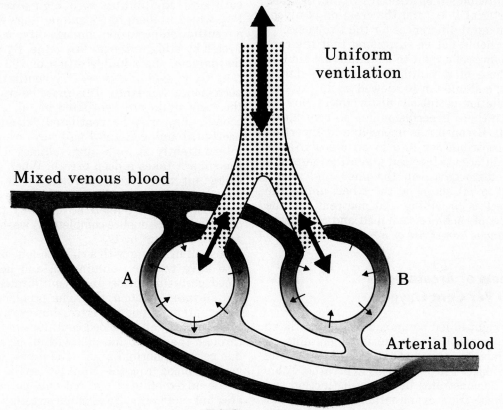

Figure 8–7. Schematic representation of the effects of a right-to-left shunt on gas exchange. (Adapted from Comroe, J. H., Jr. et al.: The Lung. Clinical Physiology and Pulmonary Function Tests. 2nd Ed. Chicago, 1962, pp. 1–390. Reprinted by permission from the authors and Year Book Medical Publishers, Inc.)

	A + B	Shunt	A + B A + B + Shunt	Units
Alveolar ventilation	4.8	0	4.8	L/min
Pulmonary blood flow	4.0	2.0	6.0	L/min
Ventilation-perfusion ratio	1.2	0	0.8	
Mixed venous P_{O_2}	40	40	40	mm Hg
Mixed venous S_{O_2}	75	75	75	per cent
Mixed venous P_{CO_2}	46	46	46	mm Hg
Alveolar P_{O_2}	114	—	114	mm Hg
Arterial P_{O_2}	114	—	59	mm Hg
Arterial S_{O_2}	98.2	—	90.5	per cent
Arterial P_{CO_2}	36	—	39	mm Hg
Alveolar-arterial P_{O_2} difference	0	—	55	mm Hg

a right-to-left shunt of one-third of the total cardiac output.

Gas exchange in Units A and B is unimpaired (see Fig. 8–7); in fact, because the individual ventilation-perfusion ratios are high, slightly more O_2 is taken up and more CO_2 is eliminated than would occur if the ratios were normal. But this slight augmentation of gas exchange does not nearly compensate for the deleterious effect of the continuous flow of mixed venous blood through the shunt. The net result from the mixing of blood from the normal and the shunt pathways is analogous to the effects of a ventilation-perfusion inequality: an inevitable reduction of arterial Po_2, an increase in arterial Pco_2, and the creation of alveolar-arterial differences for the two gases.

It should not be surprising that the consequences of a right-to-left shunt are similar to those of a ventilation-perfusion imbalance; a shunt can be viewed as an extreme ventilation-perfusion disturbance: one in which there is perfusion but no ventilation at all. Because it is impossible to apportion the contributions to a given alveolar-arterial difference between a ventilation-perfusion disturbance on the one hand and a right-to-left shunt on the other, *unless* the subject is breathing 100 per cent O_2, the effects of each are combined and considered as *venous admixture* or a "shunt-like" effect.

Effects of Breathing 100 Per Cent Oxygen

A right-to-left shunt can be differentiated from a ventilation-perfusion inequality in the laboratory and at the bedside by giving the subject 100 per cent O_2 to breathe. Table 8–3 demonstrates how this distinction can be made from examination of the alveolar and arterial gas pressures that result when

ideal lungs and lungs with either a ventilation-perfusion abnormality or a right-to-left shunt breathe 100 per cent O_2. Breathing 100 per cent O_2 ultimately replaces all the alveolar N_2 with O_2 in ventilable units, leaving only O_2, CO_2, and H_2O in the alveoli. When this occurs,

$$PA_{O_2} = PA_{TOTAL} - PA_{CO_2} - PA_{H_2O}. \quad (3)$$

Because the total or barometric pressure and H_2O vapor pressure are the same in all communicating lung units, alveolar Po_2 differs from unit to unit only by corresponding differences in alveolar Pco_2. Blood perfusing each unit equilibrates at a high alveolar Po_2, which in ideal lungs and in lungs with a ventilation-perfusion abnormality, is reflected by a high arterial Po_2 value. By this mechanism, the administration of 100 per cent O_2 is said to "correct" a ventilation-perfusion disturbance. This must be true if the lung units are ventilated at all, even though they may be ventilated extremely poorly through collateral pathways or only intermittently at high lung volumes when the subject takes a deep breath. When carrying out this study, therefore, it is obviously important to allow enough time and to insist that the subject occasionally take deep breaths to ensure complete N_2 washout and replacement by O_2.

Alveoli in a lung with a right-to-left shunt also have their N_2 eliminated, and hence blood perfusing those units equilibrates at the elevated alveolar Po_2. The problem in oxygenation is not corrected, however, because mixed venous blood continues to flow through the shunt and mix with blood that has perfused normal units. The poorly oxygenated blood from the shunt lowers the Po_2 of the mixed effluent and not only perpetuates but augments the alveolar-arterial Po_2 difference. An elevated alveolar-arterial Po_2

Table 8–3. EFFECT OF BREATHING 21 PER CENT AND 100 PER CENT O_2 ON MEAN Po_2 VALUES IN ALVEOLAR GAS AND ARTERIAL AND MIXED VENOUS BLOOD IN TWO-COMPARTMENT LUNG MODELS WITH IDEAL GAS EXCHANGE (FIG. 8–1), A VENTILATION-PERFUSION ABNORMALITY (FIG. 8–4), AND A RIGHT-TO-LEFT SHUNT (FIG. 8–7)

	Ideal		Ventilation-Perfusion Abnormality		Right-to-Left Shunt	
	21%	*100%*	*21%*	*100%*	*21%*	*100%*
Mixed venous Po_2	40	51	40	51	40	42
Alveolar Po_2	101	673	105	675	114	677
Arterial Po_2	101	673	89	673	59	125
Alveolar-arterial Po_2 difference	0	0	16	2	55	552

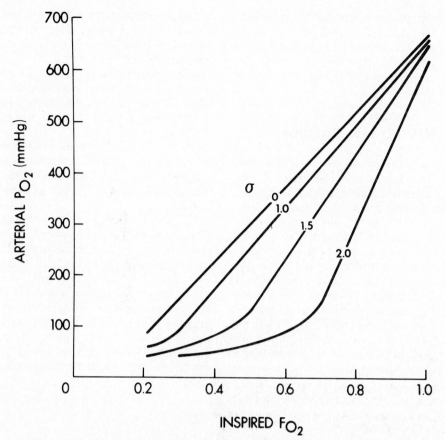

Figure 8–8. Graph showing the effects of changing inspired O_2 concentration (F_{O_2}) on arterial P_{O_2} in the presence of varying amounts of ventilation-perfusion inequality. When ventilation and perfusion are evenly matched ($\sigma = 0$), the relationship between inspired F_{O_2}, from 21 to 100 per cent, is linear. As ventilation-perfusion inequalities worsen ($\sigma = 1.0$ to 2.0), the effect of breathing a given F_{O_2} is progressively less. Note that when the ventilation-perfusion abnormality is severe ($\sigma = 2.0$), breathing gas with an F_{O_2} as high as 0.7 has little effect on arterial P_{O_2}. (Adapted and reprinted from West, J. B., and Wagner, P. D.: Pulmonary gas exchange. *In* West, J. B., and Wagner, P. D. (eds.): Bioengineering Aspects of the Lung. 1977, pp. 361–457 by courtesy of Marcel Dekker, Inc.)

difference during a properly conducted 100 per cent O_2 study signifies the presence of a right-to-left shunt, and the magnitude of the difference between the P_{O_2} value obtained and the normal value can be used to quantify the proportion of cardiac output that is shunted by using the so called "shunt equation:"

$$\frac{\dot{Q}s}{\dot{Q}_T} = \frac{Cc' - Ca}{Cc' - C\bar{v}} , \qquad (4)$$

where $\dot{Q}s/\dot{Q}_T$ is venous admixture, which is solely due to shunting when 100 per cent O_2 is breathed, and Cc', Ca, and C$\bar{v}$ are the O_2 contents of end-capillary, arterial, and mixed venous bloods, respectively. The Cc' and Ca are derived from alveolar and arterial P_{O_2} values, which are used to compute

dissolved O_2 and per cent saturation, and the subject's hemoglobin concentration. Arterial P_{O_2} is measured directly, and alveolar P_{O_2} is computed by using Equation 1. Preferably, mixed venous O_2 content is measured directly, but if appropriate samples cannot be obtained, it is often estimated by assuming an arteriovenous O_2 difference (normally 4.5 to 5.0 ml/100 ml). As a rough clinical guide, an alveolar-arterial P_{O_2} difference of 15 mm Hg while breathing 100 per cent O_2 indicates a right-to-left shunt of about 1 per cent of the cardiac output. However, this approximation is valid only when cardiac output and the arteriovenous O_2 difference are normal.

When performing the test for right-to-left shunts, it is important to administer high concentrations of O_2. As shown in Figure 8–8, the arterial P_{O_2} response of a severe ventilation-perfusion abnormality ($\sigma = 2.0$) is similar to that of a true shunt until greater than 70 per cent O_2 is breathed.[1] Even then, normal arterial P_{O_2} values do not occur until 95 or 100 per cent O_2 is administered.

Sites of Right-to-Left Shunting

When a normal young subject breathes 100 per cent O_2, an alveolar-arterial P_{O_2} difference of between 30 and 50 mm Hg can usually be detected; this demonstrates the presence of a right-to-left shunt of approximately 2 to 3 per cent of the cardiac output. Another method of quantifying the magnitude of right-to-left shunts involves the use of insoluble radioactive or measurable inert gases.[8, 10, 11] The results using these techniques differ slightly from those using the O_2 method because insoluble gases identify only shunts of blood from the systemic venous circulation through or around the lungs, whereas the O_2 method is sensitive

to venous admixture anywhere proximal to the arterial sampling site. Several studies using insoluble gases have shown virtually no right-to-left shunt (i.e., < 1 per cent) through normal lungs; these results, when combined with those from studies of shunts with 100 per cent O_2 breathing, have indicated that most of the small shunts in normal subjects occur distal to the gas exchange units.[10, 11] Thus, the normal pathways do not occur around alveoli, as shown schematically in Figure 8–7, but occur after alveoli, the *"postpulmonary shunt,"* as shown in Figure 8–9.

The chief sources of the normal postpulmonary shunt are the bronchial veins and the veins from the mediastinum that empty into pulmonary veins and the thebesian vessels of the left ventricular myocardium that empty directly into the left ventricular cavity. However, the right-to-left shunt diagramed in Figure 8–7 is not purely hypothetic; it accurately depicts the pattern of blood flow for shunts in many pathologic conditions. It is important to emphasize that

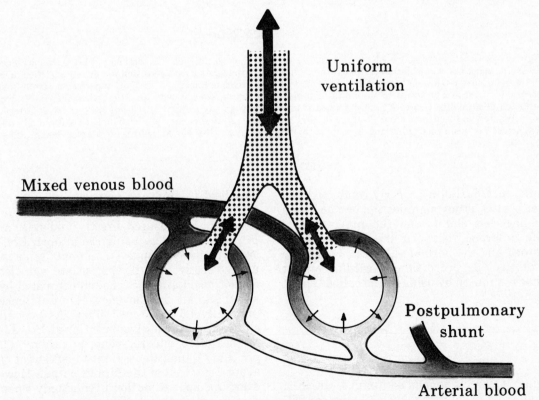

Uniform ventilation

Mixed venous blood

Postpulmonary shunt

Arterial blood

Figure 8–9. Schematic diagram showing the location of the right-to-left shunt present in normal persons. Instead of a pathway that bypasses alveoli (see Fig. 8–7), the postpulmonary shunt occurs from venous blood that mixes with arterialized blood in the pulmonary veins and left ventricular cavity. (Adapted from Comroe, J. H., Jr. et al.: The Lung. Clinical Physiology and Pulmonary Function Tests. 2nd Ed. Chicago, 1962, pp. 1–390. Reprinted by permission form the authors and Year Book Medical Publishers, Inc.)

in some instances a discrete abnormal anatomic pathway (as shown) does exist (i.e., intracardiac communications, pulmonary arteriovenous fistulae), but in other instances shunts occur through normal vessels that perfuse regions of lung that are not ventilated at all because the alveoli are filled or closed or the airways leading to the terminal units are completely obstructed (i.e., pneumonia, pulmonary edema, atelectasis). When shunts occur in patients with pulmonary disease, they are usually accounted for by the perfusion of nonventilated lung through relatively normal vascular channels.

Careful studies of right-to-left shunts in patients with lung disease and in various experimental models of acute lung injury have revealed an interesting relationship between total cardiac output and the fraction of that blood flow that is shunted (which is equal to $\dot{Q}s/\dot{Q}_T$ in Equation 4): as cardiac output increased, so did the fraction of blood flow that was shunted.[12, 13] This cannot be explained by the effect of increasing cardiac output on mixed venous O_2 content (see subsequent section), because this increase and the resulting increase in arterial O_2 content are such that the calculated shunt fraction should not change. It has been speculated that as mixed venous O_2 content increases, it causes relaxation of hypoxia-induced pulmonary arterial vasoconstriction in the nonventilated pathways; accordingly, vascular resistance decreases mainly in the nonventilated regions, which leads in turn to a preferential increase in the right-to-left shunt of blood.[14]

Effect of Changing Cardiac Output

The discussion of gas exchange thus far has dealt chiefly with the effects on gas exchange of various respiratory phenomena: alveolar ventilation, diffusion, and distribution of ventilation and blood flow, including right-to-left shunts. The single nonrespiratory factor that needs to be considered is the effect of changing cardiac output, because this affects the composition of mixed venous blood. Decreasing cardiac output causes O_2 content to decrease and CO_2 content to increase in mixed venous blood; increasing cardiac output has the opposite effect. Decreased O_2 content and increased CO_2 content in mixed venous blood usually

have little effect on arterial Po_2 and Pco_2 *in persons with normal lungs,* except in patients in shock when cardiac output is extremely low, because the amount of venous admixture is small. However, in the presence of lung disease with a substantial amount of venous admixture, resulting from either a marked ventilation-perfusion abnormality or a large right-to-left shunt, or both, the composition of mixed venous blood has considerable effect on the Po_2 and Pco_2 values of arterial blood. Figure 8–10 illustrates the interacting effects on arterial Po_2 of increasing venous admixture, shown as ventilation-perfusion mismatching of worsening severity. Except in ideal lungs ($\sigma = 0$), for a given amount of ventilation-perfusion imbalance, the lower the cardiac output, the lower the arterial Po_2.[1]

Normal Alveolar-Arterial Oxygen Difference

In studies of healthy subjects 21 to 30 years of age at rest in the seated (slightly reclining) position, a mean alveolar-arterial Po_2 difference of 8 mm Hg has been detected.[15] As indicated, the difference is due to the combined venous admixture effect from (1) mismatching of ventilation and perfusion and (2) right-to-left postpulmonary shunting of blood. Each of these mechanisms is responsible for about half of the total alveolar-arterial Po_2 difference in normal young adults. During senescence, the mean value for alveolar-arterial Po_2 difference increases to 16 mm Hg in normal persons 61 to 75 years of age;[15] this effect is mainly caused by increasing ventilation-perfusion inequalities (see Chapter 14 for details).[16] It should be noted that none of the normal alveolar-arterial Po_2 difference is caused by failure of diffusion equilibrium to occur. As emphasized earlier in this chapter, alveolar-arterial differences for O_2 from diffusion limitation do not develop in normal subjects even during heavy exercise at sea level. Diffusion disequilibrium may occur during exercise at high altitudes or in contrived experimental circumstances.

Alveolar Ventilation

The terms alveolar volume and alveolar ventilation are misnomers because the phenomena that they are supposed to designate

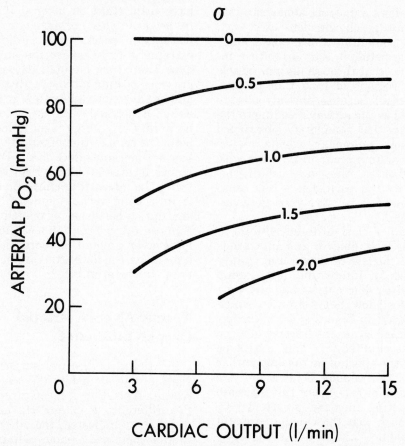

Figure 8–10. Schematic representation of the effects of changing cardiac output on arterial P_{O_2} in the presence of varying amounts of ventilation-perfusion inequality. When ventilation and perfusion are evenly matched ($\sigma = 0$), changing cardiac output has no effect on arterial P_{O_2}. As ventilation-perfusion inequalities worsen ($\sigma = 0.5$ to 2.0), arterial P_{O_2} decreases at any given cardiac output, and decreasing cardiac output decreases P_{O_2}. (Adapted and reprinted from West, J. B., and Wagner, P. D.: Pulmonary gas exchange. *In* West, J. B., and Wagner, P. D. (eds.): Bioengineering Aspects of the Lung. 1977, pp. 361–457 by courtesy of Marcel Dekker, Inc.)

take place in the entire terminal respiratory unit, i.e., alveoli, alveolar ducts, and respiratory bronchioles, not just alveoli. *Alveolar volume* is the total volume of gas in the gas exchange units at any moment, and *alveolar ventilation* is the amount of gas that moves into and out of "functioning" terminal respiratory units during a given period. The use of the word "functioning" has important implications, because measurement of alveolar ventilation depends upon the output of CO_2; a terminal respiratory unit may actually be ventilated, but if that unit is not taking up O_2 and eliminating CO_2 (e.g., a unit deprived of its blood flow), it is functionless, and the increment of fresh air it receives does not count as alveolar ventilation.

Alveolar volume is nearly the same as FRC in normal persons in the recumbent position; the slight difference between measurements of the two variables is due to the *anatomic dead space* (i.e., the volume of the nasopharynx and conducting airways), which is included in most measurements of FRC. About 35 to 40 per cent of the total alveolar volume is contained in the respiratory bronchioles and alveolar ducts, and the remainder is within true alveoli.[17] Using these values and accepting that all the structures composing the terminal respiratory unit expand and contract proportionately during breathing,[18] it is possible to estimate how each breath of fresh air is partitioned among the various anatomic units of the lungs. Assuming that a normal adult person has an anatomic dead space of 150 ml and is breathing with a tidal volume of 500 ml, an inspirate is distributed as follows: 150 ml is required to fill the anatomic dead space; the respiratory bronchioles and alveolar ducts increase their volume and accommodate 175 ml (0.35 × 500 ml); and only the remaining 175 ml, or 35 per cent of the inspirate, actually penetrates as far as alveoli.

Although the estimate in the preceding paragraph is crude and is greatly affected by the rate and depth of breathing, it supports the conclusion that only a small proportion of each new breath reaches alveoli by bulk flow through the respiratory system. As indicated in Chapter 7, incoming fresh air mixes, by molecular diffusion, extremely rapidly with the gas remaining in the terminal respiratory units after the previous breath, and convection (bulk flow) is relatively unimportant.

"Wasted" Ventilation

Alveolar ventilation cannot be measured directly but must be derived by making simultaneous measurements of two other volumes: *minute volume,* the total amount of gas inhaled through the nose or mouth, and *wasted ventilation* (also known as *physiologic dead space*)* which is considered to be that volume of each breath that is inhaled but does not reach functioning terminal respiratory units. Wasted ventilation can be viewed conceptually as the volume of gas in each breath that is literally wasted insofar as its contribution to gas exchange is concerned. The fraction of wasted ventilation per breath (V_D/V_T) is easily determined from the CO_2 pressures of simultaneously collected samples of expired air (PE_{CO_2}) and arterial blood (Pa_{CO_2}), using a modification of the Bohr equation that assumes that arterial PCO_2 is equal to alveolar PCO_2:

$$\frac{V_D}{V_T} = \frac{Pa_{CO_2} - PE_{CO_2}}{Pa_{CO_2}}. \quad (5)$$

Alveolar ventilation ($\dot{V}A$) is obtained from the total volume of gas exhaled ($\dot{V}E$) by

*Because, as Comroe used to remind us, "physiologic dead space isn't physiologic, it isn't a space, and it certainly isn't dead," wasted ventilation is the preferred term.

subtracting the fraction of the expirate that is wasted:

$$\dot{V}A = \dot{V}E\left[1 - \frac{V_D}{V_T}\right]. \quad (6)$$

This equation assumes that the volume of gas inhaled and exhaled is the same, which is not quite true. The difference can be accounted for by the fact that slightly more O_2 is removed from the inspirate than CO_2 is added to the expirate. Although the assumption of equality between arterial and alveolar PCO_2 is correct in the idealized lung, the two values differ slightly in healthy subjects and may differ considerably in patients with pulmonary disease. It should be recognized that the notion of wasted ventilation incorporates a drastic oversimplification of the physiologic events that contribute to the values obtained in the measurement. Conceptually, the lung is simply divided into two compartments: (1) an alveolar volume in which alveolar PCO_2 is everywhere equal to arterial PCO_2 and (2) a wasted ventilation volume in which there is no CO_2 whatsoever. Obviously, what actually occurs is that some terminal respiratory units are overventilated or underventilated relative to their blood flows; thus, their individual CO_2 outputs and end-capillary PCO_2 values vary a great deal. None of these individual variations can be detected by using Equation 5, because it treats the lung as consisting of only ideal alveoli and a homogeneous dead space.

Wasted ventilation, shown by the stippled region in Figures 8–1, 8–2, 8–4, 8–7, and 8–9 can be viewed as being composed of two compartments: (1) the anatomic dead space (the conducting air passages) and (2) the alveolar dead space. The latter volume is contributed to by all those terminal respiratory units that are overventilated relative to their perfusion.[19] As shown in Figure 8–11, wasted ventilation normally increases as end-inspiratory lung volume increases.[20] The observed change is primarily due to an enlargement of the anatomic dead space from the distension of airways that occurs as lung volume and transpulmonary pressure increase. Other changes in the breathing pattern, such as increasing rate and tidal volume, also cause the alveolar dead space to increase, because this breathing pattern allows less time for equilibration to occur between newly inspired fresh air and

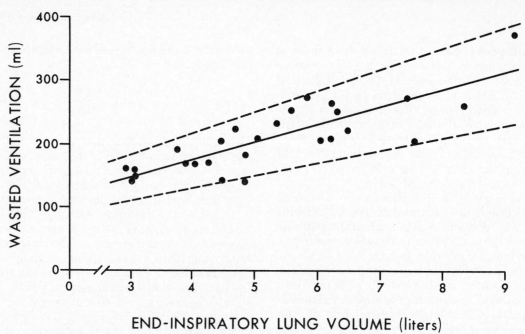

Figure 8–11. Relationship between wasted ventilation (physiologic dead space) and end-inspiratory lung volume in ten healthy young persons breathing with normal tidal volumes and respiratory frequencies. Each point represents a separate measurement. The solid line is the calculated regression line; the hatched lines were drawn by eye to define the "normal range." (Adapted and reprinted by permission from Lifshay, A. et al.: Effects of changes in respiratory pattern on physiological dead space. J. Appl. Physiol., *31*:478–483, 1971.)

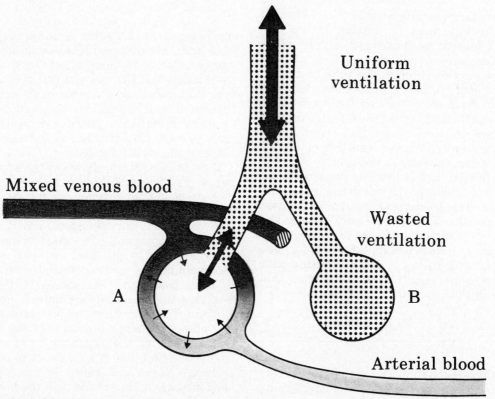

Figure 8–12. Schematic representation of a two-compartment model of the lung showing the effect of pulmonary arterial obstruction on wasted ventilation. When blood flow to Unit B ceases, any ventilation to the unit is wasted because it cannot contribute to gas exchange. Gas exchange in Unit A depends upon the amount of ventilation and blood flow to the unit. (Adapted from Comroe, J. H., Jr. et al: The Lung. Clinical Physiology and Pulmonary Function Tests. 2nd ed. Chicago, 1962, pp. 1–390. Reprinted by permission from the authors and Year Book Medical Publishers, Inc.)

residual gas in the terminal respiratory units.[20]

An increase in the alveolar component of wasted ventilation also occurs when regions of the lung are ventilated but unperfused (Fig. 8–12). This combination seldom develops in normal persons but may occur in patients with pulmonary emboli or with diseases associated with occlusion of pulmonary arteries or capillaries. Alveolus B in Figure 8–12 is stippled to show that inspired air reaching it also contributes to wasted ventilation; gas exchange is obviously impossible because there is no blood supply to the unit. Despite the theoretic challenges to its derivation, characteristic increases in wasted ventilation occur, especially during exercise, in patients with pulmonary vascular and interstitial diseases.[21, 22]

Wasted ventilation and venous admixture are both commonly employed as indexes of the presence and severity of ventilation-perfusion abnormalities. However, as already pointed out, the absolute values of both indexes can be shown to vary in the absence of any change in the distribution of ventilation and blood flow.[5] Figure 8–13 displays the results of computer analyses of a multicompartment lung model in which the amount of ventilation-perfusion inequality was held constant while ventilation was changed; under these conditions venous admixture ($\dot{Q}s/\dot{Q}T$) decreased and wasted ventilation (VD/VT) increased. An increase in total blood flow has opposite effects.[5]

OXYGEN TRANSPORT

Oxygen must be continuously supplied to all cells of the body to enable them to carry out their normal metabolic activities; this is true regardless of the specialized functions of different cell types, although some cells require more O_2 than others. The flow of O_2

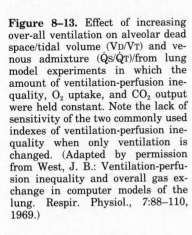

Figure 8–13. Effect of increasing over-all ventilation on alveolar dead space/tidal volume (VD/VT) and venous admixture ($\dot{Q}s/\dot{Q}T$)/from lung model experiments in which the amount of ventilation-perfusion inequality, O_2 uptake, and CO_2 output were held constant. Note the lack of sensitivity of the two commonly used indexes of ventilation-perfusion inequality when only ventilation is changed. (Adapted by permission from West, J. B.: Ventilation-perfusion inequality and overall gas exchange in computer models of the lung. Respir. Physiol., 7:88–110, 1969.)

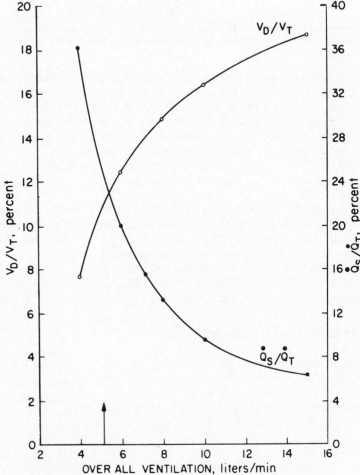

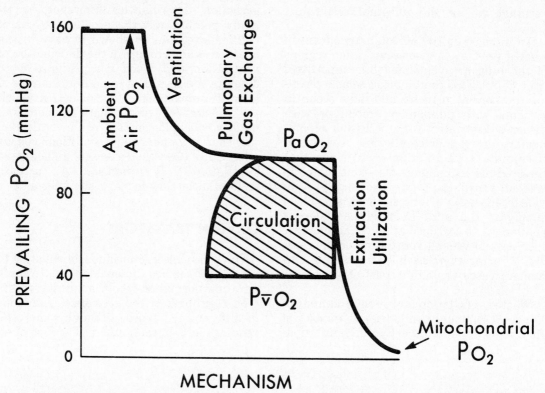

Figure 8–14. Schematic representation of the prevailing partial pressures of O_2 (Po_2) and the mechanisms causing flow of O_2 from the ambient air to the mitochondria. PaO_2 = arterial O_2 tension; $P\bar{v}O_2$ = mixed venous O_2 tension.

from ambient air to its site of consumption in intracellular mitochondria and the Po_2 values at each step in the transport chain are shown in Figure 8–14. Without O_2, a human being will lose consciousness in about 20 to 30 seconds and will die in a few minutes. The O_2 demands of a rigorous physical and metabolic existence are met by the integrated responses of the three components of the O_2 transport system: (1) the lungs, which transfer O_2 from environmental air into blood; (2) the heart and blood vessels, which circulate oxygenated blood throughout the body; and (3) the hemoglobin concentration of the blood and the affinity of hemoglobin for O_2.[23]

Definition and Determinants

Systemic O_2 transport (SO_2T), or the amount of O_2 delivered to the tissues of the body per unit time, can be calculated from the cardiac output ($\dot{Q}$) and the arterial O_2 content (CaO_2) according to the formula

$$SO_2T, \text{ ml/min} = \dot{Q}, \text{ L/min}, \times CaO_2, \text{ ml/L}. \qquad (7)$$

Because the arterial O_2 content is determined by the concentration of hemoglobin (Hgb) available for combination with O_2 and the per cent saturation of hemoglobin (SO_2), Equation 7 can be rewritten as follows:

$$SO_2T = \dot{Q} \times (\text{Hgb} \times 1.34) \times (SO_2 \div 100), \qquad (8)$$

or because per cent saturation is a function (f) of Po_2 according to the relationship defined by the oxyhemoglobin dissociation curve,*

$$SO_2T = \dot{Q} \times \\ circulatory \\ (\text{Hgb} \times 1.34) \times f(Po_2) \qquad (9) \\ erythropoietic \quad respiratory$$

The subtitles in Equation 9 identify the contributions to total O_2 transport of the three organ systems involved: the circulatory system determines cardiac output and peripheral blood flow, the erythropoietic system determines red blood cell mass and

*The affinity between O_2 and hemoglobin varies according to the influences discussed in Chapter 7.

Table 8–4. OXYGEN UPTAKE, CONSUMPTION, AND TRANSPORT AND THE COMPONENTS OF THE DELIVERY SYSTEM AT REST AND DURING EXERCISE

Variable	Rest	Exercise
O_2 uptake, consumption	250 ml/min	4000 ml/min
O_2 transport	1000 ml/min	5000 ml/min
Cardiac output	5 L/min	24 L/min
Hemoglobin concentration	15 gm/100 ml	15 gm/100 ml
Arterial blood P_{O_2}	95 mm Hg	95 mm Hg
Arterial blood O_2 content	200 ml/L	200 mg/L
Venous blood P_{O_2}	40 mm Hg	15 mm Hg
Venous blood O_2 content	150 ml/L	40 ml/L

hemoglobin concentration, and the respiratory system determines P_{O_2}. Values for O_2 uptake in the lungs, O_2 consumption in the tissues, and O_2 transport and the components of the delivery system at rest and during strenuous exercise by a well-trained athlete are shown in Table 8–4. Note that O_2 uptake and consumption are equal, which means that a steady state has been attained. The table shows that at rest, substantially more O_2 is delivered to the tissues than is used by them. Although at first glance the difference between the O_2 supplied and the O_2 consumed may appear to be an unwarranted luxury, this is not true in the case of individual organs (e.g., the heart, which uses virtually all the O_2 it receives), and the excess provides some leeway during sudden emergencies when more O_2 is needed at once by certain tissues. During progressive exercise, the amount of O_2 transported and consumed begin to approach each other.

Oxygen transport is an important physiologic variable because it sets the upper limit on the quantity of O_2 available to meet the total metabolic needs of the body. Oxygen utilization cannot exceed the supply of O_2 for very long; if it does, the deprived cells must shift from aerobic to anaerobic metabolic pathways to supply their energy needs. One of the consequences of anaerobic metabolism is the production of excess lactic acid. If not relieved, progressive acidosis ultimately disrupts intracellular metabolism and causes cellular death. Under ordinary circumstances, except at the beginning of exercise when a temporary O_2 debt is established, O_2 transport is always higher than O_2 consumption.

A narrowing of the margin between O_2 supply and demand can develop in several ways: if the demand increases, if the transport system itself is deficient, or both. Regardless of the cause, physiologic adjustments take place in an attempt to improve the balance between the amount of O_2 needed and that which is available.

Adaptations to Acute Oxygen Demands

The numerous vicissitudes of daily life are usually associated with a transient need for more O_2. Undoubtedly, the most common demand for O_2 occurs during physical activity, but increased metabolism may also be induced by fever, food intake, and administration of many drugs. Sudden needs for O_2, as well as the ordinary demands of metabolism occasioned by meals and other factors, are met chiefly by changes in cardiac output. As noted previously, cardiac output may increase four to five times its resting value; therefore, O_2 transport, by this mechanism alone, may increase to 4000 to 5000 ml/min. In addition, important regulatory mechanisms exist that serve to redistribute blood flow to exercising muscles. In most normal persons, maximal O_2 utilization during exercise is ordinarily limited by maximal cardiac output (see Chapter 11).

Minute volume of ventilation increases during exercise and serves to maintain arterial P_{O_2} at or slightly above resting values. However, increasing ventilation does not add appreciably to arterial O_2 content because of the ceiling imposed by the flat portion of the oxyhemoglobin equilibrium curve. Similarly, the slight improvement in ventilation-perfusion relationships that often occurs during exercise may raise arterial P_{O_2} a few mm Hg from its normal value at rest (about 95 mm Hg in a young healthy adult). However, inspection of the oxyhemoglobin dissociation curve (see Figure 7–7) reveals that this change causes the saturation of hemoglobin to increase from 97.2 to 97.5 per cent, and therefore adds only a trivial increment of O_2 to the blood flowing through the lungs. Although the efficiency of gas exchange cannot augment the quantity of O_2 in the bloodstream during increased metabolic needs compared with resting conditions, it should be emphasized that alveolar ventilation must at least keep up with increases in pulmonary blood flow to prevent the development of arterial hypoxia.

A red blood cell lives for about 120 days, and the turnover rate of erythrocytes is nearly 1.0 per cent of the circulating red blood cell mass per day.[24] Accordingly, it is impossible for even a marked acute increase (e.g., doubling or tripling) in red blood cell production to noticeably affect the circulating hemoglobin concentration. However, the hematocrit ratio and the hemoglobin con-

centration rise slightly in healthy subjects during severe exercise owing to a reduction in circulating plasma volume through extravasation of fluid. In an animal with a large spleen, such as a dog, the release of red blood cells that are normally sequestered in the spleen into the circulation also contributes to a rise in hemoglobin concentration.[25] Once an O_2-laden red blood cell reaches the arterial end of a tissue capillary, O_2 begins to diffuse into neighboring cells in response to the diffusion gradient between bloodstream and mitochondria. The classic concept of O_2 diffusion from capillary blood into tissue cells was originally formulated by Krough[26] and is illustrated in Figure 8–15. The diagram indicates that there is a changing gradient for diffusion of O_2 into a cylinder of tissue both along and perpendicular to the capillaries. This final link in the O_2 transport system has been recognized for many decades, during which time it has been debated whether or not these "peripheral factors" limit maximal exercise. Diffu-

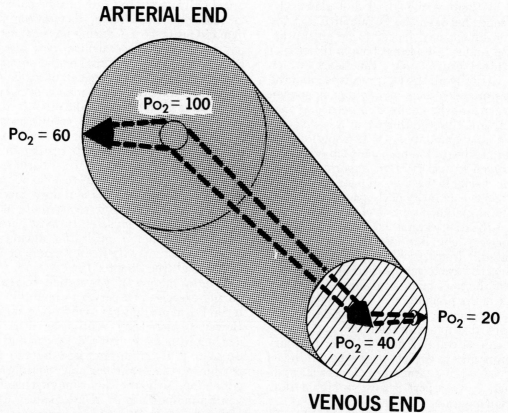

ARTERIAL END

$Po_2 = 100$

$Po_2 = 60$

$Po_2 = 20$

$Po_2 = 40$

VENOUS END

Figure 8–15. Schematic model of the diffusion gradient for O_2 along a single systemic capillary from the arterial end, where the Po_2 = 100 mm Hg, to the venous end, where the Po_2 = 40 mm Hg. Note that there is also a gradient for O_2 perpendicular to the capillary that is greater at the arterial end than at the venous end.

sion distances are affected by capillary and mitochondrial densities and, although these do not appear to limit exercise in healthy persons (see Chapter 11), their role in chronic disease states needs further investigation.

The extracellular metabolic acidosis that accompanies heavy exertion also presumably includes an increase in intracellular $[H^+]$; this serves to decrease affinity of hemoglobin for O_2 and, in effect, to increase O_2 transport because the change causes more O_2 to be released to the peripheral tissues. Although more O_2 is extracted by this mechanism, one of the consequences of its use is a decrease in capillary and venous Po_2 values, which reduces the gradient for O_2 diffusion into cells.

Adaptations to Chronic Oxygen Demands

Sustained demands for O_2 considerably in excess of ordinary metabolic needs are seldom encountered in normal subjects. However, increased O_2 consumption is a characteristic feature of certain pathologic conditions: thyrotoxicosis, acromegaly, pheochromocytoma, some malignancies, and (probably) Cushing's syndrome.[27] With excessive amounts of thyroid and growth hormones, O_2 supply is increased above normal levels by a combination of mechanisms: an increase in cardiac output and an increase in red blood cell mass. The latter effect is not always evident as a rise in hemoglobin concentration because plasma volume may also increase. (The reason for this paradoxic response of eliminating the beneficial effect of a change in red blood cell mass alone is not well understood; it presumably demonstrates dominance of volume and circulatory compensatory needs over compensation by raising hemoglobin concentration.) An increase in red blood cell DPG has been documented in patients with thyrotoxicosis, but the change is believed to be mediated by a specific effect of the excess thyroid hormone on glycolysis, rather than caused by a response to "relative" hypoxia.[28] Adaptive mechanisms in hypermetabolic disorders have not been well delineated, and whether or not changes in O_2 affinity occur needs to be examined. For the reasons discussed in the previous section, increases in ventilation keep pace with increases in cardiac output but do not add "extra" O_2 to the bloodstream.

Adaptations to Deficiencies of Oxygen Transport

Changes may occur in the circulatory, erythropoietic, and respiratory systems that seriously compromise over-all O_2 transport capabilities. When acute disturbances occur, especially in the cardiovascular system, the body is virtually defenseless, except for shifts in oxyhemoglobin affinity and in redistribution of blood flow to the heart and brain at the expense of perfusion to other organs. Compensation for decreases in O_2 transport is far more adequate in chronic than in acute disorders and in some instances restores delivery to normal. The main mechanism of adaptation is through an increase in red blood cell mass (polycythemia). At times, a shift in the oxyhemoglobin dissociation curve may contribute to O_2 utilization by making more of the delivered O_2 available to the tissues.

Chronic Circulatory Failure. Oxygen delivery is obviously reduced in conditions in which cardiac output is low. Although an increased red blood cell mass can be demonstrated in chronic disorders, hemoglobin concentration is seldom substantially elevated.[27] The main mechanism of compensation appears to be a decrease in O_2 affinity caused by an increase in red blood cell DPG concentration. The relationship between the levels of intraerythrocyte DPG and hemoglobin affinity for O_2, expressed as P_{50}, in patients with chronic cardiac disease was described earlier (see Fig. 7–9). The DPG-induced decrease in O_2 affinity becomes progressively greater as the circulatory abnormalities, reflected by a reduction in mixed venous blood O_2 saturation, worsen.[29]

Disturbances of Erythropoiesis. There is an optimum concentration of circulating red blood cells, conveniently measured as the hematocrit ratio, at which systemic O_2 transport is maximal and, not surprisingly, this occurs at the usual hematocrit levels found in the bloodstream of normal subjects (40 to 50 per cent). The relationship between acute changes of hematocrit values and O_2 transport in experimental animals is shown in Figure 8–16; also depicted is the effect of changing hematocrit on the animals' cardiac outputs.[30] As the hematocrit, and hence hemoglobin, concentrations decrease from their normal levels of 45 per cent and 15 gm/100 ml, respectively, cardiac output increases; however, the increase in blood flow is insufficient to compensate for the reduc-

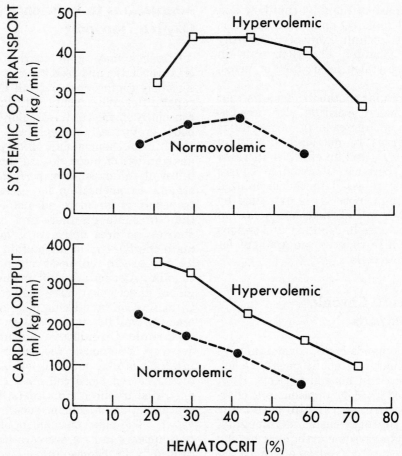

Figure 8–16. Composite graph of the effects of changes in hematocrit ratio on mean values of cardiac output and systemic O_2 transport. Results from experiments in dogs in which blood volume was held constant (normovolemic) or increased (hypervolemic). (Adapted and reprinted by permission from Murray, J. F. et al.: The circulatory effects of hematocrit variations in normovolemic and hypervolemic dogs. J. Clin. Invest., *42*:1150–1159, 1963.)

tion in hemoglobin concentration and O_2-carrying capacity, and so O_2 transport decreases. When the hematocrit is increased above about 55 per cent, viscosity causes a decrease in cardiac output that more than offsets the gain in O_2 capacity of the blood; this combination also leads to a decrease in O_2 transport. The effect of an increase in total circulating blood volume is also demonstrated in Figure 8–16; at any given hematocrit, O_2 transport and cardiac output are always higher when blood volume is expanded than when it is normal. Similar types of experiments have now been carried out in trained athletes using autotransfusions.[31] After venesection and allowing time for the blood volume and hematocrit to return to normal, expansion of blood volume by reinfusion of the athletes' own blood increased both O_2 transport and athletic performance.

In some patients with anemia, O_2 affinity is decreased, but in others it is not.[32, 33] The difference in responses may relate to the type of anemia and to whether or not intracellular alkalosis occurs. In most patients with moderate or severe chronic anemia, cardiovascular adjustments are evident and O_2 transport during moderately heavy exercise is surprisingly well maintained.[34]

Most patients with abnormal hemoglobin that is associated with either a high or a low O_2 affinity have normal O_2 transport.[35] Patients whose hemoglobin is characterized by decreased affinity are anemic, and conversely, patients whose hemoglobin reveals increased affinity are polycythemic. In both cases, tissue O_2, an important regulator of red blood cell production (see subsequent section), is virtually normal. Customarily, these patients do not have symptoms related to their hematologic disturbances, although defects in O_2 delivery might be demonstrable under maximal stress.[35]

Arterial Hypoxia. Chronic arterial hypoxia occurs in normal residents of high altitudes who breathe air that has a lower Po_2 than air at sea level. One of the main defenses against high altitude hypoxia is an increase in the O_2-carrying capacity of the bloodstream through the development of polycythemia; moreover, the magnitude of this response is related to the severity of the hypoxia, and thus is determined by the altitude at which the subject resides.[36] Figure 8–17 demonstrates the relationship between red blood cell mass and arterial O_2 saturation; the data have been compiled from studies of healthy subjects living at varying altitudes[36-40] and have been recalculated with appropriate corrections for trapped plasma and total body hematocrit.[41] The changes in circulating red blood cell mass induced by arterial hypoxia are a straightforward demonstration of the regulatory system through which available O_2 controls red blood cell production. The O_2-sensitive receptors are mainly located in the kidneys and, although there is some evidence to suggest that the juxtaglomerular cells are involved in the response, the exact cellular site(s) for the detection of hypoxia and elaboration of the regulating hormone, erythropoietin, is unknown.[42] The recent finding of nearly normal levels of *erythropoietin* in the blood of anephric patients provides persuasive evidence of an extrarenal source of the hormone.[43] When released, erythropoietin causes increased production of red blood cells by the bone marrow. The adequacy of the response depends, in part, upon the availability of iron for the synthesis of hemoglobin. An increase in circulating hemoglobin concentration means that more O_2 is carried in the bloodstream at the same Po_2, so that the receptors are "satisfied" and stop producing excess erythropoietin. It is clear that the presence of polycythemia is one of the chief mechanisms by which natives and long-term residents of high altitudes maintain O_2 transport at rest and during exercise despite severe arterial hypoxia.[44] A decrease of O_2 affinity through an increase in red blood cell DPG also occurs at high altitudes; however, the contribution of this mechanism is lim-

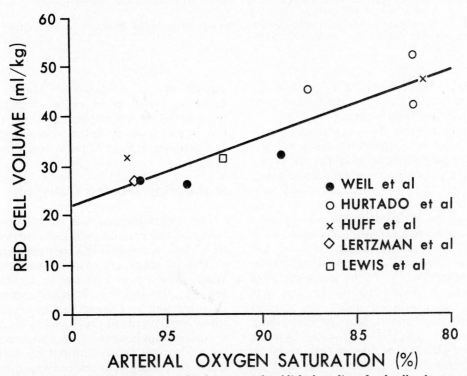

Figure 8–17. Composite graph showing results from several published studies of red cell volume and arterial oxygen saturation in normal acclimatized subjects living at various altitudes. The solid line is the regression line. The effect of hypoxia from residence at altitude is to increase red cell volume. (Adapted and reprinted by permission from Murray, J. F.: Arterial studies in primary and secondary polycythemic disorders. Am. Rev. Respir. Dis., *92*:435–449, 1965.)

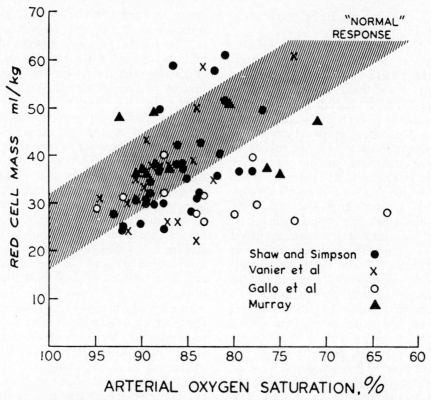

Figure 8–18. Composite graph showing results from several published studies of red cell mass (volume) and arterial oxygen saturation in patients with pulmonary disease. The shaded area delineates the normal range (mean ± two standard deviations) obtained by analysis of data in Figure 8–17. (Reprinted by permission from Murray, J. F.: Classification of polycythemic disorders with comments on the diagnostic value of arterial blood oxygen analysis. Ann. Intern. Med., *64*:892–903, 1966.)

ited because when alveolar P_{O_2} is low, O_2 loading may be impaired as much as or more than O_2 release is enhanced.[45]

Arterial hypoxia is a common consequence of many pulmonary diseases, but both the polycythemic and the DPG responses of patients are often substantially less evident than they are in healthy subjects with the same degree of hypoxia who are living at high altitudes. Using data collected from several studies, Figure 8–18 shows the poor relationship between red blood cell mass and the percentage of arterial O_2 saturation;[27, 46–48] the wide scatter of the results is obvious, as is the fact that most of the points lie below the normal range. No one knows why erythropoietic compensation in patients with hypoxia caused by pulmonary disease fails to be as good at restoring O_2 delivery as that in normal subjects at high altitudes. It may be either the effect of the disease itself on the bone marrow or red blood cell metabolism or a variety of secondary influences that

impair normal responses. Clearly, these processes need to be explored further to provide more understanding than is currently available of an important aspect of the pathophysiology of pulmonary disease.

Monitoring Oxygen Transport

The previous sections have described many of the common clinical situations in which the O_2 needs of the body are increased or the O_2 transport capacity is decreased. When an imbalance occurs in seriously ill patients, the deficit in O_2 supply can usually be corrected by enhancing any one of the three components of the O_2 delivery system: by using supplementary O_2 to increase arterial P_{O_2}, by transfusing red blood cells to increase hemoglobin concentration, or by administering drugs to increase cardiac output.

In difficult clinical circumstances it would be desirable to be able to monitor the adequacy of O_2 delivery with respect to O_2 consumption as well as the need for and the response to therapeutic interventions. What is needed is a measurement of tissue P_{O_2} levels in critical organs such as the brain and heart. Because these are not readily available, it has been customary to use mixed venous P_{O_2} as a guide to the adequacy of systemic O_2 transport. Such a relationship is predictable over a wide range of cardiac outputs because O_2 consumption is an independent variable that reflects ongoing metabolism and is not dependent on O_2 delivery once delivery exceeds a certain minimum value. Thus, other factors remaining constant, an increase or decrease in cardiac output is reflected by an increase or decrease in mixed venous P_{O_2}. However, the results of the theoretical analysis by Tenney,[49] which revealed remarkably close agreement between venous blood and mean tissue O_2 pressures *under normal resting conditions,* underscored the important discrepencies between the two P_{O_2} values that occurred when physiologic variables such as metabolic rate, hemoglobin concentration, and cardiac output were altered. Recent evidence from patients with acute lung disease[50] as well as further theoretical considerations[51] also indicate that mixed venous P_{O_2} values are not necessarily related to O_2 transport. Thus, at present there is no readily available, consistently reliable guide that indicates whether or not delivery of O_2 to the tissues is satisfactory.

REFERENCES

1. West, J. B., and Wagner, P. D.: Pulmonary gas exchange. *In* West, J. B., and Wagner, P. D. (eds.): Bioengineering Aspects of the Lung. New York, Marcel Dekker, Inc., 1977, pp. 361–457.
2. Hughes, J. M. B.: Editorial review: Pulmonary gas exchange. Clin. Sci., 58:119–125, 1980.
3. McFadden, E. R., Jr.: Respiratory heat and water exchange: physiological and clinical implications. J. Appl. Physiol., 54:331–336, 1983.
4. Comroe, J. H., Jr., Foster, R. E., II, Dubois, A. B., Briscoe, W. A., and Carlsen, E.: The Lung. Clinical Physiology and Pulmonary Function Tests. 2nd Ed. Chicago, Year Book Medical Publishers, Inc., 1962, pp. 1–390.
4a. Torre-Bueno, J. R., Wagner, P. D., Saltzman, H. A., Gale, G. E., and Moon, R. E.: Diffusion limitation in normal humans during exercise at sea level and simulated altitude. J. Appl. Physiol., 58:989–995, 1985.
5. West, J. B.: Ventilation-perfusion inequality and overall gas exchange in computer models of the lung. Respir. Physiol., 7:88–110, 1969.
6. West, J. B.: Causes of carbon dioxide retention in lung disease. New Engl. J. Med., 284:1232–1236, 1971.
7. West, J. B.: Ventilation-perfusion relationships. Am. Rev. Respir. Dis., 116:919–943, 1977.
8. Wagner, P. D., Laravuso, R. B., Uhl, R. R., and West, J. B.: Continuous distributions of ventilation-perfusion ratios in normal subjects breathing air and 100% O_2. J. Clin. Invest., 54:54–68, 1974.
9. Wagner, P. D.: Ventilation-perfusion relationships. Annu. Rev. Physiol., 42:235–247, 1980.
10. Mellemgaard, K., Lassen, N. A., and Georg, J.: Right-to-left shunt in normal man determined by the use of tritium and krypton 85. J. App. Physiol., 17:778–782, 1962.
11. Davidson, F. F., Glazier, J. B., and Murray, J. F.: The components of the alveolar-arterial oxygen tension difference in normal subjects and patients with pneumonia and obstructive lung disease. Am. J. Med., 52:754–762, 1972.
12. Lynch, J. P., Mhyre, J. G., and Dantzker, D. R.: Influence of cardiac output on intrapulmonary shunt. J. Appl. Physiol., 46:315–321, 1979.
13. Prewitt, R. M., and Wood, L. D. H.: Effect of sodium nitroprusside on cardiovascular function and pulmonary shunt in canine oleic acid pulmonary edema. Anesthesiology, 55:537–541, 1981.
14. Sandoval, J., Long, G. R., Skoog, C., Wood, L. D. H., and Oppenheimer, L.: Independent influence of blood flow rate and mixed venous P_{O_2} on shunt fraction. J. Appl. Physiol., 55:1128–1133, 1983.
15. Mellemgaard, K.: The alveolar-arterial oxygen difference: its size and components in normal man. Acta Physiol. Scand., 67:10–20, 1966.
16. Harris, E. A., Kenyon, A. M., Nisbet, H. D., Seelye, E. R., and Whitlock, R. M. L.: The normal alveolar-arterial oxygen-tension gradient in man. Clin. Sci. Mol. Med., 46:89–104, 1974.
17. Weibel, E. R., and Gomez, D. M.: Architecture of the human lung. Use of quantitative methods establishes fundamental relations between size and number of lung structures. Science, 137:577–585, 1962.
18. Klingele, T. G., and Staub, N. C.: Alveolar shape changes with volume in isolated, air-filled lobes of cat lung. J. Appl. Physiol., 28:411–414, 1970.
19. Severinghaus, J. W., and Stupfel, M.: Alveolar dead space as an index of distribution of blood flow in pulmonary capillaries. J. Appl. Physiol., 10:335–348, 1957.
20. Lifshay, A., Fast, C. W., and Glazier, J. B.: Effects of changes in respiratory pattern on physiological dead space. J. Appl. Physiol., 31:478–483, 1971.
21. Nadel, J. A., Gold, W. M., and Burgess, J. H.: Early diagnosis of chronic pulmonary vascular obstruction. Value of pulmonary function tests. Am. J. Med., 44:16–25, 1968.
22. Mohsenifar, Z., Brown, H. V., Koerner, S. K.: Abnormal wasted ventilation fraction and normal pulmonary hemodynamics during exercise in patients with exertional dyspnea. Respiration, 43:263–270, 1982.
23. Finch, C. A., and Lenfant, C.: Oxygen transport in man. New Engl. J. Med., 286:407–415, 1972.
24. Berlin, N. I., Waldmann, T. A., and Weissman, S. M.: Life span of the red blood cell. Physiol. Rev., 39:557–616, 1959.
25. Gold, P. M., and Murray, J. F.: Changes in red cell distribution, hemodynamics, and blood volume in acute anemia. J. Appl. Physiol., 26:589–593, 1969.
26. Krough, A.: The number and distribution of capil-

laries in muscles with calculation of the oxygen pressure head necessary for supplying tissue. J. Physiol., (Lond.) 52:409–435, 1918–1919B.

27. Murray, J. F.: Classification of polycythemic disorders with comments on the diagnostic value of arterial blood oxygen analysis. Ann. Intern. Med., 64:892–903, 1966.

28. Snyder, L. M., and Reddy, W. J.: Mechanism of action of thyroid hormones on erythrocyte 2,3-diphosphoglyceric acid synthesis. J. Clin. Invest., 49:1993–1998, 1970.

29. Woodson, R. D., Torrance, J. D., Shappell, S. D., and Lenfant, C.: The effect of cardiac disease on hemoglobin-oxygen binding. J. Clin. Invest., 49:1349–1356, 1970.

30. Murray, J. F., Gold, P., and Johnson, B. L., Jr.: The circulatory effects of hematocrit variations in normovolemic and hypervolemic dogs. J. Clin. Invest., 42:1150–1159, 1963.

31. Thomson, J. M., Stone, J. A., Ginsburg, A. D., and Hamilton, P.: O₂ transport during exercise following blood reinfusion. J. Appl. Physiol., 53:1213–1219, 1982.

32. Thomson, H. M., Lefrak, S. S., Irwin, R. S., Fritts, H. W., Jr., and Caldwell, P. R. B.: The oxyhemoglobin dissociation curve in health and disease. Role of 2,3-Diphosphoglycerate. Am. J. Med., 57:331–348, 1974.

33. Lichtman, M. A., Murphy, M. S., Whitbeck, A. A., and Kearney, E. A.: Oxyen binding to haemoglobin in subjects with hypoproliferative anemia, with and without chronic renal disease: role of pH. Br. J. Haematol., 27:439–452, 1974.

34. Sproule, B. J., Mitchell, J. H., and Miller, W. F.: Cardiopulmonary physiological responses to heavy exercise in patients with anemia. J. Clin. Invest., 39:378–388, 1960.

35. Stamatoyannopoulos, G., Bellingham, A. J., Lenfant, C., and Finch, C. A.: Abnormal hemoglobins with high and low oxygen affinity. Annu. Rev. Med., 22:221–234, 1971.

36. Weil, J. V., Jamieson, G., Brown, D. W., and Grover, R. F.: The red cell mass-arterial oxygen relationship in normal man. Application to patients with chronic obstructive airway disease. J. Clin. Invest., 47:1627–1639, 1968.

37. Hurtado, A., Merino, C., and Delgado, E.: Influence of anoxemia on the hemopoietic activity. Arch. Intern. Med., 75:284–323, 1945.

38. Huff, R. L., Lawrence, J. H., Siri, W. E., Wasserman, L. R., and Hennessy, T. G.: Effects of changes in altitude on hematopoietic activity. Medicine, 30:197–217, 1951.

39. Lewis, C. S., Jr., Samuels, A. J., Daines, M. C., and Hecht, H. H.: Chronic lung disease, polycythemia and congestive heart failure. Cardiorespiratory, vascular and renal adjustments in cor pulmonale. Circulation, 6:874–887, 1952.

40. Lertzman, M., Frome, B. M., Israels, L. G., and Cherniack, R. M.:Hypoxia in polycythemia vera. Ann. Intern. Med., 60:409–417, 1964.

41. Murray, J. F.: Arterial studies in primary and secondary polycythemic disorders. Am. Rev. Respir. Dis., 92:435–449, 1965.

42. Krantz, S. B., and Jacobson, L. O.: Erythropoietin and the Regulation of Erythropoiesis. Chicago, University of Chicago Press, 1970, pp. 25–46.

43. Garcia, J. F., Sherwood, J., and Goldwasser, E.: Radioimmunoassay of erythropoietin. Blood Cells, 5:405–419, 1979.

44. Lenfant, C., and Sullivan, K.: Adaptation to high altitude. New Engl. J. Med., 284:1298–1309, 1971.

45. Lenfant, C., Torrance, J. D., and Reynafarje, C.: Shift of the O₂-Hb dissociation curve at altitude: mechanism and effect. J. Appl. Physiol., 30:625–631, 1971.

46. Shaw, D. B., and Simpson, T.: Polycythaemia in emphysema. Quart. J. Med., 30:135–152, 1961.

47. Vanier, T., Dulfano, M. J., Wu, C., and Desforges, J. F.: Emphysema, hypoxia and the polycythemic response. New Engl. J. Med., 269:169–178, 1963.

48. Gallo, R. C., Fraimow, W., Cathcart, R. T., and Erslev, A. J.: Erythropoietic response in chronic pulmonary disease. Arch. Intern. Med., 113:559–569, 1964.

49. Tenney, S. M.: A theoretical analysis of the relationship of venous to average tissue oxygen pressures. Respir. Physiol., 20:283–296, 1974.

50. Danek, S. J., Lynch, J. P., Weg, J. G., and Dantzker, D. R.: The dependence of oxygen uptake on oxygen delivery in the adult respiratory distress syndrome. Am. Rev. Respir. Dis., 122:387–395, 1980.

51. Tenney, S. M., and Mithoefer, J. C.: The relationship of mixed venous oxygenation to oxygen transport: with special reference to adaptations to high altitude and pulmonary disease. Am. Rev. Respir. Dis., 125:474–479, 1982.

9

Acid-Base Equilibrium

INTRODUCTION

Maintenance of acid-base equilibrium is considered in this book on the normal structure and function of the lungs for two reasons. First, the lungs are the chief organ for the elimination of CO_2 and hence govern the amounts of H_2CO_3 in the body. Second, changes in both P_{CO_2} and acid-base equilibrium exert a profound effect on the control of breathing. This interrelationship, which is considered in greater detail in Chapter 10, normally operates to provide a physiologic safeguard against acid-base imbalances by responding in a manner that limits the severity of the changes in pH. Conversely, however, disorders of breathing are one of the major causes of acid-base disturbances encountered clinically. This chapter examines the main variables that contribute to acid-base equilibrium and how the respiratory system responds to or causes changes in blood pH.

DEFINITIONS

A lot of shorthand is used in acid-base and renal physiology. The conventional symbols, H, H^+, $[H^+]$, OH^-, $[OH^-]$, HB, B^-, and pH, are defined in Table 9–1; these definitions are used throughout this chapter and the remainder of the text.

Table 9–1. DEFINITION OF THE COMMON SYMBOLS USED TO DESCRIBE THE PROPERTIES OF ACIDS AND BASES IN PHYSIOLOGIC SOLUTIONS*

Symbol	Designation	Definition
H	Hydrogen	An atom of H existing in a combined state
H^+	Hydrogen ion Proton	The free and chemically active ionization product of H
$[H^+]$	Hydrogen ion concentration	The equivalent concentration of H^+ in a solution
HB	Acid	General designation of the chemical combination of H and its conjugate base
B^-	Conjugate base (general) H^+ acceptor Proton acceptor	General designation of the base paired with a given acid after ionization
OH^-	Hydroxyl ion	The conjugate base of H^+ present in aqueous solutions
$[OH^-]$	Hydroxyl ion concentration	The equivalent concentration of OH^- in a solution
pH	Intensity factor	Measurement of activity of $[H^+]$

*Further explanations are provided in the text.

Acids

An acid is a proton or an H^+ donor. A fundamental property of an acid (HB) is that it dissociates wholly or partly into its component ions, so that

$$HB = H^+ + B^-, \qquad (1)$$

where B^- is the conjugate base of the acid (described later).

The strength of an acid is determined by the degree to which it dissociates in solution. Correspondingly, the acidity or pH depends upon the concentration of active H^+ in a given amount of solution. Because a strong acid dissociates into its component ions considerably more than a weak one, a solution of a strong acid has more free H^+ available for immediate chemical reactions than a solution of a weak acid. But it is important to realize that if the concentrations of the two solutions (expressed as their normality) are equal, they have exactly the same *total* number of H atoms in the mixture. Thus, the principal difference between the two kinds of acids is that H is ionized and "freed" for possible reactions in the strong acid but combined and unreactive (until ionized) in the weak acid.

A distinction must be made, therefore, between the ionic and combined forms of H

that determine, respectively, the *intensity* with which the H in the solution will react and the *total quantity* of H available in the mixture.[1] The intensity factor, also called the "actual acidity," is the concentration of active H^+ in solution, or $[H^+]$, and is measured as pH. The quantity factor, also called the "titratable acidity," is the amount of H^+ in solution plus the H available for ionization over a designated physiologic pH range and is measured by titration against a base.[2] The different chemical properties of a representative strong acid and a weak acid are shown in Table 9–2.

The acids present in biologic solutions behave in the same way as those in test tubes, and it is of considerable significance that most of the acids normally present in the body are weak acids. This means that there is a great deal of combined H in body liquids but little free H^+.

Bases

A base is a proton-binder, or an H^+ acceptor. There are strong and weak bases, depending on how much H^+ the base will bind; the stronger the base, the greater its affinity for H^+. As noted in Equation 1, in the description of an acid (HB) and its ionization products H^+ and B^-, the B^- moiety is known

Table 9–2. COMPARISON OF THE CHEMICAL PROPERTIES OF 0.1 N SOLUTIONS OF A STRONG ACID AND A WEAK ACID

Acid	Dissociation Constant (Units)	Ionized H+ (mEq/L)	pH (Units)	Total H* (mEq/L)
Strong				
Hydrochloric acid	∞	0.1	1	0.1
Weak				
Acetic acid	1.8×10^{-5}	0.0013	2.9	0.1

*Titratable acidity to pH 7.0

as the *conjugate base* of that acid. Weak acids have strong conjugate bases that bind most of the available H, so that little remains in the free ionized form. This condition exists in most of the acid-base pairs of the body and is one of the reasons why the pH of body liquids is nearly neutral. As will be explained, however, there is an important and constant difference between values of intracellular and extracellular pH.

pH

The term pH was introduced by Sorensen[3] in 1909 as a convenient means of describing certain properties of chemical solutions. Although the definition has changed since Sorensen's time, the distinction he made between H+ activity and the total quantity of available H is physiologically meaningful. Within well-defined chemical limitations, pH is the negative logarithm of H+ activity (aH+):

$$pH = - \log (aH^+). \quad (2)$$

Equation 2 adds a new constraint to the measurement of acidity: not only is the number of H+ ions important but so is the designation of their chemical activity. Because the activity may vary under certain conditions, the relationship is expressed as

$$aH^+ = \gamma H^+[H^+], \quad (3)$$

where γH^+ is the activity coefficient and [H+] is the equivalent concentration of H.

During the 1960's the physiologic utility of pH was questioned, and proposals were made to substitute [H+], derived from pH using Equations 2 and 3, and to ignore the activity coefficient. These efforts resulted in a controversy over the relative usefulness of pH versus [H+] to quantify the acidity of biologic systems.[4] The chief argument for

[H+] was that it is an arithmetic function and, therefore, easier to deal with than a negative logarithm. However, of overriding importance is the fact that the behavior of a substance in a chemical system is proportional to its energy (chemical potential), and this, in turn, is a logarithmic function of the activity of the substance. A pH electrode responds to the chemical potential of H+, and thus the instrument provides a precise and readily obtained measurement of the chemical behavior of H+ in the system.[4] This information is precisely what the clinician, physiologist, and chemist need to know. Moreover, other substances can be shown to behave physiologically in logarithmic relationships to their activities, and as pointed out in Chapter 8, a logarithmic distribution seems to be the best method for describing the distributions of ventilation and perfusion in normal lungs (see Fig. 8–6). Nature may not recognize a logarithm, but it clearly responds at times in a manner that is accurately defined by logarithmic functions such as pH. Some experts, however, still perfer to use [H+], particularly to describe the relationship between [H+] and either P_{CO_2} or [HCO_3^-] over a range of acid-base disturbances.[2]

Buffer Solution

A buffer solution is a mixture of substances, usually a weak acid with its salt of a strong base, that resists a change in [H+], and therefore in pH.[2] When a strong acid or base is added to a solution containing a buffer, the change in pH is minimized compared with that which would occur if the buffer were not present. The buffers present in body liquids are extremely important because they assist the lungs and kidneys in maintenance of pH within the fairly narrow limits required by most cells to function normally.

The action of a buffer may be illustrated by showing what happens when a strong acid (e.g., HCl) or strong base (e.g., NaOH) is added to a buffer of the usual variety, consisting of a mixture of a weak acid (e.g., H_2CO_3) and its salt with a strong base (e.g., $NaHCO_3$). The buffer mixture would be as follows:

$$Na^+ + HCO_3^- + H_2CO_3 \rightleftharpoons$$
$$Na^+ + H^+ + 2HCO_3^- + \text{some } H_2CO_3. \quad (4)$$

When a strong acid (HCl) is added, the H^+ reacts with HCO_3^- in the buffer mixture:

$$H^+ + HCO_3^- \rightarrow H_2CO_3. \quad (5)$$

Equation 5 shows that the reaction product from the addition of H^+ to the buffer mixture is a weak acid (H_2CO_3). In other words, the strong acid is converted to an equivalent concentration of a weak one. In the process, free H^+ is "mopped up" as it is added to the buffer mixture, and the resulting change in pH is minimal. When a strong base (NaOH) is added,

$$H^+ + OH^- \rightarrow H_2O. \quad (6)$$

Equation 6 shows that the product of the addition of OH^- to the buffer mixture is H_2O. Thus OH^- is "mopped up" by H^+ and converted to H_2O in the process.

Blood Buffers

The amount of change in the pH of blood during a given acute alteration in acid-base equilibrium depends upon the buffering capacity of the blood. Furthermore, as implied in the general discussion of buffer solutions, large quantities of acid or base may be added to the body without producing a life-threatening alteration in pH. It is important to understand how pH is stabilized, not only to appreciate how the process operates but also to be able to identify the presence of different kinds of abnormalities and to measure their severity.

The body has several buffer systems within its extracellular and intracellular liquids. Although the extent to which each buffer contributes to the defense of body pH varies with differing kinds of acid-base disturbances (see subsequent sections), the chief buffering systems in approximate order of their importance are (1) HCO_3^- and

H_2CO_3 in plasma, interstitial, and intracellular water and carbonate in bone, (2) intracellular proteins, including hemoglobin, (3) plasma proteins, and (4) intracellular and extracellular phosphates.

The HCO_3^- system heads the list because HCO_3^- is present in appreciable quantities in nearly all body liquids and is readily available to stabilize pH. This huge reservoir of HCO_3^- has aptly been named the "alkali reserve" of the body to signify its role in the maintenance of pH.

Bicarbonate differs from other body buffers in that the product of its reaction with H^+ is a *volatile acid*, H_2CO_3. A volatile acid can be excreted in the gas with which it is in equilibrium, in this case CO_2; thus, H_2CO_3 can be viewed as having an "escaping tendency" because CO_2 leaves the body through the lungs.[1] These processes can be expressed by the following equation:

$$H^+ + HCO_3^- \rightarrow H_2CO_3 \xrightarrow{CA} H_2O + CO_2 \uparrow, \quad (7)$$

where CA indicates carbonic anhydrase, and $\uparrow$ indicates that CO_2 is eliminated by the lungs.

Equations 5 to 7 can be used to describe the changes in HCO_3^- levels, particularly plasma HCO_3^- (symbolized as $[HCO_3^-]$), when nonvolatile (sometimes called fixed) acids or bases are added to the body.* In general, the addition of nonvolatile acids lowers $[HCO_3^-]$, and the addition of bases raises $[HCO_3^-]$; moreover, the severity of the acid-base derangement is reflected, in part, in the amount by which $[HCO_3^-]$ deviates from normal values. The chief pathways of production and disposal of CO_2, H^+, and HCO_3^- are shown schematically in Figure 9–1.

Types of Acid-Base Disorders

Acid-base disturbances are traditionally differentiated into those of respiratory origin and those of metabolic origin. These two types of disorders are fundamentally different but frequently coexist. As a result, three variables (directly measured or derived) are required to describe the conditions and how they interact: arterial P_{CO_2} defines the res-

---

*It is important to specify nonvolatile acids in contrast to volatile (i.e., H_2CO_3) acids because, as will be shown, the addition and removal of these two types of acids have opposite effects on $[HCO_3^-]$.

SOURCES

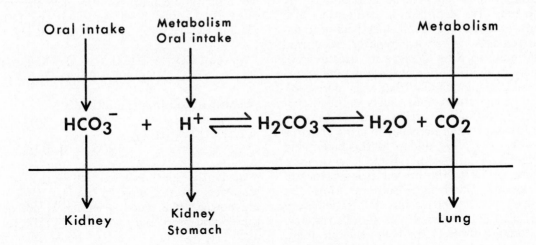

REMOVAL PATHWAYS

Figure 9–1. Schematic representation of the chief sources and removal pathways of H^+, HCO_3^-, and CO_2.

piratory component; $[HCO_3^-]$ is the most commonly used variable to describe the metabolic component; and pH (or $[H^+]$) assesses the net result of the combined effects of respiratory and metabolic disorders on acid-base equilibrium.[1, 2]

Respiratory Origin. Respiratory acid-base disorders occur when the primary cause is excessive retention or elimination of PCO_2. As emphasized in Chapter 8, arterial PCO_2 is determined by the relationship between CO_2 production ($\dot{V}CO_2$) and alveolar ventilation ($\dot{V}A$), so that

$$Pa_{CO_2} = K \frac{\dot{V}CO_2}{\dot{V}A}. \qquad (8)$$

Hyperventilation and *hypoventilation* are defined as an excess or a deficiency, respectively, of alveolar ventilation in relation to CO_2 production, normally the end product of aerobic metabolism. According to Equation 8, therefore, arterial blood PCO_2 must increase during hypoventilation and decrease during hyperventilation. *Hyperpnea* means increased breathing that may or may not be related to CO_2 production, and hence the term implies nothing about PCO_2. The presence and magnitude of a primary acute or chronic ventilatory disturbance and ac-

companying respiratory acid-base imbalance can be simply recognized and quantified by measuring arterial PCO_2. Primary metabolic acid-base disturbances cause secondary hyperventilation or hypoventilation and also may result in large deviations in arterial PCO_2. The level of PCO_2 is important because it directly determines the concentration of H_2CO_3 present in the blood, according to the following relationship:

$$H_2CO_3 = PCO_2 \times 0.0301, \qquad (9)$$

where H_2CO_3 is in mM/L or mEq/L, PCO_2 is in mm Hg, and 0.0301 is the solubility coefficient (α) of CO_2 in plasma at body temperature (37° C). Although H_2CO_3 is a weak acid, it dissociates to a limited extent and produces H^+ and HCO_3^- as follows:

$$H_2CO_3 \rightleftharpoons H^+ + HCO_3^-. \qquad (10)$$

This reaction is an important one, not only because it provides HCO_3^- for buffering and other chemical reactions but also because it shows that respiratory disturbances *per se*, by changing the amount of H_2CO_3 in the bloodstream, also change the $[HCO_3^-]$.

Metabolic Origin. Nonrespiratory or

metabolic* acid-base disorders occur when the primary cause is excessive retention or elimination of nonvolatile acid or base by the body. The definition is straightforward, but in contrast to respiratory acid-base derangements, which are readily recognized and quantified by changes in arterial P_{CO_2} and pH, identification of the kind and severity of a metabolic disturbance is more complex. As mentioned previously in the discussion of blood buffers, $[HCO_3^-]$ must decrease or increase when nonvolatile acids or bases (respectively) are added to the body, and therefore changes in $[HCO_3^-]$ serve as a useful guide to the presence or absence of metabolic acid-base disorders. However, $[HCO_3^-]$ fails to be a completely satisfactory indicator of these conditions for two reasons: (1) other buffers of the body, though quantitatively less important than HCO_3^-, are variably involved in the defense of pH, and so the effect of adding nonvolatile acid or base is not reflected solely in the HCO_3^- system, and (2) metabolic acid-base disorders frequently cause ventilation to increase or decrease, which, as just discussed (Equations 9 and 10), changes P_{CO_2} and H_2CO_3 and, therefore, the $[HCO_3^-]$. For example, if nonvolatile acid is added to the body, it "consumes" HCO_3^-; it also stimulates ventilation, which by lowering P_{CO_2} has the added effect of further reducing $[HCO_3^-]$. Indeed, the secondary hyperventilation in chronic HCl-induced metabolic acidosis can account for approximately half of the total decrement in plasma $[HCO_3^-]$, because of the effects of hypocapnia on renal acidification.[5]

These factors have led to attempts to derive a variable that would reflect the impact of a metabolic disorder on all the buffering systems of the body and would also correct for the influence of any secondary changes on $[HCO_3^-]$ from the respiratory effects of the primary disturbance; in other words, it would be a "pure" indicator of the metabolic component of an acid-base derangement.

Plasma Carbon Dioxide Content. The plasma total CO_2 content, in mM or mmol/L, is the total amount of CO_2 that can be

evolved from the plasma of a blood specimen that has been collected and centrifuged under anaerobic conditions.[6] Because the volatile H_2CO_3 has been retained, the total plasma CO_2 content ($[total\ CO_2]$) consists of

$$[Total\ CO_2] = [HCO_3^-] + [H_2CO_3], \quad (11)$$

or substituting from Equation 9,

$$[Total\ CO_2] = [HCO_3^-] + [P_{CO_2} \times 0.0301]. \quad (12)$$

A derivative measurement, which is now of historical interest only, is the CO_2-combining power.[7] If a blood specimen is not obtained and processed anaerobically, the volatile H_2CO_3 will escape; however, the plasma can be approximately "arterialized" in the laboratory by equilibrating it with 5.5 per cent CO_2 so that the P_{CO_2} is raised to about 40 mm Hg. The CO_2-combining power differs from the total plasma CO_2 content not only if the patient's P_{CO_2} differs from that which is artificially restored in the laboratory, but also because of differences between *in vivo* and *in vitro* buffering capabilities of blood.

Plasma Bicarbonate Ion Content. The actual $[HCO_3^-]$, expressed in mEq/L, can be either determined by direct measurement or derived from the familiar Henderson-Hasselbalch equation

$$pH = pK + \log \frac{[HCO_3^-]}{[H_2CO_3]}, \quad (13)$$

or by substitution from Equation 9,

$$pH = pK + \log \frac{[HCO_3^-]}{[P_{CO_2} \times 0.0301]}, \quad (14)$$

where pK, the dissociation constant, is 6.10 for plasma at 37° C. If pH and either P_{CO_2} or CO_2 content are known, $[HCO_3^-]$ can be calculated mathematically or it can be obtained from nomograms or diagrams.[8, 9]

It is important to recognize that although pH and P_{CO_2} are used to calculate and to record HCO_3^- by many automatic analyzers (according to equation 14), the derived value may not be valid in acutely ill patients, especially those in whom conditions are changing rapidly, because of reported variations in pK.[10] However, changes in pK, particularly of a clinically important mag-

---

*"Metabolic" is actually a poor term to describe all nonrespiratory causes of acid-base disturbances; for example, excessive administration of acid or alkali affects acid-base equilibrium but has nothing to do with "metabolism." However, according to present clinical usage, the generic term metabolic acid-base disorder is customarily employed, irrespective of cause, and will be used throughout this text.

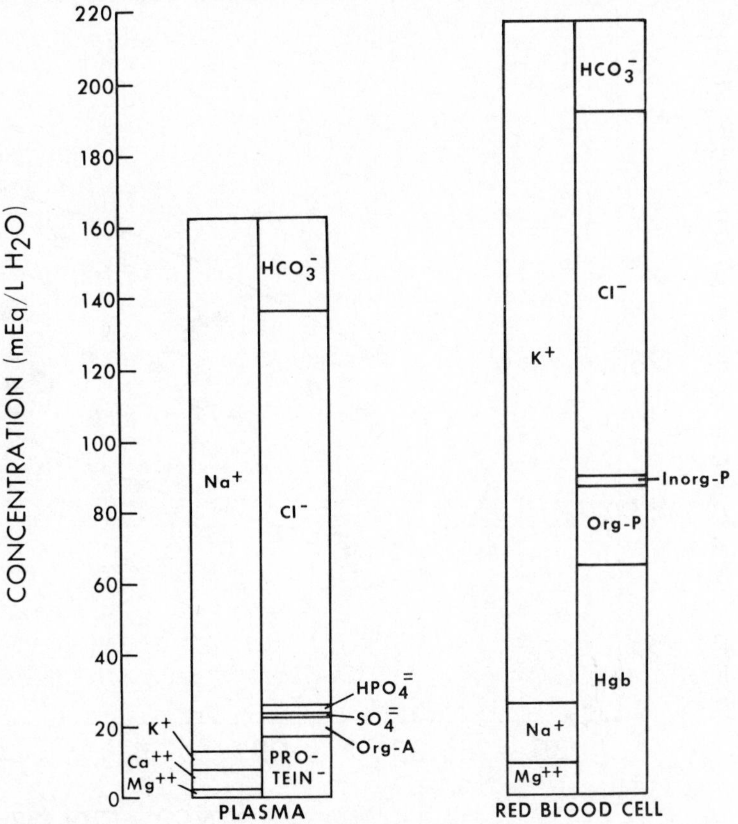

Figure 9–2. Composition of blood plasma and red blood cell intracellular liquid. Concentrations are in mEq/L of plasma and cell H_2O. The total heights of the two sets of columns differ owing to differences in the amount of H_2O in plasma (93 per cent) and in red blood cells (70 per cent).

nitude, have not been found by all investigators.

Other Variables. During the 1960's and 1970's considerable attention was directed toward finding a metabolic variable that was less affected by changes in ventilation than [HCO_3^-]. These efforts resulted in the use first of *buffer base* and then of *base excess.* Buffer base is the total quantity of all bases in whole blood that are capable of binding H^+ at the prevailing pH, expressed in mEq/L. For practical purposes, the chief buffer bases of plasma are HCO_3^- (normally about 24 mEq/L) and protein (normally about 17 mEq/L) and to a much lesser extent $HPO_4^=$ (Fig. 9–2). In contrast, cells have a different composition of buffer bases than plasma, with protein, particularly hemoglobin in red blood cells, predominating over HCO_3^- (see Fig. 9–2). Base excess is simply the difference in buffer base between the normal value expected in a given blood specimen and the value actually obtained. Neither buffer base nor base excess is measured directly; each is obtained by graphic solution of a nomogram compiled by Singer and Hastings[8] or Siggaard-Andersen,[9] respectively. However, because these metabolic variables have proved unnecessarily complex and occasionally misleading, they have largely been abandoned.[2]

Acidosis-Alkalosis

Acidosis and alkalosis are abnormal processes that result from the excessive production or elimination of acid or alkali (base) by the body and that tend to raise or lower pH.[1] To determine whether or not acidosis or alkalosis exists, it is necessary to know the normal range of the variables that are used to evaluate acid-base equilibrium. A more rigorous understanding of "normality" is now possible as a result of the studies of Madias and coworkers,[11] who documented that approximately 50 per cent of the normal variation in [HCO_3^-] is attributable to the normal variation in P_{CO_2}. Accordingly, *both* [HCO_3^-] and P_{CO_2} should be used when assessing the results of blood studies. The joint confidence region for [HCO_3^-] and P_{CO_2} that can be derived from their data is shown in Figure 9–3, and the interrelationships

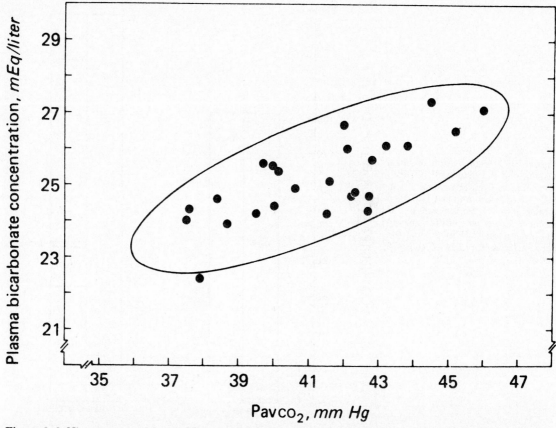

Figure 9–3. Ninety per cent joint confidence region for assessing new values for arterial Pco_2 and plasma $[HCO_3^-]$ obtained from a single arterialized venous blood specimen. A single set of acid-base data can, with 90 per cent probability, be expected to fall within this elliptical region. (From Madias, N. E., et al.: A redefinition of normal acid-base equilibrium in man: carbon dioxide tension as a key determinant of normal plasma bicarbonate concentration. Reprinted from Kidney International *16*:612–618, 1979 with permission.)

among normal values of $[HCO_3^-]$, Pco_2 and pH are presented in Table 9–3. It is also important to recognize that the pH is not necessarily above or below normal values when acidosis or alkalosis is present; whether or not pH changes depends on the adequacy of secondary mechanisms and on the presence of additional primary acid-base disorders.

Acidemia-Alkalemia

Acidemia or alkalemia is present when arterial blood pH deviates from the normal range depicted in Table 9–3. For practical clinical purposes, acidemia or alkalemia is said to occur when the arterial blood pH is less than 7.36 or greater than 7.44, respectively.[1] The arterial blood pH during the evolution of acidosis or alkalosis represents the net result of the interaction of all the

various abnormal processes and the secondary mechanisms that affect the amount of active H^+ in the bloodstream.

Extracellular-Intracellular pH

Because of the permeability of H^+ across endothelial barriers, the pH of capillary and venous blood (about 7.36) is virtually identical with that of most of the remainder of the extracellular fluid; the important exception is the pH of cerebrospinal fluid (CSF) because a relatively impermeable membrane, the blood-brain barrier, is involved (see Chapter 10). Extracellular pH also is known to differ from intracellular pH, in part because of differences in cell membrane permeability of H^+ and in part because of differing buffer systems. Intracellular pH, though difficult to determine, has been measured by a variety of techniques and has

Table 9–3. NINETY PER CENT CONFIDENCE REGION FOR PLASMA [HCO₃⁻] AND pH AT DIFFERENT LEVELS OF Pco₂ IN ARTERIALIZED VENOUS BLOOD FROM A NORMAL MAN*

P_{CO_2} (mm Hg)	$[HCO_3^-]$ (mEq/L)	pH (units)
36	22.9–23.6	7.41–7.42
37	22.6–24.7	7.39–7.43
38	22.6–25.4	7.38–7.43
39	22.8–25.9	7.37–7.43
40	23.0–26.4	7.37–7.42
41	23.4–26.8	7.36–7.42
42	23.7–27.1	7.36–7.42
43	24.2–27.4	7.36–7.41
44	24.7–27.6	7.35–7.40
45	25.2–27.8	7.35–7.40
46	26.0–27.7	7.36–7.39

*Reprinted from Madias, N. E., et al.: A redefinition of normal acid-base equilibrium in man: Carbon dioxide tension as a key determinant of normal plasma bicarbonate concentration. Reprinted from Kidney International 16:612–618, 1979 with permission).

been found in most mammals to vary from 6.8 to 7.2, depending on the species and tissues studied and the method of measurement.[12] Although the factors that control intracellular pH are poorly understood, it is recognized that changes in pH in either the intracellular or the extracellular compartment may not be reflected by parallel changes in the pH of the other compartment. In fact, in some circumstances the changes in pH in the two liquid spaces may be in opposite directions.

An important unifying concept of hydrogen ion regulation that applies to both endothermic ("warm-blooded") and ectothermic ("cold-blooded") animals and to their intracellular and extracellular systems has been proposed by Rahn and coworkers.[13] According to this theory, regulatory processes serve to maintain *intracellular* pH at or very close to the neutrality of water, the pH at which [H⁺] = [OH⁻] and at which most intermediary compounds are completely ionized and thus retained within cells because they are unable to cross cellular membranes. The pH of neutrality is 6.8 at 37° C but increases to nearly 7.5 at 0° C. Intracellular pH is anchored to the pH of neutrality—at whatever the animal's body temperature—by the compliant protein buffer imidazole of histidine. *Extracellular* pH is maintained 0.6 to 0.8 pH units higher than the prevailing intracellular pH, in other words, at a constant state of relative alkalinity, thereby providing a sink for disposing of the acid products of intracellular metabolism. Regulation of extracellular pH at a given level requires precise control of the ratio of HCO₃⁻ to H₂CO₃ by renal and ventilatory mechanisms, respectively.

How these concepts apply to humans is illustrated in Figure 9–4, which depicts the regional changes of intracellular and extracellular (blood) pH that may occur in humans during heavy exercise on a cold day. In the core of the person's body, where the temperature is 37° C, intracellular and blood pH are 6.8 and 7.4, respectively. As blood leaves the core, that flowing to exercising muscles is warmed to 41° C and that flowing to exposed skin is cooled to 25° C. These temperature changes induce a new chemical equilibrium in blood such that in the muscles its pH is 7.35 and its Pco₂ is 48 mm Hg, and in the skin blood pH is 7.60 and Pco₂ is 22 mm Hg. Despite these striking regional variations in pH and Pco₂, the CO₂ and H₂CO₃⁻ contents, the net charge of the imidazole buffer, and the relative alkalinity between cells and blood are constant throughout the body.

Based on these considerations, Rahn and coworkers[13] also proposed a useful means of solving the troublesome clinical problem of how to interpret the results of arterial blood gas and pH studies of patients who are hypothermic. The previous, and still widely used, method of correcting the measured values to the patient's body temperature requires knowledge of "normal" values for pH and Pco₂ at that particular body temperature: knowledge that simply does not exist. Rahn's solution is to warm the blood quickly and anaerobically and then to measure its pH and Pco₂ at 37° C, procedures that most analyzers do automatically. The resulting values—at 37° C—are then interpreted in the customary fashion; if pH is 7.40 and Pco₂ is 40 mm Hg, ventilation and HCO₃⁻ content are appropriate for that patient's particular temperature. This approach has been tested successfully in patients during surgical procedures that include controlled hypothermia[14] and is beginning to attract the clinical attention that it richly deserves.[15]

Normal Acid-Base Equilibrium

The chief by-products of cellular metabolic activities are water and various acids, mainly H₂CO₃ (200 mmol/kg body wt/24 hr)

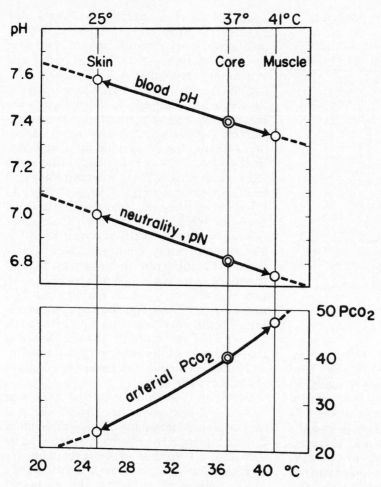

Figure 9-4. Expected changes in blood pH and Pco_2 in the arterioles of skin at 25° C and working muscle at 41° C of a healthy man with a core temperature of 37° C. (Reprinted by permission from Rahn, H.: Body temperature and acid-base regulation. Pneumonologie, *151*: 87-94, 1974.)

and acids of phosphates and sulfates (0.3 to 0.8 mEq/kg/24 hr). Under normal conditions, these residues are disposed of by the body at a rate that closely parallels their rate of formation, and intracellular and extracellular pH values are held within narrow limits (Fig. 9-5). Moreover, because the quantity of acid produced by cells may vary widely in healthy subjects, depending, for example, upon diet and physical activity, regulatory mechanisms exist that serve to govern H^+ elimination so that it keeps pace approximately with H^+ production and maintains equilibrium. Thus, the body is able to cope adequately with the usual daily vicissitudes of acid production, and it is only during abnormal circumstances that acidosis or alkalosis occurs.

Although newly produced H^+ is ultimately disposed of by the mechanisms described below, it is important to emphasize that the various responses of the body are actuated according to markedly differing time sequences. The first defense against an accumulation of H^+ and consequent lowering of pH is virtually instantaneous and consists of the sequestration or "mopping up" of H^+ by the various buffer systems throughout the body. The next defense is by the lungs, which respond within seconds to minutes to a stimulus to change CO_2 elimination. Finally, hours to days are required for completion of adjustments by the kidneys, which are aimed principally at Na^+ homeostasis with changes in plasma $[HCO_3^-]$ occurring as a by-product. Thus, acid-base "balance" must be viewed as a dynamic condition, and the factor of time must be considered when analyzing the acid-base status of a patient.

Volatile Acids

The only volatile acid produced by the body in significant quantities is H_2CO_3. Fur-

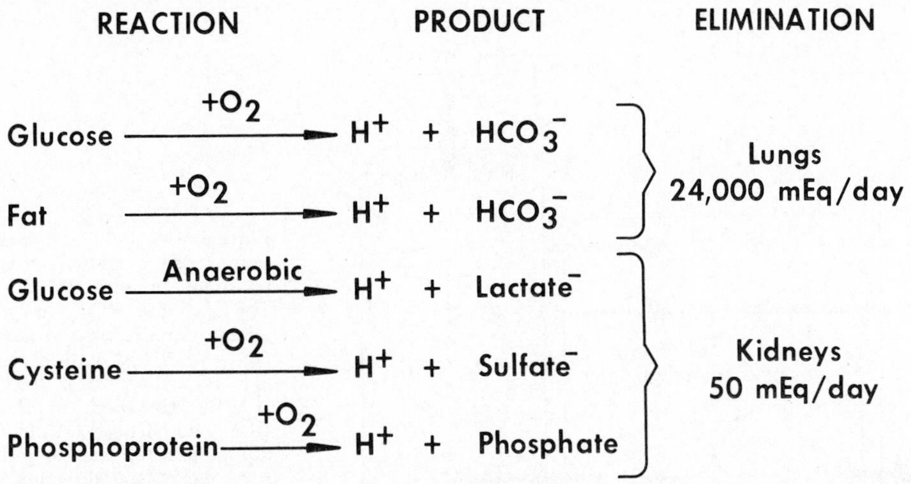

REACTION   PRODUCT   ELIMINATION

Glucose $\xrightarrow{\;+O_2\;}$ H^+ + HCO_3^- $\Big\}$ Lungs 24,000 mEq/day

Fat $\xrightarrow{\;+O_2\;}$ H^+ + HCO_3^-

Glucose $\xrightarrow{\;Anaerobic\;}$ H^+ + $Lactate^-$

Cysteine $\xrightarrow{\;+O_2\;}$ H^+ + $Sulfate^-$ $\Big\}$ Kidneys 50 mEq/day

Phosphoprotein $\xrightarrow{\;+O_2\;}$ H^+ + Phosphate

Figure 9–5. Condensed chemical reactions depicting the products of several important metabolic pathways and the routes by which H^+ is eliminated.

thermore, because CO_2 is the end product of normal oxidative metabolism, large amounts of H_2CO_3 are formed, and the rate of its production is nearly 500 times that of all other acids combined. In addition to H_2CO_3 that is formed by aerobic metabolism, H_2CO_3 may be generated by the reaction of H^+ from nonvolatile acids with HCO_3^- buffers (Equation 5); H_2CO_3 from both sources is disposed of through the elimination of CO_2 by the lungs (Equation 7). Removal of CO_2 obviously does not affect the total quantity of H in the body, but the process is an effective means of defending pH because during the chemical reactions that release CO_2 (Equation 7), active H^+ is converted to H in molecules of body water.

The mechanisms by which CO_2 is transported in the bloodstream and eliminated from the lungs are reviewed in Chapter 7. The intimate relationship between the control of breathing and the level of P_{CO_2} in arterial blood is considered in the next chapter. This relationship can be summarized by saying that the minute volume of alveolar ventilation is closely regulated by a rapidly responding system that usually holds arterial P_{CO_2} constant within normal limits (38 to 43 mm Hg) in a resting subject at sea level and allows the value to decrease somewhat during strenuous exercise (see Chapter 11). However, many peripheral and central stimuli are known to influence the control of breathing; therefore, ventilation, and hence P_{CO_2} and acid-base equilibrium, can be disturbed under both normal and pathologic conditions (see subsequent section).

Nonvolatile Acids

Nonvolatile acids are not in equilibrium with gases, so they must be removed from the body in solution by the kidneys instead of by the lungs. (Lactate and other organic acids are in part excreted in the urine and in part metabolized to CO_2 and water.) In addition to excreting H^+ formed by the production of nonvolatile acids, the kidneys also significantly influence acid-base equilibrium by regulating body stores of HCO_3^-. Bicarbonate conservation and H^+ elimination can be considered separate functions because they occur in different parts of the nephron; however, they are interrelated processes because both involve H^+ secretion by tubule cells and because together they constitute the main renal contribution to acid-base equilibrium. (The collective handling of other ions also affects acid-base balance, but this occurs indirectly through the effects on H^+-secretion.)

The regulation of HCO_3^- stores is fairly straightforward because it involves simply the reabsorption and return to the bloodstream of virtually all the HCO_3^- present in the glomerular filtrate. Because approximately 180 L of filtrate are formed each day, with a $[HCO_3^-]$ nearly equal to that in plasma, over 4000 mEq of HCO_3^- could be lost from the body in 24 hours, which would rapidly and severely deplete the HCO_3^- stores and the buffering capacity of the body. However, excessive loss is prevented by reabsorption of most of the HCO_3^- from the filtrate as it passes through the tubular

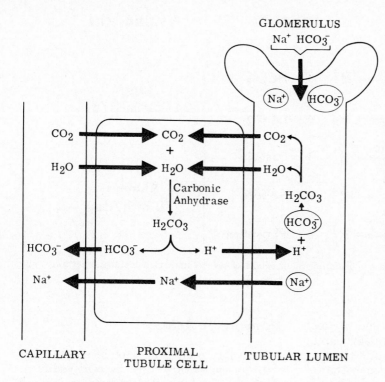

Figure 9–6. Schematic representation of the excretion of H^+ in the proximal tubules of the kidney. The Na^+ and HCO_3^- present in the glomerular filtrate are identified as Na^+ and HCO_3^- within circles. The Na^+ is reabsorbed in exchange for H^+; the H^+ then reacts with the HCO_3^- to form H_2O and CO_2 that diffuse into the tubular cell. The arrows depict the direction of movement. For further details, see text.

system. Bicarbonate ions and Cl^- are selectively reabsorbed as the principal anions that accompany Na^+ as it is actively transported from the glomerular filtrate back into the bloodstream. However, HCO_3^- is not a very diffusible ion, so it is removed from the filtrate after being transformed into the more diffusible CO_2 molecule by the process illustrated in Figure 9–6. Note that Na^+ from within the tubular lumen is exchanged for H^+ secreted by the tubule cell. The H^+ is one of the ionization products of H_2CO_3 that is formed by the hydration of CO_2 in a reaction catalyzed by carbonic anhydrase. The CO_2 and water involved may come either from metabolism within the cells or from movement into them from capillary blood or tubular filtrate. Figure 9–6 also shows that the HCO_3^- that reaches the capillary blood is another ionization product of H_2CO_3, and hence is not the original HCO_3^- that was present in the glomerular filtrate (encircled in Fig. 9–6).

The reabsorption of HCO_3^- appears to be governed in part by a threshold mechanism that serves to regulate the $[HCO_3^-]$. The process operates by the selective reabsorption of either HCO_3^- or Cl^- as the attendant anion of Na^+, depending upon whether HCO_3^- is to be conserved or wasted. Thus, there is a reciprocal and roughly equivalent relationship between the amount of HCO_3^- and Cl^- reabsorbed and the amount rejected. Although the HCO_3^- threshold may vary widely under different conditions and although the factors that control the threshold are incompletely understood, HCO_3^- reabsorption is clearly responsive to changes in arterial P_{CO_2}. This relationship is an important one because it appears to underlie the renal adaptation to primary respiratory (i.e., P_{CO_2}-dependent) acid-base disorders.

Although HCO_3^- reabsorption depends upon H^+ secretion, the H^+ involved is not lost from the body; it can be viewed as moving from cell to filtrate and back again (as H in H_2O). The excretion of surplus H^+ takes place mainly in the distal tubules and collecting ducts of the nephron. The H^+ is also formed there by the hydration of CO_2 under the influence of carbonic anhydrase and the ionization of H_2CO_3. The H^+ is then secreted into the tubular lumen in exchange for Na^+ and in the process reacts with one of three substrates, depending upon which is available in the filtrate. (1) Hydrogen ions may combine with HCO_3^- to form water and CO_2, as discussed earlier (see Fig. 9–6). Under ordinary conditions, more than half the filtered HCO_3^- is reabsorbed in the proximal tubules, and the remainder is absorbed in the distal system. (2) Hydrogen ions may

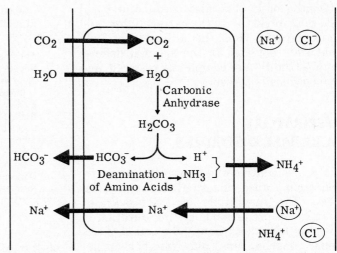

Figure 9–7. Schematic representation of the excretion of H^+ in the distal tubule of the kidney. The Na^+ and Cl^- present in the glomerular filtrate are identified as Na^+ and Cl^- within circles. Within the cell, H^+ combines with NH_3, formed by deamination of amino acids, to form NH_4^+ that is exchanged for Na^+ that is returned to the bloodstream.

CAPILLARY   DISTAL TUBULE CELL   TUBULAR LUMEN

combine with NH_3, produced by the deamidization of glutamine, to form NH_4^+ in the filtrate (Fig. 9–7). Ammonia is a strong binder of H^+, and increased NH_3 production is an important pathway of H^+ binding and elimination in states of acidosis. (3) Hydrogen ions may combine with $HPO_4^=$ to form $H_2PO_4^-$ (Fig. 9–8). The extent of this reaction is measurable as titratable acidity. Thus, in order to quantify all the H^+ excreted in the urine ([Total H^+]u), it is necessary to know the total amount of H^+ excreted in the urine as titratable acid ([TA]u) and ammonium ([NH_4^+]u):

$$[\text{Total } H^+]u = [TA]u + [NH_4^+]u. \quad (16)$$

To determine *net* renal acid loss, any HCO_3^- that appears in the urine must be subtracted from [Total H^+]u to equal Net Acid Excretion because excreted HCO_3^- represents loss of base, an effect that offsets loss of an equivalent amount of acid.

$$\text{Net Renal Acid} = [TA]u + \\ [NH_4^+]u - [HCO_3^-]u. \quad (17)$$

The excretion of surplus H^+ serves to conserve additional Na^+, but more importantly, as shown in Figures 9–7 and 9–8, the reaction generates an amount of HCO_3^- that is exactly equal to the amount of H^+ excreted and adds it to the extracellular fluid. If 100 mEq of HCO_3^- are consumed by the 100 mEq of nonvolatile acid produced by the body each day, the kidneys not only excrete

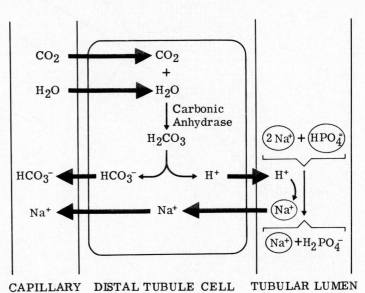

Figure 9–8. Schematic representation of the excretion of H^+ in the distal tubule of the kidney. The Na_2HPO_4 present in the glomerular filtrate ionizes into 2 Na^+ and $HPO_4^=$ shown within circles. The H^+, formed within the cell, is exchanged for one Na^+ that is returned to the bloodstream. Thus the urine contains NaH_2PO_4.

CAPILLARY   DISTAL TUBULE CELL   TUBULAR LUMEN

100 mEq of H^+ but also produce and add 100 mEq of HCO_3^- to the extracellular fluid in the process. Thus, the buffers of the body that were depleted in the original defense against the H^+ are completely restored, and homeostasis is preserved.

RESPIRATORY ACID-BASE DISORDERS

Hypoventilation and hyperventilation, by definition, cause abnormalities of arterial P_{CO_2}. The magnitude of the associated changes in pH depends on the duration of the breathing disturbance, the extent of secondary mechanisms, and whether or not coexisting disorders are present.

Respiratory Acidosis

The hallmark of respiratory acidosis is an increased arterial P_{CO_2}. Retention of CO_2 may occur in patients with normal lungs because of faulty regulation of ventilation by the central nervous system or because of impairment of respiratory muscle function. Retention of CO_2 also develops in patients with a variety of pulmonary diseases. Some

Table 9–4. COMMON CAUSES OF CO_2 RETENTION AND RESPIRATORY ACIDOSIS

With normal lungs
Anesthesia
Sedative drugs
Neuromuscular disease (poliomyelitis, myasthenia gravis, Guillain-Barré syndrome)
Obesity (Pickwickian syndrome)
Brain damage
Idiopathic
With abnormal lungs
Chronic obstructive pulmonary disease (chronic bronchitis, emphysema)
Diffuse infiltrative pulmonary disease (advanced)
Kyphoscoliosis (severe)

of the most common causes are listed in Table 9–4.

Failure to eliminate CO_2 may occur within seconds or minutes in patients undergoing anesthesia or receiving sedative drugs. A sudden depression of ventilation leads to rapid CO_2 retention and *acute* respiratory acidosis. The consequences of acute hypercapnia have been studied experimentally by exposing normal subjects to high concentrations of CO_2 in the inspired air.[16] The results of these studies are represented as line A in Figure 9–9, which extends toward the right from the point of normality

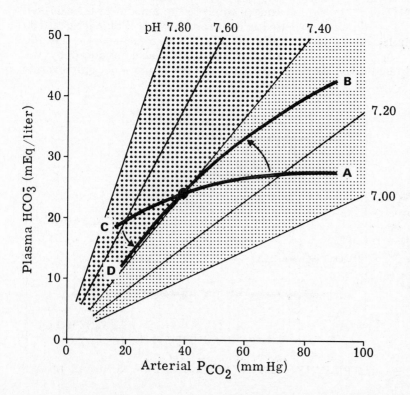

Figure 9–9. Respiratory acid-base disorders. Pooled results from several studies of the effects of acute and chronic variations in arterial P_{CO_2} on plasma HCO_3^- and pH. When P_{CO_2} is raised acutely *(acute respiratory acidosis)*, HCO_3^- and pH values lie along line A. After compensation by retention of HCO_3^- is complete *(chronic respiratory acidosis)*, values lie along line B. When P_{CO_2} is lowered acutely *(acute respiratory alkalosis)*, resulting HCO_3^- and pH values lie along line C. After compensation by rejection of HCO_3^- is complete *(chronic respiratory alkalosis)*, values lie along line D. For further details and references, see text.

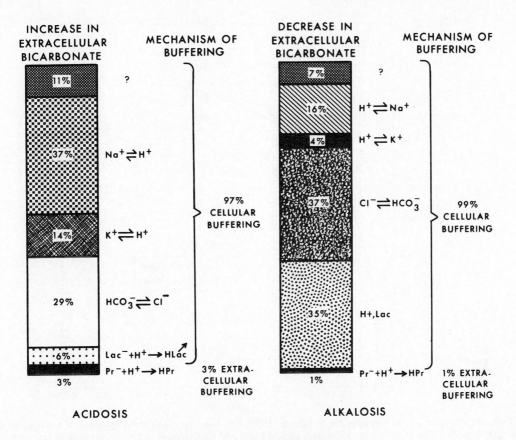

RESPIRATORY DISTURBANCES

Figure 9–10. Diagrammatic representation of the mechanisms of buffering in dogs with acute respiratory acidosis (breathing 20 per cent CO_2) and acute respiratory alkalosis (mechanical hyperventilation). Lac = lactate; Pr = protein. (Adapted from Pitts, R. F.: Physiology of the Kidney and Body Fluids. An Introductory Text. 3rd ed. Chicago, 1964, pp. 198–241. Reprinted by permission from the authors and Year Book Medical Publishers, Inc. Original data from Swan, R. C., and Pitts, R. F.: J. Clin. Invest. *34*:205, 1955, and Swan, R. C., Axelrod, D. R., Seip, M., and Pitts, R. F.: J. Clin. Invest. *34*:1795, 1955.)

($Pco_2 = 40$ mm Hg, $[HCO_3^-] = 24$ mEq/L, and pH = 7.40) and demonstrates that as Pco_2 increases, $[HCO_3^-]$ rises slightly and pH falls.

However, the acidosis that develops is less severe than that which would occur in the absence of intracellular buffering mechanisms. Figure 9–10 demonstrates how acute respiratory acidosis was defended against in dogs given 20 per cent CO_2 to breathe.[17] Entry of Cl^- into cells in exchange for HCO_3^- accounted for 29 per cent of the buffering; similarly, exchange of intracellular Na^+ and K^+ for extracellular H^+ accounted for 51 per cent; smaller increments of buffering were contributed by reactions involving lactate, plasma proteins, and an unidentified source.

If CO_2 retention persists for several days, the relationship between Pco_2 and $[HCO_3^-]$

depicted by line B (see Fig. 9–9) is observed.[18–21] In patients with *chronic* respiratory acidosis, therefore, $[HCO_3^-]$ is considerably higher than in those with acute conditions, and pH is consequently also higher (i.e., closer to normal values). The elevation in $[HCO_3^-]$ occurs through an alteration in the renal threshold, with subsequent retention of HCO_3^- and loss of an equivalent amount of Cl^-. As shown by the results depicted in Figure 9–11, it takes five to seven days for compensation by the kidney to become maximal in experimental animals.[22] Accordingly, the shift from line A to line B in humans, shown by the arrow in Figure 9–9, probably also develops over a period of several days. Although patients with chronic CO_2 retention appear to be better off with their blood pHs raised toward normal by renal compensation, the question

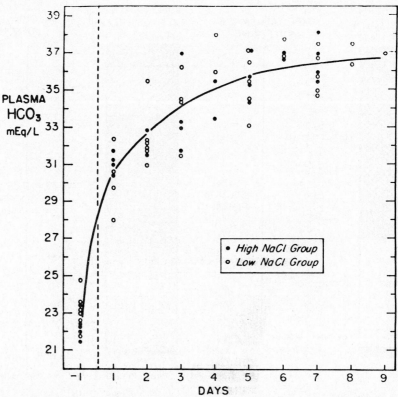

Figure 9–11. Time course of the changes in plasma HCO_3^- in response to respiratory acidosis induced in dogs constantly breathing an atmosphere containing 11 to 13 per cent CO_2. Plasma HCO_3^- continues to increase until about the fifth day after exposure. The amount of NaCl in the diet did not affect the response. (Reprinted by permission from Polak, A. et al.: Effects of chronic hypercapnia on electrolyte and acid-base equilibrium. I. Adaptation. J. Clin. Invest., *40*:1223–1237, 1961.)

still remains of why pH is not returned to normal levels in view of the kidneys' demonstrable capacity to retain additional HCO_3^- when arterial P_{CO_2} is raised even higher. Because intracellular pH has been shown to be normal in patients with chronic hypercapnia despite persistent extracellular acidosis, it was originally suggested that the effect of intracellular rather than extracellular pH governed the renal threshold for HCO_3^- reabsorption.[23] A more recent analysis of the renal responses to a multitude of chronic acid-base disturbances led to the conclusion that the disorders chiefly affect the handling of Na^+ by the nephron.[24] This in no way diminishes the importance of preserving intracellular acid-base homeostasis but implies either that there are other ways of achieving it or that Na^+ and K^+ balance has primacy over acidity.

Respiratory Alkalosis

Hyperventilation quickly lowers arterial P_{CO_2} and produces *acute* respiratory alkalosis. Hyperventilation, which is defined as a lower than normal arterial P_{CO_2}, is a common clinical finding in patients with normal lungs, and it may even occur in patients with pulmonary diseases. Some of the many causes of excessive CO_2 elimination are listed in Table 9–5. The effects of acute hyperventilation on arterial P_{CO_2}, $[HCO_3^-]$, and pH have been examined in anesthetized patients;[25] the results of these studies have led to the formulation of the relationship that is illustrated by line C in Figure 9–9. Although $[HCO_3^-]$ falls somewhat, the rise in pH becomes progressively more severe as P_{CO_2} is lowered.

The defenses against a severe change in

Table 9–5. COMMON CAUSES OF EXCESSIVE CO_2 ELIMINATION AND RESPIRATORY ALKALOSIS

With normal lungs
  Anxiety
  Fever
  Drugs (e.g., aspirin)
  Central nervous system lesions (tumors, inflammation)
  Endotoxemia
With abnormal lungs
  Pneumonia
  Diffuse infiltrative pulmonary diseases (early)
  Acute bronchial asthma
  Pulmonary vascular diseases
  Congestive heart failure

pH during acute respiratory alkalosis, like those during acute respiratory acidosis, are nearly all attributable to intracellular reactions (see Fig. 9–10). The two main mechanisms are the production of lactate to reduce the HCO_3^- content of extracellular liquids (35 per cent) and the exchange of intracellular Cl^- for extracellular HCO_3^- (37 per cent). The pH is also protected by exchanges of Na^+ and K^+ for H^+ and by an unidentified reaction.[17]

When a state of hyperventilation persists, renal mechanisms are actuated, and adaptation occurs by selective loss of HCO_3^- and retention of Cl^-. In chronic respiratory alkalosis, as in normal subjects at high altitudes, the relationship between arterial PCO_2 and $[HCO_3^-]$, which is represented by line D in Figure 9–9, is observed.[26–28] Line D is extremely close to the pH 7.40 line, indicating that compensation (renal and possibly other mechanisms) is almost perfect, and blood pH is restored to within normal values. The transition from acute to chronic respiratory alkalosis, signified by the arrow from line C to line D, is quite similar to the time course of the adjustments in chronic CO_2 retention in that both require several days to be fully developed.

METABOLIC ACID-BASE DISORDERS

Many common clinical conditions are accompanied by the addition or subtraction of acids or bases to or from body fluids. Although these disturbances often have nothing to do with the body's intrinsic metabolism, they are conventionally referred to as "metabolic" acid-base disorders.

Metabolic Acidosis

Either an increase in nonvolatile acids or an excessive loss of bases from the body can produce metabolic acidosis. These two fundamentally different causes of metabolic acidosis are often classified, as shown in Table 9–6, on the basis of whether or not they cause an increase in unmeasured anions. Although the "anion-gap" is calculated from measured constituents ($[Na^+] - [Cl^-] - [HCO_3^-]$), it reflects the concentrations and charges of unmeasured substances; thus, an increase in unmeasured anions *per se* is not specific for metabolic acidosis and, in fact, is known to occur in metabolic alkalosis.[29] The key to the recognition of metabolic acidosis lies in the demonstration of a deficit of buffer base, base excess, or $[HCO_3^-]$. A reduction of any of these components means that pH must fall and $[H^+]$ must rise. Acidosis, as mentioned, is also a potent stimulus to increased ventilation, and as a consequence PCO_2 also falls.[30] Three possible relationships between $[HCO_3^-]$ and PCO_2, depending upon the rapidity with which the acidosis develops and the magnitude of the ventilatory response, are shown by lines A, B, and C in Figure 9–12.

Note that in Figure 9–12 the axes are reversed compared with those in Figure 9–9; that is because the primary change in metabolic acid-base disturbances is an alteration in $[HCO_3^-]$. Therefore, $[HCO_3^-]$ is shown as the independent variable on the abscissa in Figure 9–12. In contrast, the primary change in respiratory disorders is reflected in PCO_2. Therefore, PCO_2 occupies the abscissa in Figure 9–9.

Metabolic acidosis is "sensed" almost im-

Table 9–6. COMMON CAUSES OF METABOLIC ACIDOSIS

Increased Unmeasured Anions (excess nonvolatile acids)
  Diabetic ketoacidosis
  Alcoholic ketoacidosis
  Lactic acidosis
  Salicylate intoxication
  Renal failure
  Methanol or ethylene glycol poisoning

Normal Unmeasured Anions (loss of bicarbonate)
  Diarrhea
  Pancreatic or biliary fistulas
  Renal tubular acidosis
  Chronic pyelonephritis
  Obstructive uropathy

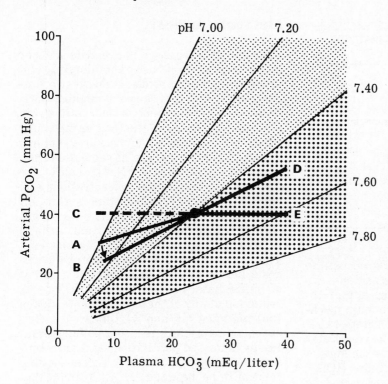

Figure 9–12. Metabolic acid-base disorders. Pooled results from several studies of the effects of variations in plasma HCO_3^- on arterial P_{CO_2} and pH. When HCO_3^- is lowered acutely *(acute metabolic acidosis)*, P_{CO_2} and pH values lie along line A. After CSF adjustments allow ventilation to increase further *(chronic metabolic acidosis)*, values lie along line B. Line C depicts the pH changes that would result from a given reduction in HCO_3^- if no increase in ventilation occurred (i.e., P_{CO_2} remained at 40 mm Hg). Two patterns of ventilation occur in response to HCO_3^- increase *(chronic metabolic alkalosis):* one with hypoventilation (line D) and one with no change (line E). For further details and references, see text.

mediately by peripheral chemoreceptors, with the result that ventilation increases and P_{CO_2} falls. The distinction between acute (line A) and chronic (line B) metabolic acidosis is determined by the magnitude of the ventilatory response, which depends in turn upon the adjustments that take place in the extracellular environment of the central chemoreceptors. As explained in detail in the next chapter, this process is reflected in the composition of cerebrospinal fluid (CSF) and requires up to one to two days for completion; until then, the ventilatory response is not fully developed because of the presence of a gradually lessening inhibitory influence that offsets part of the stimulating effect of the systemic acidosis. Line A in the figure shows the consequences of a fall in $[HCO_3^-]$ plus the immediate stimulus to respiration; hyperventilation serves to compensate partially for a reduction in $[HCO_3^-]$, but as the metabolic disorder worsens, the associated hyperventilation and reduction of P_{CO_2} becomes progressively less able to prevent pH from decreasing.

In addition to extracellular buffering by HCO_3^- and elimination of CO_2 by increasing ventilation in acute metabolic acidosis, intracellular reactions also participate in the defense of body pH. As shown by the experimental results depicted in Figure 9–13,

buffering in acute metabolic acidosis is also achieved by exchange of intracellular Na^+ (36 per cent) and K^+ (15 per cent) for extracellular H^+.[17]

Line B in Figure 9–12 depicts the relationship between $[HCO_3^-]$ and P_{CO_2} when the ventilatory response is maximal;[31] in chronic metabolic acidosis, the added effect of the secondary increase in ventilation, which is signified by the arrow, is evident in the position of line B in comparison with line A (i.e., at any given $[HCO_3^-]$, P_{CO_2} is lower, but pH is nearer to normal after respiratory adaptation occurs). Increases in the "bicarbonate space," which have been observed during metabolic acidosis, are now believed to reflect the behavior of nonbicarbonate buffers whenever plasma $[HCO_3^-]$ is low.[32] Line C shows the effect that lowering $[HCO_3^-]$ would have on pH if there were no respiratory compensation at all and if arterial P_{CO_2} remained at 40 mm Hg. It is obvious that pH changes more with a given reduction in $[HCO_3^-]$ along line C than along either line A or line B. Line C is a broken line to emphasize that it is artificial and has no clinical analogue except perhaps rarely in patients who develop metabolic acidosis but cannot augment their ventilation because of neuromuscular weakness or severe coexisting pulmonary disease.

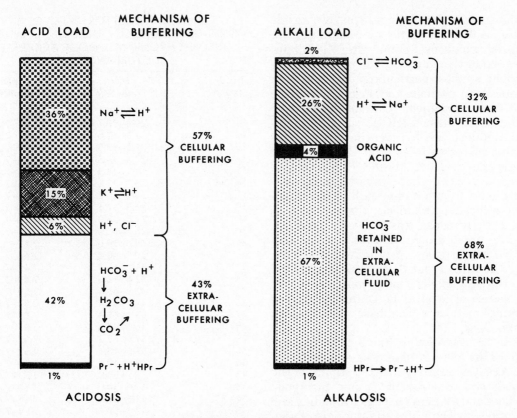

Figure 9–13. Diagrammatic representation of the mechanisms of buffering in dogs with acute metabolic acidosis (intravenous HCl) and acute metabolic alkalosis (intravenous NaHCO₃). (Adapted from Pitts, R. F.: Physiology of the Kidney and Body Fluids. An Introductory Text. 3rd ed. Chicago, 1964, pp. 198–241. Reprinted by permission from the authors and Year Book Medical Publishers, Inc. Original data from Giebisch, G., Berger, L., and Pitts, R. F.: J. Clin. Invest. *34*:231, 1955.)

Metabolic Alkalosis

Excessive elimination of nonvolatile acids or accumulation of bases produces metabolic alkalosis. Although the common causes of nonrespiratory alkalosis may involve both these processes, they are often classified into the three major categories shown in Table 9–7. Irrespective of the principal underlying cause, in patients with severe metabolic alkalosis extracellular volume is usually markedly contracted and K⁺ stores are depleted, both of which tend to worsen the alkalosis. The mechanisms by which the body defends itself against an increase in pH in acute metabolic alkalosis have been studied in dogs given large amounts of HCO₃⁻. The results of these experiments are shown in Figure 9–13. Of the total infused HCO₃⁻, two-thirds remained in the extra-

cellular spaces; P_{CO_2} (and hence H_2CO_3) doubled owing to alveolar hypoventilation. One-third of the buffering was produced by intracellular reactions, predominantly (26 per cent) an exchange of intracellular H⁺ for extracellular Na⁺.[17]

The conditions causing chronic metabolic alkalosis all produce increases in [HCO₃⁻]; however, despite similarities in [HCO₃⁻], the effect on ventilation, and hence on arterial P_{CO_2} and pH, of different causes of alkalosis has been somewhat controversial. At least two patterns of response have been demonstrated in experiments on humans and are shown in Figure 9–12.[33] Line D shows that under some circumstances, such as the administration of HCO₃⁻ or other buffers, P_{CO_2} rises, which minimizes the pH change at any given level of [HCO₃⁻]. In contrast, line E shows the presence of alkalosis from the administration of thiazide diuretics or aldosterone; no respiratory adaptation whatsoever occurs after the administration of these agents. The results of subsequent studies, particularly those of Van Ypersele de Strihou and Frans,[34] indicate that there is a linear relationship between increases in plasma [HCO_3^-] during metabolic alkalosis and hypoventilation, with resulting increases in arterial PCO_2. In other words, no evidence of line E was found. Moreover, when these investigators combined data from patients with either metabolic acidosis or alkalosis, they noted that the PCO_2 response was virtually identical over a broad range of values of plasma [HCO_3^-] from as low as 10 mEq/L to as high as 38 mEq/L. From these observations, 95 per cent confidence limits were calculated for values of arterial PCO_2 and pH during chronic metabolic acid-base disturbances (Table 9–8).

The validity of Van Ypersele de Strihou and Frans' observations was supported by the recent carefully conducted studies of the ventilatory response to chronic metabolic acidosis and alkalosis in dogs by Madias and coworkers.[35] These investigators also found a linear relationship between arterial PCO_2 and plasma [HCO_3^-], such that PCO_2 changed 0.74 mm Hg for each 1 mEq/L change in [HCO_3^-] through a wide range of bicarbonate concentrations. In dogs with metabolic alkalosis, the ventilatory response was independent of the particular mode of induction. These studies, both of humans and of dogs, have greatly clarified the continuum of ventilatory responses that occurs in chronic, otherwise uncomplicated metabolic acid-base disturbances.

Table 9–7. COMMON CAUSES OF METABOLIC ALKALOSIS

Alkalosis Secondary to Alkali Administration
    Milk-alkali syndrome
    Ingestion of sodium bicarbonate

Chloride-Responsive Alkalosis
    Gastric fluid losses
    Diuretic therapy

Chloride-Resistant Alkalosis
    Primary aldosteronism
    Bartter's syndrome

Table 9–8. VALUES FOR 95 PER CENT CONFIDENCE LIMITS OF ARTERIAL PCO_2 AND pH DURING CHRONIC METABOLIC ACID-BASE DISTURBANCES*

[HCO_3^-] (mEq/L)	PCO_2 (mm Hg)	pH (units)
10	19.5–29.7	7.33–7.15
11	20.4–30.7	7.35–7.18
12	21.3–31.6	7.37–7.20
13	22.2–32.5	7.39–7.22
14	23.2–33.4	7.40–7.24
15	24.1–34.3	7.42–7.26
16	25.0–35.2	7.43–7.28
17	25.9–36.2	7.44–7.29
18	26.8–37.1	7.45–7.31
19	27.8–38.0	7.46–7.32
20	28.7–38.9	7.47–7.33
21	29.6–39.8	7.47–7.34
22	30.5–40.8	7.48–7.35
23	31.4–41.7	7.49–7.36
24	32.4–42.6	7.49–7.37
25	33.3–43.5	7.50–7.38
26	34.2–44.4	7.50–7.39
27	35.1–45.4	7.51–7.40
28	36.0–46.3	7.51–7.40
29	37.0–47.2	7.52–7.41
30	37.9–48.1	7.52–7.42
31	38.8–49.1	7.51–7.42
32	39.7–50.0	7.53–7.43
33	40.6–50.9	7.53–7.43
34	41.5–51.8	7.54–7.44
35	42.5–52.7	7.54–7.44
36	43.4–53.7	7.54–7.45
37	44.3–54.6	7.54–7.45
38	45.2–55.5	7.55–7.46

*From Van Ypersele de Strihou, C., and Frans, A.: The respiratory response to chronic metabolic alkalosis and acidosis in disease. Clin. Sci., *45*:439–448, 1973. Copyright the Biochemical Society, London.

MIXED ACID-BASE DISORDERS

An understanding of acid-base disorders is facilitated by considering them as "pure" entities. However, this is seldom the case in clinical circumstances, in which they are often found to coexist with electrolyte and other metabolic disorders. Furthermore, the factor of time and the influence of therapy must always be included when interpreting data from patients with acid-base disturbances. Detailed consideration of these important problems is beyond the scope of this chapter, and good reviews are available elsewhere.[2, 36, 37] This chapter has emphasized the interrelationships between respiration and acid-base equilibrium and has provided a background for discussion of the control of breathing which is continued in the next chapter.

REFERENCES

1. Filley, G. F.: Acid-Base and Blood Gas Regulation. Philadelphia, Lea & Febiger, 1971, pp. 1–213.
2. Cohen, J. J., and Kassirer, J. P., (eds.): Acid-Base. Boston, Little, Brown and Co., 1982, pp. 1–510.
3. Sörensen, S. P. L.: Enzymstudien, II. Mitteilung. Über die Messung und die Bedeutung der Wasserstoffionen-konzentration bei enzymatischen Prozessen. Biochem. Z., 21:131–304, 1909.
4. Davis, R. P.: Editorial: Logland: A Gibbsian view of acid-base balance. Am. J. Med., 42:159–162, 1967.
5. Madias, N. E., Schwartz, W. B., and Cohen, J. J.: The maladaptive renal response to secondary hypocapnia during chronic HCl acidosis in the dog. J. Clin. Invest., 60:1393–1401, 1977.
6. Van Slyke, D. D., and Neill, J. M.: Determination of gases in blood and other solutions by vacuum extraction and manometric measurement. I. J. Biol. Chem., 61:523–573, 1924.
7. Van Slyke, D. D., and Cullen, G. E.: Studies of acidosis. I. The bicarbonate concentration of the blood plasma; its significance, and its determination as a measure of acidosis. J. Biol. Chem., 30:289–346, 1917.
8. Singer, R. B., and Hastings, A. B.: An improved clinical method for the estimation of disturbances of the acid-base balance of human blood. Medicine, 27:223–242, 1948.
9. Siggaard-Andersen, O.: The acid-base status of the blood. Scand. J. Clin. Lab. Invest., 15(Suppl. 70):1–134, 1963.
10. Hood, I., and Campbell, E. J. M.: Is pK OK? New Engl. J. Med., 306:864–866, 1982.
11. Madias, N. E., Androgué, H. J., Horowitz, G. L., Cohen, J. J., and Schwartz, W. B.: A redefinition of normal acid-base equilibrium in man: carbon dioxide tension as a key determinant of normal plasma bicarbonate concentration. Kidney Int., 16:612–618, 1979.
12. Roos, A., and Boron, W. F.: Intracellular pH. Physiol. Rev., 61:296–434, 1981.
13. Rahn, H., Reeves, R. B., and Howell, B. J.: Hydrogen ion regulation, temperature, and evolution. Am. Rev. Respir. Dis., 112:165–172, 1975.
14. Blayo, M. C., Lecompte, Y., and Pocidalo, J. J.: Control of acid-base status during hypothermia in man. Respir. Physiol., 42:287–298, 1980.
15. Ream, A. K., Reitz, B. A., and Silverberg, G.: Temperature correction of P_{CO_2} and pH in estimating acid-base status: an example of the emperor's new clothes? Anesthesiology, 56:41–44, 1982.
16. Brackett, N. C., Jr., Cohen, J. J., and Schwartz, W. B.: Carbon dioxide titration curve of normal man. Effect of increasing degrees of acute hypercapnia on acid-base equilibrium. New Eng.. J. Med., 272:6–12, 1965.
17. Pitts, R. F.: Physiology of the Kidney and Body fluids. An Introductory Text. 3rd Ed. Chicago, Year Book Medical Publishers, Inc., 1944, pp. 198–241.
18. Refsum, H. E.: Acid-base status in patients with chronic hypercapnia and hypoxaemia. Clin. Sci., 27:407–415, 1964.
19. Van Ypersele de Strihou, C., Brasseur, L., and de Coninck, J.: The "carbon dioxide response curve" for chronic hypercapnia in man. New Engl. J. Med., 275:117–122, 1966.
20. Dufano, M. J., and Ishikawa, S.: Quantitative acid-base relationships in chronic pulmonary patients during the stable state. Am. Rev. Respir. Dis., 93:251–256, 1966.
21. Brackett, N. C., Jr., Wingo, C. F., Muren, O., and Solano, J. T.: Acid-base response to chronic hypercapnia in man. New Engl. J. Med., 280:124–130, 1969.
22. Polak, A., Haynie, G. D., Hays, R. M., and Schwartz, W. B.: Effects of chronic hypercapnia on electrolyte and acid-base equilibrium. I. Adaptation. J. Clin. Invest., 40:1223–1237, 1961.
23. Robin, E. D., Bromberg, P. A., and Tushan, F. S.: Carbon-dioxide in body fluids. New Engl. J. Med., 280:162–164, 1969.
24. Schwartz, W. B., and Cohen, J. J.: The nature of the renal response to chronic disorders of acid-base equilibrium. Am. J. Med., 64:417–428, 1978.
25. Arbus, G. S., Hebert, L. A., Levesque, P. R., Etsten, B. E., and Schwartz, W. B.: Characterization and clinical application of the "significance band" for acute respiratory alkalosis. New Engl. J. Med., 280:117–123, 1969.
26. Severinghaus, J. W., and Carcelen, B. A.: Cerebrospinal fluid in man native to high altitude. J. Appl. Physiol., 19:319–321, 1964.
27. Pugh, L. G. C. E., Gill, M. D., Lahiri, S., Milledge, J. S., Ward, M. P., and West, J. B.: Muscular exercise at great altitudes. J. Appl. Physiol., 19:431–440, 1964.
28. Lahiri, S., and Milledge, J. S.: Acid-base in Sherpa altitude residents and lowlanders at 4880 M. Respir. Physiol., 2:323–334, 1967.
29. Madias, N. E., Ayus, J. C., and Androgué, H. J.: Increased anion gap in metabolic alkalosis: the role of plasma-protein equivalency. New Engl. J. Med., 300:1421–1423, 1979.
30. Fulop, M.: The ventilatory response in severe metabolic acidosis. Clin. Sci. Mol. Med., 50:367–373, 1976.
31. Lennon, E. J., and Lemann, J., Jr.: Defense of hydrogen ion concentration in chronic metabolic acidosis. A new evaluation of an old approach. Ann. Int. Med., 65:265–274, 1966.
32. Androgué, H. J., Brensilver, J., Cohen, J. J., and Madias, N. E.: Influence of steady-state alterations in acid-base equilibrium on the fate of administered bicarbonate in the dog. J. Clin. Invest., 71:867–883, 1983.
33. Goldring, R. M., Cannon, P. J., Heinemann, H. O., and Fishman, A. P.: Respiratory adjustment to chronic metabolic alkalosis in man. J. Clin. Invest., 47:188–202, 1968.
34. Van Ypersele de Strihou, C., and Frans, A.: The respiratory response to chronic metabolic alkalosis and acidosis in disease. Clin. Sci., 45:439–448, 1973.
35. Madias, N. E., Bossert, W. H., and Androgué, H. J.: Ventilatory response to chronic metabolic acidosis and alkalosis in the dog. J. Appl. Physiol., 56:1640–1646, 1984.
36. Narins, R. G., Jones, E. R., Stom, M. C., Rudnick, M. R., and Bastl, C.P.: Diagnostic strategies in disorder of fluid, electrolyte and acid-base homeostasis. Am. J. Med., 72:496–520, 1982.
37. Kurtzman, N. A., and Batlle, D. C., (eds.): Symposium on Acid-Base Disorders. Med. Clin. North Am., 67:751–932, 1983.

Chapter

10

Control of Breathing

INTRODUCTION

The demands of the body for uptake of O_2 and elimination of CO_2 vary considerably in normal persons during their usual daily life; O_2 consumption may increase more than tenfold, from a "basal" level during sleep to a maximal level during strenuous exercise. Remarkably, over this entire range arterial blood Po_2 remains constant within narrow limits. This constancy is made possible by a series of control mechanisms that regulate ventilation in accordance with metabolic demands and roughly in proportion to the associated increases in cardiac output.

Respiration is also governed, as discussed in Chapter 9, by alterations in the concentration of nonvolatile acids in the blood; the changes in ventilation that occur under these conditions serve to restore arterial blood pH toward a more normal value and are a principal means by which the body compensates for metabolic acid-base imbalances. Reflex hyperventilation occurs in normal persons upon ascent to high altitudes and in patients with various pulmonary diseases. Variations in the rate and depth of breathing that are not directly attributable to changes in the composition of arterial blood or to reflexes originating within the lungs are encountered in patients with a variety of common clinical disorders, such

233

as fever, metabolic diseases, and psychiatric disturbances. Besides the changes in the pattern of ventilation that occur in response to clinical or environmental abnormalities, specially coordinated respiratory movements are required for talking, singing, sniffing, coughing, hiccuping, sneezing, vomiting, and breath holding.

The multiple and diverse influences that affect breathing and gas exchange are mediated by an intricate control system that incorporates peripheral and central receptors and a complex network of nerve pathways and integrating "centers" in the brain and spinal cord. The purpose of this chapter is to examine the structure, function, and organization of the various components of the system that controls respiration in healthy humans. In addition, the mechanisms by which breathing is regulated during common physiologic stresses are also considered.

ORGANIZATION

The general pattern of organization of the neurologic respiratory control system is shown schematically in Figure 10–1. Basically, the system contains three principal interconnected components: a *controller,* which is located within the central nervous system and which initiates signals of its own in addition to integrating information from the sensing units; a group of *effectors* in the lungs, airways, and muscles of respiration that carry out commands from the controller; and different central and peripheral *sensors,* which monitor the adequacy of breathing with respect to the particular task being carried out.

The concepts that underlie the control of breathing have been developed and refined for nearly a century. Modern experimental investigations using sophisticated techniques of recording respiratory neuron ac-

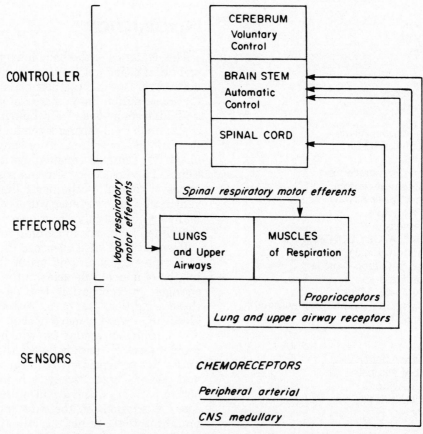

Figure 10–1. Schematic representation of the respiratory control system. The interrelationships among the central nervous system controller, effectors, and sensors, and also the connections among these components are shown. (From Berger, A. J., et al.: Regulation of respiration. By permission from New Eng. J. Med. *297*:92–97, 138–143, 194–201, 1977.)

tivity in conjunction with computerized analysis of the signals have completely changed the old belief that there are various localized centers that govern rhythmic respiration and the pattern of breathing.[1] This neurophysiologic information has been extended and amplified by the application of a variety of newly developed anatomic and histochemical methods. These studies have been particularly useful in identifying the pathways that various neurons use to transfer information from one location to another. In addition, microstimulation experiments have served to localize axonal projections of bulbospinal respiratory neurons and to permit analysis of conduction velocities in these neuronal pathways. Although much has been learned from these approaches, many questions remain unanswered because important basic information is still missing. This section provides an overview of the neuroanatomy and neurophysiology that underlie the control of breathing. Additional details are available in several excellent reviews.[2-5]

CONTROLLERS

Control of respiration by the central nervous system is functionally and anatomically partitioned: the brainstem regulates automatic respiration, whereas the cerebral cortex affects voluntary breathing. Integrating neurons in the spinal cord process efferent information from both upper and lower respiratory centers in the brain with afferent information from peripheral proprioceptors and send the final signals to the muscles of respiration. Efferent autonomic impulses also travel in the vagus nerves from the central nervous system to the airways and lung parenchyma.

Medulla

The medulla appears to be the main headquarters for spontaneous respiration in all mammals studied to date, including humans. This statement is based on two observations. (1) Rhythmic respiration continues, although the pattern of breathing is likely to change, following transection of the brain at the pontomedullary junction; this indicates that higher centers are not necessary to maintain automatic ventilatory efforts.

Moreover, transection below the medulla eliminates breathing movements. (2) Most of the neurons that demonstrate respiratory periodicity are located in the medulla.[6]

Until recently, the basic *respiratory rhythm generator* was believed to reside within inspiratory and expiratory medullary centers that were self-excitatory and mutually inhibitory. New experimental data do not support this concept, although there are still uncertainties concerning details of the origin of ventilatory oscillations.[7] The presently known medullary respiratory groups, their relationships to other neural structures, and their presumed interconnections are shown schematically in Figure 10–2. As illustrated, there are two bilateral aggregations of respiratory neurons. The *dorsal respiratory group* (DRG), situated in the ventrolateral portion of the nucleus of the tractus solitarius, consists chiefly of inspiratory neurons. The *ventral respiratory group* (VRG), located with the nucleus ambiguus and nucleus retroambiguus, contains both inspiratory and expiratory neurons.[8]

Ordinary breathing requires the orderly recruitment of *motoneurons* of the phrenic and intercostal nerves;[9] furthermore, as breathing requirements change (e.g., during progressive exercise), muscles besides the diaphragm and intercostals begin to contribute, and their motoneurons must be recruited. It seems clear that these motoneuron pools are controlled by medullary respiratory neurons located in the DRG and VRG and that axons from these sites project into the spinal cord via bulbospinal pathways. Beyond these simple statements, knowledge concerning the functions of the DRG and VRG is incomplete. Their most likely roles can be summarized as follows. The location of the DRG within the tractus solitarius, which is the recipient of incoming visceral afferent information from the ninth and tenth cranial nerves, suggests that the DRG serves to process afferent signals into a respiratory motor response. The primary site of automatic respiratory oscillations is in or extremely close to the DRG. Axons from the DRG project to inspiratory spinal motoneurons, principally the phrenic motoneurons. Neurons of the DRG project to the VRG and affect its function but not vice versa. Axons from the VRG, which is driven by the DRG, project either to certain spinal respiratory motoneurons (chiefly intercostal and abdominal) or to the accessory muscles

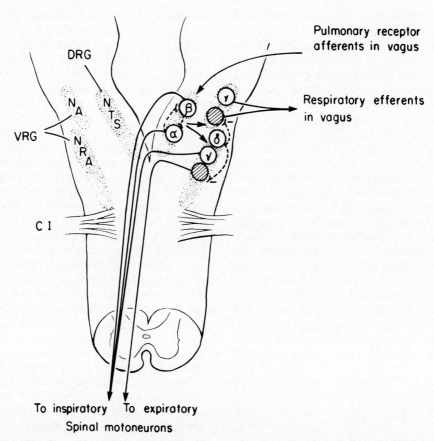

Figure 10–2. Schematic representation of the medullary respiratory neuronal groups, cell types, and suggested interconnections. The dorsal respiratory group (DRG), located in the ventrolateral nucleus of the tractus solitarius (NTS), is the site at which vagal sensory information is first incorporated into a respiratory motor response. The DRG drives the ventral respiratory group (VRG) and some spinal inspiratory motoneurons. The VRG is composed of the nucleus ambiguus (NA) and nucleus retroambiguus (NRA). Vagal respiratory motoneurons arise from NA. Axons from NRA project to some spinal inspiratory and probably all spinal expiratory motoneurons. Inspiratory cells are indicated by open circles and expiratory cells are indicated by hatched circles. Dashed lines indicate some of the proposed intramedullary neural interconnections. CI = first cervical dorsal root; α, β, γ, δ subscripts = inspiratory cell subtype designations. (From Berger, A. J., et al.: Regulation of respiration. By permission from New Eng. J. Med. 297:92–97, 138–143, 194–201, 1977.)

of respiration innervated by the vagus (e.g., sternocleidomastoid).

Pons

Neurons with respiratory activity have been identified in the pons as well as in the medulla. Pontine respiratory neurons exhibit both inspiratory and expiratory (phase-spanning) activity, and it is speculated that they may serve to smooth the transition from one phase of respiration to the next.

The pons also contains two important reg-ulatory centers: the *apneustic center* and the *pneumotaxic center*. These aggregates of neurons, presumably located in the lower and upper pons, respectively, act on medullary centers and thus modulate respiratory activity. There are rich bilateral neural connections between the pontine nuclei and both the DRG and VRG.[9] The pneumotaxic center is believed to act as a fine tuner of the pattern of breathing by influencing the response to afferent stimuli generated during hypoxia, hypercapnia, and lung inflation. The apneustic center appears to contain the normal inspiratory inhibitory mechanism. When this cutoff switch is faulty, apneusis, or sustained inspiration, results from unrestrained activity of the medullary inspiratory neurons.

Figure 10–3 shows schematically the effect on the pattern of breathing of transection at various levels of the brainstem, before and after vagotomy.[2] Transection at the junction between the pons and midbrain (level I in Fig. 10–3) does not affect normal breathing if the vagi are intact. Bilateral vagotomy plus transection at level I causes deepening and slowing of breathing, which is the usual response to vagotomy in most mammals except humans. Midpontine transection (level II), which isolates the pneumotaxic center from the lower brainstem, causes slow, deep, and regular breathing when the vagi are intact. Bilateral vagotomy in this preparation is followed by an immediate striking change in respiratory pattern to apneustic breathing (characterized by rhythmic respiration with prolonged inspiration) or to apneusis. Transection at the pontomedullary junction (level III) causes a regular type of gasping breathing that in most instances is not affected by vagotomy. Cessation of respiration follows transection at the medullospinal junction (level IV), regardless of whether or not the vagi are intact.

Higher Centers

Voluntary, or behavior-related, control of breathing resides in the cerebral cortex, although the exact sites of activity are not completely known. Stimulation of some parts of the cortex inhibits respiratory movements, whereas stimulation of other parts increases respiratory frequency. The pathways that conduct signals from the cerebral cortex to the origin of respiratory muscle motoneurons in the spinal cord are dis-

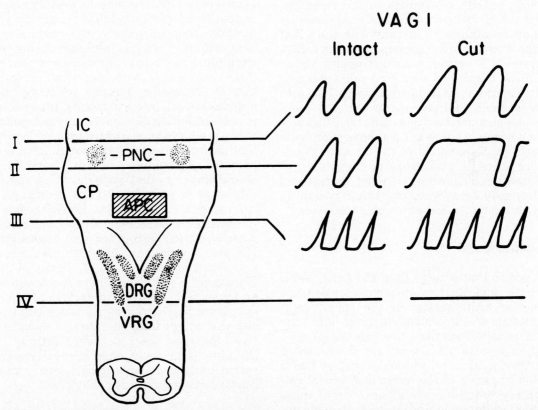

Figure 10–3. Effects of various brainstem and vagal transections on the ventilatory pattern of the anesthetized animal. On the left is a schematic representation of the dorsal surface of the lower brainstem, and on the right, a representation of tidal volume with inspiration upwards. APC = apneustic center; CP = cerebral peduncle; DRG = dorsal respiratory group; IC = inferior colliculus; PNC = pneumotaxic center; and VRG = ventral respiratory group. (From Berger, A. J., et al.: Regulation of respiration. By permission from New Eng. J. Med. *297*:92–97, 138–143, 194–201, 1977.)

tinct from those tracts concerned with automatic respiration, as dicussed subsequently (see Spinal Cord).

The importance of the voluntary control system should not be underestimated. Frequent behavior-related activities involving breathing, such as talking, crying, swallowing, and laughing, cause marked changes in ventilation that may override completely the automatic control, which responds chiefly to chemical stimuli and to changes in lung inflation. For example, during phonation, sensitivity to CO_2 decreases dramatically, and the subject tolerates considerably higher arterial P_{CO_2} values than when quiet.

Another behavior-related drive to breathing is created by the state of wakefulness, which, in turn, is a reflection of respiratory excitation by the *reticular-activating system*. These neurons are located in the reticular formation, which extends in the medial portion of the brainstem from the upper cervical cord into the diencephalon. Respiration-related activity of neurons in the reticular-activating system is markedly inhibited by light anesthesia, in keeping with the belief that these neurons contribute to the differences in breathing that distinguish wakefulness from sleep (discussed subsequently).

Respiratory-modulated activity has also been recorded from neurons in the diencephalon and mesencephalon.[10] Because section of the brain at the pontomesencephalic junction does not alter the breathing pattern, these higher neurons cannot be involved in respiratory rhythm generation; they may function to coordinate breathing with locomotor and autonomic responses.[8]

Spinal Cord

Axons that emerge from the DRG, VRG, cortex, and other supraspinal sites descend in the white matter of the spinal cord, through which central impulses influence the motoneurons that innervate the muscles of respiration. As already mentioned, there is good evidence that the descending tracts that originate in the cortex and control voluntary breathing are separate from those that originate in the brainstem and subserve involuntary breathing.[11] In support of these experimental observations, patients with neurologic deficits have been described in whom there is preservation of involuntary rhythmic control but loss of voluntary control of breathing[12] or vice versa.[13]

In addition to the separation of descending cortical and brainstem tracts, it is possible by careful sectioning in the medulla or spinal cord to selectively interrupt descending inspiratory or expiratory axons (see Berger and coworkers[2] for review and additional references). It has also been shown that the descending pathways for such nonrhythmic reflexes as cough and hiccup that involve respiratory muscles are distinct from those influencing rhythmic breathing.[14]

The abundant neural traffic in the descending tracts is integrated with local reflex information at the level of the spinal cord from which the segmental motoneurons that innervate respiratory muscles emerge. The integrative processes at the segmental level are complex and probably differ in various respiratory muscles (see section on Muscle Receptors).

There are also differences among various respiratory muscle groups in the mechanisms of agonist-antagonist activation. Electrophysiologic studies of intercostal nerves have revealed that inspiratory alpha motoneuron activity is inhibited during expiration and, conversely, that expiratory motoneuron activity is inhibited during inspiration. The obvious physiologic benefit of these responses is to prevent reflex contraction of antagonist muscles when agonist muscles are actively contracting. Intercostal muscle inhibition does not occur via a spinal reflex mechanism, as it presumably does in limb skeletal muscles, but through the influence of descending central respiratory neural impulses that act by exciting spinal inhibitory interneurons.[2] Thus, central control rather than local reflex activity ensures uncontested contraction of the intercostal muscles during inspiration and expiration. However, the manner in which diaphragm antagonist muscles influence activity of the diaphragm is unknown. There appears to be an unusual distribution of segmental afferent nerves from diaphragm antagonist muscles that might influence phrenic motoneurons. Moreover, because motor activity in the phrenic nerve extends into early expiration, continued diaphragmatic contraction counteracts and retards exhalation.

EFFECTORS

The main effectors of breathing are obviously the muscles of respiration. Because the anatomy and function of the respiratory muscles have been discussed in Chapter 5, only certain additional aspects will be considered here. Besides the nervous control of the classic respiratory muscles, other central neural mechanisms regulate both the participation in breathing of skeletal muscles in the upper airways and the responses of smooth muscle and mucous glands within the tracheobronchial system.

Lungs and Upper Airways

During normal awake breathing, resistance to airflow through the upper airways decreases slightly during inspiration and increases slightly during expiration. Because of these counteracting mechanisms, overall resistance remains nearly constant. During sleep, in contrast, mean overall upper airway resistance increases because, compared with the awake pattern of breathing, inspiratory resistance does not decrease as much, whereas expiratory resistance increases more (see subsequent section on Sleep). These observations can be explained by the influence of central neural control mechanisms on the state of contraction of skeletal muscles in the upper airways, including those supporting the tongue and larynx.

In healthy subjects, a tonic level of electromyographic activity is detectable in the genioglossus muscle that increases phasically during inspiration;[15] the genioglossus is an important muscle because it protrudes the tongue and opens the upper airway. Similarly, in careful studies of upper airway muscles of lightly anesthetized rabbits, inspiration-related electromyographic activity was recorded from nearly all the upper airway muscles including the glossal, suprahyoid, infrahyoid, and pharyngeal muscles;[16] the only exceptions were the inferior pharyngeal constrictors, which demonstrated expiration-related activity, and the stylohyoid and digastric muscles, which had no demonstrable activity. Thus the phenomenon of contraction during inspiration appears to involve most upper airway muscles. Widening the oropharynx and larynx makes good sense during inspiration because it serves to decrease resistance to airflow and the work of breathing. But it is not so clear why upper airway resistance increases during expiration. Neurally mediated narrowing of the upper airway slows expiratory airflow and contributes, along with antagonistic contraction of the diaphragm, to the

fact that exhalation through the intact larynx is slower than when the larynx is bypassed experimentally and the lungs empty passively.[17] Additional laboratory studies have shown that expiratory "braking" is a reproducible phenomenon under a variety of conditions.[18] These results suggest that the brain monitors expiratory airflow and makes necessary corrections to maintain a "desired" rate of emptying, even though the physiologic utility of the process is uncertain.

In addition to the central nervous system output just described that innervates skeletal muscles of the upper airway, preganglionic efferent fibers travel in the vagus nerves from the medulla to aggregates of small ganglia situated in and around extrapulmonary and intrapulmonary airways.[19] Postganglionic fibers travel to smooth muscle and glands located in bronchi. Bronchioles do not contain glands, and the bronchiolar smooth muscle in humans, in contrast with that in dogs, does not appear to be innervated.[20] When stimulated, vagal efferent fibers cause smooth muscle contraction and release into the lumen of glandular contents, which may or may not be accompanied by cough. As described in Chapter 3, this response is part of an important protective reflex designed to keep the lungs and air passages free of noxious substances, but it is not part of normal respiration. Recently, however, it has been possible to demonstrate phasic activity of tracheobronchial smooth muscle during quiet breathing manifested by inspiratory contraction and expiratory relaxation.[21] Thus, both skeletal and smooth muscle components of the effector system shown in Figure 10–1 are continuously modulated by neural output from the controller, such that the muscles contract (predominantly) during inspiration. Remarkably, however, the effects on airway resistance are opposite: contraction of upper airway skeletal muscles opens the oropharynx and larynx and decreases resistance to airflow, whereas contraction of tracheobronchial smooth muscle narrows airways and increases resistance.

Muscles of Respiration

The actual amount of ventilation at any time depends on the needs of the moment as determined by voluntary and involuntary centers in the controller. The integrated output from supraspinal and spinal pathways is transmitted to the muscles of respiration through the alpha motoneurons that innervate the contractile fibers of a particular muscle. Peripheral nerves also contain gamma motoneurons that innervate the muscle fibers within muscle spindles, which are part of the system of sensors (see section on Muscle Receptors).

The strength of contraction depends not only on the intensity of the stimulus reaching the muscle but on many intrinsic properties of the muscle itself (e.g., initial fiber length, presence of fatigue, etc.), as discussed in Chapter 5. Under ordinary conditions of progressive exercise, there is a coordinated strengthening of contraction of muscle fibers within a particular muscle and recruitment of additional muscle groups in response to needs for increased O_2 uptake and CO_2 elimination by the lungs. The factors that control breathing during exercise are reviewed in Chapter 11. Ventilatory responses to other normal and abnormal physiologic stresses are discussed at the end of this chapter. But it must always be remembered that a neurally mediated change in breathing requires a signal of central origin that reaches respiratory muscles capable of responding to that command. Abnormalities either of the muscles themselves or of the respiratory system (i.e., the lungs and chest wall) may have a considerable effect on the final response. This subject is dealt with further in the section on Tests of Respiratory Control.

SENSORS

In a system that must be as responsive as breathing to varying needs for ventilation it is obviously desirable to have suitable sensors to initiate changes and to monitor whether or not the correction is appropriate. Accordingly, the respiratory system is equipped with four sets of well-characterized sensors, each of which will be described. In addition, because the symptom of breathlessness conveys information about the state of breathing, this poorly understood sensation will also be briefly discussed.

Peripheral Chemoreceptors

Immediate hyperventilation is one of the principal compensatory responses to sudden hypoxemia. This reaction, which appears in all mammalian species, depends on specialized chemoreceptors that monitor the chemical composition of arterial blood. In 1930, Heymans and coworkers[22] discovered the chemoreceptor activities of the *carotid bodies*, and in 1939, Comroe[23] established that the *aortic bodies* also function as chemoreceptors.

The carotid bodies are nestled in the bifurcation of the common carotid arteries. They are extremely well vascularized, and their blood flow is high relative to their size; in addition, they have one of the highest metabolic rates of any organ of the body. The carotid bodies contain two main cell types—type I cells (also called glomus cells, chief cells, and enclosed cells) and type II cells (also called supporting cells, sheath cells, enclosing cells, and sustentacular cells)—that are interspersed among numerous axons and their terminals and abundant blood vessels (Fig. 10–4). There has been a controversy about the innervation of the carotid body and how nerve stimuli affect the function of the oxygen. Recent information about the ultrastructure and neurophysiologic responses of the carotid body suggests that virtually all the nerve endings in contact with glomus cells are axons of afferent sensory nerves that travel in a branch of the carotid sinus nerve and reach the brain in the glossopharyngeal (ninth cranial) nerve (Fig. 10–5).[24] The few terminals on glomus cells that appear to be efferent (5 per cent of the total) are from sympathetic fibers that reach the carotid body from the superior cervical ganglion. Other sympathetic nerves from the same source innervate blood vessels within the carotid body. The only efferent nerves that travel with the afferent axons in the sinus nerve are preganglionic parasympathetic fibers that innervate blood vessels.

The structure and function of aortic chemoreceptors vary in different species. In cats a few discrete organs that resemble tiny carotid bodies have been identified, and in dogs aggregates of glomus cells in varying numbers and distributions near the aorta have been reported (Fig. 10–6).[25] Remarkably little is known about the location of aortic bodies in humans. Because of the observation that the ventilatory response to hypoxia in humans is abolished by carotid body resection or denervation, it has been concluded that the chemoreceptor activity of aortic bodies is slight or nil;[26] hence in-

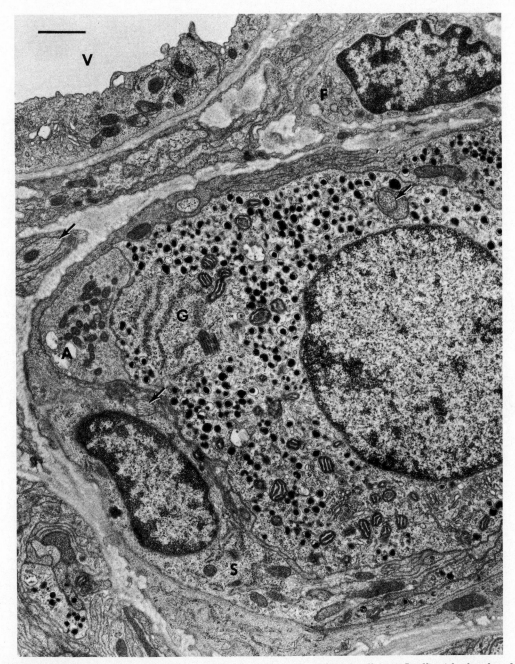

Figure 10–4. Electron micrograph of the carotid body of a cat. G = glomus cell (type I cell) with abundant large dense-cored vesicles; S = sheath cell (type II cell); A = afferent nerve ending with numerous synaptic vesicles; V = blood vessel; F = fibroblast (probable); and arrows = axons. Horizontal bar = 1 μm. (× 12,800. Courtesy of Dr. Donald McDonald.)

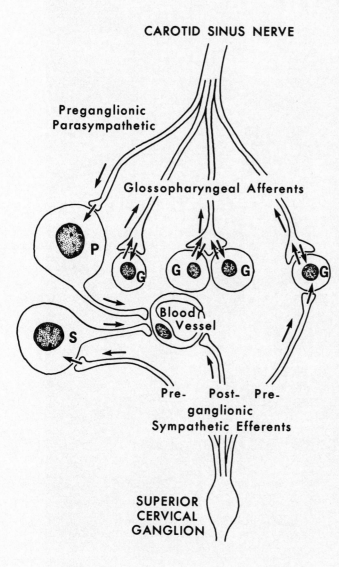

CAROTID SINUS NERVE

Preganglionic
Parasympathetic

Glossopharyngeal Afferents

P

G G G G G G

Blood
Vessel

S

Pre- Post- Pre-
ganglionic
Sympathetic Efferents

SUPERIOR
CERVICAL
GANGLION

Figure 10–5. Schematic representation of the innervation of the carotid body. Afferent fibers of the glossopharyngeal (IX) nerve form reciprocal synapses with glomus cells (G); blood vessels are innervated by postganglionic fibers of parasympathetic (P) and sympathetic (S) origin; occasional preganglionic sympathetic fibers synapse with glomus cells. Arrows indicate the direction of impulses. (Adapted from information supplied by Dr. Donald McDonald.)

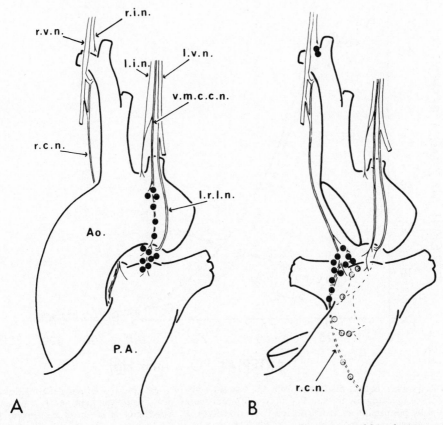

A   B

Figure 10–6. Location of 34 aortic bodies identified in 23 dogs by microdissection and histologic examination. *A*, Bodies innervated by the left vagus; *B*, bodies innervated by the right vagus. Ao = aorta; P.A. = pulmonary artery; r.v.n., l.v.n. = right and left vagus nerves; r.i.n., l.i.n. = right and left innominate nerves; l.r.l.n. = left recurrent laryngeal nerve; r.c.n. = recurrent cardiac nerve; v.m.c.c.n. = ventromedial cervical cardiac nerve. (Reprinted from Coleridge, H. M. et al.: Thoracic chemoreceptors in the dog. A histological and electrophysiological study of the location, innervation and blood supply of the aortic bodies. Circ. Res., *26*:235–247, 1970 by permission of The American Heart Association, Inc.)

terest in these structures is correspondingly minimal. Afferent nerve impulses from aortic chemoreceptors travel to the brain in the vagus nerves.

Response to Stimulation. Chemoreceptor activity from the carotid bodies is increased by decreased arterial Po_2, increased arterial Pco_2, or decreased arterial pH. The aortic body chemoreceptors in many mammals other than humans behave somewhat differently: activity increases in response to decreased Po_2 and increased Pco_2 but no change or depression accompanies decreased pH. The circulatory responses actuated by the two sets of peripheral chemoreceptors differ considerably. Stimulation of the carotid body causes bradycardia and hypotension, whereas stimulation of the aortic bodies provokes tachycardia and hypertension.[27]

The peripheral chemoreceptors are tonically active in normal persons breathing ambient air at sea level, and this activity can be suppressed by breathing high concentrations of O_2. Although the effect of hyperoxia on ventilation is small and difficult to demonstrate, the response to hypoxia is usually considerable and readily demonstrable. These differences are shown in Figure 10–7, which is a plot of the relationship between carotid chemoreceptor nerve activity and arterial Po_2.[28] As Po_2 decreases below 500 mm Hg, there is only a slight increase in impulse activity; in contrast, as Po_2 goes below 100 mm Hg, the increase is striking. Below 30 mm Hg, the initial marked increase in impulse activity is not sustained, and it gradually declines. Whereas the chemoreceptor response to changing arterial Po_2 is remarkably alinear, the response to

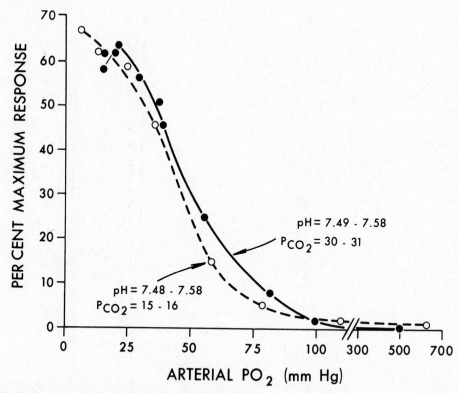

Figure 10–7. Average neural discharge from the carotid body of a cat, plotted as per cent maximum activity, showing response to changing arterial P_{O_2} at two different values of P_{CO_2}; pH was kept nearly constant. (Adapted and reprinted by permission from Hornbein, T. F., and Roos, A.: Specificity of H ion concentration as a carotid chemoreceptor stimulus. J. Appl. Physiol., *18*:580–584, 1963.)

changing P_{CO_2} from 20 to 60 mm Hg and pH from 7.20 to 7.60 is nearly linear. When two stimuli affect the peripheral chemoreceptors simultaneously, the effects are synergistic; in other words, the resulting increase in nerve activity is greater than the sum of the two separate responses. Besides responding to changes in P_{O_2}, P_{CO_2}, and pH, chemoreceptor activity is provoked by decreases in blood flow, such as may occur when systemic blood pressure falls or when sympathetic activity causes vasoconstriction of vessels in the carotid bodies.

Studies in humans have revealed that the carotid bodies are entirely responsible for hypoxic ventilatory drive, account for about 30 per cent of the response to breathing increased CO_2, and produce all the ventilatory compensation for the acute metabolic acidosis of exercise.[29] Breath-holding time is prolonged after bilateral carotid body resection, especially during hypoxia.

Mechanisms for Chemoreception. The mechanisms by which chemical stimuli change the frequency of neural impulses in the efferent nerves from the peripheral chemoreceptors are speculative. An interesting model based on the presence of high- and low-affinity cytochrome a_3 has been proposed.[30] Similarly, the actual chemosensitive elements within the carotid bodies are not known. Originally, it was believed that the glomus cells were the actual sensors, but recent evidence argues against this. Today's prevailing theory suggests that the *afferent nerve terminals* within the carotid body are the receptors, a notion based in part on the observation that neuromas that form on the cut end of the carotid sinus nerve are chemosensitive in the absence of carotid body tissue.[31] In addition, the afferent nerve fibers have been shown to form reciprocal synapses with the glomus cells. Because glomus cells exhibit vivid fluorescence, they are believed to contain catecholamines, especially dopamine, which may serve as the neurotransmitter. Collectively, these findings led McDonald[32] to suggest that the glomus cell is a dopaminergic inhibitory interneuron that modulates the generation of impulses in the afferent nerve terminal. According to this theory, chemical stimulation of the sensory nerve endings in the carotid bodies generates impulses directed toward the brainstem and also provokes secretion of a neurotransmitter that causes release of dopamine from glomus cells. Dopamine, in turn, modulates chemoreceptor sensitivity by acting on receptors mediating excitation and inhibition of the sensory nerves. It is also possible that regulatory processes originating in the brainstem rather than the carotid body could affect peripheral chemoreceptor sensitivity.

Central Chemoreceptors

Total denervation of the peripheral chemoreceptors abolishes the hyperpnea of acutely induced hypoxia but does not eliminate, although it reduces slightly, the ventilatory responses to increases in arterial P_{CO_2}. This demonstration of the existence of respiratory chemoreceptors that are anatomically distinct from the carotid and aortic bodies initiated a number of ingenious experiments that have established the location of chemosensitive regions within the central nervous system and the way in which these neurons respond to certain chemical changes in their environment.

The location and behavior of central chemoreceptors were clarified considerably by the important contributions of Leusen.[33, 34] He showed that changes in the composition of artificial cerebrospinal fluid (CSF) used experimentally to perfuse the brain from the third or lateral cerebral ventricles to the cisterna magna (ventriculocisternal perfusion) had a marked influence on ventilation: increasing [H$^+$] stimulated ventilation, whereas lowering [H$^+$] depressed it. These results have been confirmed and extended by many investigators and form the basis of the belief that the chemosensitive elements of the central nervous system are within "reach" of the CSF.

The results of a variety of neurophysiologic studies have demonstrated three bilateral areas in the medulla that are involved in central chemosensitivity. The best established of these is the chemosensitive region located by Mitchell[35] on the ventrolateral medullary surface lateral to the pyramids and medial to the roots of the seventh through tenth cranial nerves. Another chemosensitive area is caudal to the first one, lateral to the pyramids, but medial to the root of the twelfth nerve. A third region, which is not itself chemosensitive, is located between the other two. The importance of this third area can be demonstrated by the nearly complete loss of CO_2-induced ventilatory responses when it is electrocoagulated; this observation has led to the conclusion that afferent fibers from the two chemosensitive regions enter the middle region, from which neurons then project to the respiratory integrating sites elsewhere in the medulla. It should be emphasized that a large amount of evidence has been accumulated in recent years to suggest that central chemosensitivity does not arise from brainstem respiratory neurons in the DRG and VRG but originates instead from distinct aggregates of medullary chemoreceptor cells.[2] However, histologic identification of these cells has proved elusive, and there is no information whatsoever about their final neuronal projections.

Response to Stimulation. Experiments carried out in the 1920's revealed that intravenous administration of HCl caused hyperpnea, and although blood pH decreased, CSF pH increased. Similarly, administration of NaHCO$_3$ caused an increase in arterial pH but a decrease in CSF pH.[36] The changes in CSF and arterial pH in *opposite* directions during infusion of nonvolatile acids or bases differed strikingly from the demonstration that pH values in both CSF and blood change in the *same* direction when P_{CO_2} is altered. These observations indicate that the ventilatory responses in patients with acute metabolic acidosis or alkalosis are not mediated by central chemoreceptors, because changes in CSF pH are in the wrong direction and therefore must be attributed to chemosensitive mechanisms located elsewhere, presumably in the carotid bodies.

These paradoxic phenomena were explained by the earlier experiments of Jacobs[37, 38] on the relative diffusibilities of CO_2, H$^+$, and HCO_3^- across biologic membranes. It is known that CO_2 diffuses readily across cell membranes and, consequently, a change in P_{CO_2} promptly affects intracellular pH. In contrast, because H$^+$ and HCO_3^- diffuse poorly, adding them to the bloodstream has only a small immediate effect on intracellular pH. The rapid diffusion of CO_2 and the slow diffusion of H$^+$ and HCO_3^- were believed to account for the different acute ventilatory stimuli that reach central chemoreceptors in patients with respiratory and metabolic acid-base disorders. More recent data, however, suggest that this may not necessarily be the case. When pH in intracerebral interstitial fluid—the medium that actually bathes the chemosensitive cells—and cisternal CSF was measured while blood pH was changed by infusions of HCl or $NaHCO_3$, acute changes in blood pH were reflected by changes in interstitial fluid pH within 30 minutes, whereas cisternal CSF pH was unchanged.[39] Similar findings have been reported by others, but the results are not entirely consistent (for references, see review by Nattie[40]). These observations certainly raise the possibility that fairly rapid (10 to 40 minutes) changes in cerebral interstitial fluid pH may occur when blood pH is altered and thus that central chemoreceptors may contribute more to the ventilatory responses to metabolic acid-base disturbances than previously suspected (see section on Integrated Responses). The results of measurements of tissue pH and brain surface pH reinforce the concept that some sort of regulation occurs at the *blood-brain barrier* because the changes in the brain are less than those in blood. Furthermore, the constancy of CSF pH while intracerebral interstitial fluid pH is changing emphasizes that these two fluid compartments are not in equilibrium during acute acid-base changes.

It should also be pointed out that the transient ventilatory response to a step change in alveolar CO_2 concentration in humans has a time constant of as high as 89 seconds.[41] This means that the central chemoreceptors reach equilibration with arterial blood much more slowly than the peripheral chemoreceptors, which equilibrate virtually instantaneously. These observations underscore the differences in the time course of the responses, depending on whether the stimulus is P_{CO_2} or $[H^+]$, between the peripheral chemoreceptors on the one hand and the central chemosensitive cells on the other.

Cerebrospinal Fluid. The data summarized in the preceding discussion support the concept that the central chemoreceptors are responsive to $[H^+]$ in the surrounding cerebral (medullary) interstitial fluid. Furthermore, during a steady state, in contrast to acutely changing conditions, cerebral interstitial fluid $[H^+]$ is supposedly in equilibrium with CSF $[H^+]$.[40] This provides the rationale for sampling and analyzing CSF

to find out what is "going on" centrally. It is essential, therefore, to have some understanding of CSF formation, its chemical composition, and the effects of various systemic disturbances of CSF pH. For details, the reader is referred to reviews by Leusen[42] and Nattie.[40]

It has been generally agreed that CSF is formed mainly in the choroid plexus of the lateral cerebral ventricles; however, recent attention has been directed toward another important cerebral source, probably the capillary endothelial cells.[43] The fluid produced by the choroid plexus flows through the ventricles and aqueduct into the subarachnoid spaces surrounding the brain and spinal cord. The CSF is absorbed into the bloodstream through arachnoid villi that protrude into cerebral venous sinuses.

The composition of newly formed choroidal CSF is determined solely by choroid plexus ion transport processes. In contrast, the composition of cerebral interstitial fluid is more complex, being determined by exchange across the blood-brain barrier, by exchange across the brain cells, and by exchange with CSF itself. Thus, the relationship between brain interstitial fluid and CSF is complicated and not well understood. But it is easy to infer that changes in the composition of one fluid compartment could affect the composition of the other, and this must be kept in mind when using CSF as a mirror of interstitial fluid.

The composition of CSF has been thoroughly studied in many animals, including humans (Table 10–1). Noteworthy differences from plasma composition include a much lower CSF protein concentration, a higher Cl^- and P_{CO_2}, and a lower pH. The major secretory process includes active movement of Na^+ by means of the enzyme adenosine triphosphatase, with related movements of K^+, Cl^-, and HCO_3^-. The enzyme carbonic anhydrase is also involved because when its action is inhibited, the rate of formation of CSF decreases.

Most previous studies of CSF regulation assumed some sort of dependency on plasma $[H^+]$, $[HCO_3^-]$, or pH. Now the concept is being increasingly accepted that changes in CSF $[H^+]$ and $[HCO_3^-]$ that occur independent of changes in P_{CO_2} must be accompanied—if not caused—by changes in strong ions.[44] The strong ion difference in CSF may be approximated as $[Na^+] - [Cl^-]$. This means that CSF pH may change primarily

Table 10–1. NORMAL VALUES (MEAN ± SD) FOR THE COMPOSITION OF CEREBROSPINAL FLUID (CSF) AND ARTERIAL BLOOD

Substance	CSF	Arterial Blood
Na	141.2 ± 6.0 mEq/L	140.6 ± 7.2 mEq/L
K	2.96 ± 0.45 mEq/L	4.46 ± 0.45 mEq/L
Ca	2.43 ± 0.05 mEq/L	5.23 ± 0.27 mEq/L
Mg	2.40 ± 0.14 mEq/L	1.94 ± 0.15 mEq/L
Cl	127 ± 3 mEq/L	103 ± 3 mEq/L
HCO_3	21.5 ± 1.2 mEq/L	24.8 ± 1.4 mEq/L
Protein	15–45 mg/100 ml	6.6–8.6 gm/100 ml
Glucose	45–70 mg/100 ml	70–105 mg/100 ml
P_{CO_2}	50.2 ± 2.6 mm Hg	39.5 ± 1.2 mm Hg
pH	7.336 ± 0.012	7.409 ± 0.018

because of changes in CSF strong ion composition or that pH variations may be triggered by input of $[H^+]$, $[HCO_3^-]$, or P_{CO_2}.[44] Of the strong ions that might be involved in CSF acid-base regulation, the most important seem to be Cl^-, lactate, hydroxybutyrate, and other inorganic and organic anions with high dissociation constants.[40] Remarkably few experimental studies have been done to analyze CSF strong ion responses to induced acid-base disturbances; such data coupled with measurements of CSF $[H^+]$ and $[HCO_3^-]$ should provide a better understanding than exists at present about CSF acid-base regulation.

Lungs and Upper Airways

The lungs and upper airways are equipped with a multitude of receptors that, when stimulated, have profound effects on breathing as well as on the circulation and other visceral and somatic systems.[45] The three main lower airway and pulmonary receptor networks—the stretch receptors, the irritant receptors, and the C-fibers, including the J-receptors—are fully discussed in Chapter 3. These receptors all have their afferent pathways in the vagus nerve and their central terminals in the tractus solitarius. As stated, because the DRG is located within the tractus solitarius, there is good reason to believe that the DRG processes incoming afferent information into a respiratory motoneuron response.

Other cranial nerves, as well as the vagus, serve as afferent pathways for receptors in the upper airway.[46] When stimulated chemically or mechanically, receptors in the nose send signals by way of the trigeminal and olfactory nerves. Responses to nasal stimulation include sneezing, apnea, and bradycardia. Stimulation of receptors in the epipharynx causes the sniff or aspiration reflex; afferent fibers from these receptors travel in the glossopharyngeal nerve, which also has its central terminals in the tractus solitarius. Finally, there are numerous receptors in the larynx that are functionally similar to irritant receptors in that they respond to mechanical or chemical stimuli, but the reflex effects are variable. Among the possible responses are coughing, slow deep breathing, apnea, bronchoconstriction, and hypertension.

Muscle Receptors

There are four main types of muscle receptors: (1) free nerve terminals, (2) encapsulated nerve endings, (3) Golgi tendon organs, and (4) muscle spindles. Whether or not the first two types are present in respiratory muscles is not well established, and their role, if any, in the control of breathing is unknown. This discussion, therefore, will concentrate on tendon organs and muscle spindles, which are better characterized, although information about them is incomplete.

In comparison with other skeletal muscles, including the intercostals, the diaphragm is poorly supplied with both Golgi tendon organs and muscle spindles; there appear to be more of the former than the latter. In contrast, the intercostal muscles are relatively well supplied with both tendon organs and spindles, and the spindles predominate. There is, however, a greater density of spindles in inspiratory than in expiratory intercostal muscles, and the number in both groups is greater in muscles in the upper (cephalad) compared with the lower portion of the chest wall. Information from these sensors is mainly integrated at the spinal segmental level and may contribute to agonist-antagonist muscle behavior;[47] however, as already discussed, direct supraspinal control seems to dominate this relationship.

It is also evident that some afferent impulses travel to the brain in ascending spinal tracts. But the influence of these signals on the control of breathing is far from clear. It appears that the contribution of inspiratory afferent information from the diaphragm, and possibly from the intercostals as well, to tidal volume regulation is negligible.[48] It is also possible that supraspinal projections of muscle sensors play a more important role in regulation of posture than of respiration. Muscle sensors have also been linked to the pathogenesis of dyspnea by Campbell,[49] but much needs to be done to support this theory.

Breathlessness

The symptom of breathlessness means different things to different people, and there is no universally accepted definition.[50] *Dyspnea,* which to many is synonymous with breathlessness, implies not only the concept of awareness of breathing but that the sensation is unpleasant. Breathlessness develops when healthy persons undertake progressively increasing exercise, and it finally causes them to stop or slow down.[51] The same or a similar disagreeable sensation occurs in patients with a variety of underlying diseases at a less than normal level of activity, and under these circumstances is pathologic. Like other sensations, such as pain, breathlessness is difficult to quantify, and its perception and description will vary from person to person and from situation to situation. Dyspnea is also like pain in that some sort of receptor system is presumably involved. There is no doubt that the sensation of breathlessness makes one consciously aware of breathing; accordingly, there must be sensors that monitor the act of ventilation and are able to perceive when the demand to breathe is somehow not satisfied.[51]

But despite a considerable amount of investigation concerning the neural mecha-

nisms that subserve dyspnea, the location, stimuli, and neural pathways of the putative receptor(s) are virtually unknown. Furthermore, the search for a single common physiologic abnormality that is associated with breathlessness in the many conditions in which it occurs has been fruitless. It seems likely that there may be several different neurogenic systems, each with its own receptor, that may lead to dyspnea. Thus, chemoreceptors may react to chemical stimuli, intrapulmonary mechanoreceptors may react to deformation, and receptors in the muscles of breathing may react to stretch. According to the conditions of the moment, each of these receptors could be "set" to respond to stimuli at an increased or decreased intensity. Clearly, much more work needs to be done to disentangle the complexities of breathlessness as it occurs in health and disease.

TESTS OF RESPIRATORY CONTROL

A variety of tests have been developed to evaluate the control of breathing in both normal persons and patients with respiratory disorders. In general, each of these measures one or more variables related to the act of breathing, such as minute volume, frequency, tidal volume, or developed pressure, under resting conditions and in response to a stimulus to augment ventilation. Given the complexity of the control system, it is often difficult to sort out the precise role of each of the component parts. However, the two old and three relatively new tests of breathing, which will be reviewed in this section, have provided important insights into the mechanisms underlying breathing abnormalities in many different diseases. Further information is available in a report of a symposium on clinical methods for the study of the regulation of ventilation.[52]

Response to Hypoxia

When a normal person breathes a low concentration of O_2, the resulting decrease in arterial Po_2 of the blood flowing through the carotid bodies stimulates an increased frequency of impulses in the sinus nerve. After central processing, the signals actuate an effector response consisting of increased ventilation, cardiac output, and blood pressure. By gradually decreasing the concentration of O_2 in the inspired mixture and measuring corresponding changes in ventilation, it is possible to evaluate a subject's response to hypoxia. The relationship between arterial P_{O_2} and ventilation (Fig. 10–8A) is hyperbolic and differs depending on whether arterial P_{CO_2} is allowed to fall, as it normally does when ventilation increases, or is held constant by adding CO_2 to the inspired mixture, as is the case during an *isocapnic hypoxia response test*. Because hyperbolic curves are cumbersome to analyze, the response to hypoxia is now often expressed as the relationship between expired ventilation and arterial O_2 saturation, monitored with an ear oximeter (Fig. 10–8B). Under these circumstances, hypoxic sensitivity is reported as the slope of the line ($\Delta \dot{V}/1\%$ desaturation). Ventilatory responses to isocapnic hypoxia vary widely, with nearly a tenfold variation in $\Delta \dot{V}/1\%$ desaturation having been observed in normal subjects.[53] Hypoxic sensitivity, as discussed in greater detail subsequently, decreases with increasing age and is characteristically depressed or even absent in long-term residents of high altitudes.[54] Furthermore, blunted responses to hypoxia contribute to the pathophysiologic abnormalities of patients with severe chronic bronchitis or massive obesity or after the administration of opiates and other sedative drugs.

Response to Carbon Dioxide

The ideal test of central chemoreceptor sensitivity would measure the changes in ventilation that result from a given change in $[H^+]$ within the chemosensitive cells, but there are many theoretic and practical reasons why such a test cannot be designed. One approach to the problem has been through the use of *carbon dioxide response tests*, which although useful, have certain limitations. (1) The stimulus cannot be quantified precisely because it is impossible

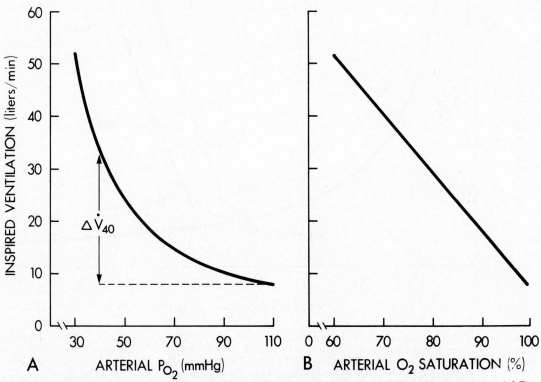

Figure 10–8. Typical hypoxic response curves of a normal person at sea level, at standard constant arterial P_{CO_2}. *A,* The hyperbolic relationship between arterial P_{O_2} and ventilation is shown; also indicated is the hypoxic sensitivity index. ($\Delta \dot{V}40$). *B,* The relationship becomes linear when inspired ventilation is plotted against increasing arterial desaturation. (From Berger, A. J., et al.: Regulation of Respiration. Reprinted by permission from New Eng. J. Med. *297*:92–97, 138–143, 194–201, 1977.)

to measure pH in or even near the central receptors; (2) the peripheral chemoreceptors and other CO_2-sensitive sites as well as the central chemoreceptors are stimulated by the effects on pH of breathing CO_2; (3) there is a wide range of "normality"; and (4) the response is modified, and thus difficult to interpret, by changes in the mechanics of breathing.

Two types of CO_2 response tests are available: the steady-state method, in which the subject breathes air enriched with different concentrations of CO_2, usually 0, 3, 5, and 7 per cent for approximately ten minutes each before measurements are made; and the rebreathing method, in which the subject breathes from a bag prefilled with 7 to 8 per cent CO_2 and excess O_2 (40 to 93 per cent),

while ventilatory volume and end-tidal CO_2 concentration are recorded continuously. The rebreathing method has virtually replaced the steady-state method because it yields similar information and is much easier and faster for the subject to perform.

A plot of the relationships between ventilation and end-tidal P_{CO_2} obtained by the steady-state and rebreathing techniques is shown in Figure 10–9. After a few breaths, the rebreathing curve is parallel to the steady-state curve but displaced about 8 mm Hg to the right. The CO_2 sensitivity is reported as the slope of the curve ($\Delta\dot{V}$/mm Hg). Normal values in healthy adults range from 2 to 5 L/min × mm Hg.

The ventilatory response to CO_2 decreases with age, but not as much as the response

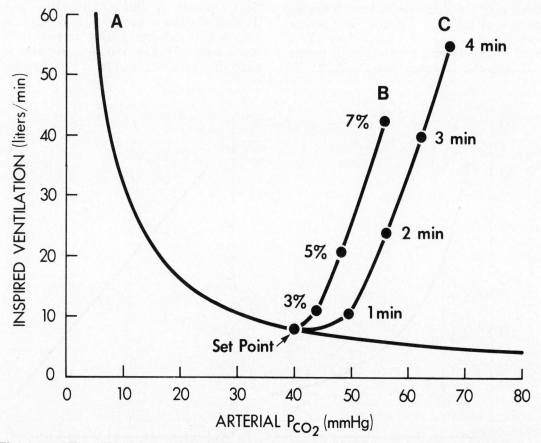

Figure 10–9. Three CO_2 response curves relating inspired ventilation (BTPS) to arterial P_{CO_2} of a normal person at sea level. Curve A approximates the metabolic hyperbola, a reciprocal relation between alveolar P_{CO_2} and alveolar ventilation when inspired gas contains no CO_2. Curve A assumes that dead space is 30 per cent of the total ventilation. Curve B is the steady-state ventilatory response to elevated arterial P_{CO_2} obtained by breathing CO_2 mixtures (e.g., 3 per cent, 5 per cent, and 7 per cent) for at least 10 minutes each. Curve C is the rebreathing CO_2 response, obtained by rebreathing from a bag of 5 to 7 L prefilled with 7 per cent CO_2 in 40 to 93 per cent O_2 for about four minutes. The overall "gain" of the respiratory control system is the ratio of the slope of B to the slope of A at the set point, which is about −10. (From Berger, A. J., et al.: Regulation of Respiration. By permission from New Eng. J. Med. *297*:92–97, 138–143, 194–201, 1977.)

to hypoxia. Sensitivity to CO_2 is also blunted in certain endurance athletes and can be severely depressed by a variety of sedatives, narcotics, and anesthetic agents. Important differences in CO_2 sensitivity can be demonstrated in patients with obstructive pulmonary disease and these can be reproduced in normal persons when they are breathing with added mechanical loads.[55] Thus, it is difficult to interpret the results of CO_2 response tests in patients with mechanical disturbances of their lungs or chest wall.

Occlusion Pressure

The tests of ventilatory responses to hypoxia and CO_2 provide useful information about chemosensitivity, but interpretation is necessarily limited because both tests are influenced by mechanical abnormalities anywhere in the respiratory system. Recently the test of mouth occlusion pressure as a measurement of respiratory center output, the so-called respiratory drive, was described that avoids many of the problems inherent in other methods.[56]

The test is performed by having a subject breathe through a mouthpiece with separate inspiratory and expiratory valves. During expiration at a time unknown to the subject, the operator closes the inspiratory valve so that the subject begins the next breath in the usual way, unaware that the airway has been occluded. Instead of inhaling air, negative pressure is generated in the mouthpiece until the subject notices that the airway is occluded and makes conscious efforts to resist. However, the pressure generated during the initial 0.2 to 0.3 seconds of occlusion represents the force developed by the inspiratory muscles in response to the same total respiratory neural drive as in a normal breath. Because there is no flow of gas and because lung volume scarcely changes during inspiration against an occlusion, the pressure generated is virtually unaffected by the mechanical properties of the respiratory system and by the force-velocity relationships of the muscles. However, because of the effects of variable length-tension relationships of the respiratory muscles, the measurements are influenced by changes in lung volume, and thus serial studies must be made at the same volume, preferably with the subject in the supine position.[57]

Provided certain relatively simple techniques nical considerations are observed, the pressure developed during the first 0.1 second after occlusion, often called the $P_{0.1}$, reflects both the neuronal drive to the muscles of inspiration and the contractile capabilities of these muscles. Additional information can be provided by performing a series of occlusion pressure measurements while CO_2 is added to the inspired gas. From these observations the relationship between changes in $P_{0.1}$ and alveolar (actually end-tidal) P_{CO_2} can be derived $(\Delta P_{0.1}/\Delta PA_{CO_2})$. Although measurement of occlusion pressure is a relatively new test, it appears to be a useful way of assessing respiratory drive and respiratory muscle capabilities.

Breathing Cycle Timing

Beginning with Haldane and Priestly[58] in 1905, most workers used pulmonary ventilation, measured as minute volume, to determine the output of the respiratory centers. Twenty-six years later Barcroft and Margaria[59] tried to emphasize that more complete understanding of the control of breathing was available through knowledge of inspiratory and expiratory timing and of flow rates. This work was largely ignored until the publication by Clark and von Euler[60] reopened interest in the systematic study of the breathing cycle and its accompanying flow rates. Much use is now being made of the following equation to analyze ventilation ($\dot{V}$):

$$\dot{V} = (V_T/T_I) \times (T_I/T_{TOT}), \qquad (1)$$

where V_T is tidal volume, T_I is the duration of inspiration, and T_{TOT} is the duration of inspiration and expiration. Thus, V_T/T_I is mean inspiratory flow, which is a measure of *inspiratory drive,* and T_I/T_{TOT} is the ratio of inspiratory to total cycle duration, or the *duty cycle,* which is a reflection of *respiratory timing.*[61] These are easy measurements to make and useful to have, but it should be noted that mean inspiratory flow rate is influenced by the mechanical properties of the respiratory system. Application of these techniques helped to solve the long-standing mystery concerning why some patients with chronic obstructive pulmonary disease retain CO_2 and others do not. Both groups have equally enhanced drive to breathe but their tidal volumes and inspiratory timing are different.[62]

Electromyography and Electroneurography

The use of electrical signals to represent the output of the respiratory control system is attractive because they are independent of the mechanical properties of the effectors and thus are a big step closer to the "source" than measurements of ventilation. Two general types of recordings are available: electromyograms from one or more of the respiratory muscles, often the diaphragm, and electroneurograms from one of the nerves innervating a respiratory muscle, usually the phrenic.

These methods have their greatest value in detecting *changes* in respiratory center output during a single experiment. Given both technical and inherent physiologic variations, both electromyography and electroneurography have limited value in comparing one person with another or even in differentiating abnormal from normal. Improvements in technology are bound to come that will enable more use to be made of these fundamentally attractive techniques.

INTEGRATED RESPONSES

Breathing is regulated on a moment to moment basis, primarily in response to changing metabolic needs, the most studied of which is exercise (see Chapter 11). Changes in the control of breathing also occur in normal persons during sleep, and when this system is faulty, severe patho-

physiologic disturbances may result. The regulatory systems also adjust breathing to minimize the effects of stresses that threaten the O_2, CO_2, and H^+ composition of blood and tissue, such as breathing air with a low Po_2 and respiratory and metabolic acid-base disturbances. This section will review how breathing is regulated during sleep, at high altitude, and in certain common acid-base abnormalities.

Sleep

Recent investigations of respiratory control during sleep have shown striking differences from the awake state. However, these studies also indicate that the changes observed differ among the various phases of sleep (Table 10–2). Sleep is not a uniform state but a recurring cyclic pattern of sequential stages with a periodicity in adults of approximately 90 minutes. Two distinctive sleep states have been defined in humans and in other animals on the basis of behavioral, electroencephalographic, electromyographic, and electrooculographic criteria: *rapid eye movement* (REM) or active sleep and *nonrapid eye movement* (nonREM) or quiet sleep. NonREM sleep is subdivided into four stages of progressively deepening sleep, of which the deepest two (stages 3 and 4) are often called *slow wave* sleep because of the characteristic electroencephalographic pattern that develops.

During the lighter stages (1 and 2) of nonREM sleep, the pattern of breathing is regular and periodic. Tidal volume and res-

Table 10–2. SUMMARY OF RESPIRATORY CONTROL MECHANISMS WHILE AWAKE AND DURING SLEEP*

| Mechanism | Awake | | Non-REM Sleep | | REM Sleep |
	Inactive	Active	Stages 1 and 2	Stages 3 and 4	
Dominant influence on breathing	Metabolic	Behavior	Metabolic	Metabolic	Nonmetabolic
Pattern of breathing	Regular	Irregular	Periodic	Regular	Irregular
Apnea					
Occurrence	Absent	Absent	Often	Absent	Frequent
Duration	—	—	≤15 sec	—	≤15 sec
Mechanism	—	—	Δ state	—	REM activity
Response to metabolic stimuli	Present	Decreased	Present	Decreased	Further decreased
Chest wall movement	Phasic	Phasic	Phasic	Phasic	Paradoxic

*Data from Philipson, E. A.: Control of breathing during sleep. Am. Rev. Respir. Dis., *118*:909–939, 1978.
Abbreviations: Non-REM = non-rapid-eye-movement; REM = rapid-eye-movement; Inactive = absence of behavioral ventilatory activity; Active = presence of behavioral ventilatory activity; Metabolic = metabolic respiratory control system; Behavioral = behavioral respiratory control system; Δ state = changing state between wakefulness and sleep.

piratory rate vary and there may be brief episodes of apnea (*Cheyne-Stokes* breathing). The changes in breathing pattern correspond to fluctuations between wakefulness and sleep. The extent of periodic breathing varies in normal subjects but increases in persons older than 40 years and is almost invariable at high altitudes. Breathing becomes regular during slow wave sleep, but because the component of ventilatory drive related to behavioral activities, including the state of wakefulness from reticular-activating system stimuli, is withdrawn, minute volume is usually somewhat less than while quietly awake. Accordingly, arterial P_{CO_2} increases 4.1 to 6.5 mm Hg, P_{O_2} decreases 3.5 to 9.4 mm Hg, and pH decreases 0.03 to 0.05 units.[65]

Breathing during REM sleep is characteristically irregular and not periodic, with brief periods of apnea up to 15 and sometimes 20 seconds or even longer in normal adults and children and 10 seconds in infants. Irregular breathing often coincides with bursts of REM and other muscle activity. At other times, chest wall motion is paradoxic and there are marked fluctuations in the smooth muscle tone of airways. In view of the characteristic irregularity of breathing during REM sleep, it is difficult to obtain steady-state measurements. On average (i.e., when the variations are smoothed out), both ventilation and arterial blood gas values are about the same during REM sleep as during slow wave sleep.[66]

The ventilatory response to CO_2 is decreased during slow wave sleep compared with that during wakefulness and further decreased during REM sleep.[67] Although the results are not always consistent,[68] similar progressive decreases from wakefulness to slow wave sleep to REM sleep in the ventilatory response to hypoxia have been reported.[69] Of note is the observation that *arousal* from sleep is preserved during hypercapnia but markedly impaired during hypoxia.[68]

The responses during the various phases of sleep to stimulation of intrapulmonary receptors (i.e., stretch receptors, irritant receptors, and C-fibers) in humans have not been fully worked out. In general, it appears that reflex stimulation of breathing is diminished during sleep and that the effects are more marked on the muscles that control upper airway patency than on the inspiratory activity of the diaphragm. This imbalance coupled with the gravitational effects of the supine posture usually adopted for sleep tends to promote upper airway obstruction, a phenomenon of great importance in the pathogenesis of the *sleep apnea syndrome*.[66]

Hypoxia

The effects on ventilation of breathing a hypoxic gas mixture have been divided into three phases depending on the duration of exposure: acute hypoxia (up to 1 hr), short-term hypoxia (1 hr to days), and long-term hypoxia (years to generations).[70] Each phase will be briefly reviewed.

Acute Hypoxia. The usual response to acutely induced hypoxia has already been described. As inspired P_{O_2} is gradually reduced from its normal sea level value, little increase in ventilation occurs until arterial P_{O_2} decreases below 100 mm Hg, and the increase usually does not begin until the value is below 60 mm Hg; thereafter worsening hypoxemia to an arterial P_{O_2} of about 30 mm Hg evokes a progressively greater and greater increase in ventilation. Below 30 mm Hg, the ventilatory response diminishes. It is generally agreed that the stimulus to increase breathing during acute hypoxia in humans is mediated chiefly by the carotid chemoreceptors. Local production of lactic acid or suprapontine influences may augment the effects of carotid body stimulation. Among the consequences of acute hypoxia-induced hyperventilation are a decrease in P_{CO_2} and an increase in pH in arterial blood and CSF, both of which serve to inhibit ventilation. These inhibitory influences may explain why the ventilatory response to acute hypoxia is not as brisk as the response to short-term hypoxia several hours or a few days later.

Short-Term Hypoxia. The immediate ventilatory response to acute hypoxia is followed by a subsequent gradual increase in ventilation that is reflected in arterial blood by an increase in P_{O_2} and further decrease in P_{CO_2}. The differences between the acute and short-term responses to hypoxia can be easily demonstrated by administering high concentrations of O_2, thus removing the hypoxic stimulus, during the two conditions. In acute hypoxia breathing is restored to normal, but after short-term acclimatization is complete, only a slight decrease in ventilation occurs. This means that breathing has been "reset" at a new level that tends to be maintained even when the original stimulus is withdrawn.

It was originally postulated that the increase in breathing during short-term hypoxia was caused by a return of blood and CSF [H+] to normal values by compensatory adjustments in [HCO$_3$-], which removed the inhibitory effects of acutely induced alkalinization in the two compartments. However, the results of the rigorous experiments of Dempsey and coworkers[71] showed that the increases in ventilation during short-term acclimatization bore no consistent relationship to changes in blood or CSF [H+]. It is now believed that the changes in blood and CSF PO$_2$, PCO$_2$, and pH are the result, and not the cause, of the increase in ventilation. Moreover, the mechanisms that underlie the breathing responses during short-term adaptation to hypoxia are unknown.

Long-Term Hypoxia. People who have lived for many years at high altitudes, the so-called highlanders, exhibit certain ventilatory characteristics that differ from newly acclimatized sojourners to the same altitudes. When the groups are compared, many highlanders can be shown to have lost their ventilatory response to acutely induced hypoxia and, in addition, they ventilate less at rest, during exercise, and when breathing CO$_2$. Long-term ventilatory insensitivity to hypoxia is clearly an acquired and not a genetic trait, because babies born at high altitudes have normal responses to induced hypoxia during infancy but lose them during childhood.[72] Although children who move to high altitudes may become insensitive to hypoxia more quickly than adults, studies of adults after arrival at high altitudes show a steady decrease of hypoxic

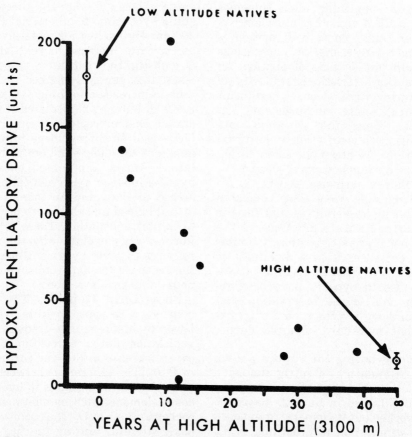

Figure 10–10. Effect of time spent at high altitude (3100m) on hypoxic ventilatory drive. The data suggest that loss of hypoxic ventilatory responsiveness is a function of time spent at high altitude. After 25 years, hypoxic ventilatory drive is usually depressed to values found in high-altitude natives. (From Weil, J. V., et al.: Acquired attenuation of chemoreceptor function in chronically hypoxic man at high altitude. J. Clin. Invest., 50:186–195, 1971. Copyright permission from The American Society for Clinical Investigation.)

responsiveness that is more marked during the first ten years than thereafter, but the change continues for up to 30 years (Fig. 10–10).[54]

The mechanisms by which the ventilatory responses to hypoxia are attenuated in highlanders are unknown. There is indirect evidence that chemoreceptor function may be faulty, but other evidence suggests that abnormal suprapontine modulation may be responsible (for review and additional references, see Dempsey and Forster[70]).

Respiratory Acidosis

The renal response to acute and chronic respiratory acidosis, produced either by increased endogenous CO_2 loads (i.e., respiratory failure) or by exogenous CO_2 loads (i.e., breathing a gas mixture enriched with CO_2), has been reasonably well worked out (see Chapter 9). In both types of respiratory acidosis HCO_3^- is generated, some acutely and some through the delayed conservation of HCO_3^- by the kidneys, and blood pH returns toward normal. But ventilatory control obviously differs depending on the source of the CO_2. When arterial PCO_2 increases in the presence of an endogenous CO_2 load, regardless of whether or not CO_2 production is increased, alveolar ventilation is insufficient to eliminate that quantity of CO_2 and, by definition, *respiratory failure* results (see Equation 2, Chapter 8); this, in turn, implies that an abnormality exists with one or more components of the respiratory control system: sensors, controllers, or effectors. In contrast, when CO_2 is administered to healthy humans or to experimental animals, a brisk ventilatory response occurs that indicates how the normal respiratory control operates under the stress of that particular stimulus. When patients with lung disease breathe added CO_2, the overall ventilatory response is often abnormal. Such information, however, does not indicate the location of the defects of respiratory control caused by different diseases.

The results of studies of chronic CO_2 exposure reveal an acute increase in ventilation that appears to be sustained or even to increase as exposure continues (for review and additional references, see Dempsey and Forster[70]). Blood pH decreases acutely and then gradually increases during the next few days as renal compensation occurs. Ar-

terial PCO_2 remains elevated throughout but is higher during chronic exposures than during acute exposures. The changes in human CSF $[H^+]$ and $[HCO_3^-]$ are not as well defined as those in the blood and, as discussed (see section on Cerebrospinal Fluid), there is considerable uncertainty as to whether the changes in CSF pH actually reflect the $[H^+]$ stimulus in the interstitial fluid surrounding the central chemosensitive cells. The CSF pH during chronic exposure to CO_2 becomes normal, or it may remain slightly on the acid side of control values. The change toward or to normal of CSF pH is related to an increase in CSF $[HCO_3^-]$, which has a different time course than the accompanying increase in plasma $[HCO_3^-]$ (Fig. 10–11).[73]

Because both blood and CSF $[H^+]$ decrease and may even normalize during the first few days of CO_2 exposure—at a time when the hyperpnea is sustained or increasing—it is evident that neither peripheral nor central chemoreceptors can account for the chronic ventilatory response to CO_2 exposure. It is not at all clear, however, what other mechanisms supervene and perpetuate the hyperpnea. The system that causes the response is durable because after the chronic CO_2 stimulus is removed, hyperpnea may continue for as long as two weeks.

Respiratory Alkalosis

Respiratory alkalosis typically occurs in healthy persons living at high altitudes and in women during pregnancy, and it is a relatively common finding in patients with certain kinds of lung disease (e.g., pulmonary vascular diseases and interstitial infiltrative diseases). The *sine qua non* of respiratory alkalosis is a lower than normal value of arterial PCO_2. Blood pH will vary, depending on whether the process is acute (alkalemia) or chronic (normal).

Control of breathing in respiratory alkalosis is complex, but the presence of hyperventilation obviously represents net dominance of the composite stimuli to increase breathing (e.g., hypoxia, progesterone, reflexes of intrapulmonary origin) over those that act to decrease breathing (e.g., decreased blood and CSF PCO_2 and $[H^+]$). During chronic respiratory alkalosis induced by exposure to simulated high altitude, CSF pH remained on the alkaline side of nor-

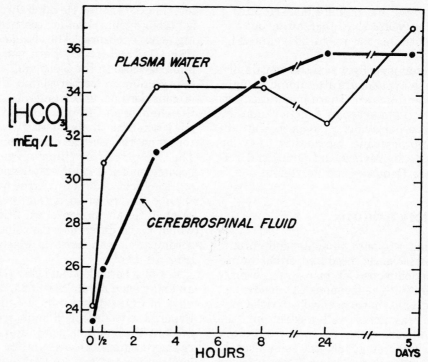

Figure 10–11. Time course of the changes in the concentration of bicarbonate in cerebrospinal fluid and in plasma water before (zero time) and during exposure to 12 per cent CO_2. (From Bleich, H. L. et al.: The response of cerebrospinal fluid composition to sustained hypercapnia. J. Clin. Invest., 43:1–16, 1964. By copyright permission of the American Society for Clinical Investigation.)

mal.[74] The decrease in CSF [HCO_3^-] that occurs in compensated respiratory alkalosis is presumably attributable to changes in CSF chloride and lactate concentrations, but the relative importance of each is not known and probably varies, depending on the type, duration, and severity of the underlying abnormality.[40] Once the changes have occurred, as with respiratory acidosis, ventilation gets "set" at a new level that tends to be sustained, even when the original stimulus is eliminated.

Metabolic Acidosis

As pointed out (see Chapter 9), the extent of respiratory compensation for metabolic acidosis and alkalosis has been carefully documented by van Ypersele de Strihou and Frans.[75] In stable metabolic acidosis they reported striking interindividual consistency in the arterial P_{CO_2} response to variations in [HCO_3^-], which averaged 1.2 (range 0.9 to 1.5) mm Hg decrease in P_{CO_2} for each 1 mEq/L decrease in [HCO_3^-]. There seems to be a clear time-dependent ventila-

tory response to prolonged administration of a given metabolic acid load: about one-half of the chronic ventilatory response occurs acutely and the remainder chronically (up to two to three days). A similar time course of gradually decreasing ventilation has been observed in humans whose metabolic acidosis has been rapidly corrected.

The receptors that mediate hyperventilation in metabolic acidosis are not known with certainty. Some believe that both the peripheral and central chemoreceptors are stimulated by changes in [H^+] of blood and CSF,[76] whereas others propose that only the [H^+] in the interstitial fluid environment of the medullary chemosensitive cells is important.[77] Nearly all studies of CSF pH in acute metabolic acidosis have revealed paradoxical alkalosis related to a decrease in P_{CO_2}. The situation in chronic acidosis, however, is controversial: some authors report normal values for CSF pH; others find values on the acid side of normal.[71] The limitations of using CSF pH as an index of medullary interstitial fluid pH as well as the different time courses of pH changes in these two compartments in induced metabolic acid-base disturbances have already been emphasized. Moreover, it is difficult to evaluate to what extent the choroid plexus and the blood-brain barrier contribute to the regulation of CSF and interstitial fluid pH in metabolic acidosis.[40]

Metabolic Alkalosis

Van Ypersele de Strihou and Frans[75] also studied respiratory regulation in stable metabolic alkalosis. They reported an interindividual variation of 0.9 (range 0.8 to 1.2) mm Hg increase in PCO_2 for each 1 mEq/L increase in [HCO_3^-]. The consistency of results is in part explained by the fact that most patients had chronic renal failure, and it was possible to adjust their plasma [HCO_3^-] values by varying the concentrations of chloride and acetate in the dialysate. Others have shown that the ventilatory response to induced metabolic alkalosis is quite variable, depending on whether or not potassium is lost in the process.[78] When potassium depletion accompanies metabolic

alkalosis (e.g., following administration of aldosterone or thiazide diuretics), no ventilatory compensation occurs. In contrast, when metabolic alkalosis is induced by a method that conserves potassium (e.g., following administration of buffers), a predictable decrease in ventilation and an increase in arterial PCO_2 result.

The ventilatory responses of dogs to chronic metabolic acidosis and chronic metabolic alkalosis of graded severity and of various causes were considerably clarified by the recent report of Madias and coworkers.[79] These investigators found that the magnitude of the ventilatory response was remarkably uniform throughout a wide range of chronic metabolic acid-base disturbances ([HCO_3^-] from 14.3 to 35.6 mEq/L) and, in contrast with the findings in humans noted above, did not depend on how the disorder was induced. On average, arterial PCO_2 changed 0.74 mm Hg for a 1 mEq/L chronic change in [HCO_3^-].

The effects of chronic metabolic alkalosis on CSF pH in humans, like the effects in chronic metabolic acidosis, are inconsis-

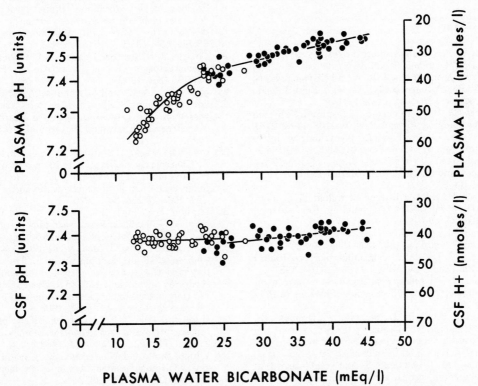

Figure 10–12. Cerebrospinal fluid (CSF) and plasma pH and H⁺ activity in metabolic acidosis (○) and alkalosis (●) and their relation to plasma bicarbonate in dogs. (Replotted and reprinted by permission from Chazan, J. A. et al.: Effects of chronic metabolic acid-base disturbances on the composition of cerebrospinal fluid in the dog. Clin. Sci., *36*:345–358, 1969.)

tent.[71] The results of experiments in dogs in which particular care was taken to ensure that a steady state was present are shown in Figure 10–12. Values of CSF pH were unchanged from normal during chronic metabolic acidosis but rose slightly during chronic alkalosis.[80] Changes of this magnitude could easily be overlooked in studies of patients, given the inherent difficulties of establishing steady-state clinical conditions and of measuring pH in poorly buffered CSF.

Summary

Some progress has been made during the last decade in unravelling the complex mechanisms that regulate ventilation in sleep, at high altitude, and during acid-base disturbances. The ventilatory responses to acute perturbations are reasonably well understood, but how ventilation is sustained at a given level during chronic exposure or persistent stimulation is still uncertain. Clearly, much more needs to be learned about the control of breathing in health and disease.

REFERENCES

1. Pitts, R. F.: Organization of the respiratory center. Physiol. Rev., 26:609–630, 1946.
2. Berger, A. J., Mitchell, R. A., and Severinghaus, J. W.: Regulation of respiration. New Engl. J. Med., 297:92–97, 138–143, 194–201, 1977.
3. Cohen, M. I.: Neurogenesis of respiratory rhythm in the mammal. Physiol. Rev., 59:1105–1173, 1979.
4. Kalia, M.: Central respiratory rhythmicity. Introductory remarks. Fed. Proc., 40:2363–2394, 1981.
5. Hornbein, T. F. (ed.): Regulation of Breathing. Parts I and II. New York, Marcel Dekker, 1981, pp. 1–1436.
6. Batsel, H. L.: Localization of bulbar respiratory center by microelectrode sounding. Exp. Neurol., 9:410–426, 1964.
7. Merrill, E. G.: Where are the real respiratory neurons? Fed. Proc., 40:2389–2394, 1981.
8. Cohen, M. I.: Central determinants of respiratory rhythm. Annu. Rev. Physiol., 43:91–104, 1981.
9. Kalia, M. P.: Anatomical organization of central respiratory neurons. Annu. Rev. Physiol., 43:105–120, 1981.
10. Vibert, J. F., Caille, D., Bertrand, F., Gromysz, H., and Hugelin, A.: Ascending projection from the respiratory centre to mesencephalon and diencephalon. Neurosci. Lett., 11:29–33, 1979.
11. Aminoff, M. J., and Sears, T. A.: Spinal integration of segmental, cortical and breathing inputs to thoracic respiratory motoneurones. J. Physiol. (Lond.), 215:557–575, 1971.
12. Newsom Davis, J.: Control of the muscles of breathing. In Widdicombe, J. G. (ed.): Respiratory Phys-

iology: MTP International Review of Science. Ser. 1, Vol. 2. London, Butterworth, 1974, pp. 221–246.
13. Severinghaus, J. W., and Mitchell, R. A.: Ondine's curse—failure of respiratory center automaticity while awake. Clin. Res., 10:122, 1962.
14. Newsom Davis, J., and Plum, F.: Separation of descending pathways to respiratory motoneurons. Exp. Neurol., 34:78–94, 1972.
15. Sauerland, E. K., and Harper, R. M.: The human tongue during sleep: electromyographic activity of the genioglossus muscle. Exp. Neurol., 51:160–170, 1976.
16. Orem, J., Norris, P., and Lydic, R.: Laryngeal abductor activity during sleep. Chest, 73(2 Suppl):300–301, 1978.
17. Rothstein, R. J., Narce, S. L., deBerry-Borowiecki, B., and Blanks, R. H. I.: Respiratory-related activity of upper airway muscles in anesthetized rabbit. J. Appl. Physiol., 55:1830–1836, 1983.
18. Bartlett, D., Jr., and Remmers, J. E.: Reflex control of expiratory airflow and duration. J. Physiol. (Lond.), 247:22P–23P, 1975.
19. Richardson, J. B.: Nerve supply to the lungs. Am. Rev. Respir. Dis., 119:785–802, 1979.
20. Doidge, J. M., and Satchell, D. G.: Adrenergic and non-adrenergic inhibitory nerves in mammalian airways. J. Auton. Nerv. Syst., 5:83–99, 1982.
21. Mitchell, R. A., Herbert, D. A., and Baker, D. G.: Inspiratory rhythm in airway smooth muscle tone. J. Appl. Physiol., 58:911–920, 1985.
22. Heymans, C., Bouckaert, J. J., and Dautrebande, L.: Sinus carotidien et réflexes respiratoires. II. Influences respiratoires réflexes de l'acidose, de l'alcalose, de l'anhydride carbonique, de l'ion hydrogène et de l'anoxémie. Sinus carotidien et échanges respiratoires dans les poumons et au dela des poumons. Arch. Int. Pharmacodyn. Ther., 39:400–450, 1930.
23. Comroe, J. H., Jr.: The location and function of the chemoreceptors of the aorta. Am. J. Physiol., 127:176–191, 1939.
24. McDonald, D. M., and Mitchell, R. A.: The innervation of glomus cells, ganglion cells, and blood vessels in the rat carotid body: a quantitative ultrastructural analysis. J. Neurocytol., 4:177–230, 1975.
25. Coleridge, H. M., Coleridge, J. C. G., and Howe, A.: Thoracic chemoreceptors in the dog. A histological and electrophysiological study of the location, innervation and blood supply of the aortic bodies. Circ. Res., 26:235–247, 1970.
26. Lugiani, R., Whipp, B. J., Seard, C., and Wasserman, K.: Effect of bilateral carotid-body resection on ventilatory control at rest and during exercise in man. New Engl. J. Med., 285:1105–1114, 1971.
27. Comroe, J. H., Jr., and Mortimer, L.: The respiratory and cardiovascular responses of temporally separated aortic and carotid bodies to cyanide, nicotine, phenyldiguanide and serotonin. J. Pharmacol. Exp. Ther., 146:33–41, 1964.
28. Hornbein, T. F., and Roos, A.: Specificity of H ion concentration as a carotid chemoreceptor stimulus. J. Appl. Physiol., 18:580–584, 1963.
29. Whipp, B. J., and Wasserman, K.: Carotid bodies and ventilatory control dynamics in man. Fed. Proc., 39:2668–2673, 1980.
30. Mills, E., and Jobsis, F. F.: Mitochondrial respiratory chain of carotid body and chemoreceptor response to changes in oxygen tension. J. Neurophysiol., 35:405–428, 1972.

31. Mitchell, R. A., Sinha, A. K., and McDonald, D. M.: Chemoreceptive properties of regenerated endings of the carotid sinus nerve. Brain Res., 43:681–685, 1972.
32. McDonald, D. M.: Regulation of chemoreceptor sensitivity in the carotid body: the role of presynaptic sensory nerves. Fed. Proc., 39:2627–2635, 1980.
33. Leusen, I. R.: Chemosensitivity of the respiratory center. Influence of CO_2 in the cerebral ventricles on respiration. Am. J. Physiol., 176:39–44, 1954.
34. Leusen, I. R.: Chemosensitivity of the respiratory center. Influence of changes in the H^+ and total buffer concentrations in the cerebral ventricles on respiration. Am. J. Physiol., 176:45–51, 1954.
35. Mitchell, R. A., Loeschcke, H. H., Massion, W. H., and Severinghaus, J. W.: Respiratory responses mediated through superficial chemosensitive areas on the medulla. J. Appl. Physiol., 18:523–533, 1963.
36. Gesell, R., and Hertzman, A. B.: The regulation of respiration. IV. Tissue acidity, blood acidity and pulmonary ventilation; effects of semipermeability of membranes and the buffering action of tissues with the continuous method of recording changes in acidity. Am. J. Physiol., 78:610–629, 1926.
37. Jacobs, M. H.: To what extent are the physiological effects of carbon dioxide due to hydrogen ions? Am. J. Physiol., 51:321–331, 1920.
38. Jacobs, M. H.: The production of intracellular acidity by neutral and alkaline solutions containing carbon dioxide. Am. J. Physiol., 53:457–463, 1920.
39. Davies, D. G., and Nolan, W. F.: Cerebral interstitial fluid acid-base status follows arterial acid-base perturbation. J. Appl. Physiol., 53:1551–1555, 1982.
40. Nattie, E. E.: Ionic mechanisms of cerebrospinal fluid acid-base regulation. J. Appl. Physiol., 54:3–12, 1983.
41. Gelfond, R., and Lambertsen, C. J.: Dynamic respiratory response to abrupt change of inspired CO_2 and normal and high Po_2. J. Appl. Physiol., 35:903–913, 1973.
42. Leusen, I.: Regulation of cerebrospinal fluid composition with reference to breathing. Physiol. Rev., 52:1–56, 1972.
43. Eisenberg, H. M., Suddith, R. L., and Crawford, J. S.: Transport of sodium and potassium across the blood-brain barrier. In Eisenberg, H. M., and Suddith, R. L. (eds.): The Cerebral Microvasculature. New York, Plenum, 1980, pp. 57–67.
44. Stewart, P. A.: How to Understand Acid-Base. A Quantitative Acid-Base Primer for Biology and Medicine. New York, Elsevier, 1981.
45. Pack, A. I.: Sensory inputs to the medulla. Am. Rev. Physiol., 43:73–90, 1981.
46. Richardson, P. S., and Peatfield, A. C.: Reflexes concerned in the defense of the lungs. Bull. Europ. Physiopathol. Respir., 17:979–1012, 1981.
47. Newsom Davis, J.: Spinal control. In Campbell, E. J. M., Agostoni, E., and Newsom Davis, J. (eds.): The Respiratory Muscles: Mechanics and Neural Control. London, Lloyd-Luke, 1970, pp. 205–233.
48. Duron, B.: Intercostal and diaphragmatic muscle endings and afferents. In Hornbein, T. F. (ed.): Regulation of Breathing. Part I. New York, Marcel Dekker, 1981, pp. 473–540.
49. Campbell, E. J. M.: The relation of the sensation of breathlessness to the act of breathing. In Howell, J. B. L., and Campbell, E. J. M. (eds.): Breathlessness. Oxford, Blackwell Sci. Pub., 1966, pp. 55–65.
50. Workshop report: Exercise testing in the dyspneic patient. Am. Rev. Respir. Dis., 129(Suppl): S1–S100, 1984.
51. Wasserman, K.: Physiology of gas exchange and exertional dyspnea. Clin. Sci., 61:7–13, 1981.
52. Lourenco, R. V. (ed.): Clinical methods for the study of the regulation of breathing. Chest, 70(Suppl): 109–195, 1976.
53. Rebuck, A. J., and Woodley, W. E.: Ventilatory effects of hypoxia and their dependence on Pco_2. J. Appl. Physiol., 38:16–19, 1975.
54. Weil, J. V., Byrne-Quinn, E., Sodal, I. E., Filley, G. R., and Grover, R. F.: Acquired attenuation of chemoreceptor function in chronically hypoxic man at high altitude. J. Clin. Invest., 50:186–195, 1971.
55. Eldridge, F., and Davis, J. M.: Effect of mechanical factors on respiratory work and ventilatory responses to CO_2. J. Appl. Physiol., 14:721–726, 1959.
56. Whitelaw, W. A., Derenne, J. P., and Milic-Emili, J.: Occlusion pressure as a measure of respiratory center output in conscious man. Respir. Physiol., 23:181–199, 1975.
57. Milic-Emili, J., Whitelaw, W. A., and Derenne, J. P.: Occlusion pressure—a simple measure of the respiratory center's output. New Engl. J. Med., 293:1029–1030, 1975.
58. Haldane, J. S., and Priestley, J. G.: The regulation of the lung—ventilation. J. Physiol. (Lond.), 32:225–266, 1905.
59. Barcroft, J., and Margaria, R.: Some effects of carbonic acid on the character of human respiration. J. Physiol. (Lond.), 72:175–185, 1931.
60. Clark, F. J., and von Euler, C.: On the regulation of depth and rate of breathing. J. Physiol. (Lond.), 222:267–295, 1972.
61. Milic-Emili, J., and Grunstein, M. M.: Drive and timing components of ventilation. Chest, 70(Suppl): 131–133, 1976.
62. Sorli, J., Grassino, A., Loranze, G., and Milic-Emili, J.: Control of breathing in patients with chronic obstructive lung disease. Clin. Sci. Mol. Med., 54:295–304, 1978.
63. Sharp, J. T., Druz, W., Damon, J., and Kim, M. J.: Respiratory muscle function and the use of respiratory electromyography in the evaluation of respiratory regulation. Chest, 70(Suppl):150–154, 1976.
64. Eldridge, F. L.: Quantification of electrical activity in the phrenic nerve in the study of ventilatory control. Chest, 70(Suppl):154–157, 1976.
65. Philipson, E. A.: Control of breathing during sleep. Am. Rev. Respir. Dis., 118:909–939, 1978.
66. Cherniack, N. S.: Sleep apnea and its causes. J. Clin. Invest., 78:1501–1506, 1984.
67. Philipson, E. A.: Respiratory adaptations in sleep. Am. Rev. Physiol., 40:133–156, 1978.
68. Hedemark, L. L., and Kronenberg, R. S.: Ventilatory and heart rate responses to hypoxia and hypercapnia during sleep in adults. J. Appl. Physiol., 53:307–312, 1982.
69. Douglas, N. J., White, D. P., Weil, J. V., and Zwillich, C. W.: Hypoxia ventilatory response decreases during sleep in normal man. Am. Rev. Respir. Dis., 125:286–289, 1982.
70. Dempsey, J. A., and Forster, H. V.: Mediation of ventilatory adaptations. Physiol. Rev., 62:262–346, 1982.

71. Dempsey, J. A., Forster, H. V., and DoPico, G. A.: Ventilatory acclimatization to moderate hypoxemia in man. J. Clin. Invest., *53*:1091–1100, 1974.
72. Lahiri, S., Brody, J. S., Motoyama, E. K., and Velasquez, T. M.: Regulation of breathing in newborns at high altitude. J. Appl. Physiol., *44*:673–678, 1978.
73. Bleich, H. L., Berkman, P. M., and Schwartz, W. B.: The response of cerebrospinal fluid composition to sustained hypercapnia. J. Clin. Invest., *43*:11–16, 1964.
74. Fencl, V., Gabel, R. A., and Wolfe, D.: Composition of cerebral fluids in goats adapted to high altitude. J. Appl. Physiol., *47*:508–513, 1979.
75. Van Ypersele de Strihou, C., and Frans, A.: The respiratory response to chronic metabolic alkalosis and acidosis in disease. Clin. Sci., *45*:439–448, 1973.
76. Mitchell, R. A., and Singer, M. M.: Respiration and cerebrospinal fluid in metabolic acidosis and alkalosis. J. Appl. Physiol., *20*:905–911, 1965.
77. Fencl, V., Vale, J. R., and Broch, J. A.: Respiration and cerebral blood flow in metabolic acidosis and alkalosis in humans. J. Appl. Physiol., *27*:67–76, 1969.
78. Goldring, R. M., Cannon, P. J., Heinemann, H. O., and Fishman, A. P.: Respiratory adjustment to chronic metabolic alkalosis in man. J. Clin. Invest., *47*:188–202, 1968.
79. Madias, N. E., Bossert, W. H., and Androgué, H. J.: Ventilatory response to chronic metabolic acidosis and alkalosis in the dog. J. Appl. Physiol., *56*:1640–1646, 1984.
80. Chazan, J. A., Appleton, F. M., London, A. M., and Schwartz, W. B.: Effects of chronic metabolic acid-base disturbances on the composition of cerebrospinal fluid in the dog. Clin. Sci., *36*:345–358, 1969.

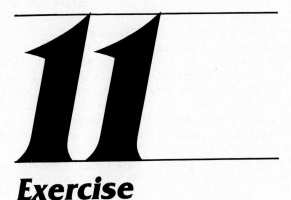

Chapter

Exercise

INTRODUCTION

Movement from one place to another (locomotion) is a characteristic of all members of the animal kingdom. In higher animals the ability to obtain food and to avoid predators, which usually requires rapid motion, is essential for survival. Although human beings are undoubtedly more sedentary now than in the past, ordinary daily life consists of a variety of activities that involve muscular effort. This type of physical exercise requires a complex physiologic interplay between the respiratory and circulatory systems that enables them to meet the increased gas exchange requirements of contracting muscles. A variety of other mechanisms mobilize energy substrates to provide the fuel that sustains metabolic needs.

This chapter will briefly review the biochemical events that underlie muscle contraction and that, in turn, create a need for more O_2 and for elimination of newly produced CO_2. The discussion will mainly focus on how these demands, which can be viewed as a local problem in gas transport, are solved by interacting physiologic mechanisms. As has been the policy elsewhere in this book, the technical details of laboratory evaluation, in this case of exercise testing, will not be considered. Excellent reviews of this clinically important subject are available.[1, 2]

261

ENERGETICS

Exercise, whether for health purposes or not, can be differentiated clearly from the resting state by the simple fact that during exercise various skeletal muscles are actively contracting under the influence of neurogenic stimuli. In complete rest, on the other hand, with the exception of those muscles engaged in quiet breathing, skeletal muscles are relaxed.[3] Even in the resting state, skeletal muscles, which constitute approximately 40 per cent of body weight in normal humans, account for 35 to 40 per cent of the "basal" O_2 consumption.[4] Although appreciable, this value may increase to 95 per cent or more of a considerably augmented O_2 consumption during strenuous exercise.

The chemical energy that enables the contractile elements within muscle cells to shorten and to perform work comes from ingested food substrates, chiefly carbohydrates and fatty acids; these provide the fuel for the formation of high-energy adenosine triphosphate (ATP). The concentration of ATP in resting muscle cells is relatively low to begin with and decreases slightly during exercise. The amount of ATP initially present is only sufficient to sustain the energy requirements of contraction for less than one second and thus must be quickly and steadily replenished.[1] At the onset of exercise, initial energy needs are met by the regeneration of ATP from intracellular stores of creatine phosphate. But as exercise continues and increases in intensity, the concentration of creatine phosphate decreases; thereafter, the maintenance of intramuscular ATP supplies depends on the catabolism of available fuel substrates, which occurs in a triphasic sequence: first muscle glycogen, then blood glucose, and finally free fatty acids.[4]

The generation of ATP takes place predominantly in the mitochondria of muscle cells and chiefly by the energy-yielding electron transport chain, which requires O_2 as the terminal oxidant. This *aerobic* reaction is characterized by the consumption of O_2 and the production of CO_2 in a fractional quantity that varies from 0.7 (fatty acids) to 1.0 (carbohydrates), depending on the substrates utilized. Because there is very little O_2 available in the interior of cells, a new supply of O_2 must be continuously delivered to the mitochondrial transport chain for oxidation. Similarly, the H^+ derived from the production of CO_2 and the formation of H_2CO_3 must be removed from the cells to permit metabolism to continue.

Three general physiologic adjustments provide the necessary O_2 to support aerobic metabolism and to eliminate the excess CO_2 produced in the process of muscle contraction: (1) increased ventilation, (2) increased cardiac output, and (3) redistribution of blood flow to the working muscles. The linkages among these essential elements of gas transport are shown in Figure 11–1.

When O_2 supplies are inadequate or when other essential metabolic requirements are

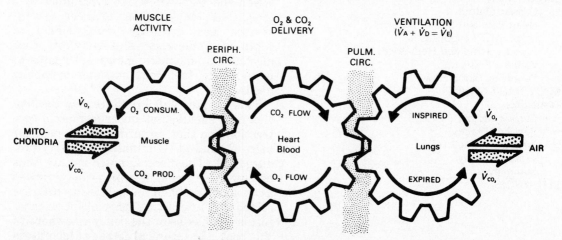

Figure 11–1. Schematic diagram of interaction among physiologic mechanisms during exercise. Gears represent the coupling between each of the gas transport mechanisms between the ambient air and the mitochondria within the muscle cells. CONSUM. = consumption; PROD. = production; CIRC. = circulation; PERIPH. = peripheral; and PULM. = pulmonary. (From Wasserman, K.: Physiology of gas exchange and exertional dyspnea. Clin. Sci., 61:7–13, 1981. Copyright © 1981, The Biochemical Society, London.)

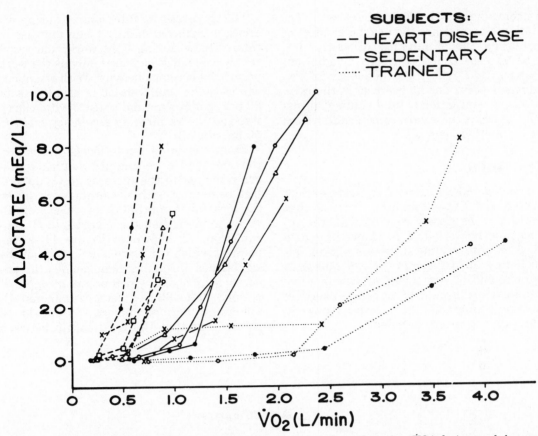

Figure 11–2. Change (Δ) in lactate concentration plotted against O_2 consumption ($\dot{V}O_2$) during graded exercise testing in patients with heart disease (primarily of the mitral valve), sedentary subjects, and well-trained normal subjects. Anaerobic metabolism with production of excess lactate occurs at low work loads in the patients, at moderate loads in the sedentary persons, and only at high loads in the trained athletes. (Reprinted by permission from Wasserman, K., and Whipp, B. J.: Exercise physiology in health and disease. Am. Rev. Respir. Dis., *112*:219–249, 1975.)

exceeded, *anaerobic* metabolism ensues and contributes to the generation of ATP. Anaerobic chemical reactions do not consume O_2, carbohydrate is the obligatory substrate, lactic acid is the end-product, and ATP production is much lower, approximately nineteen-fold lower, than the amount of ATP produced by aerobic metabolism of an equivalent amount of carbohydrate. Newly generated lactic acid is buffered by HCO_3^- stores, thereby producing CO_2 and H^+ that must be removed for metabolism to continue. The appearance of excess CO_2 and H^+ in the bloodstream stimulates a further increase in ventilation (see Chapter 10). Thus, as discussed in greater detail subsequently, the onset of lactic acid production is signaled by a detectable augmentation in ventilatory volume, which is customarily measured as expired minute ventilation.

The level of exercise at which aerobic metabolism is no longer sufficient to meet all the energy requirements and at which

anaerobic metabolism supervenes has been called by Wasserman and coworkers[6] the *anaerobic threshold.* As illustrated in Figure 11–2, the anaerobic threshold varies with the amount of exercise conditioning and can be used as a measure of physical fitness. However, according to a recent analysis by Jones,[7] the relationships among lactic acid generation, increased CO_2 output, and increased minute ventilation may be in part coincidental and caused by the interplay of several factors. In other words, more than lactic acid production alone may be involved in the mechanisms underlying the "anaerobic threshold" in the continuum of ventilatory responses to progressive exercise.

GAS EXCHANGE

As shown in Figure 11–1, the first step in the series of linked reactions in the flow of O_2 from the ambient air to the mitochondria of exercising muscles is an increase in ventilation; this also has the beneficial effect of increasing the elimination of newly produced excess CO_2 from the body. In addition, changes that reflect the efficiency of gas exchange occur during exercise in the ratio of wasted ventilation to tidal volume, diffusing capacity, alveolar-arterial differences for O_2 and CO_2, and pH.

Ventilation

The demands of exercise for increased O_2 uptake and CO_2 elimination require that ventilation be closely coupled with the intensity of the work load. As shown in Figure 11–3, minute volume increases almost immediately upon the initiation of muscular exercise and reaches a plateau within a few minutes during mild to moderate exercise; however, minute volume increases progressively during severe exercise.[8]

The increased minute volume during exercise is achieved mainly by an increase in tidal volume during light work, and respiratory frequency increases only as the work performed becomes heavier. With strenuous exercise, the tidal volume is usually about 50 per cent of a normal person's vital capacity, and the respiratory frequency is 40 to 50 breaths/min.[9]

From rest to moderate levels of exercise, the increase in ventilatory volume is linearly related to the increase in O_2 uptake. But beginning with moderate work loads, the increase in ventilation becomes progressively greater than the increase in O_2 consumption. As shown in Figure 11–4, the point at which ventilation departs from the established linear segment defines the anaerobic threshold, which occurs at approximately 50 to 60 per cent of maximal O_2 uptake in normal subjects. It should be pointed out that the relationship between

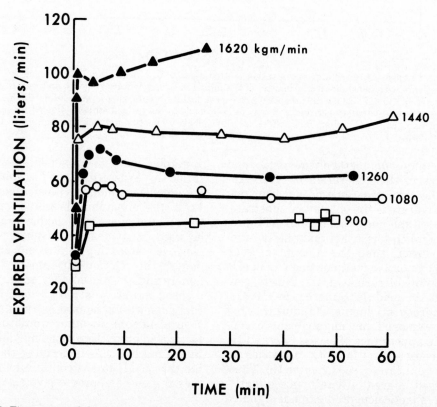

Figure 11–3. Time course of changes in expired ventilation at different work intensities. (Data from Nielsen, M.: Untersuchungen über die Atemregulation beim Menschen. Skandinav. Arch. Physiol., 74 (Suppl. 10):82–208, 1936. Reprinted by permission from Asmussen, E.: Muscular Exercise. In Fenn, W. O., and Rahn, H. (eds.): Handbook of Physiology, Section 3. Respiration. vol. II. Washington, D.C., American Physiological Society, 1965, pp. 939–978.)

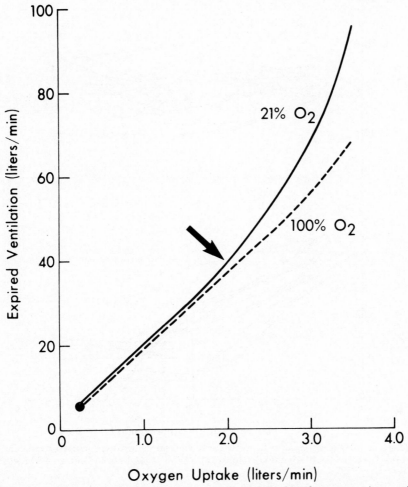

Figure 11–4. Effect of increasing O_2 uptake by exercise (measured with a bicycle ergometer) on expired ventilation while breathing room air (21% O_2) and 100% O_2. The arrow on the room air curve indicates the anaerobic threshold: the point at which ventilation is no longer linearly related to O_2 uptake. (Adapted from Asmussen, E., and Nielsen, M.: Studies on the regulation of respiration in heavy work. Acta Physiol. Scand., *12*:171–188, 1946.)

CO_2 output and expired ventilation is even more uniform than that between O_2 uptake and ventilation. The additional "drive" to ventilation reflects mainly the progressive accumulation of lactic acid in the bloodstream. The contribution of anaerobic metabolism and lactate production has been demonstrated by experiments using supplemental O_2;[10] breathing air mixtures enriched with O_2 lowered ventilation during heavy work but had no effect in the same subjects at rest or during light work (see Fig. 11–4). Further discussion of the factors that initiate and regulate the amount of ventilation during exercise follows in the next section.

Wasted Ventilation to Tidal Volume Ratio

The volume of anatomic dead space usually increases slightly during exercise because of the distension of airways that accompanies deep breathing (see Fig. 8–11); in contrast, the volume of alveolar dead space normally present at rest decreases. Thus, because the two components of (total) wasted ventilation change in opposite directions, the absolute values of wasted ventilation are nearly constant during exercise (Fig. 11–5A). However, because tidal volume increases considerably in response to increasing work loads, the ratio of wasted

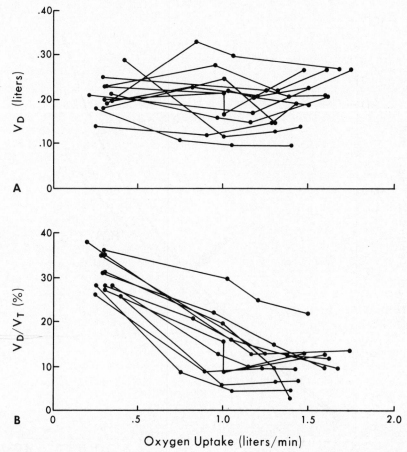

Figure 11–5. Effect of increasing O_2 uptake by exercise (measured with a bicycle ergometer) on *A*, wasted ventilation (V_D) and *B*, wasted ventilation:tidal volume ratio (V_D/V_T). (Data from Glazier, J. B., and Murray, J. F.: Unpublished observations, 1974.)

ventilation to tidal volume normally decreases from approximately 30 per cent to 10 to 15 per cent during exercise (Fig. 11–5*B*). By this mechanism, alveolar ventilation increases from about 70 per cent of minute volume at rest to about 85 to 90 per cent of minute volume during heavy exercise.[12]

Diffusing Capacity

The changes in intravascular pressures within the pulmonary artery and left atrium during exercise serve both to recruit previously closed pulmonary capillaries and to distend capillaries that had been perfused but not maximally dilated. The consequences of these phenomena are (1) a better matching of ventilation and perfusion, with resulting improvement of gas exchange, and

(2) increases in pulmonary capillary blood volume and membrane-diffusing capacity.[13]

In most but not all studies, pulmonary diffusing capacity for CO has been found to increase linearly and continuously as O_2 uptake increases to maximal values during exercise. In contrast, it has been shown that pulmonary diffusing capacity for O_2 reaches its maximal level at submaximal work loads.[14] These studies, however, are difficult to perform, and the results must be considered equivocal. Whether or not diffusing capacity reaches a plateau during exercise is an important question that needs to be investigated further.

As stressed in Chapter 8, pulmonary diffusion does not limit exchange of O_2 and CO_2 in healthy resting subjects at sea level; in fact, there is considerable utilizable reserve in this function, so that large reductions in diffusing capacity must occur before differences become apparent between the

Po_2 of alveolar gas and that of red blood cells at the end of their passage through pulmonary capillaries. The increase in diffusing capacity during exercise serves to promote O_2 uptake and to ensure that alveolar-end-capillary Po_2 differences remain negligible. It is possible that regional variations in the transit times of red blood cells at high rates of exercise could result in insufficient time for O_2 equilibrium to occur in some gas exchange units; whether or not this occurs has not been settled. Therefore, during exercise at sea level, pulmonary diffusing capacity is adequate to maintain equilibrium at the completion of gas exchange across the air-blood barrier except possibly during maximal or near-maximal work loads. In normal persons living at high altitudes, however, owing to the low Po_2 in the inspired air, the total amount of O_2 that can diffuse into the blood per unit time is reduced despite the presence of a perfectly normal alveolar-capillary membrane and normal or even increased pulmonary capillary blood volume. The reduction in diffu-

sion of O_2 is of little consequence at rest, but it does reduce maximal O_2 uptake and thereby reduces maximal attainable work loads. The higher the altitude, the greater the diffusion limitation.[15] Similarly, the presence of pulmonary abnormalities that impair diffusion is seldom important in resting patients, but they may impose serious limitations on gas transfer during exercise, which is evidenced by a reduction in maximal O_2 uptake and work capacity.

Alveolar-Arterial Oxygen Tension

Despite the considerable increases in O_2 consumption, minute volume of ventilation, and cardiac output during exercise, alveolar and arterial Po_2 compositions remain remarkably constant. Figure 11–6 depicts the mean alveolar and arterial values of both O_2 and CO_2 at rest and during progressively increasing work loads in the upright position (bicycling); the alveolar-arterial Po_2 difference during exercise initially de-

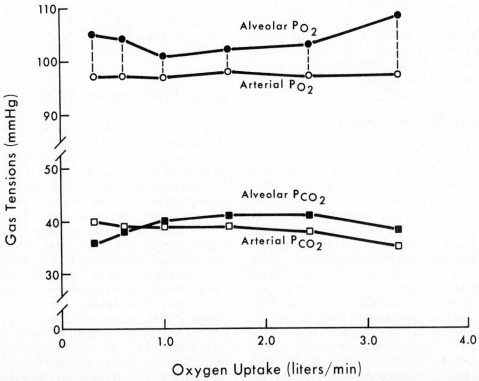

Figure 11–6. Effect of increasing O_2 uptake by exercise (on a bicycle ergometer) on alveolar and arterial Po_2 and Pco_2. Mean values from studies in five healthy subjects. The vertical dashed line represents the alveolar-arterial Po_2 difference. (Data from Whipp, B. J., and Wasserman, K.: Alveolar-arterial gas tension differences during graded exercise. J. Appl. Physiol., 27:361–365, 1969.)

creases slightly from the resting value and then increases at very high work loads.[16]

The resting alveolar-arterial P_{O_2} difference of 8 mm Hg, as discussed in Chapter 8, results from slight mismatching of ventilation and perfusion and from a small postpulmonary right-to-left shunt. The ventilation-perfusion imbalance is mainly due to the effects of gravity on the distribution of pulmonary blood flow. At rest in the upright position, blood flow is several times greater to the base than to the apex of each lung, but during exercise, the increase in pulmonary artery pressure causes blood flow to become more uniformly distributed throughout the lungs;[17] this improves the matching of ventilation and blood flow and, consequently, reduces the alveolar-arterial P_{O_2} difference. (This phenomenon is reflected in the decreased height of the vertical dashed lines in Fig. 11–6.) At very high levels of work, the alveolar-arterial P_{O_2} difference increases to a value greater than that at rest (also shown in Fig. 11–6). The mechanism of the increase is not known, but two possibilities have been suggested: (1) a decrease in the O_2 content of mixed venous blood, which has the effect of worsening the decrease in arterial P_{O_2} from whatever venous admixture already exists (see Fig. 8–10), and (2) a limitation of diffusion so that complete equilibration of O_2 between alveolar gas and pulmonary capillary blood does not occur.

Alveolar-Arterial Carbon Dioxide Tension

Figure 11–6 also shows the relationship between mean alveolar and arterial P_{CO_2} values at rest and during exercise. The fact that alveolar P_{CO_2} is lower than arterial P_{CO_2} at rest may at first seem surprising, but it is accounted for by the poor perfusion of the upper regions of the lungs that results from the gravitational distribution of blood flow. Mean alveolar P_{CO_2} reflects gas composition in those air spaces in which CO_2 uptake has occurred as well as in the apices that are ventilated but poorly perfused. This so-called alveolar dead space effect disappears during exercise, owing to the improved perfusion of the upper regions of the lungs, and thus alveolar P_{CO_2} becomes equal to or slightly higher than arterial P_{CO_2}. The latter discrepancy reflects increased CO_2 de-

livery to the lungs and oscillation of alveolar and arterial values around slightly different mean levels.[18]

During heavy exercise, both alveolar and arterial P_{CO_2} values begin to fall, because of the hyperventilation that occurs in response to the lactic acid that begins to accumulate at these work intensities (see Fig. 11–4); the fall in alveolar P_{CO_2} is associated with the rise in alveolar P_{O_2}, as shown in Figure 11–6. In exhaustive work, alveolar P_{CO_2} may decrease to about 30 mm Hg.[10]

pH

At light work loads, arterial pH and P_{CO_2} are normal. Even at moderately heavy work loads above the anaerobic threshold, pH remains virtually normal because of the buffering of lactic acid by HCO_3^- and because the added increment of ventilation eliminates the CO_2 liberated in the reaction. However, at increasingly heavy and exhausting work loads, pH begins to decrease and may decline to values as low as 7.25 to 7.30 despite further hyperventilation and a reduction in P_{CO_2}. Thus, respiratory compensation for the steadily worsening metabolic (lactic) acidosis is at first nearly perfect but then gradually fails to keep pace, and acidemia supervenes.

REGULATION OF VENTILATION

Arterial P_{O_2} and P_{CO_2} are almost exactly the same during mild and moderate exercise as at rest. Simply maintaining arterial blood gases at their resting levels may not sound like much of an adjustment, yet this constancy can be achieved only by a remarkable correspondence between the intensity of work on the one hand and the amount of ventilation on the other. Despite extensive investigation, the mechanisms that couple alveolar ventilation to increases in O_2 consumption and CO_2 production are still poorly understood. The search for the primary stimulus to increased ventilation during exercise—the stimulus that is linked tightly to, is actuated by, and responds to variations in metabolic activity—has led to two different principal hypotheses, although these are not mutually exclusive and may coexist. According to one theory, the stimulus is chemically mediated; in the other, it occurs by means of a reflex pathway. (The interested reader is referred to the reasoned analysis by Dempsey and coworkers[19] of the arguments for and against each theory and to the recent comprehensive review by Whipp[20] of all the possibilities.)

Role of Carbon Dioxide

Since Haldane and Priestley[21] studied the problem in the early 1900's, much attention has been directed toward the role that CO_2 plays in the regulation of ventilation during exercise. Carbon dioxide has always been a logical choice as a regulator because its production parallels the severity of muscular work and because the medullary chemoreceptors are able to respond quickly to new levels of CO_2 in the brain and CSF. Although the CO_2 theory has been found deficient in part, it is a convenient place to begin an examination of the factors involved in the control of breathing during exercise.

As discussed in Chapter 8, arterial P_{CO_2} varies directly with CO_2 production and inversely with alveolar ventilation (see Equation 8–2); accordingly, at any constant CO_2 production, the relationship between alveolar ventilation, or the more commonly measured total expired ventilation, and arterial P_{CO_2} is expressed by a hyperbolic curve similar to those shown in Figure 11–7; the lower curve defines possible values for arterial P_{CO_2} and expired ventilation at resting CO_2 production, and the upper curve depicts the same variables during mild exercise, when CO_2 production is quadrupled. Normal values for resting arterial P_{CO_2} and expired ventilation are 40 mm Hg and 8 L/min, respectively (point A, Fig. 11–7); however, if ventilation is either suppressed (e.g., by sedative drugs) or stimulated (e.g., by apprehension or anxiety), the resulting values of arterial P_{CO_2} and expired ventilation will be *on the curve*, but to the right or left (respectively) of point A. Similarly, if ventilation is abnormally high or low while exercising, the resulting arterial P_{CO_2} will differ from the normal value of 40 mm Hg and will lie to the right or left of point B on the upper curve.

If the change in ventilation during exercise were due solely to the ventilatory drive from newly produced CO_2 that begins to accumulate in the bloodstream, the response

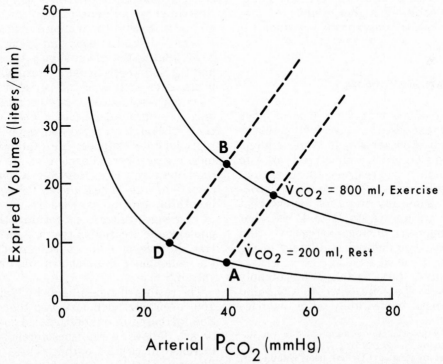

Figure 11–7. Relationship between expired ventilation and arterial P_{CO_2} when CO_2 output is 200 ml (rest) and 800 ml (exercise). The dashed lines represent "normal" CO_2 response curves. For details, see text.

would be determined by the subject's sensitivity to CO_2.* Normal CO_2 responsiveness is shown by the dashed line moving up and to the right from point A in Figure 11–7 (see Chapter 10 for discussion of CO_2 response lines). The CO_2 response line intersects the exercise CO_2 production curve at point C and thereby defines the arterial P_{CO_2} and expired ventilation values that should occur during exercise if the patient's sensitivity to CO_2 were the *only* mechanism controlling breathing. Although the differences between the arterial P_{CO_2} and minute ventilation values represented by points B and C are small, they are readily detectable. Thus, because the effect of CO_2 alone sets conditions at point C rather than point B, other stimuli must be present to account for the observed increment in ventilation during exercise.

The results of recent studies have provided further support for the concept that the resting level of arterial P_{CO_2}, the so-called *set point*, establishes the value that is maintained during exercise at mild to moderate work loads; in other words, if resting (steady-state) arterial P_{CO_2} is lower or higher than normal to begin with, the same value will be sustained during exercise.[24] This means that the ventilatory response during exercise will differ, depending on the P_{CO_2} to be achieved: higher minute volumes are required if the set point is low than if it is high.

Nonmetabolic Factors

One way of reaching point B is to move along the exercise CO_2 production curve from C to B. Another way is to move along the resting CO_2 production curve from A to D and then up a CO_2 response line of normal sensitivity from D to B. Although it is controversial, some investigators believe that the latter process (A to D to B) is what actually happens during exercise[22, 25] and that at least two distinct regulatory mechanisms are involved.[26]

1. The first (fast) factor is presumably nonmetabolic (i.e., unrelated to CO_2) and occurs almost immediately after exercise begins. The rapid effect of this stimulus suggests strongly that it is reflex in origin. The nonmetabolic factor causes ventilation to increase, and because CO_2 production has not had time to rise, the values of arterial P_{CO_2} and expired ventilation change from those at point A to those at point D (see Fig. 11–7).

2. The second (slow) factor is presumably metabolic in origin and requires seconds to minutes to exert its complete effect on ventilation. The time sequence suggests that this factor is humorally mediated, and metabolically produced CO_2 provides a straightforward explanation for the shift from point D to point B. The subsequent hyperventilation that occurs during strenuous work has been related to lactic acid (or other products of anaerobic metabolism) acting mainly on the carotid chemoreceptors.

Role of Reflexes

An extensive search has been made to identify the nonmetabolic stimulus to ventilation. The evidence available at present favors a reflex mechanism that originates from the exercising muscles and limbs. Experiments have demonstrated (1) that passive movements of the limbs of humans or experimental animals cause ventilation to increase, (2) that the increase in ventilation is almost instantaneous and is not affected by occluding the blood supply to the limb, and (3) that the ventilatory response disappears after section of the peripheral nerve or dorsal root subserving the muscle and during spinal anesthesia. These observations, although controversial and not always reproducible,[27] support the contention that mechanoreceptors of some type are situated in skeletal muscles. However, a major deficiency in the reflex theory of control of breathing during exercise is the lack of convincing evidence concerning the morphology and location of the presumed receptors. Muscle spindles, once candidates for the role, have been shown not to be involved.[28]

The results of experiments by Wasserman and coworkers[29] demonstrated that ventilation increased in unanesthetized dogs in the breath following an isoproterenol-induced increase in cardiac output. These findings illustrate that ventilation rapidly adjusts to changes in cardiac output or one of its de-

*Evidence supporting the assumption that ventilatory response to metabolically produced CO_2 is the same as that to inhaled CO_2 has been obtained in humans;[22] additional studies have recently been reviewed.[23]

rivatives, and led to the theory of "cardiac hyperpnea" or "CO_2 flow." Furthermore, the response was shown not to be mediated by the carotid or aortic bodies and to be linked closely to the level of the alveolar, and hence arterial, CO_2. Thus, it was proposed that rapidly responding CO_2 receptors might be responsible for the prompt increase in ventilation at the onset of exercise and that other sources of reflex stimulation might be relatively unimportant. However, the results of more recent investigations, which showed that alveolar and arterial P_{CO_2} values transiently changed in the wrong direction at the onset of exercise,[30] are damaging to the "CO_2 flow" theory.

Other Factors

The main stimulus to ventilation during exercise results from the interaction of presumed chemical and neurogenic influences. However, other factors, especially those related to temperature regulation and conditioned responses, are known to be important.

Ventilation is closely linked to temperature regulation in animals in which the chief mechanism of excess heat elimination is panting. The extent to which this highly complex system, presumably involving hypothalamic and medullary interconnections, is present in humans has not been fully established. The data that are available from hypothermia experiments suggest that normal subjects do not rely on their respiratory systems to regulate body temperature during short episodes of mild exercise.[31] It is likely, however, that the effects of temperature on ventilation would be more discernible during prolonged or heavy exercise, because elevated body temperature increases CO_2 production and CO_2 sensitivity, both of which should increase ventilation.

Psychogenic influences, particularly conditioned responses, may profoundly affect ventilation before and during exercise; for example, it is well known that dogs trained to run on a treadmill anticipate the stress of exercise and change their breathing pattern before the treadmill is actually turned on. Undoubtedly, similar influences operate in humans under certain conditions. Fur-

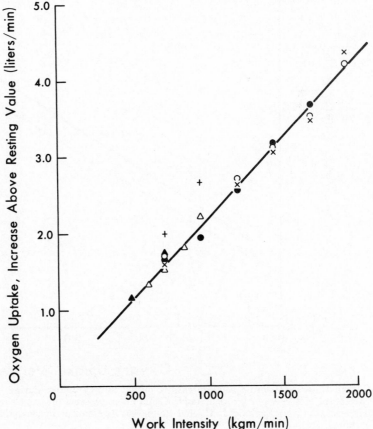

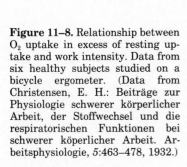

Figure 11–8. Relationship between O_2 uptake in excess of resting uptake and work intensity. Data from six healthy subjects studied on a bicycle ergometer. (Data from Christensen, E. H.: Beiträge zur Physiologie schwerer körperlicher Arbeit, der Stoffwechsel und die respiratorischen Funktionen bei schwerer köperlicher Arbeit. Arbeitsphysiologie, 5:463–478, 1932.)

thermore, breathing is often modified to suit the rhythmic pattern of the exercise being undertaken; thus, the swimmer and the cross-country runner, at the same work intensity, demonstrate different combinations of tidal volumes and breathing frequencies.

CIRCULATION

As already emphasized, contracting muscles require additional O_2, and it is generally recognized that the increase in O_2 consumption that occurs during exercise is the best available measurement of the total muscular effort expended (Fig. 11–8). Increased O_2 demands can be satisfied either by an increase in O_2 transport or by an increase in O_2 extraction; during muscular exercise, the additional O_2 requirements are met by increases in *both* transport to and extraction by the working muscles.

Cardiac Output

Systemic O_2 transport, as defined and discussed in Chapter 8, depends upon the total blood flow to the tissues of the body (the cardiac output) and the content of O_2 in arterial blood (which is determined by arterial P_{O_2}, the amount of hemoglobin available, and the affinity of hemoglobin for O_2). In normal subjects, the elevated O_2 transport during exercise is achieved almost entirely by an increase in cardiac output, and a well-defined relationship has been established between cardiac output and O_2 consumption or O_2 uptake (the variable that is actually measured) during exercise. This relationship is linear at progressively greater intensities of exercise, but ultimately a plateau is reached that is called maximal O_2 uptake.[32] When studies are properly conducted, this level is a stable and reproducible physiologic characteristic of the subject being tested.[33]

The magnitude of the increase in cardiac output as work load is steadily increased is shown in Figure 11–9. The figure also indicates that cardiac output at a given level of exercise will be 1 to 2 L/min higher if the exercise is performed while the person is supine compared with the value in the upright position.[34] The influence of posture is

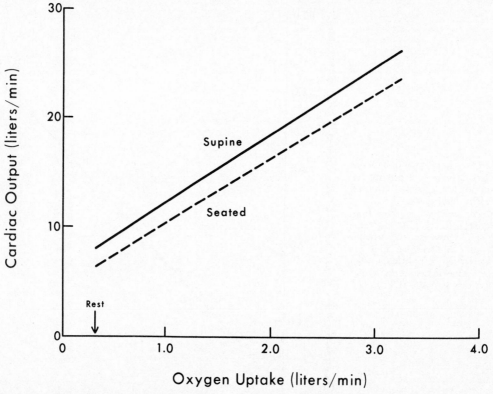

Figure 11–9. Relationship between cardiac output and O_2 uptake during exercise. The dashed line represents normal subjects in seated position, and the solid line represents the same subjects supine. (Adapted and reprinted by permission from Ekelund, L. G., and Holmgren, A.: Central Hemodynamics during exercise. Circ. Res., *20 & 21*(Suppl. 1):33–43, 1967.)

primarily attributable to the effects of gravity on venous return to the heart; cardiac filling and, consequently, right and left ventricular volumes and stroke volume are all greater when subjects are supine than when they are upright.

Another important determinant of the cardiac output response to exercise is the age of the subject. Older persons have lower cardiac outputs at a given work load than younger persons in both the supine and upright positions.[34] Changes are known to occur in cardiac biochemistry during aging, but the molecular mechanisms responsible for them are unknown (see Chapter 14 for further discussion). The effect of aging on hemodynamics is reflected in a reduction in heart rate and usually stroke volume at any O_2 uptake.

Heart Rate and Stroke Volume

An increase in cardiac output can result from an increase in either heart rate or stroke volume or both. Although the rate of cardiac contractions increases linearly with O_2 consumption during muscular work (Fig. 11–10), the magnitude of the change in rate (i.e., the slope of the line) is determined by the size of the stroke volume: the smaller the stroke volume, the greater the increase

in heart rate.[35] Stroke volume may vary under different circumstances and depends upon the physical condition of the subject, the mass of muscles that are performing the work, and the distribution of blood flow.[9] Each of these affects the ventricular volumes and the filling and emptying conditions of the heart. These factors also account for the variations in stroke volume encountered in patients with various diseases.

In general, when progressively increasing exercise is performed in the upright position, stroke volume increases initially to a value comparable to that in the resting supine position; thereafter, stroke volume remains relatively constant. Superior athletes, in contrast to untrained subjects, have considerable reserve stroke volume because their hearts are enlarged. During exhausting exercise, stroke volumes greater than 200 ml have been measured in highly trained athletes; these volumes, by comparison, exceed the usual end-diastolic volumes of untrained persons during maximal exercise.[36]

Normally, most of the increase in cardiac output during exercise depends on an increase in heart rate, which has an age-dependent maximum. The increased heart rate is caused chiefly by increased sympathetic and decreased parasympathetic cardiac efferent activity. Several reflexes pre-

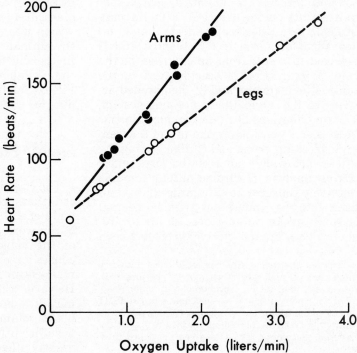

Figure 11–10. Relationship between heart rate and O_2 uptake in the same subject during work with the arms and with the legs. (Adapted and reprinted by permission from Asmussen, E., and Hemmingsen, I.: Determination of maximum working capacity at different ages in work with the legs or with the arms. Scand. J. Clin. Lab. Invest., *10*:67–71, 1958.)

sumably interact to cause these effects. Well-trained athletes have lower resting heart rates than untrained subjects. Thus, even though maximal heart rates are the same in the two groups, trained persons have a greater *range* of heart rate increase available to them. This reserve, coupled with their greater reserve stroke volume, accounts for the large cardiac outputs that enable athletes to supply their muscles with the O_2 needed for championship performances.

Myocardial Responses

Muscle contractility is an elusive but important physiologic phenomenon that can be defined as "an increase in the force developed during isometric contraction at constant muscle length and stimulus." Myocardial contractility, according to this definition, can be measured with precision only under highly artificial laboratory conditions, and its assessment in humans presents formidable problems. There are, however, several indexes related to contractility* that can be derived from measurable variables in normal subjects at rest and during exercise. Regardless of which index is used, there is abundant evidence that myocardial contractility increases during exercise.[37, 38] Presumably, two separate components interact to augment myocardial contractility during exercise: (1) an increase in heart rate (the treppe effect) that is independent of adrenergic influences and is believed to result from an increase in the rate of interaction of specific sites in the contractile elements and (2) heightened activity of the sympathetic nervous system. The contributions of these two mechanisms have been separated by the use of β-adrenergic blocking drugs and cardiac pacing.[38]

It is not widely appreciated that under *resting* conditions, cardiac output remains relatively constant despite large changes in heart rate (e.g., induced by artificial pacing) because stroke volume goes down as frequency goes up and vice versa. It has been

*Indexes of contractility can be divided into two categories: (1) the rate of change of pressure with respect to time during isovolumic contraction (e.g., dP/dT/IT, where IT equals developed pressure at dP/dT minus end-diastolic pressure), and (2) derivatives of contractile element shortening velocity (e.g., circumferential shortening rate at a given developed pressure).

shown experimentally that cardiac output remained within ±20 per cent of control levels when heart rate was varied from less than 50 to greater than 200 per cent of control values, because stroke volume changes proportionately in the opposite direction.[39] This means that during *exercise*, because stroke volume is always higher than it would be at the same heart rate under resting conditions, other mechanisms are actuated that maintain or even increase stroke volume. One of these is the Frank-Starling mechanism, through which the extra stretch imparted to the muscle fibers of the ventricles consequent to the increased filling of the heart causes stroke volume to increase; thus, at any given heart rate, end-diastolic volume (i.e., initial myocardial fiber length) and stroke volume are both larger during exercise than at rest. Normally, the increase in contractility and the Frank-Starling effect are complementary and interact during exercise to raise cardiac output, but when one of the mechanisms cannot be utilized, as may result from disease, drugs, or experimental intervention, the heart makes greater use of the other to increase blood flow. A good example of the heart taking advantage of its available resources for increasing cardiac output is shown by experiments in trained greyhounds that had their adrenergic-mediated contractility mechanisms eliminated by surgical cardiac denervation.[40] The total cardiac output response to racing after denervation was the same as before; but because the animals could not reflexly increase their myocardial performance during exercise, they simply relied more heavily on the Frank-Starling mechanism than when cardiac nervous activity was intact.

Blood Volume and Hematocrit

The changes in blood volume and hematocrit that accompany exercise are variable and depend upon the severity and duration of the work load and the physical condition of the subject. Maximal exercise usually causes a reduction in plasma volume and an increase in hematocrit ratio (8 per cent).[41] However, the magnitude of any change that may develop in hemoglobin concentration or blood volume during submaximal exercise is sufficiently small that O_2 transport is not greatly affected by this mechanism.

Extremely hard exercise, particularly in a hot environment, may be associated with minor amounts of hemolysis. In contrast, severe exercise by well-trained athletes or workers accustomed to it does not produce detectable changes in either blood volume or hemoglobin concentration;[42] the constancy of blood volume may reflect the effects of conditioning, because it is well established that highly trained persons have larger total amounts of hemoglobin and greater circulating blood volumes and heart volumes than unconditioned persons of similar body build.

The importance of hemoglobin concentration, which sets one limit to arterial O_2 transport (see Chapter 8 for further discussion), was nicely demonstrated by Buick and coworkers.[43] These investigators studied highly trained athletes in a series of experiments that included venesection and freezing the blood for storage, waiting until total blood volume was replenished, and then increasing hemoglobin concentration by transfusing each subject with his own blood. In all instances, maximal O_2 uptake, endurance capacity, heart rate, and peak lactic acid concentrations at a fixed level of submaximal exercise indicated *improved* performance after hemoglobin concentration was elevated by transfusion. These results also demonstrate the close link between O_2 transport on the one hand and maximal aerobic exercise capacity on the other.

Vascular Pressures

Systolic, diastolic, and mean systemic arterial blood pressures increase gradually during exercise and in the steady state bear a relationship to the intensity of the work performed (Fig. 11–11). At very heavy work loads, especially in untrained subjects, systolic pressures above 200 mm Hg are common. Systolic, diastolic, mean pulmonary arterial, and wedge pressures also increase linearly with increasing levels of exercise (Fig. 11–12).

Because systolic pressures in both pulmonary and systemic arterial systems increase during exercise, there must be

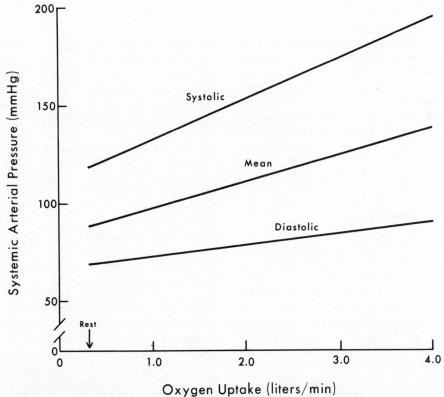

Figure 11–11. Relationship between systolic, diastolic, and mean systemic arterial pressures and O_2 uptake during exercise in the supine position. (Data from Ekelund, L. G., and Holmgren, A.: Central hemodynamics during exercise. Circ. Res., *20 & 21*(Suppl. 1):33–43, 1967.)

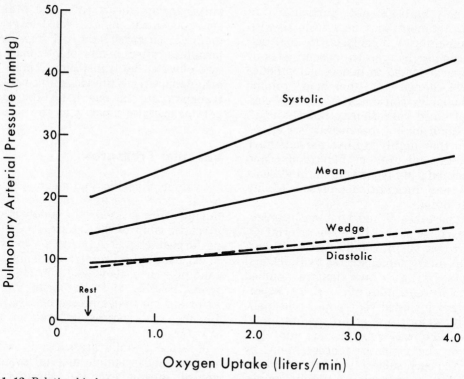

Figure 11–12. Relationship between systolic, diastolic, mean, and "wedge" pulmonary arterial pressures and O₂ uptake during exercise in the supine position. (Data from Ekelund, L. G., and Holmgren, A.: Central hemodynamics during exercise. Circ. Res., *20 & 21*(Suppl. 1):33–43, 1967.)

corresponding changes in right and left ventricular systolic pressures. However, the diastolic pressure responses differ in the two ventricular cavities: right ventricular end–diastolic pressure decreases, but left ventricular end–diastolic pressure increases (as indicated by the elevated pulmonary arterial wedge pressure). These responses must reflect differences in the distensibilities of right and left ventricular myocardiums.

Peripheral Blood Flow

The discussion in the previous sections has centered on how cardiac output and systemic O_2 transport are increased during exercise. But it is obvious that for the increased flow of O_2 to be useful it has to reach the capillary beds perfusing the active muscle groups. Redistribution of peripheral blood flow is achieved by *vasodilatation* in the working muscles, including the muscles of respiration and to some extent the skin, and *vasoconstriction* in the viscera and nonworking muscles. These variations in regional blood flow are produced by a complex interplay of local vasodilator and general vasoconstrictor mechanisms, the exact causes of which are unknown. Vasoconstriction in the splanchnic and renal vascular beds redistributes 70 to 80 per cent of the resting blood flow (or about 2.2 L/min) from these organs to exercising muscles.[32] The increase in cardiac output above the resting value is distributed mainly (80 to 90 per cent) to the working muscles, including those of respiration.

The importance of the O_2 requirements of the respiratory muscles has only recently been appreciated. Although their O_2 needs are small at rest, they are appreciable at the minute volumes necessary to support strenuous exercise (see Fig. 5–9). Bye and coworkers[44] calculated that blood flow to respiratory muscles may reach 8 L/min and that their O_2 requirements could represent at least 25 per cent of maximal O_2 uptake. Whether or not the O_2 needs of the respiratory muscles ever limit maximal exercise capacity in healthy persons is far from clear, although it probably happens in patients whose work of breathing is increased.

Because vasodilatation in the large work-

Table 11–1. COMPARISON OF THE MEAN HEMODYNAMIC RESPONSES TO MAXIMAL EXERCISE IN HIGHLY TRAINED ATHLETES AND MIDDLE-AGED WOMEN*

Group	Cardiac Output (L/min)	Blood Pressure (mm Hg)	Peripheral Vascular Resistance (units)
Athletes	36.0	116	3.2
Women	11.5	164	14.3

*Data from Ekblom, B., and Hermansen, L.: Cardiac output in athletes. J. Appl. Physiol., *25*:619–625, 1968 and Kilbom, A., and Åstand, P. O.: I. Physical training with submaximal intensities in woman. II. Effect on cardiac output. Scand. J. Clin. Lab. Invest., *28*:163–175, 1971.

ing muscle groups outweighs vasoconstriction that occurs in most other organs, peripheral vascular resistance decreases and becomes an important mechanism governing the magnitude of the cardiac output response during exercise. This relationship is dramatically illustrated by the data shown in Table 11–1. Highly trained athletes are able to increase their cardiac outputs substantially with only a slight increase in mean systemic arterial blood pressure; this means that their peripheral vascular resistance decreases remarkably.[45] In contrast, untrained persons such as the subjects reported in Table 11–1, middle-aged women, achieve only modest increases in cardiac output and their arterial pressure increases appreciably;[46] accordingly, their mean peripheral vascular resistance was 4.5 times greater than that of the athletes.

BODY TEMPERATURE

The exercising body resembles a machine in the sense that only a fraction of the total energy produced by the consumption of fuel is transformed into useful work. The quantity of energy that is not converted into mechanical work degenerates into heat. The heat production of an exercising subject has a particular value for a given work intensity and during strenuous exercise may reach values 15 to 20 times the value at rest. Some of the extra heat is stored in the body and raises its temperature (Fig. 11–13), and

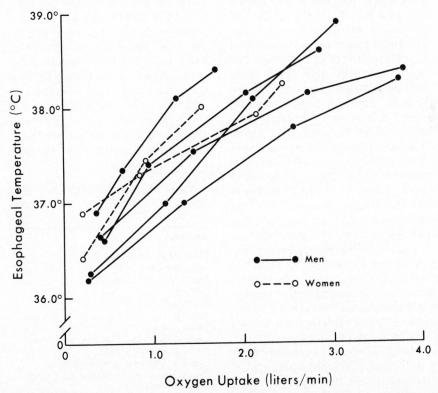

Figure 11–13. Effect of increasing O₂ uptake by exercise (measured with a bicycle ergometer) on esophageal temperature. Individual measurements in seven healthy subjects. (Adapted and reprinted by permission from Saltin, B., and Hermansen, L.: Esophageal, rectal, and muscle temperature during exercise. J. Appl. Physiol., *21*:1757–1762, 1966.)

the remainder is dissipated.[47] Once the body temperature is elevated to the steady-state value that corresponds to the amount of work being performed, all the heat produced by the muscles subsequently must be eliminated. In humans, heat dissipation occurs mainly through the skin, and this process requires a considerable increase in blood flow to the body surface. During heavy exercise in hot and humid environments where heat loss is impaired, an unusually large amount of blood flow must be diverted to the skin, which presents the body with simultaneous demands for blood flow to working muscles and to the skin. These demands may be met by a further increase in cardiac output and by redistribution of visceral blood flow; when these reserves are exhausted, certain compromises occur that, in general, limit maximal O_2 uptake.[48]

TRAINING

The effects of training are remarkably complex and have been the subject of countless investigations. However, it should be emphasized at the outset of a discussion about the topic that it is virtually impossible to design suitable experiments that will answer some of the important and unsolved questions about the effects of training. For example, five outstanding men cross-country skiers had an average maximal O_2 uptake of 5.6 L/min, and two champions had values above 6.0 L/min; in contrast, sedentary men had maximal O_2 uptakes of about 3.0 L/min.[49] Clearly, there is a remarkable difference in maximal O_2 uptake, transport, and utilization between top athletes and untrained men. Some of these differences are due to the fact that exceptional athletes have large hearts, increased blood volumes and red blood cell masses, and greater than "normal" pulmonary diffusing capacity measurements. What is not known is whether these attributes are inherited and champions are genetically endowed with superior ability or whether these so-called dimensional characteristics of athletic prowess are acquired through years of rigorous exercise. Training has been shown to improve several circulatory and respiratory physiologic variables related to exercise performance; however, training has not been demonstrated to have an effect on several of the critical physical dimensions that govern maximal O_2 uptake and delivery during exercise.

The chief difficulty in designing experiments lies in the selection of appropriate subjects. The person who is willing to be a test subject in a strenuous physical conditioning program is highly motivated and is likely to manifest an interest in athletics by a certain degree of physical conditioning at the outset. In contrast, the unfit person has already demonstrated a lack of interest in athletic activities; accordingly, it is difficult to enroll him in a serious physical training program and to maintain his enthusiastic participation throughout. Furthermore, some of the variables that are being measured, especially the dimensional characteristics, may require years to change or may be changeable only during growth of the subject, and experiments of sufficient duration with suitable control subjects are obviously difficult to carry out.

Despite the problems of experimental design and interpretation, it is widely recognized that it is possible to increase the maximum amount of muscular exercise that a person can perform by a period of physical training. A rigorously conducted exercise conditioning program of sufficient duration improves principally the O_2 transport capacity of the circulatory system and the oxidative metabolic capacity of the skeletal muscle cells. These physiologic qualities are, in turn, reflected in a measurable increase in maximal O_2 uptake and in lesser changes (i.e., "demands") in obligatory circulatory and metabolic adjustments, compared with those required in the pretraining state.[50] The physiologic variables that have been examined to determine whether they con-

Table 11–2. SUMMARY OF THE EFFECTS OF TRAINING ON CIRCULATORY AND RESPIRATORY FUNCTION DURING PHYSICAL EXERCISE

Variable	Response
Maximal O_2 uptake	Increased
Work output	Increased
Mechanical efficiency	Unchanged
Cardiac output	Increased
Maximal heart rate	Unchanged
Heart rate at submaximal loads	Decreased
Stroke volume	Increased
Arteriovenous O_2 difference	Increased
Hemoglobin, hematocrit	Unchanged
Blood lactate level at maximal loads	Increased
Blood lactate level at submaximal loads	Decresed
Maximal ventilation	Unchanged
Ventilation at submaximal loads	Decreased
Pulmonary diffusing capacity	Unchanged
Capillary density in muscles	Increased
Oxidative enzymes in muscles	Increased

tribute to the increased work capacity that follows training are summarized in Table 11–2. It should be emphasized that not all of those that may change actually do change in a given person. There appears to be considerable individual variation in the response to exercise training that depends, in part, upon the subject's physical fitness at the time training begins.

Cardiac Factors

The results of nearly all studies of healthy subjects have indicated that the increased maximal O_2 uptake observed during training is consistently related to an increase in maximal cardiac output.[50] Depending on whether or not mixed venous O_2 content also decreases, the increase in cardiac output accounts for between 50 and 100 per cent of the increase in maximal O_2 uptake. It is well established that heart rate at maximal O_2 uptake is unchanged by training, which means that stroke volume must increase. Accordingly, at a given level of submaximal exercise, cardiac output and heart rate are lower and stroke volume is higher after training compared with the pretraining values.

Mean arterial blood pressure does not change with training, indicating that systemic vascular resistance at maximal O_2 uptake is decreased. This important change is presumably related to augmented vasodilatation in working muscles (discussed subsequently) and may contribute to the improvement in cardiac performance by decreasing afterload and allowing the heart to empty more completely (thus increasing stroke volume). In addition, myocardial contractility is enhanced by training.

Peripheral Factors

Although less well documented than the systemic hemodynamic responses, training induces several adaptations in the working muscle groups that enable them to receive more blood flow and to utilize more O_2. The biochemical basis of the training-induced changes in skeletal muscle cells that increase their oxidation capacity have recently been reviewed.[51]

Muscle Blood Flow. It is widely accepted that the greater part of the increase in maximal cardiac output that results from training is directed toward active muscle groups, but little direct proof of this assumption exists.[50] It must be remembered also that the muscles of respiration are part of the working muscle groups during exercise and that the O_2 requirements of ventilation increase at a greater rate than the quantity of air inhaled. This means that a steadily increasing proportion of the increased capacity to transport O_2 must be distributed to the respiratory muscles.

The mechanisms by which training increases blood flow to working muscle groups are not known with certainty. It appears that the generalized sympathetic vasoconstrictor response during exercise, which is offset to some extent by local mechanisms in working muscles thereby increasing their blood flow, is attenuated by training; by this means blood flow to active muscles is able to increase above pretraining levels.[50]

It has been demonstrated that repetitive exercise has an important effect on the density of muscle capillaries in experimental animals. In guinea pigs made to run on a treadmill, the number of capillaries increased in muscles whose work output increased (heart and gastrocnemius) compared with those muscles that were not exercised (masseter).[52] An increased density of capillaries would have the obvious advantage of improving the diffusion of O_2 and other metabolic substrates by effectively shortening the distance for transfer between the capillary lumens and the mitochondria and other sites of utilization within the contracting fibers. In contrast with the results in experimental animals, it was originally claimed that training did not affect the capillary density in human skeletal muscles.[53] This conclusion needs to be reevaluated in the light of the results of Anderson's more recent study[54] that showed an increase in the number of capillaries per square millimeter and an increase in the ratio between the number of capillaries and the number of muscle cells.

Oxygen Extraction. As previously mentioned, the increase in cardiac output during training acounts for 50 to 100 per cent of the increase in maximal O_2 uptake. Viewed another way, from 0 to 50 per cent of the increase in maximal O_2 uptake can be attributed to increased O_2 extraction, which has been shown to occur in working muscle groups. A reduction in venous O_2 content indicates an adaptation by which muscles can function at a lower than usual Po_2, presumably as a result, in part, of changes in oxidative enzyme capacity as well as the previously noted increase in capillary density.

Maximal O_2 extraction from blood would be enhanced by a shift to the right of the oxyhemoglobin equilibrium curve, although the extent to which this occurs is not clear. A rightward shift, which was not associated with an increase in erythrocyte DPG (see Chapter 7), was observed in world-class competitive athletes[55] but is not a constant systemic effect of training. Local factors such as increases in temperature and acidity decrease the O_2 affinity of blood perfusing exercising muscles and thus contribute to increased O_2 extraction.

Oxygen Utilization. Exercise training programs can be designed specifically to increase either aerobic or anaerobic work capacity. However, in most physical conditioning programs both capacities increase to some degree and are reflected by changes in the blood level of lactate and the muscle cell biochemical composition. After training, the level of lactate in the blood is lower at a given submaximal work load than it was before.[50] The reduced blood levels at submaximal exercise are probably caused by an increase in the amount of energy produced aerobically, because training has been shown to increase oxidative capacity.[56] Long-term exercise induces muscle mitochondrial proliferation, increases the concentration of oxidative enzymes, and increases the synthesis of glycogen and triglyceride, which are important intracellular energy sources.[57] Although it is likely that the observed increase of mitochondria and enzymes could allow the muscle to function at a lower Po_2, this explanation for the increased O_2 extraction after training remains speculative.

Respiratory Factors

Maximal ventilation in some normal subjects is unchanged by physical training.[58] In other subjects, however, ventilation increases after training, corresponding to the increase in maximal O_2 uptake that occurs.[49] At submaximal exercise loads, ventilation is always less after training than before.

The pulmonary diffusing capacity of competitive athletes, especially swimmers, is higher than that of nonathletes.[59] Although

this difference is caused by a higher pulmonary capillary blood volume in the athletes, the basic explanation for its occurrence is unknown. Most studies of the effect of training on pulmonary diffusing capacity have failed to demonstrate any changes attributable to short-term exercise programs.[60] These investigations, however, did not rule out the possibility that training of longer duration—for example, beginning in childhood—could lead to improvements in diffusing capacity; such an increase, if it did develop, might be related to the large total blood volumes, especially red blood cell masses, that athletes characteristically have.[61] The other explanation is, of course, that athletes are endowed by heredity and then selected on the basis of their superior physical attributes.

Studies of ventilatory control in athletes revealed a marked depression of hypoxic and hypercapnic responses at rest.[62] These results indicate diminished chemoreceptor function and, because they were also observed in other (nonathletic) members of the same family, probably are genetic in origin.

Work Efficiency

The efficiency of individual muscle fibers (measured as the amount of work performed related to the total energy consumed) does not appear to be influenced by training. This has been demonstrated for simple physical acts such as walking on level ground. However, the results of training involving more complicated physical maneuvers, such as treadmill exercise and bicycling, often reveal that the same amount of work can be performed at a lower O_2 uptake. This should not be interpreted as indicating increased muscle efficiency but that learning and practice have resulted in a more coordinated relaxed movement; because fewer muscles (agonists and antagonists) are participating, the motion requires less O_2 to perform.

Summary

There has been a long-standing debate concerning whether the maximal O_2 uptake is limited by the capacity of the cardiovascular system to deliver O_2 to the working muscles or by the capacity of the muscle fibers to utilize O_2. The evidence seems now to favor the cardiovascular system as the more important limiting factor. There is little reason to believe that the lungs of ordinary healthy persons ever limit maximal gas exchange. However, the role played by the respiratory muscles is coming under increasing scrutiny, and it is conceivable that their needs for blood flow and O_2 can restrict the blood flow and O_2 available to other muscles, especially in highly trained athletes undergoing strenuous exercise.

REFERENCES

1. Wasserman, K., and Whipp, B. J.: Exercise physiology in health and disease. Am. Rev. Respir. Dis., 112:219–249, 1975.
2. Jones, N. L., and Campbell, E. J. M.: Clinical Exercise Testing. Philadelphia, W. B. Saunders Co., 1982, pp. 1–268.
3. Asmussen, E.: Exercise: general statement of unsolved problems. Circ. Res., 20 & 21(Suppl. 1):2–5, 1967.
4. Felig, P., and Wahren, J.: Fuel homeostasis in exercise. New Engl. J. Med., 293:1078–1084, 1975.
5. Wasserman, K.: Physiology of gas exchange and exertional dyspnea. Clin. Sci., 61:7–13, 1981.
6. Wasserman, K., Whipp, B. J., Koyal, S. N., and Beaver, W. L.: Anaerobic threshold and maximal oxygen uptake for three modes of exercise. J. Appl. Physiol., 41:544–559, 1973.
7. Jones, N. L.: Editorial review: Hydrogen ion balance during exercise. Clin. Sci., 59:85–91, 1980.
8. Nielsen, M.: Untersuchungen über die Atemregulation beim Menschen. Skandinav. Arch. Physiol., 74(Suppl. 10):83–208, 1936.
9. Asmussen, E.: Muscular exercise. In Fenn, W. O., and Rahn, H. (eds.): Handbook of Physiology, Section 3. Respiration. Vol. II. Washington, D.C., American Physiological Society, 1965, pp. 939–978.
10. Asmussen, E., and Nielsen, M.: Studies on the regulation of respiration in heavy work. Acta Physiol. Scand., 12:171–188, 1946.
11. Glazier, J. B., and Murray, J. F.: Unpublished observations, 1974.
12. Jones, N. L., McHardy, G. J. R., Naimark, A., and Campbell, E. J. M.: Physiological dead space and alveolar-arterial gas pressure differences during exercise. Clin. Sci., 31:19–29, 1966.
13. Johnson, R. L., Jr., Spicer, W. S., Bishop, J. M., and Forster, R. E.: Pulmonary capillary blood volume, flow and diffusing capacity during exercise. J. Appl. Physiol., 15:893–902, 1960.
14. Shepard, R. H., Varnauskas, E., Martin, J. E., and Riley, R. L.: Relationship between cardiac output and apparent diffusing capacity of the lung in normal man during treadmill exercise. J. Appl. Physiol., 13:205–210, 1958.
15. Torre-Bueno, J. R., Wagner, P. D., Salzman, H. A., Gale, G. E., and Moon, R. E.: Diffusion limitation in normal humans during exercise at sea level and simulated altitude. J. Appl. Physiol. 58:989–995, 1985.
16. Whipp, B. J., and Wasserman, K.: Alveolar-arterial gas tension differences during graded exercise. J. Appl. Physiol., 27:361–365, 1969.
17. West, J. B.: Distribution of gas and blood in the normal lungs. Brit. Med. Bull., 19:53–58, 1963.
18. Staub, N. C.: Alveolar-arterial oxygen tension gradient due to diffusion. J. Appl. Physiol., 18:673–680, 1963.
19. Dempsey, J. A., Vidruk, E. H., and Mastenbrook, S. M.: Pulmonary control systems in exercise. Fed. Proc., 39:1498–1505, 1980.
20. Whipp, B. J.: Ventilatory control during exercise in humans. Annu. Rev. Physiol., 45:393–413, 1983.
21. Haldane, J. S., and Priestley, J. G.: The regulation of the lung—ventilation. J. Physiol. (Lond.), 32:225–266, 1905.
22. D'Angelo, E., and Torelli, G.: Neural stimuli increasing respiration during different types of exercise. J. Appl. Physiol., 30:116–121, 1971.
23. Flenley, D. S., and Warren, P. M.: Ventilatory responses to O_2 and CO_2 during exercise. Annu. Rev. Physiol., 45:415–426, 1983.
24. Oren, A., Wasserman, K., Davis, J. A., and Whipp, B. J.: Effect of CO_2 set point on ventilatory response to exercise. J. Appl. Physiol., 51:185–189, 1981.
25. Bainton, C. R.: Effect of speed vs. grade and shivering on ventilation in dogs during active exercise. J. Appl. Physiol., 33:778–787, 1972.
26. Kao, F. F.: An experimental study of the pathways involved in exercise hyperpnea employing cross-circulation techniques. In Cunningham, D. J. C., and Lloyd, B. B. (eds.): The Regulation of Human Respiration. Philadelphia, F. A. Davis Company, 1963, pp. 461–502.
27. Weissman, J. L., Whipp, B. J., Huntsman, D. J., and Wasserman, K.: Role of neural afferents from working limbs in exercise hyperpnea. J. Appl. Physiol., 49:239–248, 1980.
28. Horbein, T. F., Sorensen, S. C., and Parks, C. R.: Role of muscle spindles in lower extremities in breathing during bicycle exercise. J. Appl. Physiol., 27:476–479, 1969.
29. Wasserman, K., Whipp, B. J., and Castagna, J.: Cardiodynamic hyperpnea: hyperpnea secondary to cardiac output increase. J. Appl. Physiol., 36:457–464, 1974.
30. Favier, R., Desplanches, D., Frutoso, J., Grandmontagne, M., and Flandrois, R.: Ventilatory and circulatory transients during exercise: new arguments for a neurohumoral theory. J. Appl. Physiol., 54:647–653, 1983.
31. Christensen, E. H.: Beiträge zur Physiologie schwerer körperlicher Arbeit, der Stoffwechsel und die respiratorischen Funktionen bei schwerer körperlicher Arbeit. Arbeitsphysiologie, 5:463–478, 1932.
32. Rowell, L. B.: Human cardiovascular adjustments to exercise and thermal stress. Physiol. Rev., 54:75–159, 1974.
33. Hermansen, L.: Oxygen transport during exercise in human subjects. Acta Physiol. Scand. (Suppl.) 399:1–104, 1973.
34. Ekelund, L. G., and Holmgren, A.: Central hemodynamics during exercise. Circ. Res., 20 & 21(Suppl. 1):33–43, 1967.
35. Asmussen, E., and Hemmingsen, I.: Determination of maximum working capacity at different ages in work with the legs or with the arms. Scand. J. Clin. Lab. Invest., 10:67–71, 1958.
36. Folkow, B., and Neil, E.: Circulation. Oxford University Press, London, 1971, pp. 170–198.
37. Sonnenblick, E. H., Braunwald, E., Williams, J. F., Jr., and Glick, G.: Effects of exercise on myocardial

force-velocity relations in intact unanesthetized man: relative roles of changes in heart rate, sympathetic activity, and ventricular dimensions. J. Clin. Invest., *44*:2051–2062, 1965.

38. Braunwald, E., Sonnenblick, E. H., Ross, J., Jr., Glick, G., and Epstein, S. E.: An analysis of the cardiac response to exercise. Circ. Res., *20 & 21*(Suppl. 1):44–58, 1967.

39. Bristow, J. D., Ferguson, R. E., Mintz, F., and Rapaport, E.: The influence of heart rate on left ventricular volume in dogs. J. Clin. Invest., *42*:649–655, 1963.

40. Donald, D. E., and Shepherd, J. T.: Response to exercise in dogs with cardiac denervation. Am. J. Physiol., *205*:393–400, 1963.

41. Van Beaumont, W., Greenleaf, J. E., and Juhos, L.: Disproportional changes in hematocrit, plasma volume, and proteins during exercise and bed rest. J. Appl. Physiol., *33*:55–61, 1972.

42. Astrand, P. O., and Saltin, B.: Plasma and red cell volume after prolonged severe exercise. J. Appl. Physiol., *19*:829, 832, 1964.

43. Buick, F. J., Gledhill, N., Froese, A. B., Spriet, L., and Meyers, E. C.: Effect of induced erythrocythemia on aerobic work capacity. J. Appl. Physiol., *48*:636–642, 1980.

44. Bye, P. T. P., Farkas, G. A., and Roussos, C.: Respiratory factors limiting exercise. Annu. Rev. Physiol., *45*:439–451, 1983.

45. Ekblom, B., and Hermansen, L.: Cardiac output in athletes. J. Appl. Physiol., *25*:619–625, 1968.

46. Kilbom, A., and Astrand, I.: Physical training with submaximal intensities in woman. II. Effect on cardiac output. Scand. J. Clin. Lab. Invest., *28*:163–175, 1971.

47. Saltin, B., and Hermansen, L.: Esophageal, rectal, and muscle temperature during exercise. J. Appl. Physiol., *21*:1757–1762, 1966.

48. Nadel, E. R.: Circulatory and thermal regulation during exercise. Fed. Proc., *39*:1491–1497, 1980.

49. Saltin, B., and Astrand, P. O.: Maximal oxygen uptake in athletes. J. Appl. Physiol., *23*:353–358, 1967.

50. Hurley, B. F., Hagberg, J. M., Allen, W. K., Seals, D. R., Young, J. C., Cuddihee, R. W., and Holloszy, J. O.: Effect of training on blood lactate levels during submaximal exercise. J. Appl. Physiol., *56*:1260–1264, 1984.

51. Holloszy, J. O.: Adaptations of muscular tissue to training. Prog. Cardiovasc. Dis., *18*:445–458, 1976.

52. Petrén, T., Sjöstrand, T., and Sylvén, B.: Der Einfluss des Trainings auf die Häufigkeit der Capillaren in Herz und Skeletmuskulatur. Arbeitsphysiologie, *9*:376–386, 1936.

53. Hermansen, L., and Wachtlova, M.: Capillary density of skeletal muscle in well-trained and untrained men. J. Appl. Physiol., *30*:860–863, 1971.

54. Anderson, P.: Capillary density in skeletal muscles of man. Acta Physiol. Scand., *95*:203–205, 1975.

55. Rand, P. W., Norton, J. M., Barker, N., and Lovell, M.: Influence of athletic training on hemoglobin-oxygen affinity. Am. J. Physiol., *224*:1334–1337, 1973.

56. Gollnick, P. O., Armstrong, B., Sanbert, C. W., Piehl, K., and Saltin, B.: Effect of training on enzyme activity and fiber composition of human skeletal muscle. J. Appl. Physiol., *34*:107–111, 1973.

57. Morgan, T. E., Cobb, L. A., Short, F. A., Ross, R., and Gunn, D. R.: Effects of long-term exercise on human muscle mitochondria. *In* Pernow, B., and Saltin, B. (eds.): Muscle metabolism during exercise. New York, Plenum, 1971, pp. 87–95.

58. Douglas, F. G. V., and Becklake, M. R.: Effect of seasonal training on maximal cardiac output. J. Appl. Physiol., *25*:600–605, 1968.

59. Mostyn, E. M., Helle, S., Gee, J. B. L., Bentivoglio, L. G., and Bates, D. V.: Pulmonary diffusing capacity of athletes. J. Appl. Physiol., *18*:687–695, 1963.

60. Anderson, T. W., and Shephard, R. J.: Physical training and exercise diffusing capacity. Int. Z. Angew, Physiol., *25*:198–209, 1968.

61. Bevegård, S., Holmgren, A., and Jonsson, B.: Circulatory studies in well-trained athletes at rest and during heavy exercise, with special reference to stroke volume and the influence of body position. Acta Physiol. Scand., *57*:26–50, 1963.

62. Byrne-Quinn, E., Weil, J. V., Sodal, I. E., Filley, G. F., and Grover, R. F.: Ventilatory control in the athlete. J. Appl. Physiol., *30*:91–98, 1971.

Chapter

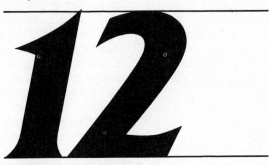

Metabolic Functions and Liquid and Solute Exchange

INTRODUCTION

The emphasis in all of the chapters in this book so far has been on respiration, which has been defined as the processes of gas exchange between an organism and its environment. The structure and function of the lungs themselves, the anatomy and physiology of the skeletal muscles of respiration, the control of breathing, and how these processes are integrated during exercise have been considered in detail. In this and the next chapter (Defense Mechanisms) some other important functions of the lungs that do not involve gas exchange, the so-called nonrespiratory functions, are reviewed. This chapter deals with the expanding field of information concerning the roles of the lungs as a metabolic organ, as an endocrine organ, as a site for the production or transformation of a variety of biologic substances, and as a site for the formation and removal of large quantities of liquid and solute. Each of these activities presumably contributes to the maintenance of physiologic homeostasis, although in many instances a full understanding of how and why

283

is lacking. Given these limitations, knowledge concerning the clinical implications of the nonrespiratory functions of the lungs, except for the formation of pulmonary edema and pleural effusion, is even more rudimentary; however, some speculations about these exciting subjects are offered when warranted.

METABOLIC FUNCTIONS

The lungs are made up of more than 40 different types of cells, each with its own resting energy requirements. The specialized functions of certain cells require "extra" energy to sustain such activities as contraction of tracheobronchial and pulmonary vascular smooth muscle, beating of cilia, bronchial gland secretion, transformation of chemical substances, and the synthesis of surfactant and connective tissue proteins. This section will consider the overall metabolism of the lungs and the metabolic pathways that underlie two of their most important synthetic processes.

Oxygen Utilization and Energy Production

The study of metabolism, whether of the whole organism or its separate components, begins with quantification of O_2 consumption. However, precise measurement of the O_2 requirements of the lungs is difficult, and the results using different types of preparations (isolated perfused organ, tissue slices, tissue homogenates, and isolated cells) are quite variable.[1] The technical problem stems from the fact that the lungs have two blood supplies (pulmonary and bronchial) and, most importantly, from the fact that they remove O_2 from the inspired air to supply the metabolic needs of the rest of the body. For this reason the tiny fraction of O_2 actually utilized by lung tissue is "lost" in the much larger quantity supplied for consumption by systemic organs.

Bearing in mind the uncertainties imposed by these technical constraints, the O_2 consumption of isolated perfused lungs of rabbits has been reported as 39 μL/min × g dry wt[2] and of dogs as 48 μL/min × g dry wt.[3] Measurements made from lung slices tend to be higher and much more variable.[1] The limited available data that permit comparison between the O_2 consumption of the lungs and other organs are shown in Table 12–1. When compared with organs with a high rate of O_2 uptake (heart, kidney, thyroid, brain, and liver), the lungs' utilization is much lower and comparable to that observed in intestine and resting skeletal muscle. From other available data, it is also possible to approximate the lungs' contribution to whole-body O_2 consumption, which has been calculated to be about 1 per cent of total O_2 expenditure in resting humans.[1]

Thus the quantity of O_2 consumed by the lungs is relatively low compared with that of other organs. But this generalization overlooks the fact that some cells (e.g., type II epithelial cells) may be much more metabolically active than others.

Substrate Utilization. The utilization of energy-producing substrates appears to be uniquely important for the lungs. This is because, in contrast with other organs, the lung parenchyma and smaller airways obtain adequate O_2 for their metabolic needs from the inspired air and are not dependent on O_2 supplied through the bloodstream. Thus, whether or not lung tissue death (pulmonary infarction) follows pulmonary arterial occlusion from embolization or other causes probably depends more on the interruption of a supply of substrates, such as glucose, fatty acids, and amino acids, rather than on an insufficient supply of O_2.[5]

Both tissue slices and perfused lungs are able to consume large quantities of glucose. However, the precise metabolic fate of glucose and its importance as a metabolic substrate are not completely established. It appears that glucose metabolism is central to

Table 12–1. COMPARISON OF O_2 CONSUMPTION OF VARIOUS DOG ORGANS STUDIED *IN SITU**

Organ	O_2 Consumption (μl/min · g dry wt)
Heart	283–788
Kidney	259–527
Thyroid	421
Brain	200–350
Liver	192
Intestine	54
Skeletal muscle (resting)	9–59
Isolated lung	48

*Data from Weber, K. C., and Visscher, M. B.: Metabolism of the isolated canine lung. Am. J. Physiol., *217*:1044–1052, 1969 and Altman, P. L., and Dittmer, D. S. (eds.): Biological Handbook: Metabolism. Bethesda, Maryland, Fed. Am. Soc. Exp. Biol., 1968, pp. 379–385.

energy production in the lung, although stores of carbohydrate are limited; furthermore, glucose is taken up by the lungs in quantities comparable to those in other organs, and it is metabolized by the usual biochemical pathways.[6]

There is good evidence that fatty acids can also serve as a metabolic substrate in lungs. The fatty acid supplies may derive either from plasma lipids or from intrapulmonary stores that, in contrast with carbohydrate stores, are sufficient to meet energy needs for several hours. Radioautography has demonstrated that the type II epithelial cell is extremely active in lipid metabolism.[7]

Surfactant Synthesis

The cellular source (Chapter 1), role in parenchymal support (Chapter 2), and contribution to elastic recoil (Chapter 4) of pulmonary surfactant have already been described. The term surfactant refers to the complex mixture of surface-active material (i.e., a substance capable of lowering surface tension), chiefly phospholipids and proteins, present at the air-liquid interface of the terminal respiratory units (see Table 1–4).[8] Given the physiologic importance of surfac-

tant, it is not surprising that compared with tissues from other organs, lung tissue is particularly active in lipid synthesis, much of which is directed toward the production of surfactant.[9] Many studies of surfactant formation have been done to examine the biochemical pathways that lead to the formation of dipalmitoylphosphatidylcholine (DPPC), because this substance is surface active and it is one of the principal components of pulmonary surfactant. It should be pointed out, however, that more than just DPPC is required to produce all of the remarkable surface-active properties exhibited by normal lungs.

Phosphatidylcholines are found elsewhere in the body, but those in the lungs are unique in that approximately 35 per cent are disaturated. Several possible pathways for the synthesis of phosphatidylcholine and its subsequent saturation in the lungs have been demonstrated *in vitro*, but which one or more are active *in vivo* is uncertain. Figure 12–1 illustrates some of the proposed routes for the synthesis of disaturated phosphatidylcholine.[10] As shown, phosphatidylcholine can be formed from either phosphatidic acid or CDP-choline. The last step is the remodeling of unsaturated phosphatidylcholine through the intermediary lyso-

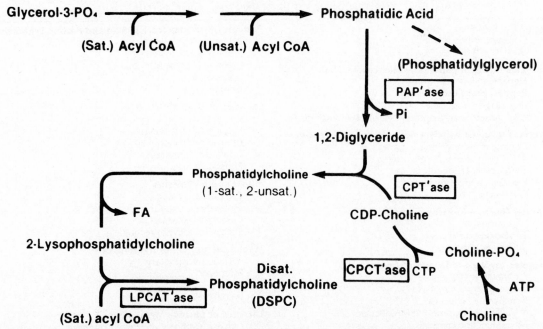

Figure 12–1. Route of synthesis of disaturated phosphatidylcholine (DSPC). Abbreviations used for enzymes: PAP'ase = phosphatidate phosphatase; CPT'ase = phosphatidate cytidylytransferase; CPCT'ase = cholinephosphate cytidylytransferase; LPCAT'ase = lysophosphatidylcholine acyltransferase. For discussion of pathways, see text. (Reprinted by permission from Rannels, D. E., et al.: Use of radioisotopes in quantitative studies of lung metabolism. Fed. Proc., *41*:2833–2839, 1982.)

phosphatidylcholine and the addition of a fatty acid by acylation of the CoA derivative to form disaturated phosphatidylcholine (DSPC in Fig. 12–1). Further details about the composition of surfactant,[11] the role of type II epithelial cells in its formation,[12] and the metabolism and regulation of phospholipid synthesis in the lungs are provided in recent reviews.[9, 13]

Protein and Connective Tissue Synthesis

The structural and functional complexities of the lungs are obvious; accordingly, they should be expected to contain a large number of diverse proteins. As shown in Table 12–2, the spectrum of proteins described in lungs can be subdivided into numerous functional types (for review and additional references, see Collins and Crystal[14]). Some of these proteins, such as the enzymes that participate in energy production, are also found in cells throughout the body, where they subserve general metabolic needs. Other proteins, such as collagen and elastin, are also found in other organs but often in different amounts from those that occur in the lungs. The apoprotein of pulmonary surfactant appears to be unique to the lungs.

Protein Synthesis. Protein synthesis begins in the nucleus and involves the transcription of specific regions of genetically determined DNA to form messenger RNA that is coded for the particular protein to be synthesized. Translation of messenger RNA and final assembly of the constituent amino acids occur on membrane-bound ribosomes in the cytoplasm. Each of the many steps of protein synthesis is under the control of a specific enzyme.[14]

Although all cells must synthesize proteins to some extent, autoradiographic studies of the lung parenchyma after the intravenous administration of radiolabeled amino acid precursors revealed incorporation chiefly in the cytoplasm of type II epithelial cells.[15] The free amino acids used in normal protein synthesis come from a variety of intracellular and extracellular pools as well as from protein degradation.[10] Recent data indicate that circulating amino acids are necessary for normal protein synthesis by the lungs[16] and that turnover is depressed during starvation.[17]

Connective Tissue Synthesis. Collec-

Table 12–2. THE SPECTRUM OF PROTEINS DESCRIBED IN THE LUNGS*

Structural Proteins
  Collagen, Types I–IV
  Elastin
	Proteins Involved in Nucleic Acid and Protein Synthesis
	  Adenosine deaminase
	  tRNA methyltransferase
	  Aminoacyl-tRNA synthetases
	  Histones
	  Uridine kinase

Enzymes Modifying Structural Macromolecules
  Heparin sulfate sulfotransferase
  Peptidyl prolyl hydroxylase
  Procollagen peptidase
  UDP galactose: glycoprotein galactosyl transferase
	Enzymes of Lipid Metabolism
	  Choline kinase
	  Lysolecithin transacylase
	  Choline phosphotransferase
	  Fatty acid synthetase
	  Phospholipases

Proteins Involved with Hormones and Active Peptides
  Angiotensin-converting enzyme
  11β-hydroxysteroid dehydrogenase
  Glucocorticoid receptors
  Prostaglandin synthetase
  Guanyl cyclase
	Mitochondrial Proteins
	  Cytochrome c & c_1
	  Monoamine oxidase
	  Cytochrome oxidase
	  Succinate dehydrogenase

Special Function Proteins
  γ-globulins
  Superoxide dismutase
  Surfactant apoprotein
	Lysosomal and Other Hydrolases
	  Alkaline phosphatase
	  Esterases
	  ATPase
	  Lysozyme

Proteins Involved in Drug Metabolism
  Alcohol dehydrogenase
  N-hydroxyamine oxidase
  Benzpyrene reductase
  NADPH: cytochrome P450 reductase
  Mixed function oxidases
	Enzymes of Glucose Metabolism
	  Glucose-6-phosphate dehydrogenase
	  Glycogen phosphorylase
	  Lactic dehydrogenase

*Reprinted from Collins, J. F., and Crystal, R. G.: Protein synthesis. In Crystal, R. G. (ed.): The Biochemical Basis of Pulmonary Function. New York, 1976, pp. 171–212, by courtesy of Marcel Dekker Inc.

Table 12–3. RELATIONSHIP OF LUNG CELLS TO LUNG CONNECTIVE TISSUE SYNTHESIS*

| Structure | Specific Cell Type | Collagen Synthesis | | | | Elastic Fiber Synthesis |
		Type I	Type II	Type III	Type IV	
Parenchyma						
	Types I & II	Yes	?	Yes	?	?
	Endothelial	Yes	?	Yes	Yes	?
	Mesenchymal	Yes	No	Yes	Yes	Prob
Blood Vessels						
	Smooth Muscle Cell	Prob	?	Prob	?	Prob
Airways						
	Chondroblast	No	Prob	?	?	?
Pleura						
	Mesothelial Cell	Yes	No	Prob	Prob	Yes

*Update from Hance, A. J., and Crystal, R. G.: The connective tissue of lung. Am. Rev. Respir. Dis., 112:657–711, 1975; Crystal, R. G.: personal communication, 1984.

tively, collagen and elastin are the most abundant proteins in human lungs, and there is more of the former than the latter. As described in Chapter 2, these fibers make up the connective tissue network that serves to support the lungs, contributes to pulmonary elastic recoil, and limits the extent of inflation. It is not surprising, therefore, that collagen and elastin are found in most component structures of the lungs, including the parenchyma, airways, blood vessels, and pleura.

The cellular sources of pulmonary collagen and elastin are shown in Table 12–3. As can be seen, in many instances the exact cell type responsible for connective tissue synthesis is unknown. Cells of mesenchymal origin, including smooth muscle cells and chondroblasts, are principally involved, but type I and type II epithelial cells and endothelial cells also contribute to collagen synthesis.

Of the more than eight kinds of collagen that have been identified in connective tissues, five have been detected in lungs. Type I is the most abundant and is found in most connective tissue; type II is present chiefly in the cartilages of the trachea and bronchi; type III is usually associated with type I; and type IV is a major constituent of basement membranes.[18] Small amounts of type V (not shown in Table 12–3) may be associated with type IV in basement membranes. The various types of collagen differ from each other in the amino acid sequences of the three alpha chains that comprise the basic tropocollagen molecule.[19] A schematic illustration of the steps in the biosynthesis of collagen is shown in Figure 12–2. As indicated in general terms previously, transcription of DNA to form collagen-specific

messenger RNA (mRNA) takes place inside the nucleus (step a, Fig. 12–2); subsequent translation of a particular type of alpha chain is directed by a distinct mRNA. Thereafter, collagen mRNA moves from nucleus to cytoplasm (step b), where translation (step c) and hydroxylation (step d) on membrane-bound ribosomes result in formation of a pro-α-chain of suitable structure for the type of collagen being produced. Stabilization takes place first by disulfide bond linkage and later by helix formation (step f). After glycosylation (step g), the molecule is secreted from the cell (step h). Tropocollagen, which is formed by enzymatic cleavage of the peptide extensions at each end of the pro-α-molecule (step i), is then free to polymerize with other tropocollagen, resulting in collagen fibril formation (step j). The fibril is subsequently reinforced by intermolecular and intramolecular cross-links to form mature collagen.[20]

Formation of elastic tissue involves the biosynthesis of two distinct substances, tropoelastin and microfibrils, which then combine to form an elastic fiber. These processes are illustrated in Figure 12–3A. The mesenchymal cell first synthesizes the microfibrils, which are elongated, beaded structures oriented in a semiparallel fashion. Sometime later, the same cell synthesizes chains of tropoelastin, which contain frequent lysyl residues. The enzyme lysyl oxidase converts some of the available residues to aldehydes to form the cross-linked product called elastin. The fully developed elastin fiber is formed when elastin invests the microfibrils. Figure 12–3B depicts the formation of a desmosine cross-link between two tropoelastin chains through the action of lysyl oxidase as described above. Other

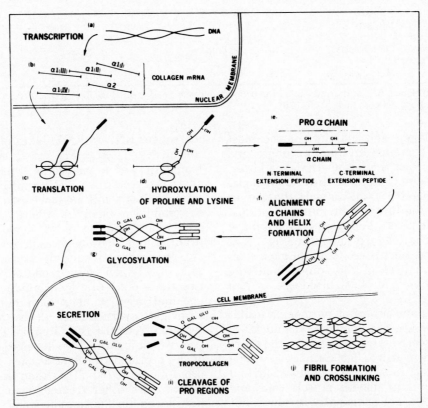

Figure 12–2. Schematic illustration of the steps in the biosynthesis of collagen. (a) Transcription of collagen structural genes in DNA results in formation of collagen mRNA; subsequent translation of each chain type is presumably directed by a distinct mRNA. (b) Collagen mRNAs move from nucleus to cytoplasm. (c) to (e) Translation of collagen mRNA on membrane-bound ribosomes and subsequent hydroxylation of some prolyl and lysyl residues result in formation of pro-α-chain. The pro-α-chain contains an N-terminal precursor region, an α-chain "helical" region, and a C-terminal precursor region. Under normal conditions, hydroxylation is completed near the time of release of newly synthesized pro-α-chain from the ribosome. (f) Three pro-α-chains of appropriate type are aligned and their association stabilized first by disulfide bond formation within the C-terminal precursor region and subsequently by helix formation of the α-chain portion. (g) Prior to secretion, some hydroxylysine residues are glycosylated with the monosaccharide galactose (GAL) or the disaccharide glucosylgalactose (GLU-GAL). Glycosylation of hydroxylysine begins during translation of the nascent pro-α-chain but may continue after helix formation. (h) The completed protropocollagen is secreted from the cell. (i) After secretion , the N- and C-terminal extension peptides are removed sequentially, which probably requires the action of two separate proteolytic enzymes. The resulting tropocollagen then polymerizes with other tropocollagens, resulting in collagen fibril formation. (j) The fibril is subsequently reinforced by inter- and intramolecular crosslinks. (Reprinted from Hance, A. J., and Crystal, R. G.: *In* Crystal, R. G. (ed.): The Biochemical Basis of Pulmonary Function. New York, 1976, pp. 215–271, by courtesy of Marcel Dekker, Inc.)

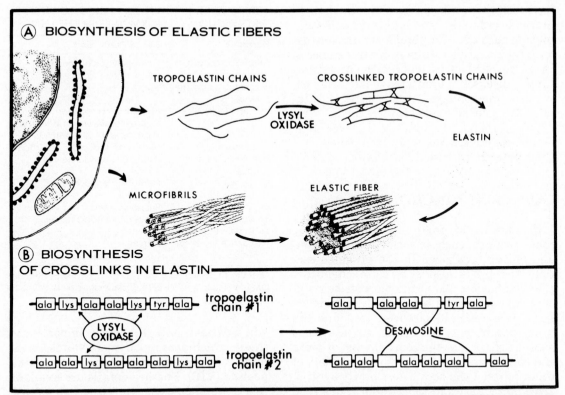

Figure 12–3. Biosynthesis of the elastic fiber and elastic crosslinks. *A*, A mesenchymal cell first synthesizes the microfibrils. These are elongated, beaded structures that lie in semiparallel array. At some later point, the cell synthesizes tropoelastin chains. The enzyme, lysyl oxidase, converts selected lysyl residues in the tropoelastin to aldehydes that subsequently form crosslinks. The crosslinked amorphous component (elastin) invests the microfibrils to form the mature elastic fiber. It is not known whether the conversion of tropoelastin to elastin occurs before or after the association with the microfibrils. *B*, An example of the formation of a desmosine crosslink between two tropoelastin chains. The lysyl residues are surrounded by alanine residues. Although it has been proposed that as many as four tropoelastin chains could be held together by a single desmosine crosslink, only the configuration shown here has, as yet, been demonstrated. (Reprinted by permission from Hance, A. J., and Crystal, R. G.: The connective tissue of lung. Am. Rev. Respir. Dis., *112*:657–711, 1975.)

types of cross-links have been described and are discussed in detail in recent references.[19, 21]

Clinical Significance. The normal aging process is associated with changes in the elastic properties of normal lungs (see Chapter 14 for details), which must be related in some way to alterations in collagen or elastic tissue. To date, no quantitative relationships between structure and function have been detected that explain the changes in elasticity. In fact during senescence, the quantity of lung elastin increases whereas the amount of collagen is unchanged; neither finding explains the constant decrease of elastic recoil that accompanies old age. Similarly, no changes in total collagen or elastin have been consistently observed in any lung disease.[20] These observations have led to the speculation that the normal age-related changes in pulmonary mechanics and the abnormalities that are found in pulmonary diseases such as emphysema are caused by local rather than generalized changes in connective tissue.[22] Thus, alterations in the extent of cross-linking may stiffen or relax collagen and elastic fibers. Furthermore, in diseases like interstitial fibrosis, remodeling of the lungs by changing the sites of deposition of collagen, not increasing the total quantity, may be responsible for the profound abnormalities of pulmonary mechanics.[23]

Many of the interstitial fibrotic diseases are characterized by increased numbers of fibroblasts, which are presumably the source of the abnormal deposits of collagen. Because the number of pulmonary mesenchymal cells is controlled, in part, by an *alveolar macrophage-derived growth factor,* studies have been carried out in patients with fibrotic disorders in search of a growth-stimulating substance for fibroblasts. In contrast with the negative results in control subjects, in 82 per cent of patients with interstitial lung diseases bronchoalveolar lavage yielded macrophages that were spontaneously releasing a growth factor that causes fibroblasts to replicate.[24] These interesting findings need to be confirmed, but their pathogenetic implications are obvious.

ENDOCRINE FUNCTIONS

In addition to producing substances for their own use, such as surfactant, collagen, and elastin, described in the previous section, the lungs also synthesize chemicals that can be detected in the bloodstream and that may affect the behavior of distant organs. It is difficult, however, to define the lungs as an endocrine organ in the classic sense of serving as the source of one or more internal secretions that regulate or control other parts of the body. Most newly synthesized pulmonary substances appear destined for local regulatory processes and those that appear outside the lungs may represent "spill-over" into blood or lymph. The present evidence indicates that the lungs synthesize substances that act directly on the cells that produced them in the first place (autocrine function), or adjacent cells (paracrine function), or on adjacent neurons (neurocrine function). Probably the earliest example of a true pulmonary endocrine function was the demonstration that the isolated perfused lungs of sensitized guinea pigs release histamine and slow-reacting substance of anaphylaxis when challenged with specific antigen. Other examples are the humoral syndromes that are caused by small cell or carcinoid bronchogenic carcinomas.[25] (It is of interest that the progenitor cell for these two malignancies is the Kulchitsky cell [see Fig. 2–6], which has also been called the pulmonary endocrine cell.) But these humoral events take place in pathologic situations and the role of the lungs as an endocrine organ in the maintenance of normal physiologic homeostasis remains to be established.

The humoral substances that are believed to be synthesized in the lungs, rather than being produced elsewhere and stored in the lungs, are listed in Table 12–4. This section

Table 12–4. KNOWN OR SUSPECTED SITE OF PRODUCTION OF HORMONES IN THE LUNGS*

Hormone	Site of Production
Adrenocorticotropic hormone	Pulmonary endocrine cell(?)
Arachidonic acid metabolites	
Prostaglandins	Alveolar macrophages, endothelium, fibroblasts, smooth muscle, type II cells, platelets
Leukotrienes	Mast cells, basophils, neutrophils
Bombesin-like peptides	Pulmonary endocrine cell
Calcitonin	Pulmonary endocrine cell
Histamine	Mast cell
Opiate peptides	Pulmonary endocrine cell
Serotonin	Pulmonary endocrine cell
Substance P	Nerves
Vasoactive intestinal peptide	Nerves

*Data from Becker, K. L., and Gazdar, A. F.: The Endocrine Lung in Health and Disease. Philadelphia, W. B. Saunders Co., 1984, pp. 7–24.

will consider only the most important of these: arachidonic acid metabolites, histamine, substance P, and vasoactive intestinal peptide (VIP). Further details are available in a comprehensive review that has recently been published.[26]

Arachidonic Acid Metabolites

The generation of arachidonic acid metabolites begins with the liberation of the parent compound through the action of the enzyme phospholipase A_2 on membrane-bound phospholipid (Fig. 12–4). This is not only the first but the rate-limiting step in the biosynthesis of all arachidonic acid products.[27] There are two major synthetic pathways through which arachidonic acid is converted to pharmacologically active substances: each of the pathways bears the name of the enzyme that catalyzes the initial reaction. The *cyclooxygenase pathway* generates unstable endoperoxides, from which the "primary" prostaglandins—PGD_2, PGE_2, $PGF_{2\alpha}$, PGI_2 (prostacyclin), and thromboxane A_2—are derived. The *lipoxygenase pathway* leads to the formation of 5-hydroperoxy-eicosatetraenoic acid (5-HPETE), from which the leukotrienes—LTB_4, LTC_4, LTD_4, and LTE_4—are derived. As indicated in Table 12–4, the major tissue sources of cyclooxygenase products are alveolar macrophages, fibroblasts, smooth muscle cells, and type II epithelial cells;

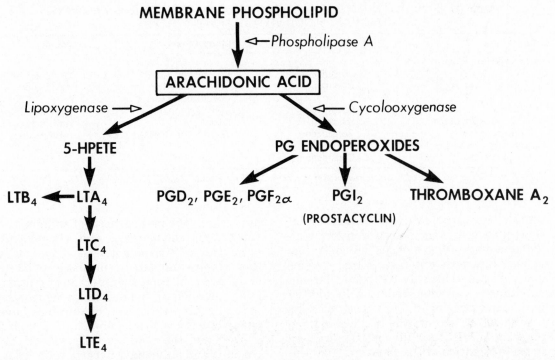

Figure 12–4. Pathways of arachidonic acid metabolism. Prostaglandins (PGD_2, PGE_2, $PGF_{2\alpha}$, and PGI_2) and thromboxane A_2 are generated via the cyclooxygenase pathway; the leukotrienes (LTB_4, LTC_4, LTD_4, and LTE_4) are generated via the lipoxygenase pathway.

endothelial cells are rich sources of prostacyclin, and platelets are active producers of thromboxane A_2. The most important cellular sites of lipoxygenase reactions are mast cells, basophils, and neutrophils. As will be emphasized in the next section, the lungs also serve as an important site for the inactivation of many of these products.

There is no doubt that the active products of membrane-derived arachidonic acid have remarkable biologic potency. But the regulation of the system is poorly understood. The physiologic consequences appear to depend on which cell types are activated and which enzymatic pathways are utilized. Not only are different tissues endowed with different enzymes that lead to the synthesis of various tissue-specific end-products, but disease states, injury, and stress may alter enzymatic activity and favor the generation of mediators not usually associated with a particular tissue. To complicate the problem further, there are important variations among species. An immense amount of work on arachidonic acid metabolites has been carried out during the last decade and several reviews of component subjects are available.[27-30] The following is a brief survey of

the actions of these lipid mediators on pulmonary tissues, with emphasis on the normal human lung when data are available; Table 12–5 summarizes the findings.

Cyclooxygenase Pathway. In general, prostaglandins of the D and F series are constrictors, whereas those of the E series are dilators. PGE_2 is, in part, an exception to this generality because, although it is a vasodilator in the fetus and newborn, it is a weak vasoconstrictor in the adult; PGE_1 (not shown in Table 12–5) is a potent vasodilator of the pulmonary circulation. Prostaglandins also have profound effects on platelet activity, some enhancing and others inhibiting aggregation. In contrast to the leukotrienes, which also act on pulmonary vascular and airway smooth muscle, prostaglandins neither increase vascular permeability nor promote chemotaxis.

Because arachidonic acid metabolites are not stored in tissues, their appearance reflects *de novo* synthesis in response to some sort of stimulus. Prostaglandins are released from the lungs during anaphylaxis, inflammation, hypoxia, pulmonary edema, and mechanical stimulation.[29] However, the precise role of these end-products in mediating the

Table 12–5. *IN VIVO* EFFECTS OF ARACHIDONIC ACID METABOLITES ON AIRWAYS, PULMONARY BLOOD VESSELS, AND PLATELETS*

Product	Airways	Blood Vessels	Platelets
Cyclooxygenase Pathway			
PGD$_2$	Constriction	Constriction	Unknown
PGE$_2$	Dilatation	Dilatation (Fetus)	Aggregation
		Constriction (Adult)	
PGF$_{2\alpha}$	Constriction	Constriction	No effect
PGI$_2$ (Prostacyclin)	Dilatation	Dilatation	Antiaggregation
Thromboxane A$_2$	Constriction	Constriction (weak)	Aggregation
Lipoxygenase Pathway			
Leukotrienes	Constriction	Constriction	No effect

*Data from Hyman, A. L. et al.: Prostaglandins and the lung. Am. Rev. Respir. Dis., *117*:111–136, 1978.

overall reaction to various stimuli is unclear. Because of the interaction of prostaglandins with other biologic cascades, such as the kallikrein-kinin and clotting systems, it is difficult to identify the particular contribution of a specific mediator. In addition to the conditions mentioned, prostaglandins may have a role in the pathogenesis of bronchoconstriction in allergic asthma[31] and in the adaptation of the fetal and maternal circulations during gestation;[28] their withdrawal after birth contributes to the closure of the ductus arteriosus in the newborn[32] (see Chapter 1).

Lipoxygenase Pathway. The principal products of the lipoxygenase pathway are the leukotrienes: LTB$_4$, LTC$_4$, LTD$_4$, and LTE$_4$. Of these, three are sulfidopeptide leukotrienes (LTC$_4$, LTD$_4$, and LTE$_4$) and comprise the mediator originally described as slow-reacting substance of anaphylaxis (SRS–A). Accordingly, these compounds evoke slow, sustained bronchospasm that is greater in peripheral than in central airways[33] and may play an important role in bronchial asthma. In addition, the sulfidopeptide leukotrienes have been implicated as a cause of the bronchial hyperresponsiveness that characterizes the asthmatic condition.[34] Bronchoconstriction and bronchial hyperresponsiveness may be quite separate phenomena, in view of the recent demonstration that there are at least two distinct sulfidopeptide leukotriene receptors.[35] The same leukotrienes mediate increased vascular permeability in certain tissues, such as guinea pig skin, hamster buccal mucosa, and human skin (see Lewis and Austen[30] for review and additional references), but their role in the lungs is uncertain. Leukotriene B$_4$ is a potent chemotactic agent and also has endothelial cell adherence activity.

In addition to probably playing an important role in the pathogenesis of asthma, the vasoactive, edemagenic, and chemotactic properties of the leukotrienes have made them likely candidates as mediators of many of the essential components of inflammation. Other pulmonary conditions in which abnormal concentrations of leukotrienes have been found are cystic fibrosis (LTB$_4$ and LTD$_4$)[36] and the syndrome of postnatal hypoxemia and pulmonary hypertension (LTC$_4$ and LTD$_4$).[37]

Mast Cell Mediators

The human lung contains abundant mast cells that have been identified chiefly within the bronchial mucosa and within the deeper connective tissues surrounding pulmonary venules. Some are also situated in the lung parenchyma, which is presumably the origin of the mast cells that are routinely recovered by bronchopulmonary lavage. Mast cells can be recognized by their characteristic granules, which stain metachromatically with toluidine blue for visualization by light microscopy and which have variable staining characteristics of electron microscopy (see Fig. 2–10).

Recently, it has been demonstrated that there are at least two separate populations of rat mast cells, presumably of distinct cellular origins, with different mediator products, receptor targets, and functions. Although less well characterized, human mast cells exhibit similar heterogeneity as shown by both functional and histochemical studies. Circulating basophils, which are a cell line distinct from mast cells, may be recruited to the lungs, where they participate in various immunologic reactions.

When stimulated by IgE-mediated immediate hypersensitivity reactions, mast cells release both preformed and newly generated biologically active substances. Rat mast cell granules, which are the most thoroughly studied, contain several preformed mediators: histamine, serotonin, eosinophil chemotactic factor of anaphylaxis (ECF–A), ECF-oligopeptides, high molecular weight neutrophil chemotactic factors, chymase, and macromolecular heparin (for review and additional references, see Lewis and Austen[38]). Stimulated mast cells also release newly synthesized mediators, including the sulfidopeptide leukotrienes, which are also called slow-reacting substance of anaphylaxis (i.e., LTC_4, LTD_4, and LTE_4, see previous section), a platelet-activating factor, and a lipid chemotactic factor.

Histamine. The best known and most thoroughly studied mast cell mediator is histamine, which has long been believed to play an important role in IgE-mediated immediate hypersensitivity reactions. Now it appears that other mast cell mediators are as important as or even more important than histamine in accounting for the full spectrum of pulmonary abnormalities encountered in human asthma. The biologic effects of histamine in an intact mammalian lung include increased airway resistance and contraction of airway smooth muscle, both of which are attributable to direct and reflex effects.[39] Histamine causes constriction of vascular smooth muscle, particularly in veins, and induces a transient increase in endothelial permeability.[40] The constrictor effects of histamine on smooth muscle are readily reversed by specific antagonists and dilator drugs. As stated (see Chapter 6), histamine is one of the leading candidates as the mediator of the pulmonary arterial vasoconstrictor response to hypoxia.[41]

Other Mediators. Much more is involved in bronchial asthma, particularly severe refractory asthma (i.e., *status asthmaticus*), than reversible contraction of smooth muscle and mucosal edema. Accordingly, mediators other than just histamine must be involved. Among these, recent evidence points persuasively at mast-cell generated leukotrienes[33, 34] and at neutrophil chemotactic factors.[42] Further advances in this rapidly expanding field can be expected to clarify remaining uncertainties.

Vasoactive Peptides

Normal mammalian lungs contain or may synthesize several vasoactive peptides (see Table 12–4). Many similar substances have been identified in the upper gastrointestinal tract; this is not surprising because both the lungs and the gastrointestinal system develop from the embryonic foregut. The physiologic action of some of the pulmonary vasoactive peptides has been established mainly through *in vitro* studies of various tissue preparations. Accordingly, the role of these substances in health and disease is speculative.

Neuropeptides. Pulmonary vasoactive intestinal peptide (VIP) and substance P are principally located in nerves supplying airways and pulmonary blood vessels; VIP has also been identified in mast cells from the rat (for review and additional references, see Said[43]). Whereas VIP relaxes airway and pulmonary vascular smooth muscle, substance P causes smooth muscle contraction in airways and blood vessels. It is also possible that both VIP and substance P may serve as neurotransmitters or neuromodulators in the lungs and other organs.

Other Peptides. Bradykinin may be formed in the lungs through the action of kallikrein on tissue kininogen; bradykinin is also inactivated in the lungs. Angiotensin II is generated in the pulmonary endothelium by the same enzyme that inactivates bradykinin. These two vasoactive peptides, which have opposite effects on both the systemic and pulmonary circulations, are considered further in the next section. A bombesin-like peptide, which has spasmogenic activity on airway and pulmonary vascular smooth muscle, has been identified in the Kulchitsky, or endocrine, cells of fetal but not adult lungs.[43]

Endocrine Cell Products

As shown in Table 12–4, the pulmonary endocrine cell is believed to synthesize several humoral substances. This cell has a variety of names but has been referred to earlier in this book as the Kulchitsky cell (see Fig. 2–6). The pulmonary endocrine cell is a member of the APUD (*A*mine content, amine *P*recursor *U*ptake, amino acid *D*ecarboxylase) family of cells that are also found in other organs and that share certain biochemical and histochemical properties. Pulmonary endocrine cells may occur singly or in groups called neuroepithelial bodies (see Fig. 3–17) in the epithelium of airways. For unexplained reasons, there are many more endocrine cells in the lungs of fetal and newborn animals than in children or adults. Both Kulchitsky cells and neuroepithelial bodies appear to be innervated, judging from the frequent presence of adjacent unmyelinated axons, although these are less common in humans than in other mammals.[44] Pulmonary endocrine cells may be the site of production of adrenocorticotrophic hormone or its precursors. These cells have been shown more convincingly to contain bombesin-like peptides, calcitonin, opiate peptides, and serotonin (for review and additional references, see Becker and Gazdar[26]). As is the case with other humoral agents known to be synthesized by normal lungs, the physiologic roles of these substances are completely unknown but possibly important.

TRANSFORMATION OF BIOCHEMICAL SUBSTANCES

Probably the first observation that the lungs are capable of removing vasoactive substances from the blood was made by Starling and Verney[45] in 1925; these investigators reported that they were unable to maintain adequate perfusion of an isolated kidney unless the lungs were in the circuit to remove a potent vasoconstrictor substance. It was not until 1948 that Rapport and coworkers[46] discovered that serotonin (5-hydroxytryptamine) was the likely vasoconstrictor substance, and seven years later, Gaddum and coworkers[47] demonstrated that serotonin was indeed inactivated during perfusion through the lungs. Important information was added during the 1960's, especially by Vane[48] and associates, who initiated a systematic study of the role of the lungs in the transformation of biochemical substances. Since then considerable progress has been made, particularly concerning the disposition of certain peptides, amines, steroids, and xenobiotic (foreign) substances within the pulmonary circulation (Table 12–6). However, it should be pointed out that these substances are relatively easy to measure in blood, and virtually no information is available about the processing of other hormones of interest for which precise functional assays are not available: parathormone, ACTH, gastrin, proinsulin, insulin, and C-peptide.[49] There is no doubt that much remains to be learned about the bio-

Table 12–6. SUMMARY OF THE FATE OF CIRCULATING SUBSTANCES DURING A SINGLE PASSAGE THROUGH THE INTACT PULMONARY CIRCULATION

Substance	Fate
Amines	
Acetylcholine	Uncertain
Serotonin	Almost completely removed
Norepinephrine	Up to 30% removed
Epinephrine	Not affected
Dopamine	Not affected
Histamine	Not affected
Peptides	
Bradykinin	Up to 80% inactivated
Angiotensin I	Converted to angiotensin II
Angiotensin II	Not affected
Vasopressin	Not affected
Arachidonic Acid Metabolites	
Prostaglandin E_2	Almost completely removed
Prostaglandin $F_{2\alpha}$	Almost completely removed
Prostaglandin A_2	Not affected
Prostacyclin (PGI$_2$)	Not affected
Thromboxane	Unknown
Leukotrienes	Almost completely removed
Adenine Nucleotides	
Adenosine triphosphate	Almost completely removed
Adenosine monophosphate	Almost completely removed

chemical functions of the pulmonary circulation.

Amines

Several vasoactive amines have been shown to be inactivated to some extent during a single passage through the pulmonary circulation, but several others are unaffected. Whether or not a substance is degraded depends not only on the presence of the necessary enzyme but also on the uptake or carrier system that permits contact between enzyme and substrate.

Acetylcholine. It was originally believed that the lungs inactivated acetylcholine almost completely.[50] The results of more recent experiments, however, did not confirm these findings (unpublished observations cited by Alabaster[51]). Thus, the role of the pulmonary circulation in the removal of acetylcholine must be regarded as uncertain.

Serotonin. When small amounts of serotonin are administered by continuous intravenous infusion, nearly all (as much as 98 per cent) is removed during passage through the pulmonary circulation. When serotonin is given by bolus injection, smaller amounts (as low as 33 per cent) are inactivated.[52] The removal of serotonin depends first on cellular uptake followed by rapid enzymatic degradation by monoamine oxidase. Of the two processes the rate-limiting step is uptake by the cell, which may be inhibited by drugs such as cocaine or tricyclic antidepressants. Cellular uptake and degradation of serotonin in the pulmonary circulation occur in endothelial cells, especially those within arterioles and capillaries.[53] Some serotonin is also taken up by platelets and neurons, but in these cells, in contrast with those in the endothelium, serotonin is stored in membrane-bound granules and not degraded. As mentioned previously, serotonin is found in pulmonary endocrine cells, especially those in neuroepithelial bodies. These cells synthesize their own serotonin and do not contribute to its removal from the bloodstream.[52]

Catecholamines. A good example of the exquisite selectivity of the pulmonary handling of vasoactive substances is shown by the catecholamines. Approximately 30 per cent of norepinephrine is removed by the pulmonary circulation by a process that depends on cellular uptake and enzymatic degradation by monoamine oxidase. In contrast, neither epinephrine nor dopamine is removed by the pulmonary circulation (*in vivo*), even though both are substrates for monoamine oxidase, and all three catecholamines (including norepinephrine) have been shown to be altered by passage through other organs such as the heart.[54] The location of preferential uptake of norepinephrine, like serotonin, is the vascular endothelium of the pulmonary circulation. However, evidence from pharmacologic studies suggests that the sites of removal of norepinephrine are distinct from those of serotonin.[55]

Histamine. As mentioned in the previous section, pulmonary mast cells and circulating basophils contain preformed histamine that is released in IgE-mediated immediate hypersensitivity reactions. Furthermore, mammalian lungs contain histamine-metabolizing enzymes. However, judging from the results of most of the studies that have examined the possibility, histamine is not removed from the bloodstream during passage through the lungs,[52] probably because there is no carrier mechanism that permits its entry into the cells and provides access to the enzymes.

Peptides

The biochemical transformations in the lungs that have been studied more intensively than any other are probably those of bradykinin and angiotensin I. This is in part because the reactions are carried out by the same enzyme, and in part because control of these two circulating peptides provides an opportunity to regulate systemic blood pressure.

Bradykinin. Experiments have revealed 80 per cent or greater removal of bradykinin during its passage through the lungs of several mammalian species.[52] Bradykinin is one of the potent endogenous vasodilator products of the kininogen-kinin system and is believed to play a role in inflammatory responses, hereditary angioneurotic edema, and neonatal circulatory adjustments. Bradykinin is inactivated in the lungs through the action of a dipeptidylcarboxypeptidase, which probably has free access to the pulmonary circulation because of its location on the luminal surface membrane of endothelial cells. The same enzyme converts angiotensin I to angiotensin II and is known as *angiotensin-converting enzyme.* Although the lungs contain other kinases, the action of angiotensin-converting enzyme is by far the most important and is the rate-determining step in the inactivation of bradykinin and other vasodilator peptides in the lungs.

Angiotensin. The decapeptide angiotensin I is formed in the bloodstream from an L-globin precursor by the action of the enzyme renin. Angiotensin I has relatively little vasomotor potency, but it is rapidly converted to the highly active octapeptide angiotensin II by angiotensin-converting enzyme. This enzyme is found to some extent in peripheral vascular endothelium, but its localization to the immense endothelial surface of the pulmonary circulation (Fig. 12–5A) causes more rapid conversion of angiotensin I to II in the lungs than elsewhere.[57] Furthermore, because the entire cardiac output flows through the pulmonary circulation, the lungs are the most important site of generation of angiotensin II. Angiotensin I may also be converted in the

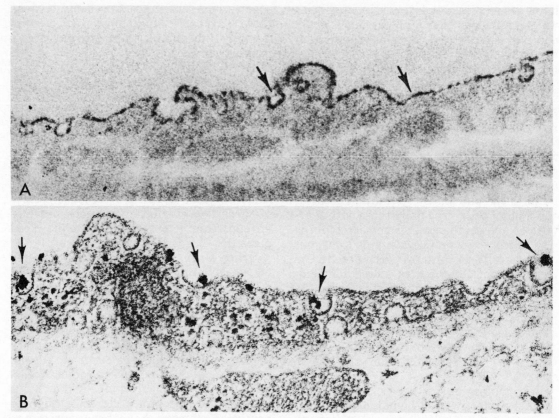

Figure 12–5. *A,* Section of rat pulmonary capillary endothelium prepared to demonstrate the location of angiotensin-converting enzyme. The electron-dense reaction product (arrows) is located on the plasma membrane and caveolae intracellulare facing the vascular lumen (original magnification × 76,000). (Reprinted by permission from Ryan, U. S., et al.: Localization of angiotensin converting enzyme (Kininase II), II Immunocytochemistry and immunofluorescence. Tis. Cells, *8:*125–146, 1976.) *B,* Cytochemical localization of 5′- nucleotidase in blood-free rat lung. Some of the pinocytotic vesicles facing the lumen of the vessel wall contain an electron-dense reaction product (arrows), which does not appear on other membranes or organelles (original magnification × 95,000). (Reprinted by permission from Smith, U., and Ryan, J. W.: Pinocytotic vesicles of the pulmonary endothelial cell. Chest, *59:*12S–15S, 1971.)

lungs to angiotensin III, which when compared with angiotensin II is more active in stimulating the release of aldosterone but less active in increasing blood pressure.[58] No appreciable metabolic breakdown of angiotensin II occurs in the lungs unless unphysiologic quantities of substrate are provided.

Other Peptides. Although endothelial cells in culture inactivate substance P, whole lungs do not. Neither do the lungs degrade or modify other vasoactive peptides such as vasopressin, oxytocin, and vasoactive intestinal peptide.[52]

Arachidonic Acid Metabolites

As described in the previous section, the lungs are an important source of synthesis of arachidonic acid metabolites, through both the cyclooxygenase and lipoxygenase pathways. As will be pointed out in this section, the lungs also have an important function in the inactivation of these products, although their degradation is highly selective.

Cyclooxygenase Products. Between 60 and 90 per cent of the vasoactive prostaglandins E_2 and $F_{2\alpha}$ are degraded during a single passage through the pulmonary circulation.[29] In contrast, prostaglandin A_2 (not a "primary" prostaglandin but a metabolite of E_2) and prostacyclin (PGI_2) are unaffected by the lungs. The fate of thromboxane A_2 is not known with certainty. The selectivity of prostaglandin removal is not attributable to enzymatic activity because the key inactivating enzyme, 15-OH prostaglandin dehydrogenase, does not have substrate specificity.[52] The selectivity of pulmonary removal appears to reside in the dependence on cellular uptake through a carrier-mediated, energy-dependent process, which can be suppressed by various pharmacologic substances. The localization of 15-OH prostaglandin dehydrogenase within the lungs is not known, but clearly it exists somewhere with access to the pulmonary circulation.

Lipoxygenase Products. All four leukotrienes (see Fig. 12–4) are inactivated by neutrophils, and the three sulfidopeptide leukotrienes (i.e., SRS-A) are also catabolized by eosinophils.[31] In addition, SRS-A loses its biologic potency during a single passage through the pulmonary circulation,[59] although the site and mechanism of this inactivation are unknown.

Adenine Nucleotides

The adenine nucleotides adenosine triphosphate and adenosine monophosphate are almost completely removed during a single passage through the pulmonary circulation. Cellular uptake is not necessary, and the relevant phosphate esterase enzymes have been shown to be situated preferentially in *caveolae intracellulare* that are often open to the vascular lumen (Fig. 12–5B).

Clinical Implications

The role of the lungs in the transformation of biologic substances is indisputable, and the pulmonary vascular bed is ideally located and equipped for metabolic functions. First, the lungs are interposed between the systemic venous and arterial circulations. This means that the lungs receive virtually the entire venous drainage and have access to all products elaborated in the body or absorbed from the gastrointestinal tract. Consequently, the lungs are strategically located to degrade or modify circulating substances and thereby control the composition of blood entering the systemic circulation. Second, the enormous surface area of the pulmonary vascular bed is enlarged even further by endothelial projections (Fig. 12–6A) and depressions, the caveolae (Fig. 12–6B). This immense endothelial surface is studded with superficial enzymes and equipped with carrier sys-

tems that allow entry of selected products for intracellular processing. Presumably, such an elaborate system that handles remarkably potent compounds would be expected to have important and discernible clinical effects. As yet, however, these have proved difficult to document.[63] Part of the problem lies in the fact that many of the substances that the lungs degrade are also produced in the lungs, where they apparently serve as "local" hormones. Furthermore, there are back-up enzymatic pathways in the bloodstream and other organs that can perform the same metabolic functions as the lungs.

The most obvious systemic function of the lungs' metabolic activities is in blood pressure control. However, although circulating levels of angiotensin-converting enzyme may be increased or decreased in various pulmonary disorders, there is no clear association between these changes and blood pressure. Complete inhibition of angiotensin-converting enzyme, although it lowers blood pressure in patients with hypertension, is certainly compatible with life, and no adverse consequences seem to appear. Enzymatic activity in the lungs is also known to be suppressed by hypoxia, hyperoxia, and certain drugs.[54] Although the contribution of the altered concentrations of vasoactive substances has been evaluated to some extent in animal models,[64] few studies have been performed in humans. Until more results are available, definite comment concerning the clinical relevance of the metabolic functions of the lungs is unwarranted.

Another activity of the lungs that is just beginning to attract the attention it deserves concerns the pulmonary uptake and disposition of therapeutic agents and other chemicals. It is clear from the limited data available that the lungs have an important role not only in the handling of natural endogenous substances but also of foreign exogenous substances (xenobiotics).[65] However, the clinical significance of the lungs' contribution to the pharmacology and toxicology of a steadily growing list of xenobiotics is totally unknown.

LIQUID AND SOLUTE EXCHANGE

Among the significant developments of the past decade are the results of investigations concerning both the anatomy and

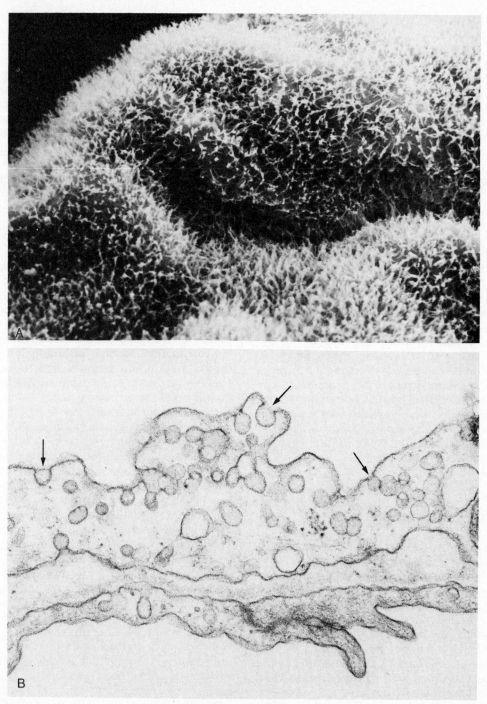

Figure 12–6. *A,* Scanning electron micrograph of the luminal surface of the pulmonary artery of the rat. Endothelial projections protrude towards the lumen with the effect of increasing the surface area of the endothelial cell that is exposed to circulating substrates. ($\times$ 3000.) (Reprinted with permission from Ryan, U. S., and Ryan J. W.: Vasoactive substances and the lungs: Cellular mechanisms. *In* Saldeen T. (ed.): The Microembolism Syndrome. Stockholm, Amqvist and Wiksell, 1979, pp. 223–232.) *B,* Transmission electron micrograph, showing a capillary endothelial cell with large numbers of caveolae. Caveolae may occur at the luminal surface and may be spanned by a delicate diaphragm (arrows). In section, vesicles appear to occur in the cytoplasm singly or fused in groups, or may show evidence of a supportive stomal ring. ($\times$ 47,000.) From Ryan, U. S.: Structural basis for metabolic activity. Ann. Rev. Physiol., *44*:223–239, 1982. Reproduced, with permission from the Annual Reviews Inc.)

physiology of liquid and solute movement in the lungs. These data provide a firm foundation regarding the basic mechanisms involved in the formation and removal of extravascular extracellular liquid in the lungs and how disturbances in these processes cause pulmonary edema (defined as an abnormal accumulation of extravascular liquid). The new formulation has resulted in a drastic revision of the old concept that the lungs are "dry" organs. Now we known that, in proportion to their weight, the lungs are as "wet" or even wetter than most organs in the body.

The principal site of liquid filtration under normal conditions is the pulmonary capillary endothelium, but arterioles and venules are involved to some extent as well. Collectively, the vessels from which the fluid is filtered are called the *microvasculature* of the lungs. Normally, there is net outward filtration of liquid, which cannot be measured directly in humans, but which is estimated to be 10 to 20 ml/hr in adults.[66] Normally, a similar amount is removed from the lungs through the pulmonary lymphatic circulation to prevent the retention of excessive liquid. Pulmonary edema nearly always represents an enhancement of the processes favoring liquid filtration, but it can only occur when the rate of filtration exceeds the rate of removal.

Anatomic Considerations

The interalveolar septum, it will be recalled (Chapter 2), is composed of several pulmonary capillaries that are supported within the septal wall and lined by alveolar epithelium on both sides (Fig. 12–7). Each capillary consists of a tube of endothelial cells supported by a basement membrane. The endothelium is primarily a thin cytoplasmic layer because nuclei compose only a small portion of the surface area covered by each cell. It can be seen in Figure 12–7 that the basement membranes of the endothelium and epithelium appear to be fused over about half of the capillary perimeter, but that elsewhere the two basement membranes are separated by an interstitial space that contains chiefly connective tissue elements and an occasional macrophage or fibroblast. The region where the basement membranes are fused is called the thin portion of the alveolar-capillary septum, or the

air-blood barrier, and because of its narrowness must be the chief location for the diffusion of gases into and out of the bloodstream; conversely, the region that contains the interstitial space is called the thick portion of the septum and presumably is the major site of liquid and solute exchange. This is a beneficial arrangement because, as can be visualized in Figure 12–7, the spatial separation of functions means that the interstitial space of the interalveolar septum may accommodate increased amounts of fluid without necessarily impairing gas exchange. Moreover, as will be discussed in greater detail later, physical forces exist that drain liquid from the interstitial space of the thick portion of the septum into the interstitial spaces surrounding conducting airways and blood vessels; this mechanism also serves to limit liquid accumulation in the terminal respiratory units and the possible interference of edema with gas transfer.

Adjacent cells in both endothelium and epithelium either abut bluntly or overlap each other and produce in both instances a narrow cleft between cells (Fig. 12–8). However, the results of both physiologic and anatomic experiments indicate that there is a difference in the permeability of the microvascular endothelium on the one hand and the alveolar epithelium on the other.[67] Part of the explanation probably lies in the complexity of the intercellular junctions of the two membranes. Ultrastructural studies using freeze fracture techniques have demonstrated that pulmonary endothelial junctions are composed of one or sometimes two strands, which may have a beaded appearance in some regions and are discontinuous in other regions (Fig. 12–9A). In contrast, epithelial cell junctions are considerably more complex and consist of an intricate network of interconnecting junctional strands (Fig. 12–9B). The junctions form a continuous belt-like region surrounding both type I and type II epithelial cells and resemble those described in other "tight" epithelial barriers.

The different rates of movement of small and large molecules through membranes are often explained by assuming that pores with varying dimensions exist; however, the anatomic counterparts of the postulated pore system in the alveolar-capillary membrane are not known and, at least in other organs, the pore theory failed to account satisfactor-

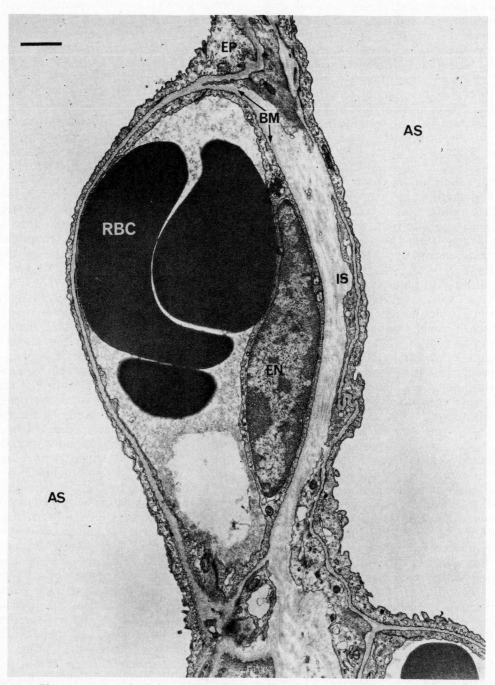

Figure 12–7. Electron micrograph of a human lung. Two capillaries containing red blood cells (RBC) are suspended in the interalveolar septum between two alveolar spaces (AS). The basement membranes (BM) of the epithelium (EP) and endothelium (EN) appear to be fused over the thin portion of the septum (or air-blood barrier) and are separated over the thick portion of the septum containing the interstitial space (IS). Horizontal bar = 1 μm. ($\times$ 11,000. Courtesy of Dr. Ewald R. Weibel.)

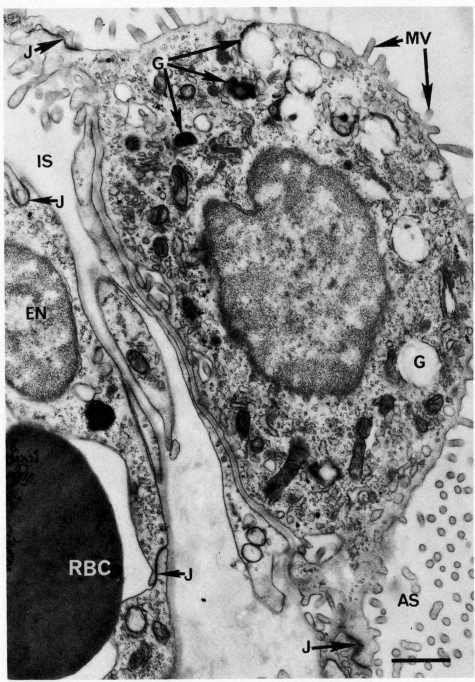

Figure 12–8. Electron micrograph of the alveolar-capillary membrane from an adult man showing alveolar epithelium composed of a type II cell, recognized by its characteristic inclusions (G) and microvilli (MV), that abuts type I cells at intercellular junctions (J). Two junctions (J) between adjacent endothelial cells (EN) are also demonstrated. RBC = red blood cell; IS = interstitial space; AS = alveolar space. Horizontal bar = 1 μm. (× 16,000. Courtesy of Dr. Donald McKay.)

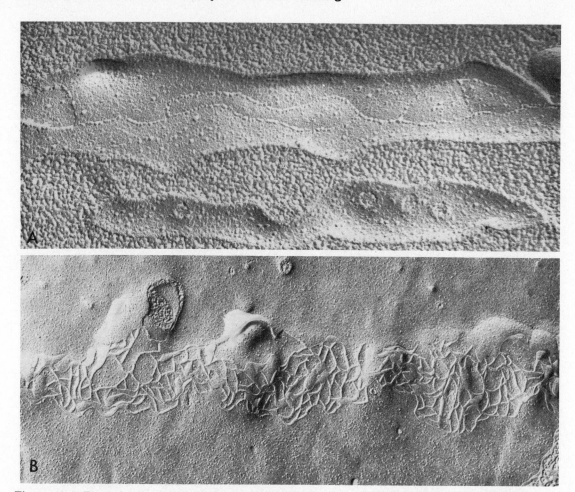

Figure 12–9. Freeze fracture studies of the intercellular junctions between (A) pulmonary capillary endothelial cells (original magnification × 118,000) and *(B)* alveolar epithelial cells (original magnification × 48,000). Note that the endothelial junction consists of one or two beaded strands, whereas the epithelial junction is composed of numerous interconnected and continuous strands. The complexity of the junctions reflects, and may determine, the relative permeabilities of the two cellular barriers to liquid and solute movement. (Courtesy of Dr. E. 6chneeberger.)

ily for the results of experimental studies of molecular transport.[67a] It is generally believed that liquid and solutes pass from the bloodstream into the interstitial space of the interalveolar septum through interendothelial junctions, which restrict the passage of protein-sized, lipid-insoluble molecules; thereafter, liquid is prevented from entering alveolar spaces by the presence of the relatively tighter interepithelial junctions. The transport of proteins and other macromolecules is poorly understood and highly controversial.[68] Ultrastructural studies clearly show the entrance of macromolecules into endothelial pinocytotic vesicles,[69] but the contribution of the vesicular system to overall protein transport is uncertain. Recent evidence summarized by Schneeberger[68] indicates that plasma proteins interact with the glycoprotein layer on the surface of endothelial cells to form another barrier that may be responsible for some of the molecular sieving properties of the endothelium. Not only is the alveolar epithelium a tighter barrier to liquid and solute filtration than the microvascular endothelium, but it is more restrictive to protein movement as well.

Once filtered, liquid does not accumulate in the pericapillary interstitial space of the interalveolar septum. Instead, liquid flows into the interstitial spaces surrounding airways and blood vessels where, as described in Chapter 3, the lymphatic capillaries are located through which liquid is removed from the lungs. The continuity between the perimicrovascular and peribronchovascular interstitial spaces provides the necessary pathway for the movement of filtered liquid from its site of formation to its site of removal from the lungs through the pulmonary lymphatics. As will be explained, there is a built-in pressure difference between the two spaces that provides the driving force that causes liquid to flow from one location to the other. As pulmonary edema occurs, substantial volumes of liquid accumulate in the peribronchovascular spaces, which can be viewed as a large reservoir that must first be filled before liquid overflows into the alveolar spaces. Although liquid is normally cleared from the distal peribronchovascular space by lymphatic capillaries, when edema accumulates more proximally around large airways and blood vessels, it is removed by the bloodstream, chiefly the bronchial circulation.

Physiologic Factors

The amount of extravascular liquid in the lungs at a given moment obviously depends upon the balance between the rate of formation of liquid and the rate of its removal. Net liquid flow ($\dot{Q}f$) across an endothelial barrier can be described by the classic Starling equation,

$$\dot{Q}f = Kf[(Pmv - Ppmv) - \sigma(\pi mv - \pi pmv)], \quad (1)$$

where Kf is the filtration coefficient, which describes the permeability characteristics of the endothelial membrane through which exchange occurs; Pmv and Ppmv are the hydrostatic pressures in the microvascular and permicrovascular interstitial spaces, respectively; πmv and πpmv are the colloid osmotic (oncotic) pressures in the plasma and interstitial liquids; and σ is the colloid reflection coefficient, a term that defines the effectiveness of the membrane in preventing the flow of colloid compared with the flow of H_2O. From the results of recent experiments, it is now possible to describe with reasonable precision the magnitude of the pressures that presumably operate within and around the microvasculature of the normal human lungs and hence that govern liquid and solute filtration; these are shown in Table 12–7.

Permeability of the Microvascular Membrane

Permeability in a biologic system denotes the ease with which substances cross membranes, including the pulmonary vascular endothelium and the alveolar epithelium. As stated previously, all molecules do not move across pulmonary capillaries with equal freedom; some are more selectively retained within the bloodstream than others. In general, low molecular weight substances cross more readily than those with high molecular weights, but lipid solubility, electrical charge, and molecular orientation are also important. In the Starling equation, the filtration coefficient describes the porosity, or leakiness, of the capillary endothelium for water. When the permeability of the membrane increases, the filtration coefficient increases, and the reflection coefficient decreases. Accordingly, more liquid is filtered at any given balance of forces across the membrane, and large molecules in the blood have freer access to the interstitial

Table 12–7. MEAN VALUES OF HYDROSTATIC PRESSURES (P), COLLOID OSMOTIC PRESSURES (π), AND REFLECTION COEFFICIENTS (σ) IN THE PULMONARY CIRCULATION AND IN THE PERIMICROVASCULAR INTERSTITIAL SPACE AND THE CONTRIBUTIONS OF ARTERIOLES, CAPILLARIES, AND VENULES TO OVERALL FILTRATION*

	Pulmonary Artery	Arterioles	Capillaries	Venules	Pulmonary Veins
Intravascular (mm Hg)					
P	14.0	11.0	9.0	7.0	5.0
π	24.3	24.3	24.3	24.3	24.3
Endothelium (mm Hg)					
σ	–	0.9	0.85	0.8	–
Interstitial (mm Hg)					
P	–	–5.0	–2.0	–5.0	–
π	–	10.0	14.6	15.6	–
Per cent of Total (%)					
Filtrate	–	7	66	27	–

*Modified from Staub, N. C.: Pathophysiology of pulmonary edema. *In* Staub, N. C., and Taylor, A. E. (eds.): Edema. New York, Raven Press, 1984, pp. 719–746.

space than when permeability is normal. Because the alveolar epithelium is normally much less permeable than the vascular endothelium, the liquid that constantly flows into the perimicrovascular interstitial space is prevented from continuing into the alveolar space.

It should be pointed out that the filtration coefficient does not include the dimensions of the membrane through which filtration occurs. If the surface area doubles and other conditions are unchanged, filtration will also double. Because of the complexity of the system, quantification of the permeability characteristics of the barriers to liquid and solute movement in the lungs in health and disease has proved extremely difficult.

Hydrostatic and Osmotic Forces

The values in Table 12–7 for intravascular and interstitial hydrostatic and colloid osmotic pressures are generalizations of data obtained mainly by micropuncture techniques in isolated dog lungs.[71, 72] Pressure in the pulmonary veins has been set at a normal value and blood flow through the vasculature has been adjusted to simulate conditions at rest. Thus the data are realistic approximations of the hydrostatic forces that act across the endothelium throughout the microvasculature. The other values will be commented on. It is clear from the Starling equation that the pressures on both sides of the membrane must be known to calculate the effective pressure, the so-called *transmural pressure,* serving to cause filtration.

Intravascular Forces. The data for the distribution of intravascular pressures (see Table 12–7) have been modified from those actually obtained by Bhattacharya and Staub[71] (see Fig. 6–7) for convenience of modeling. From arterioles to venules, hydrostatic pressure decreases from 11.0 to 7.0 mm Hg, which acknowledges that nearly half of the resistance to blood flow through the pulmonary circulation resides within the capillaries, and of the remainder, more resistance is located on the arterial side than on the venous side of the capillary bed. Note that the intravascular colloid osmotic pressure, which is mainly due to the effects of circulating proteins, especially albumin, is constant within all pulmonary blood vessels. This is because the small extravasation

of protein that occurs as blood flows through either normal or leaky lungs does not perceptibly affect the plasma concentration.[73]

Interstitial Forces. It should be mentioned at the outset that it is extremely difficult to obtain values for either colloid osmotic pressure or hydrostatic pressure within the interstitial spaces of the lung, particularly the narrow space within the interalveolar septum. Moreover, available values from measurements of interstitial hydrostatic pressure vary greatly, and there is no unanimity about which method is best for the purpose.[74]

The hydrostatic pressures shown in Table 12–7 were obtained by micropuncture studies.[72] No data exist on either regional colloid osmotic pressure or endothelial reflection coefficients, and the values shown are estimations based on the results of many other studies.[70] The slightly subatmospheric value of hydrostatic pressure reflects the contribution of the film of surfactant, which tends to recoil toward the alveolus (see Fig. 6–4). The derivation of the more negative pressure surrounding arterioles and venules has already been discussed (see Fig. 6–5), and direct measurements support the notion that peribronchovascular interstitial pressure is about the same as pleural pressure at low lung volumes and becomes more negative at high lung volumes.[75] It should be recognized that other techniques of measuring interstitial hydrostatic pressure in the lungs usually yield values that are systematically more negative than those shown in the table.[74]

The changing values of estimated interstitial colloid osmotic pressure reflect the fact that the osmotic reflection coefficient is also changing along the vascular endothelium. The data show that the arterioles have a higher reflection coefficient, and hence lower interstitial colloid osmotic pressure, than those that occur in veins, with the values for capillaries lying in between. The colloid osmotic reflection coefficients shown in the table are substantially higher than those directly measured for several proteins.[76]

To calculate the volume of liquid filtered at the arterioles, capillaries, and venules, it is necessary to know the filtration coefficient and the total surface area of each vascular bed. When these unknown variables are approximated, it appears that about two-thirds of the total filtrate comes from the capillaries, 27 per cent comes from venules, and only 7 per cent comes from arterioles.[70]

Lymphatic Removal

As already stated, once liquid has been filtered across the microvascular endothelium into the perimicrovascular space, it does not enter the alveolar spaces but instead flows into the peribronchovascular spaces from which it is removed. The continuity between the two interstitial spaces provides the necessary pathway for the movement of liquid from its major site of filtration to its site of removal from the lungs through the pulmonary lymphatics. The driving force for liquid translocation is created by the difference in hydrostatic pressures in the two interstitial spaces: the pressure in the peribronchovascular interstitium is always more negative (-5 mm Hg) than that in the pericapillary interstitium (-2 mm Hg).

The anatomy and some functional characteristics of the pulmonary lymphatic circulation are described in Chapter 3. The lymph capillaries provide the chief disposal mechanism for much of the liquid, virtually all of the proteins and other macromolecules and, at times, even particles.[77] It is believed that the filtrate that reaches the peribronchovascular interstitial space has free access to the lumen of the lymphatic capillaries, presumably through gaps between adjacent cells; the openings in the discontinuous basal lamina may facilitate vesicular transport of macromolecules.[78] But it is less certain how the liquid, once it enters capillaries, is forced into the lymphatic collecting vessels that have continuous walls and contain valves. There does appear to be a pressure gradient that favors lymph flow from the periphery of the lung to the hilus. As liquid accumulates in the interstitium and distends the bronchovascular space, lymph capillaries are not collapsed, as might be expected because of their delicate structure, but are pulled open by the tension exerted on the tethers that connect the outer walls to the surrounding connective tissue sheath (see Fig. 3–5).

Lymph flow in large collecting ducts seems mainly dependent on contraction of smooth muscle in the vessel walls,[79] but the propulsive force in smaller channels is less obvious and ventilatory movements and circulatory pulsations probably contribute. The bicuspid funnel-shaped valves throughout the lymphatic circulation ensure a one-way flow of lymph into collecting vessels. Although no data are available in humans, judging from observations in experimental animals, lymphatic removal capacity can increase at least five- to tenfold above basal rates.

Pulmonary Edema

A thorough discussion of the pathophysiology of pulmonary edema is beyond the scope of a book on normality. But since pulmonary edema represents an abnormality of one or more of the many processes that govern fluid handling in normal lungs, certain essential features will be briefly mentioned. As stated previously, pulmonary edema occurs *only* when the rate of filtration exceeds the rate of removal of liquid. There are certain disorders of impaired lymphatic function that are associated with clinical pulmonary edema, but these are rare and will not be considered. Accordingly, it is necessary to review only the two fundamental processes that cause increased filtration—an increase in net driving pressure and an increase in microvascular permeability—and the sequence of fluid accumulation in the various tissue spaces of the lungs.

High-Pressure Edema. The net driving pressure for liquid filtration represents the sum of the two pairs of transmural hydrostatic and osmotic pressures, which are often referred to as "Starling forces,"[73] shown in Equation 1. Transmural hydrostatic pressure normally serves to cause outward filtration, and transmural colloid osmotic pressure acts to retain liquid in the bloodstream. Thus, more liquid is filtered when intravascular hydrostatic pressure goes up,[80] as in heart failure, or when perimicrovascular pressure goes down, as when alveolar surface tension is increased.[81] In either situation, if the barrier function of the microvasculature is retained, the liquid that extravasates is unusually low in protein; the newly formed liquid either dilutes or washes out the proteins already present in the interstitial space, thereby increasing the transmural colloid osmotic pressure difference and decreasing the net driving pressure. For every 2 mm Hg increase in intravascular hydrostatic pressure there is approximately a 1 mm Hg decrease in interstitial colloid osmotic pressure.[80] In other words, half of the effect of increasing transmural hydrostatic pressure is offset by this mechanism.

A decrease in plasma protein concentration, with consequent lowering of intravascular colloid osmotic pressure, does not by itself cause pulmonary edema, presumably because the lymphatics can deal with whatever extra filtrate is formed. But the change does affect the hydrostatic pressure threshold at which edema accumulation begins, as shown by Guyton and Lindsey[82] and as illustrated in Figure 12–10. It is worth emphasizing that when protein concentration and permeability are normal, edema does not occur until intravascular hydrostatic pressure is raised to about 25 mm Hg; even though filtration must increase considerably at lower pressures, the lungs do not become edematous because of the dilution of inter-

stitial proteins and the availability of reserve lymphatic removal capacity.

Increased Permeability Edema. The other major category of pulmonary edema is that due to increased permeability of the microvascular membrane to liquid and protein.[84] Increased permeability pulmonary edema underlies the clinical disorder called the adult respiratory distress syndrome[83] and can be produced in animal models by a variety of experimental interventions. Common to all these situations is some sort of injury to the microvascular endothelium that allows extravasation of *protein-rich* liquid into the interstitial spaces and in many instances into the alveolar spaces. It follows from this discussion that the two basic types of pulmonary edema can be differentiated by the ratio of protein concentration in the edema fluid relative to that in plasma: high-pressure edema has a low ratio (<0.6), whereas increased permeability edema has

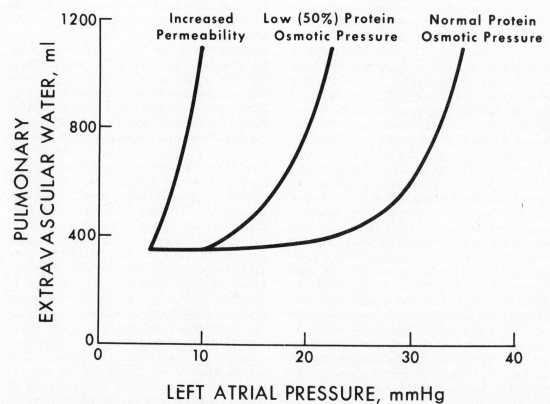

Figure 12–10. Relationship between pulmonary extravascular water content and left atrial pressure. Curve at right represents conditions of normal capillary permeability and plasma protein osmotic pressure; middle curve represents normal permeability and plasma protein osmotic pressure of 50 per cent normal; left curve shows relationship when permeability of capillary is increased, regardless of plasma protein osmotic pressure. Curves represent a conceptualization derived from data from multiple sources. (Reprinted by permission from Hopewell, P. C., and Murray, J. F.: Adult respiratory distress syndrome. *In* Moser, K. M., and Spragg, R. G. (eds.): Respiratory Emergencies. 2nd Ed. St. Louis, C. V. Mosby Co., 1982, pp. 94–122.)

a high ratio (>0.6).[82] Once the membrane is damaged and its permeability is increased, the amount of liquid filtered is extremely sensitive to changes in hydrostatic pressure. Small increases in intravascular hydrostatic pressure cause large leaks of fluid,[85] as shown in Figure 12–10.

Sequence of Formation of Pulmonary Edema. When filtration across the pulmonary microvascular endothelium increases, whether from increased pressure or increased permeability, some of the excess water appears in the pericapillary interstitial space. However, only a small amount of liquid is accommodated in the interalveolar septum because of the ease with which water moves from the pericapillary into the peribronchovascular interstitial space. The extra liquid in the interalveolar septum cannot be recognized by light microscopy and accounts for a gain in weight of the lung of only a few per cent. In contrast, substantial volumes of pulmonary edema can accumulate in the peribronchovascular interstitial space when the rate of filtration exceeds the rate of removal. This process produces the "cuffs" that are visible by light microscopy. The bronchovascular space can accommodate an increase in weight of up to 30 to 35 per cent of the lungs, which in the normal adult represents 300 to 350 ml of liquid.

Alveolar flooding occurs after both the pericapillary and bronchovascular interstitial spaces are filled and the rate of filtration continues to exceed that of removal. However, the actual site of the leak that allows interstitial liquid to enter alveoli is not known. What is known is that alveoli are completely filled with either liquid or air, except for small amounts of liquid in the corners of alveoli; partial filling and gas trapping are never prominent in histologic studies of edematous lungs. The most likely pathway for alveolar flooding is between or across epithelial cells, but no breaks in the continuity of the normally tight membrane can be demonstrated by ultrastructural studies. It has been speculated that the liquid flows peripherally from a leak or some site of communication proximal to alveoli, but this theory needs to be confirmed. Foam clearly means that air and liquid have intermixed, probably in airways. It should be emphasized that the presence of alveolar flooding with foam represents the last stage in the sequence of pathophysiologic events culminating in clinically apparent pulmonary edema. Because accumulation of substantial excess interstitial liquid precedes alveolar flooding, efforts at early recognition of pulmonary edema are directed toward detecting the stage of interstitial edema.

Exchange Across the Pleura

The pleural spaces lie between the mesothelial surfaces of the visceral and parietal pleuras in each hemithorax. Normally, the pleural spaces are empty except for a small amount of liquid in each cavity (0.1 to 0.2 ml/kg body weight),[86] which is spread out in a thin film perhaps 10 to 20 μm in thickness over the external surface of the lobes and which extends into the fissures. The layer of liquid is thick enough to prevent the visceral and parietal pleural surfaces from touching each other (Fig. 12–11), thus strengthening the notion that pleural surface and liquid pressures are similar (i.e., there is no loss of pressure from deformation at points of contact; see Chapter 4).

The parietal pleura receives its blood supply from systemic sources, which means that the average hydrostatic pressure in the parietal pleural microvessels is about 25 mm Hg. The most remarkable features of the parietal surface are the lymphatic stomata (Fig. 12–12) that communicate with underlying lymphatic lakes and that give rise, in turn, to collecting lymphatic channels.[87] In contrast with the parietal pleura, the visceral pleura is not of uniform thickness and has no stomata. The blood supply to the visceral pleura in humans is from the bronchial circulation, so that the average hydrostatic pressure in the visceral pleural microcirculation is probably only a little less than that in the neighboring parietal pleural vessels; the slightly lower pressure on the side of the visceral pleura occurs because much of the bronchial blood supply drains into the low-pressure pulmonary venous system. According to Staub and coworkers,[88] the principal function of the pleural spaces and the lubricating liquid they contain is not to couple the lungs to the chest wall but rather to facilitate rapid and extensive movement of the lungs against the chest wall.

The Starling forces acting across the pleural membranes are not fully known. The intravascular pressures must be about the same as in systemic microvessels elsewhere, with allowances for the vertical gradient of

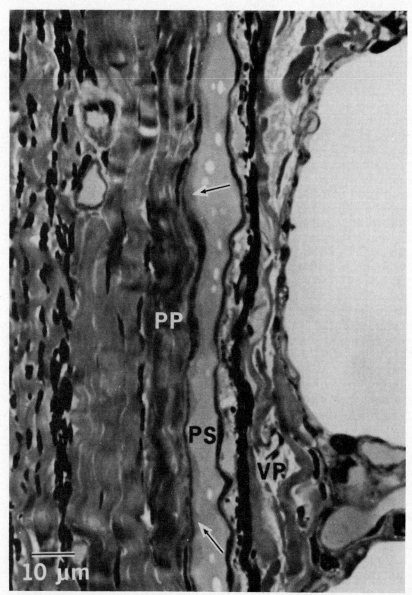

Figure 12–11. Light micrograph of a 1 μm thick section from a block of freeze-substituted tissue from a sheep, whose chest wall and lung were frozen intact. The mesothelial cells, with their bent microvilli (arrows), of both the parietal pleura (PP) and the visceral pleura (VP), are visible. Between these two cell layers is the pleural space (PS). Its average width is 10 μm; the opposing microvilli do not touch. The density in the pleural space is due to stained protein in the pleural liquid. (Reprinted from Staub, N. C., et al.: Transport through the pleura: Physiology of normal liquid and solute exchange in the pleural space. *In* Chretien, J., et al. (eds.): The Pleura in Health and Disease. New York, in press, by courtesy of Marcel Dekker, Inc.)

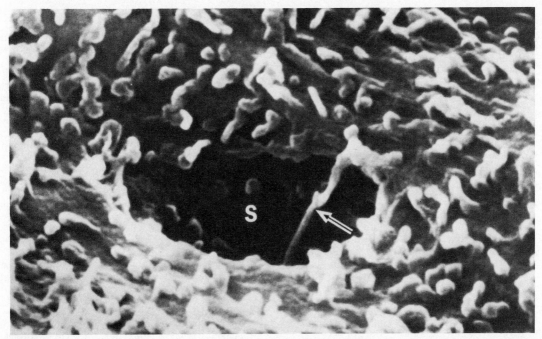

Figure 12–12. Scanning electron micrograph of a stoma (S) in the parietal pleura of a sheep. The stomata occur as openings in the layer of mesothelial cells, which have few, stubby microvilli. A cellular bridge (arrow) crosses this stoma. (× 14,820.) (Reprinted by permission from Albertine, K. H., et al.: The structure of the parietal pleura and its relationship to pleural liquid dynamics in sheep. Anat. Rec., 208:401–409, 1984.)

pressure in the thorax and the lower mean pressures in the bronchial circulation. The interstitial pressures are those in the pleural space itself: hydrostatic pressure varies as pleural liquid pressure, and colloid osmotic pressure is a function of the low protein concentration (1.5 g/100 ml). When approximations of these values are used in the Starling equation, it appears that there must be forces serving to promote filtration from *both* surfaces, but more from the parietal than visceral pleura. This analysis contradicts the long-standing belief that liquid is filtered from the parietal pleura and absorbed from the visceral membrane. Furthermore, if true, it means that there must be another site for reabsorption of pleural liquid: the lymphatic stomata could fulfill this function nicely. However, neither the new theory nor the conventional explanation is supported by the results of recent experiments that indicate that the *pulmonary* microvascular endothelium determines the rate of formation and composition of pleural liquid.[89] Clearly, we need to know more about liquid turnover in the pleural space under normal conditions before we can understand the perturbations that lead to pleural effusion in disease.

REFERENCES

1. Fisher, A. B.: Oxygen utilization and energy production. *In* Crystal, R. G., (ed.): The Biochemical Basis of Pulmonary Function. New York, Marcel Dekker, Inc., 1976, pp. 75–104.
2. Koga, H.: Studies of the function of isolated perfused mammalian lung. Kumamoto Med. J., 11:1–11, 1958.
3. Weber, K. C., and Visscher, M. B.: Metabolism of the isolated canine lung. Am. J. Physiol., 217:1044–1052, 1969.
4. Altman, P. L., and Dittmer, D. S. (eds.): Biological Handbook: Metabolism. Bethesda, Maryland, Fed. Am. Soc. Exp. Biol., 1968, pp. 379–385.
5. Tierney, D. F.: Lung metabolism and biochemistry. Annu. Rev. Physiol., 36:209–231, 1974.
6. Tierney, D. F., and Levy, S. E.: Glucose metabolism. *In* Crystal, R. G., (ed.): The Biochemical Basis of Pulmonary Function. New York, Marcel Dekker, Inc., 1976, pp. 105–125.
7. Darrah, H. K., and Hedley-Whyte, J.: Rapid incorporation of palmitate into lung: site and metabolic fate. J. Appl. Physiol., 34:205–213, 1973.
8. King, R. J., and Clements, J. A.: Surface active materials from dog lung. II. Composition and physiologic correlations. Am. J. Physiol., 223:715–726, 1972.
9. Mason, R. J.: Lipid metabolism. *In* Crystal, R. G. (ed.): The Biochemical Basis of Pulmonary Function. New York, Marcel Dekker, Inc., 1976, pp. 127–169.
10. Rannels, D. E., Low, R. B., Youdale, T., Volkin, E., and Longmore, W. J.: Use of radioisotopes in quan-

titative studies of lung metabolism. Fed. Proc., 41:2833–2839, 1982.

11. Clements, J. A., and King, R. J.: Composition of surface active material. In Crystal, R. G. (ed.): The Biochemical Basis of Pulmonary Function. New York, Marcel Dekker, Inc., 1976, pp. 363–387.

12. King, R. J.: Utilization of alveolar epithelial type II cells for the study of pulmonary surfactant. Fed. Proc., 38:2637–2643, 1979.

13. Rooney, S. A.: The surfactant system and lung phospholipid biochemistry. Am. Rev. Respir. Dis., 131:439–460, 1985.

14. Collins, J. F., and Crystal, R. G.: Protein synthesis. In Crystal, R. G. (ed.): The Biochemical Basis of Pulmonary Function. New York, Marcel Dekker, Inc., 1976, pp. 171–212.

15. Massaro, G. D., and Massaro, D.: Granular pneumocytes. Electron microscopic radioautographic evidence of intracellular protein transport. Am. Rev. Respir. Dis., 105:927–931, 1972.

16. Besterman, J. M., Watkins, C. A., and Rannels, D. E.: Regulation of protein synthesis in lung by amino acids and insulin. Am. J. Physiol., 245:E508–E514, 1983.

17. Rannels, D. E., Sahms, R. E., and Watkins, C. A.: Effects of starvation and diabetes on protein synthesis in lung. Am. J. Physiol., 236:E421–E428, 1979.

18. Prokop, D. J., and Kivirikko, K. I.: Heritable diseases of collagen. New Engl. J. Med., 311:376–386, 1984.

19. Hance, A. J., and Crystal, R. G.: The connective tissue of lung. Am. Rev. Respir. Dis., 112:657–711, 1975.

20. Hance, A. J., and Crystal, R. G.: Collagen. In Crystal, R. G. (ed.): The Biochemical Basis of Pulmonary Function. New York, Marcel Dekker, Inc., 1976, pp. 215–271.

21. Horwitz, A. L., Elson, N. A., and Crystal, R. G.: Proteoglycans and elastic fibers. In Crystal, R. G. (ed.): The Biochemical Basis of Pulmonary Function. New York, Marcel Dekker, Inc., 1976, pp. 273–311.

22. Sandberg, L. B., Soskel, N. T., and Leslie, J. G.: Elastin structure, biosynthesis, and relation to disease states. New Engl. J. Med., 304:566–579, 1981.

23. Fulmer, J. D., Bienkowski, R. S., Cowan, M. J., Breul, S. D., Bradley, K. M., Ferraus, V. J., Roberts, W. C., and Crystal, R. G.: Collagen concentration and rates of synthesis in idiopathic pulmonary fibrosis. Am. Rev. Respir. Dis., 122:289–301, 1980.

24. Bitterman, P. B., Adelberg, S., and Crystal, R. G.: Mechanisms of pulmonary fibrosis. Spontaneous release of the alveolar macrophage—derived growth factor in the interstitial lung disorders. J. Clin. Invest., 72:1801–1913, 1983.

25. Odell, W. D., and Wolfsen, A. R.: Humoral syndromes associated with cancer. Annu. Rev. Med., 29:379–406, 1978.

26. Becker, K. L., and Gazdar, A. F.: The Endocrine Lung in Health and Disease. Philadelphia, W. B. Saunders Co., 1984.

27. Said, S. I.: Pulmonary metabolism of prostaglandins and vasoactive peptides. Annu. Rev. Physiol., 44:257–268, 1982.

28. Mathé, A. A., Hedqvist, P., Strandberg, K., and Leslie, C. A.: Aspects of prostaglandin function in the lung. New Engl. J. Med., 296:850–855, 910–914, 1977.

29. Hyman, A. L., Spannhake, E. W., and Kadowitz, P. J.: Prostaglandins and the lung. Am. Rev. Respir. Dis., 117:111–136, 1978.

30. Lewis, R. A., and Austen, F. A.: The biologically active leukotrienes: biosynthesis, metabolism, receptors, functions, and pharmacology. J. Clin. Invest., 73:889–897, 1984.

31. Hardy, C. C., Robinson, C., Tattersfield, A. E., and Holgate, S. T.: The bronchoconstrictor effect of inhaled prostaglandin D_2 in normal and asthmatic men. New Engl. J. Med., 311:209–213, 1984.

32. Coceani, F., and Olley, P. M.: The response of the ductus arteriosus to prostaglandins. Can. J. Physiol. Pharmacol., 51:220–225, 1973.

33. Weiss, J. W., Drazen, J. M., Coles, J., McFadden, E. R., Jr., Weller, P. F., Corey, E. J., Lewis, R. A., and Austen, K. F.: Bronchoconstrictor effects of leukotriene C in humans. Science, 216:196–198, 1982.

34. Griffin, M., Weiss, J. W., Leitch, A. G., McFadden, E. R., Jr., Corey, E. J., Austen, K. F., and Drazen, J. M.: Effects of leukotriene D on the airways in asthma. New Engl. J. Med., 308:436–439, 1983.

35. Krilis, J., Lewis, R. A., Corey, E. J., and Austen, K. F.: Specific receptors for leukotriene C_4 on a smooth muscle cell line. J. Clin. Invest., 72:1516–1517, 1983.

36. Cromwell, O., Walport, M. J., Morris, H. R., Taylor, G. W., Hodson, M. E., Batten, J., and Kay, A. B.: Identification of leukotrienes D and B in sputum from cystic fibrosis patients. Lancet, 2:164–165, 1981.

37. Stenmark, K. R., James, S. L., Voelkel, N. F., Toews, W. H., Reeves, J. T., and Murphy, R. C.: Leukotrienes C_4 and D_4 in neonates with hypoxemia and pulmonary hypertension. New Engl. J. Med., 309:77–80, 1983.

38. Lewis, R. A., and Austen, K. F.: Nonrespiratory functions of pulmonary cells: the mast cell. Fed. Proc., 36:2676–2683, 1977.

39. Nadel, J. A.: Autonomic regulation of airway smooth muscle. In Nadel, J. A. (ed.): Physiology and Pharmacology of the Airways. New York, Marcel Dekker, Inc., 1980, pp. 217–257.

40. Brigham, K. L., and Owen, P. J.: Increased sheep lung vascular permeability caused by histamine. Circ. Res., 37:647–657, 1975.

41. Fishman, A. P.: Vasomotor regulation of the pulmonary circulation. Annu. Rev. Physiol., 42:211–220, 1980.

42. Lee, T. H., Nagakura, T., Papageorgiou, N., Iikura, Y., and Kay, A. B.: Exercise-induced late asthmatic reactions with neutrophil chemotactic activity. New Engl. J. Med., 308:1502–1505, 1983.

43. Said, S. I.: Pulmonary metabolism of prostaglandins and vasoactive peptides. Annu. Rev. Physiol., 44:257–268, 1982.

44. Lauweryns, J. M., Peuskens, J. C., and Cokelaere, M.: Argyrophil, fluorescent and granulated (peptide and amine producing?) AFG cells in human infant bronchial epithelium. Light and electron microscopic studies. Life Sci., 9:1417–1429, 1970.

45. Starling, E. H., and Verney, E. B.: The secretion of urine as studied in the isolated kidney. Proc. R. Soc. Lond. (Biol.), 97:321–363, 1925.

46. Rapport, M. M., Greene, A. A., and Page, I. H.:

Serum vasoconstrictor (serotonin). J. Biol. Chem., *176*:1243–1251, 1948.

47. Gaddum, J. H., Hibb, C. O., Silver, A., and Swan, A. A. B.: 5-hydroxytryptamine. Pharmacological action and destruction in perfused lungs. Q. J. Exp. Physiol., *38*:255–262, 1953.

48. Vane, J. R.: The release and fate of vasoactive hormones in the circulation. Brit. J. Pharmacol., *35*:209–242, 1969.

49. Ryan, J. W.: Processing of endogenous polypeptides by the lungs. Annu. Rev. Physiol., *44*:241–255, 1982.

50. Eiseman, B., Bryant, L., and Waltuch, T.: Metabolism of vasomotor agents by the isolated perfused lung. J. Thorac. Cardiovasc. Surg., *48*:798–806, 1964.

51. Alabaster, V. A.: Inactivation of endogenous amines in the lungs. *In* Bakhle, Y. S., and Vane, J. R. (eds.): Metabolic Functions of the Lung. New York, Marcel Dekker, Inc., 1977, pp. 3–31.

52. Said, S. I.: Metabolic functions of the pulmonary circulation. Circ. Res., *50*:325–333, 1982.

53. Strum, J. M., and Junod, A. F.: Radioautographic demonstration of ^{3}H-5-hydroxytryptamine uptake by pulmonary endothelial cells. J. Cell. Biol., *54*:456–467, 1972.

54. Gillis, C. N., and Pitt, B. R.: The fate of circulating amines within the pulmonary circulation. Annu. Rev. Physiol., *44*:268–281, 1982.

55. Iwasawa, Y., and Gillis, C. N.: Pharmacological analysis of norepinephrine and 5-hydroxytryptamine removal from the pulmonary circulation: differentiation of uptake sites for each amine. J. Pharmacol. Exp. Ther., *188*:386–393, 1974.

56. Ryan, U. S., Ryan, J. W., Whitaker, C., and Chin, A.: Localization of angiotensin converting enzyme (Kininase II), II. Immunocytochemistry and immunofluorescence. Tissue Cell, *8*:125–146, 1976.

57. Longenecker, G. L., and Huggins, C. G.: Biochemistry of the pulmonary angiotensin-converting enzyme. *In* Bakhle, Y. S., and Vane, J. R. (eds.): Metabolic Functions of the Lung. New York, Marcel Dekker, Inc., 1977, pp. 55–83.

58. Ryan, J. W., and Ryan, U. S.: Pulmonary endothelial cells. Fed. Proc., *36*:2683–2691, 1977.

59. Piper, P. J., Tippins, J. R., Samhoun, M. N., Morris, H. R., Taylor, G. W., and Jones, C. M.: SRS-A and its formation by the lung. Bull. Eur. Physiopathol. Respir. *17*:571–583, 1981.

60. Smith, U., and Ryan, J. W.: Pinocytotic vesicles of the pulmonary endothelial cell. Chest, *59*:12S–15S, 1971.

61. Ryan, U. S., and Ryan, J. W.: Vasoactive substances and the lungs: cellular mechanisms. *In* Saldeen, T. (ed.): The Microembolism Syndrome. Stockholm, Amqvist and Wiksell, 1979, pp. 223–232.

62. Ryan, U. S.: Structural basis for metabolic activity. Annu. Rev. Physiol., *44*:223–239, 1982.

63. Block, E. R., and Stalcup, S. A.: Metabolic functions of the lung. Of what clinical relevance? Chest, *81*:215–223, 1982.

64. Pitt, B. R.: Metabolic functions of the lung and systemic vasoregulation. Fed. Proc., *43*:2573–2574, 1984.

65. Brandenburger-Brown, E. A.: The localization, metabolism and effects of drugs and toxicants in the lung. Drug Metab. Rev., *3*:33–87, 1974.

66. Staub, N. C.: Pulmonary edema. Physiologic approaches to management. Chest, *74*:559–564, 1978.

67. Schneeberger, E. E.: Structural basis for some permeability properties of the air-blood barrier. Fed. Proc., *37*:2471–2478, 1978.

67a. Renkin, E. M.: Capillary transport of macromolecules: pores and other endothelial pathways. J. Appl. Physiol., *58*:315–325, 1985.

68. Schneeberger, E. E.: Proteins and vesicular transport in capillary endothelium. Fed. Proc., *42*:2419–2424, 1983.

69. Palade, G. E., Simionescu, M., and Simionescu, N.: Structural aspects of the permeability of the microvascular endothelium. Acta Physiol. Scand. (Suppl.), *463*:11–32, 1979.

70. Staub, N. C.: Pathophysiology of pulmonary edema. *In* Staub, N. C., and Taylor, A. E. (eds.): Edema. New York, Raven Press, 1984, pp. 719–746.

71. Bhattacharya, J., and Staub, N. C.: Direct measurements of microvascular pressures in the isolated perfused dog lung. Science, *210*:327–328, 1980.

72. Bhattacharya, J., Gropper, M. A., and Staub, N. C.: Interstitial fluid pressure gradient measured by micropuncture in excised dog lung. J. Appl. Physiol., *56*:271–277, 1984.

73. Staub, N. C.: The pathogenesis of pulmonary edema. Prog. Cardiovasc. Dis., *23*:52–80, 1980.

74. Parker, J. C., and Taylor, A. E.: Comparison of capsular and intra-alveolar fluid pressures in the lung. J. Appl. Physiol., *52*:1444–1452, 1982.

75. Lai-Fook, S. J.: Perivascular interstitial fluid pressure measured by micropipettes in isolated dog lung. J. Appl. Physiol., *52*:9–15, 1982.

76. Parker, J. C., Parker, R. E., Granger, D. N., and Taylor, A. E.: Vascular permeability and transvascular fluid and protein transport in dog lung. Circ. Res., *48*:549–561, 1981.

77. Lauweryns, J. M., and Baert, J. H.: State of the art. Alveolar clearance and the role of the pulmonary lymphatics. Am. Rev. Respir. Dis., *115*:625–683, 1977.

78. Leak, L. V.: The structure of lymphatic capillaries in lymph formation. Fed. Proc., *35*:1863–1871, 1976.

79. Reddy, N. P., and Staub, N. C.: Intrinsic propulsive activity of thoracic duct perfused in anesthetized dogs. Microvasc. Res., *21*:183–192, 1981.

80. Erdmann, A. J., III., Vaughan, T. R., Jr., Brigham, K. L., Woolverton, W. C., and Staub, N. C.: Effect of increased vascular pressure on lung fluid balance in unanesthetized sheep. Circ. Res., *37*:271–284, 1975.

81. Albert, R. K., Lakshminarayan, S., Hildebrandt, J., Kirk, W., and Butler, J.: Increased surface tension favors pulmonary edema formation in anesthetized dogs' lungs. J. Clin. Invest., *63*:1015–1018, 1979.

82. Guyton, A. C., and Lindsey, A. W.: Effect of elevated left atrial pressure and decreased plasma protein concentration on the development of pulmonary edema. Circ. Res., *7*:649–657, 1959.

83. Hopewell, P. C., and Murray, J. F.: Adult respiratory distress syndrome. *In* Moser, K. M., and Spragg, R. G. (eds.): Respiratory Emergencies. St. Louis, 2nd. Ed., C. V. Mosby Co., 1982, pp. 94–122.

84. Staub, N. C.: Pulmonary edema due to increased microvascular permeability to fluid and protein. Circ. Res., *43*:143–151, 1978.

85. Huchon, G. J., Hopewell, P. C., and Murray, J. F.: Interactions between permeability and hydrostatic pressure in perfused dogs' lungs. J. Appl. Physiol., 50:905–911, 1981.
86. Wiener-Kronish, J. P., Albertine, K. G., Licko, V., and Staub, N. C.: Protein egress and entry rates in pleural fluid and plasma in sheep. J. Appl. Physiol., 56:459–463, 1984.
87. Albertine, K. H., Wiener-Kronish, J. P., and Staub, N. C.: The structure of the parietal pleura and its relationship to pleural liquid dynamics in sheep. Anat. Rec., 208:401–409, 1984.
88. Staub, N. C., Wiener-Kronish, J. P., and Albertine, K. H.: Transport through the pleura: physiology of normal liquid and solute exchange in the pleural space. In Chretien, J., Bignon, J., Hirsch, A., and Huchon, G. J. (eds.): The Pleura in Health and Disease. New York, Marcel Dekker, Inc., (in press).
89. Kinasewitz, G. T., Groome, L. J., Marshall, R. P., and Diana, J. N.: Permeability of the canine visceral pleura. J. Appl. Physiol., 55:121–130, 1983.

Chapter

13

Defense
Mechanisms

INTRODUCTION

The body is in direct contact with its external environment through the air inhaled during breathing. Each day the tracheobronchial tree and terminal respiratory units are exposed to more than 10,000 L of ambient air that may contain infectious microorganisms and hazardous dusts or chemicals. There is no doubt that a wide variety of pulmonary or systemic infections, inflammatory lung disorders, and malignancies may result from airborne exposure. There is also no double that, for the most part, the lungs are able to prevent the development of disease. The medical and socioeconomic importance of inhalation pulmonary diseases has resulted in a large amount of research on how the lungs defend themselves against the continuous onslaught of the various noxious substances it may encounter during normal breathing. A large amount of valuable information has resulted from these investigations, and it is now possible to assemble the various elements that contribute to pulmonary defenses and to understand how the lungs resist development of disease from infectious agents, chemicals, physical injury, immunologic phenomena, and neoplasia. In addition, insight has been gained into how specific defects in the lungs' defense mechanisms lead to pulmonary injury and disease.

The separate roles of the numerous components of the system of defenses that interact to protect the lungs and the rest of the body against injury and disease are too complex (and often poorly understood) to review in detail here. This chapter will consider briefly the main determinants that affect the outcome of the battle between the beleaguered human host, who is constantly being challenged in the process of breathing, and an endless array of potentially harmful microorganisms and chemical substances. Thus, it is necessary to examine how certain particles and vapors are removed from the airstream within the normal respiratory tract, and once deposited, how some substances are handled by nonspecific (i.e., nonimmunologic) defense mechanisms of the respiratory tract and others are handled by cell-mediated and antibody-mediated immunologic responses. The components of the nonspecific and immunologic defense mechanisms that will be considered successively in this chapter are given in Table 13–1.

A distinction should be made between use of the general term *immunity* and the specific term *immunologic*. Immunity means a condition of being exempt from injury or harmful influences (diseases, taxes, military conscription), and immunologic denotes highly specific biologic phenomena characterized by recall or memory and the capability of mounting an anamnestic reaction.

DEPOSITION OF PARTICLES AND VAPORS

To have an effect in the lungs or the rest of the body, inhaled substances must first of all be removed from the airstream by either depositing on the mucosal surface or dissolving in the epithelial lining. This section will consider the factors that affect the deposition and uptake of particles and vapors in the respiratory tract.

Aerosols

The term aerosol is used to describe any system of liquid droplets or solid particles dispersed in air (or some other gas) that remains airborne for a reasonable length of time.[1] The essential requirements of an aerosol are for the particles to be so small that they settle slowly and for the aerial suspension to be stable. Because large particles tend to settle rapidly, clinically important aerosols, whether industrial, natural, or therapeutic, are composed mainly of particles less than 10 μm in diameter.

Particles are removed from the airstream the instant they contact any portion of the lining of the respiratory tract. Furthermore, once a particle has touched the epithelial surface, it ordinarily is not resuspended in the airstream and must be cleared from the body by some other means. The three principal forces that govern the deposition of particles in the airways and airspaces—inertia, sedimentation, and diffusion—are illustrated in Figure 13–1.[2] The effects of charge and interception are much less important and will not be considered.

Inertia. During inhalation, particles are forced to change their directions repeatedly as they travel through the numerous curves and branches in the nasopharynx and tracheobronchial tree. However, once in motion, a particle tends to move in the same direction, owing to inertial forces. This means that if a particle continues in its original direction when it should turn, it

Table 13–1. MECHANISMS THAT CONTRIBUTE TO THE DEFENSE OF THE RESPIRATORY TRACT

Nonspecific defense mechanisms
  Clearance
    Nasal clearance
    Tracheobronchial clearance
    Alveolar clearance
  Secretions
    Tracheobronchial lining (mucus)
    Alveolar lining (surfactant)
    Lysozyme
    Interferon
    Complement
  Cellular defenses
    Nonphagocytic
      Airway epithelium
      Terminal respiratory epithelium
    Phagocytic
      Blood phagocytes (polymorphonuclear neutrophilic leukocytes, monocytes)
      Tissue phagocytes (alveolar macrophages)
  Biochemical defenses
    Antiproteolytic enzymes
    Antioxidants
Specific defense (immunologic) mechanisms
  Antibody-mediated (B lymphocyte–dependent) immunologic responses
    Serum immunoglobulins
    Secretory immunoglobulins
  Cell-mediated (T lymphocyte–dependent) immunologic responses
    Lymphokine-mediated
    Direct cellular cytotoxicity

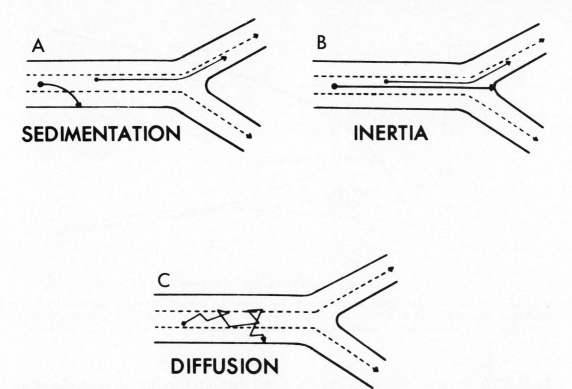

Figure 13–1. Schematic representation of the three main mechanisms of aerosol particle deposition. Particles (solid symbols and lines) cross streamlines of inspired airflow (dashed lines) and deposit on the airway surface because of sedimentation from gravity *(A)*, inertial impaction *(B)*, and diffusion from brownian movement *(C)*. (Reprinted by permission from Brain, J. D., and Volberg, P. A.: State of the art. Deposition of aerosol in the respiratory tract. Am. Rev. Respir. Dis., *120*:1325–1373, 1979.)

will touch and hence be deposited upon the epithelial surface. Because inertial forces increase with air velocity, inertial deposition of particles is greater in the upper than in the lower airways and is enhanced by increased frequency of breathing. Impaction is the essential mechanism of deposition of particles greater than 10 μm; hence it is most important in the nasopharynx. Impaction, however, remains an appreciable force, causing 19 per cent of total tracheobronchial deposition of particles as small as 2.0 μm.[3]

Sedimentation. Although an aerosol is a reasonably stable suspension, the particles are under the influence of gravity and will settle if given enough time. The speed at which a particle settles is determined by the density of the particle and the square of its diameter; accordingly a silica particle settles faster than a grain of pollen the same size. Deposition by sedimentation occurs more readily in relatively still air and thus is greater toward the peripheral units than in central airways. For similar reasons, at a given minute volume, sedimentation is augmented by breathing slowly and deeply.

Sedimentation is the most important mechanism of deposition of particles between 5.0 and 0.2 μm and occurs mainly distal to the fifth bronchial division.[4]

Diffusion. Aerosol particles may demonstrate random (brownian) motion if the particles are small enough to be influenced by the continuous bombardment of the surrounding gas molecules. Consequently, deposition by diffusion is negligible for particles larger than 0.5 μm and is important only in the terminal respiratory units, where the mass movement of air is trivial. Brownian motion is the most important mechanism of respiratory tract deposition of particles 0.1 μm and smaller.[4] It will be recalled (Chapter 7) that the mixing of newly inspired fresh air with air remaining from the previous breath takes place in the distal units by diffusion of gas molecules rather than by bulk flow; however, owing to differences in size, the diffusion of gas molecules is orders of magnitude faster than the diffusion of particles.

Whether or not a particle is deposited in the respiratory tract depends upon the air-

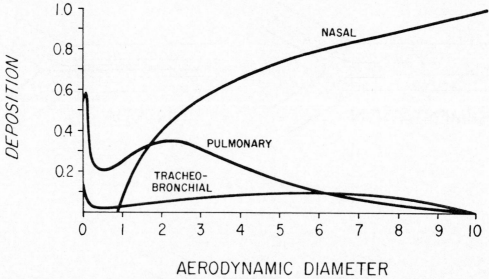

Figure 13–2. Nasal, tracheobronchial, and pulmonary deposition as a function of particle size at a breathing pattern of 15 breaths/min, 750 ml tidal volume. (Reprinted by permission from Task Group on Lung Dynamics: Deposition and retention models for internal dosimetry of the human respiratory tract. Health Phys., *12*:173–207, 1966.)

flow at different levels within the system and the size, density, and shape of the particle. It is obviously desirable to know both the distribution and deposition of particles in order to understand the pathogenesis of various pneumoconioses and the mode of action of therapeutic aerosols. It is possible to calculate airflow velocity at a given tidal volume and respiratory frequency from the dimensions of the airways and terminal respiratory units; from these data, the behavior of varying-sized spherical particles of unit density can be approximated. An example of the deposition of different-sized particles during normal quiet breathing (tidal volume 750 ml, 15 breaths/min) through the nose is shown in Figure 13–2. Although the distribution of aerosols is difficult to examine precisely in humans, the results of most studies support the calculations diagrammed in Figure 13–2.[5]

The following conclusions are warranted about the differing characteristics of particle trapping at various levels within the respiratory system.[6]

1. Almost all particles larger than 10 μm are deposited in the nasal passages and hence do not penetrate as far as the tracheobronchial tree. Conversely, the efficiency of nasopharyngeal filtering decreases as particle size decreases and becomes negligible at about 1 μm.

2. Accordingly, the percentage of parti-

cles that penetrate into the terminal respiratory units rises from essentially zero with particles 10 μm and above to a maximum with particles 1 μm and below.

3. On a scale of graded particle sizes (see Fig. 13–2) those about 2 μm in aerodynamic diameter demonstrate a peak of deposition within terminal respiratory units; larger particles are trapped in the airways, and smaller particle retention decreases because impaction in alveoli decreases down to a particle size of about 0.5 μm.

4. Particles smaller than 0.5 μm are also retained in considerable numbers, owing to a relative increase in the force of impaction by diffusion with decreasing particle size.

It should be emphasized that these statements apply only to "idealized" aerosols that contain spherical particles of unit density. When considering the distribution and retention behavior of irregularly shaped materials of varying densities, appropriate mathematical corrections must be introduced. Better yet, the aerodynamic behavior of an aerosol can be directly measured with available instruments to determine the equivalent aerodynamic mass median diameter of the particles. It must be remembered, however, that particles may change size as they move through the upper respiratory passages if they are sensitive to moisture (hygroscopic), and thus gain or lose water.

Gases (Vapors)

According to toxicologic nomenclature, gases are classified into three main groups:[7] therapeutic, inert, and toxic. Therapeutic gases include O_2 and inhalation anesthetics and occasionally CO_2. Inert gases are normally of no physiologic consequence, but they are frequently used under controlled conditions in the laboratory to study various aspects of respiratory function. Toxic gases produce undersirable physiologic effects that are usually accompanied by pathologic responses. Sometimes gases must be classified in more than one category; for example, a therapeutic gas may also be toxic (O_2 in high concentrations), and an inert gas may be therapeutic (He). Because this chapter is concerned with the defenses of the lung, only the deposition and fate of toxic gases will be considered. The respiratory handling of O_2 and CO_2 has already been discussed (Chapter 7), and excellent reviews are available on the behavior of inert gases.[8, 9]

The penetration into and retention within the respiratory tract of toxic gases is exceedingly variable and depends upon the physical properties of the gas, its concentration in the inspired air, and the rate and depth of ventilation. Inhalation of a noxious gas usually has an immediate and profound effect on the pattern of breathing.[10] Reflexes are triggered by chemical stimulation of receptors located in the nose (sneezing, laryngeal closure[11]), larynx (coughing, laryngeal closure, slowing of breathing[11, 12]), airways (coughing, laryngeal narrowing, hyperpnea, bronchoconstriction[13, 14]), and lung parenchyma (rapid shallow breathing[12]). When the entire system is activated, breathing consists of a variable mixture of sneezes, coughs, wheezes, gasps, grunts, and pants.

As indicated earlier, a force is required to impact a particle on the respiratory surfaces. In contrast, part of the airstream containing an inhaled toxic gas is always in contact with the moist epithelial lining of the nasopharynx, conducting airways, and distal airspaces. Therefore, some of the foreign gas is absorbed as the mixed inspirate flows through the upper air passages, and the amount removed varies according to the solubility of the gas. Highly water-soluble gases like SO_2 and ozone, when present in low concentrations, are completely extracted during passage through the nose of healthy subjects during brief exposures;[15] in contrast, insoluble gases like phosgene, NO_2, and Cl_2 are removed much less completely and hence penetrate deeper into the respiratory tract. The amount of water-soluble gas that can be contained in tissues is limited, and saturation occurs quickly, unless the amount already dissolved is removed by blood flow or chemical degradation. This means that if a highly soluble gas is present in high concentrations, the absorptive capacity of the nasal passages becomes overwhelmed, and the gas penetrates deep into the tracheobronchial tree. Less soluble gases that are poorly extracted in the conducting airways reach and mix with the air contained in distal respiratory units, and a fraction of the foreign gas is absorbed immediately. The amount taken up is proportional not only to the solubility and alveolar concentration of the foreign gas but also to the volume of tissue to which the gas is exposed. Because the alveolar surface is so extensive, large amounts of a toxic gas may be extracted by the lung even though the solubility of the gas is relatively low.

Temperature and Humidity

Inspired air is brought to body temperature (37° C) and saturation (PH_2O 47 mm Hg) by the time it reaches the terminal respiratory units. It was formerly believed that conditioning was complete by the time the inspirate reached the larynx or upper trachea.[16] Now it is recognized that much more of the tracheobronchial system may be involved in the conditioning process. Heat exchange and humidification begin the moment inspired air enters the body. During quiet breathing of ordinary ambient air, conditioning is completed in the upper airways. But when the heat-exchanging capacity of the nasopharynx is overtaxed by decreasing the temperature of the inspirate or by increasing minute volume, incompletely conditioned air may reach peripheral airways, and the temperature of central airways may decrease substantially.[17]

Changing from nasal breathing to mouth breathing also shifts the chief site of temperature control and humidification to a more distal location; bypassing the upper airway with an endotracheal tube or tracheostomy cannula moves the site entirely into the trachea and bronchi. The heat loss from and cooling of the upper respiratory tract associated with breathing cool air at high minute volumes seems clearly linked to the pathogenesis of exercise-induced asthma.[17] Similarly, thermal injuries of the upper respiratory tract may occur from the inhalation of extremely hot air or especially of steam. When thermal injuries of the trachea and bronchi are present, superficial burns of the face and nose are apt to be particularly severe and indicate the difference in the intensity of heat that contacts the surface of the body and that which reaches the airways.

NONSPECIFIC DEFENSE MECHANISMS

The filtering system of the respiratory tract is not perfect, and a certain amount of potentially harmful material is deposited within the airways or airspaces during ordinary daily activities. To guard itself and the rest of the body, the respiratory system is normally furnished with several different nonspecific defense mechanisms, including clearance pathways, secretions with antimicrobial properties, and systems of cells that either impose physical barriers or actively phagocytose particles. The processes are nonspecific because they are effective against a variety of substances, not just specific ones (for comparison see the subsequent section on immunologic mechanisms). Moreover, all nonspecific defenses are present from birth, and because they are not acquired by exposure, they are sometimes referred to as innate responses.

Clearance

Highly water-soluble gases and liquid particles are absorbed at the sites of contact with the epithelial lining of the respiratory tract. Less soluble substances may be either eliminated or absorbed, depending upon the balance between the effectiveness of the clearance mechanisms and the rate of solution of the substance. The physiologic and pathologic consequences of absorption are determined by how much cellular damage and malfunction result from the biochemical reactions produced by the toxic substance and may vary from mild to lethal.

The fate of solid (insoluble) particles is considerably different. Coarse particles are filtered in the nose; finer ones are trapped in the nasopharynx and along the airways.

Only very small particles (see Fig. 13–2) penetrate to the terminal respiratory units, where some are deposited and the remainder are exhaled. Almost all of the solid particles that impact in the airways and lung parenchyma are ultimately eliminated from the body, but the mechanisms involved and the time required for complete removal vary greatly, depending upon the chemical properties of the particles and how far into the respiratory tract they penetrate before impacting. There are two interdigitating clearance systems that serve to remove particles deposited in different locations: clearance from the nasopharynx and tracheobronchial tree is achieved by *mucociliary transport,* and clearance from the terminal respiratory units is by *macrophage transport.* The efficiency of these processes can be appreciated by recognizing that residents of most cities inhale several hundred grams of solid particles over their lifetimes, yet analysis of their lungs after death reveals only a few grams of mineral ash.[6] The efficiency of clearance is also believed to be crucial to the pathogenesis of the slowly developing pneumoconioses because the severity of these diseases depends not only upon the quantity of dust initially deposited, but also upon its subsequent removal.[6]

Nasal Clearance. The anatomy, physiology, and contributions of the nose to the defense of the lungs have recently been reviewed by Proctor.[18] The nose is structured anatomically so that most of the particulate matter that is inhaled through it impacts near the front on nonciliated epithelium where the passages are narrow and tortuous and where hairs are located; deposition of particles anteriorly facilitates their removal by nose blowing and sneezing.[19] Particles deposited more posteriorly are swept backward over the mucus-lined, ciliated epithelium to the nasopharynx where they are swallowed. Nasal clearance occurs at an average rate of approximately 6 mm per minute, but there is an inexplicably wide range of clearance among apparently healthy persons. It is uncertain whether slowing of nasal mucociliary clearance results from an abnormality of either the physicochemical properties of mucus or the action of cilia, although the former seems more likely.[18]

Tracheobronchial Clearance. As in the posterior nasopharynx, removal of particles from the entire system of conducting airways is carried out by mucociliary clearance: a film of mucus is continuously impelled proximally by the beating motion of cilia that cover most of the surface of the tracheobronchial epithelium. Any particles that deposit on the film of mucus are carried along with it to the oropharynx, where they are swallowed or expectorated.

The number of cilia on the surface of each ciliated cell varies from one species to another; human ciliated cells have approximately 200.[20] A characteristic of ciliated cells, as shown in Figure 13–3, is their numerous mitochondria, which cluster beneath the basal bodies of the cilia and are

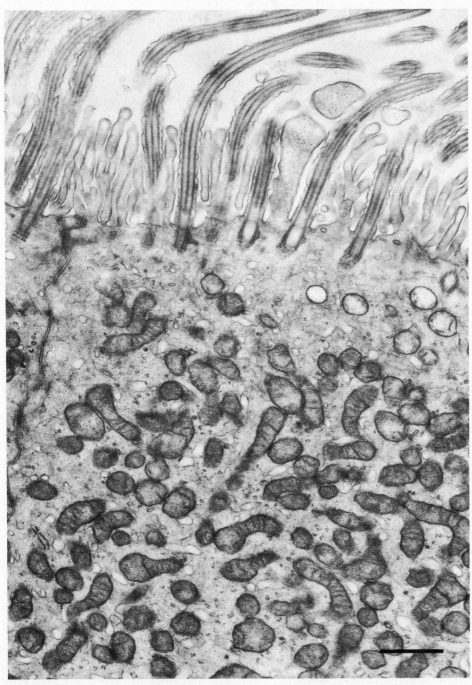

Figure 13–3. Electron micrograph of the luminal portion of a ciliated epithelial cell. Numerous mitochondria cluster beneath the basal bodies of the cilia. Horizontal bar = 1 μm. (× 12,500. Courtesy of Dr. Donald McKay.)

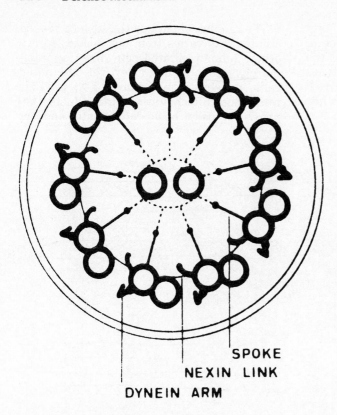

SPOKE
NEXIN LINK
DYNEIN ARM

Figure 13–4. Schematic cross-sectional diagram of a cilium showing its main structural components. From Palmbald, J., et al.: Ultrastructural, cellular, and clinical features of the immotile-cilia syndrome. Ann. Rev. Med., *35*:481–492, 1984. Reprinted, with permission from Annual Reviews Inc.)

presumably the chief sites of energy production from ATP for ciliary activity. A cilium is a complex structure that contains two central and nine microtubular fibrilar doublets, on each of which there are two dynein arms (Fig. 13–4).[21] There is still some uncertainty about exactly how cilia move, but unquestionably there is sliding of the subfibers and bridging of the spaces between adjacent microtubules by the dynein arms appears essential. Impaired ciliary motion associated with ultrastructural defects is now known to predispose to multiple respiratory infections and bronchiectasis, and causes the immotile cilia (or ciliary dyskinesia) syndrome.[22] The cilia of a single cell and those of contiguous cells, though not anatomically connected, appear to be coordinated so that a metachronal wave of effective surface motion spreads in a proximal direction. Cilia beat rapidly with a characteristic biphasic stroke—a fast forward flick followed by a slow backward recovery.

The mucous lining throughout most of the airways is composed of a double (sol-gel) layer on the surface of the bronchial epithelium, depicted in Figure 13–5.[23] The inner layer, in which the cilia beat, is the periciliary liquid or sol phase of the transport medium, and the outer layer is the viscous or gel phase. The viscous layer is nonabsorbent to water and presumably serves to protect the sol phase from desiccation; moreover, the tips of the beating cilia just strike the innermost portion of the gel covering them, thus facilitating proximal movement of the layer. There is still no resolution to the long-standing argument over whether the mucous blanket is continuous or composed of scattered plaques.[24]

Because of the obvious difficulty in conducting suitable *in vivo* studies of mucociliary function in humans, most of the available information has been derived from experimental animals. In the rat, for example, cilia have been observed to beat at a frequency of 1300 beats/min and to move the overlying mucous film at an average rate of about 13.5 mm/min.[25] Judging from studies in humans, employing direct observations of small plastic disks through a cinebronchofiberscope, the speed of tracheobronchial clearance is almost twice as fast (21.5 mm/min).[26] However, clearance is distinctly slower in the bronchioles (0.5 to 1 mm per min) compared with that in the trachea and main bronchi (5 to 20 mm/min).[4] Even though the rate of mucociliary trans-

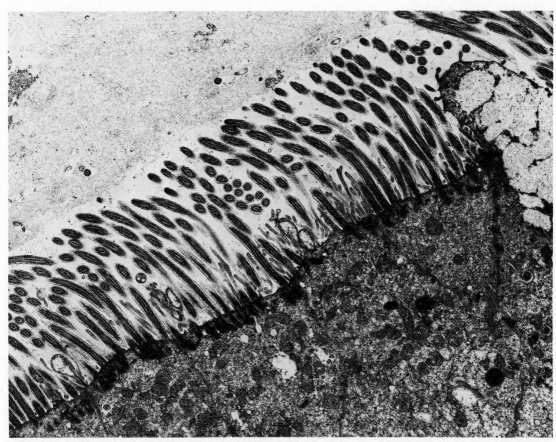

Figure 13–5. Electron micrograph of the mucociliary apparatus of the rat bronchus fixed with glutaraldehyde and osmium vapor. Ciliated cells and one goblet cell (right side) are seen in the epithelial layer. The tips of the cilia, which lie in the sol layer, just touch the base of the mucous (gel) layer (original magnification × 6,600). (Reprinted by permission from Yoneda, K.: Mucous blanket of the rat bronchus. An ultrastructural study. Am. Rev. Respir. Dis., *114*:837–842, 1976.)

port increases as the streams converge, there remains a problem concerning the fate of all the secretions. The thickness of the mucous layer is fairly constant throughout the airways, whereas the surface area of the bronchioles is more than 2000 times that of the trachea (see Fig. 2–2). Thus, there should be considerable piling-up of mucus as it moves centrally. If the mucous layer were discontinuous, as has been proposed, consolidation and speeding-up of the plaques would prevent thickening of the layer, but this needs to be established. Mucociliary clearance varies widely, even in normal healthy persons; in 14 nonsmokers, the mean 90 per cent clearance time of a radio-labeled aerosol was 494 min, but the standard deviation was 130 min.[27]

Alveolar Clearance. The fate of solid particles that settle on the alveolar surface differs from that of particles deposited on the airway surface. The majority of the particulate load from both surfaces reaches the gastrointestinal tract via the mucociliary escalator and by swallowing. Some alveolar particles remain sequestered within the lung parenchyma, some particles reach intrapulmonary, hilar, or other lymph nodes, and some enter the bloodstream and may circulate to any organ in the body;[28] which of these pathways is utilized depends upon the quantity and physicochemical properties of the substances deposited and the capabilities of the host's removal mechanisms.

Particles may traverse these routes in either the naked state or, more commonly, within phagocytes. Thus, considerable variation is possible in the means of removing substances from the alveolar surface, and this is reflected in the enormous range of alveolar clearance half-times that may occur (<1 day to >1400 days).[5]

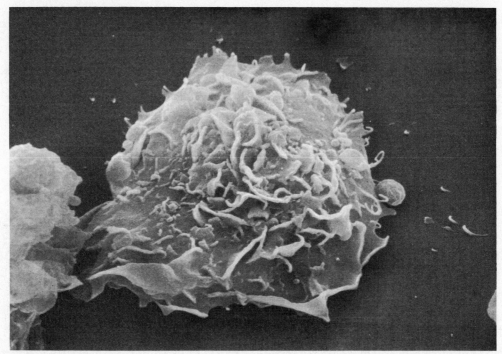

Figure 13–6. Scanning electron micrograph of a rat macrophage. Characteristic ruffles (lamellipodia) facilitate enfolding of particles during phagocytosis. (× 7400. Courtesy of Marguerite M. Kay, National Institute of Aging.)

1. Under normal conditions in which the aggregate dust load is light, almost all of the particles are phagocytosed by alveolar macrophages (Fig. 13–6), which then eliminate the particle either by digesting it or by carrying it along the alveolar surface to the beginning of the mucociliary transport system.[29] From there, both the macrophage and its particulate contents are propelled centrally to the oropharynx, where they are swallowed.

2. The second pathway of alveolar clearance also depends upon macrophages for phagocytosis and transport, although it is unknown whether the particle is phagocytosed on the alveolar surface or after crossing the epithelial lining. In either case, instead of moving along the alveolar surface the particle-laden macrophage moves through the interstitial space of the interalveolar septum until it reenters the lumen of the airspaces, often at the site of or actually through the lymphatic aggregates at the junctions of respiratory and terminal bronchioles or through the more proximally located bronchus-associated lymphoid tissues.[28] Septal transport represents a "short cut" from alveolus to respiratory bronchiole compared with surface transport but takes longer to traverse. The time course of this pathway varies from 1 to 14 days.

3. Some of the particles that reach the peribronchovascular interstitial space enter lymphatic capillaries instead of reentering bronchioles. Once inside the lymphatic system, the particle has access to more centrally located lymph channels and lymph nodes. If the particle successfully navigates these sites of possible retention, it reaches the bloodstream, through which it may circulate to other organs.

It is generally agreed that unless the particle load is heavy and macrophage transport via surface and septal pathways is overwhelmed, little, if any, of the inhaled material reaches the hilar lymph nodes or bloodstream. However, with increasing exposure and saturation of phagocytic capacity, more and more particles can be found in regional lymph nodes and elsewhere in the body.

4. Some of the particles originally deposited in alveoli may be sequestered in the lung parenchyma by a tissue reaction. This reaction is complex, and many details about the mechanisms involved are lacking. The pathogenesis of the response clearly relates to the cytotoxicity of the inhaled substance.

For example, silica (SiO_2) particles are usually lethal to the macrophages that engulf them; the dead cells (or their products) may give rise to a tissue reaction that prevents further ingestion or the silica particles may be recycled from one macrophage to another. Further discussion about the biology and multiple functions of alveolar macrophages is provided later in this chapter.

Secretions

The respiratory tract distal to the larynx is normally sterile. The absence of culturable microorganisms depends not only upon the swift and efficient mucociliary and alveolar clearance mechanisms but also upon the constituents of the secretions that overlie the respiratory epithelium. Thus, defense against penetration into the lung's interior is imposed by the physical and chemical barriers of the surface film and the epithelial lining and is enhanced by the presence in the secretions that cover the epithelium of several antimicrobial substances, such as lysozyme, lactoferrin, and interferon, that serve to destroy or inhibit many bacteria and viruses.

Tracheobronchial Lining. The layer of liquid that normally lines the tracheobronchial tree has different constituents and derives from several cell types. The lining of terminal bronchioles probably originates from Clara cells or from the secretions of type II alveolar cells. The two-phase sol-gel lining layer may begin in more proximal (i.e., not terminal) bronchioles in which goblet cells, the most peripherally located mucus-secreting cells, are situated. As mentioned, bronchial glands only contribute secretions to the mucous layer in bronchi. The structure and function of each of these mucus-secreting constituents is described in Chapter 2. Further details about the chemistry,[30] rheology,[31] and mechanisms of clearance[32] of mucus are available.

Much less is known about the cellular origin, composition, regulatory mechanisms, and fate of periciliary fluid, the "other" vital component of the two-phase liquid layer. In most secretory epithelia the movement of water is governed by local osmotic gradients created by active ion transport. The studies of Olver and colleagues[33] have shown that the same process occurs in the tracheal epithelium of dogs in response to the active secretion of Cl^- toward the luminal surface

and of Na^+ in the other direction. These findings have been confirmed in other mammalian species (see Nadel and coworkers[34] for review and additional references), and additional details are now available about the intracellular activities associated with Cl^- secretion.[35] The cell type(s) responsible for active ion transport in intact epithelium have not been identified, and both surface epithelial cells and submucosal gland cells may be involved. Because ion fluxes occur in animals whose tracheal epithelium has no glands, surface epithelial cells alone are capable of active transport.[34]

The composition and physical properties of the mucous layer are known to change dramatically in various bronchopulmonary and cardiac diseases; whether or not the characteristics of the periciliary layer change is not known and should be studied. Inflammatory processes, allergic reactions, cystic fibrosis, circulatory failure, and respiratory tract neoplasms all usually increase the volume and change the character of the secretions from those normally produced. Furthermore, a striking increase or decrease in mucus viscosity affects mucociliary clearance,[36] and this is probably one reason why there is such a high incidence of pulmonary infections in patients with these diseases.

For obvious clinical reasons, there is considerable interest in the regulatory mechanisms that control respiratory tract secretions in healthy lungs, the types of abnormalities that occur in various diseases, and how these disturbances can be manipulated by pharmacologic and other means. We seem to be on the threshold of important advances in understanding these complex processes.

Alveolar Lining. Studies in experimental animals have revealed marked variations in the rates at which different species of bacteria are killed after inhalation (Fig. 13–7). Part of the variation may be attributed to the capacity of some bacteria to multiply within the respiratory tract[37] and another part to the varying bactericidal activity of alveolar macrophages.[38] Although the alveolar lining liquid contains immunoglobulins G and A and small amounts of complement (each discussed subsequently), functionally the liquid is weak in opsonins, substances that facilitate phagocytosis by coating bacteria. Recent data indicate that alveolar surfactant serves as an opsonin and enhances *in vitro* phagocytosis and intracel-

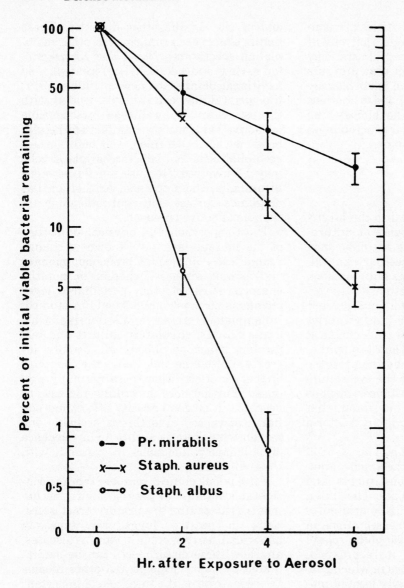

Figure 13–7. Clearance of *Proteus mirabilis, Staphylococcus aureus,* and *Staphylococcus albus* by normal mouse lung. (Reprinted by permission from Green G. M., and Kass, E. H.: The influence of bacterial species on pulmonary resistance to infection in mice subjected to hypoxia, cold stress, and ethanolic intoxication. Br. J. Exp. Pathol., *46*:360–366, 1965.)

lular killing of *Staphylococcus aureus* by alveolar macrophages.[39]

Lysozyme. The enzyme lysozyme is one of the most well-characterized antimicrobial substances found in respiratory tract secretions and other tissues and fluids of humans. Lysozyme attacks muramic acid, a constituent of all bacterial cell walls. When the antimicrobial activity of lysozyme is studied in the absence of other factors normally present in respiratory secretions, it is found to be more effective against gram-positive than against gram-negative bacteria; the decreased susceptibility of gram-negative organisms is a consequence of the outer, mainly lipoprotein layers of their cell walls, which protect the inner muramic acid–containing portion.[40] The activity of lyso-zyme against gram-negative bacteria is enhanced in the presence of antibody and activated complement. The combined action of antibody and complement on the outer wall of the bacterium exposes the inner layers to the enzymatic action of lysozyme.

Lysozyme is also one of the important hydrolytic enzymes contained in lysosomes, the membrane-bound intracellular structures that participate in the killing of bacteria after phagocytosis. For example, lysozyme has been demonstrated in large quantities within alveolar macrophages from patients with tuberculosis and probably represents an important adaptive host response in the defense against spread of the infection.

Interferon. In 1957, Isaacs and

Lindemann[41] reported the discovery of a potent antiviral substance that they called interferon. Since then, interferons have been the subject of intensive investigations that have progressed to the stage of clinical trials of the treatment of viral diseases and malignancies, with initially promising results.[42]

Interferons are a family of related glycoproteins rather than single homogeneous molecules and constitute part of the natural defense system of vertebrate species from the teleost fishes up to and including humans. In general, there is limited cross-reactivity among interferons from different species, and interferons are most effective in the cells of the same animal species that produced them. The chief natural stimulus for *in vivo* interferon production appears to be a viral infection; however, a variety of biologic and synthetic materials can also provoke cells to synthesize large amounts of interferon.

There are several types of human interferons that are designated by the cell types from which they are produced *in vitro*: human leukocyte interferon, fibroblast interferon, lymphoblastoid interferon, and immune interferon, which can be distinguished physicochemically and antigenically. Interferons are extremely potent substances and, in addition to their antiviral effects, have antiproliferative, antitumor, and immunoregulatory actions.[43]

The exact sequence of intracellular biochemical events that culminate in increased resistance to viral infection is not known but appears to incorporate two separate processes. The first step entails the synthesis and release of interferon by infected cells, and the second step involves the stimulation by interferon of an intracellular antiviral polypeptide that protects uninfected cells. The second step is necessary because interferon has no antiviral activity *per se* and can only act in the cells that it contacts by enhancing the production of antiviral substances.

Although human cells, in general, are not as efficient synthesizers of interferons as cells from other vertebrates, interferon has been found in secretions from the respiratory tract and is known to be produced by alveolar macrophages.[44] Interferon is also one of the biologically active factors called *lymphokines* released by sensitized lymphocytes during cell-mediated immunologic reactions; it is of interest that macrophages, one of the chief effectors of cell-mediated immunity, are able to transfer the information for interferon production to lymphocytes.[45] As further information is gained concerning how interferons contribute to pulmonary defenses, effective therapeutic use can be made of the various biologic products that are becoming available in increasing quantities.

Complement. The activity of complement was once believed to be limited mainly to its role as an essential cofactor that allowed certain antigen-antibody reactions to reach completion. At present complement is known to be an important mediator of various aspects of the inflammatory response such as enhancement of vascular permeability and chemotaxis of polymorphonuclear leukocytes. These multiple functions have recently been reviewed.[46, 47]

The complement system is composed of more than 20 component plasma proteins that participate in a sequential, or "cascading," reaction that results in active products that are both cell bound and in the liquid phase. The cell-bound complexes contribute to membrane lysis and cell death, and the liquid phase ingredients contribute to the humorally mediated portion of the inflammatory response.

It is well established that the complement system has two major pathways (Fig. 13–8) and that either can cause activation of the final products.[47] Activation of the *classical pathway* is initiated by the union of antigen and antibody, which then binds to and activates the C1 complex. In contrast, activation of the *alternative pathway* is initiated by direct contact with viable bacteria, both gram-positive and gram-negative, fungi, endotoxins, certain immune complexes, and other substances. Because activation of the alternative pathway leads to opsonization of the microorganisms in the absence of specific antibody, this system has been called the body's "first line of defense" against certain infections.

The main biologically active products of the complement system include C3b, C3a, and C5a (see Fig. 13–8). As indicated, C3b promotes phagocytosis; C3a and C5a possess anaphylatoxin activity (i.e., they cause release of histamine from mast cells and increase vascular permeability); and C5a also is chemotactic, increases the adhesiveness of polymorphonuclear leukocytes, and promotes release of their lysosomal enzymes.

Only small amounts of complement com-

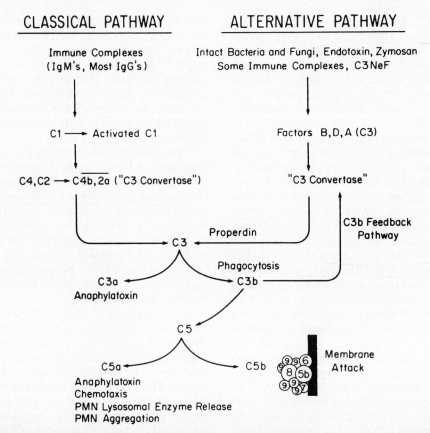

Figure 13–8. Pathways of complement activation leading to generation of biologically active peptides and the actions of the peptides are shown. (Adapted and reprinted with permission from Perez, H. D.: Biologically active complement (C5)-derived peptides and their relevance to disease. Rev. Oncol/Hematol., *1*:199–225, 1984. Copyright CRC Press, Inc., Boca Raton, FL)

ponents have been found in respiratory tract secretions or in bronchoalveolar lavage liquid obtained from normal persons. However, when vascular and epithelial membrane permeability are increased (e.g., during inflammation), it is possible that complement constituents of plasma have less restrained access to the interstitial tissues, alveolar spaces, and airways, and in this manner may contribute to the local defenses of the lungs.

Cellular Defenses

In addition to the antimicrobial substances that are naturally present in the secretions lining the respiratory tract, both nonphagocytic and phagocytic cell populations also contribute to the defense of the lungs and the rest of the body.

Nonphagocytic Cells. The surface epithelium and basement membrane of the airways and terminal respiratory units im-

pose a physical barrier that guards the interior of the lungs, and hence their lymphatic channels and blood vessels, from penetration by infectious agents and toxic substances. Furthermore, even if harmful materials reach the interior of the epithelial cells, the cells are probably capable of some inactivation by intracellular neutralization or digestion. The efficacy of this physical defense system is demonstrated by the increased susceptibility to pyogenic respiratory tract infections after injury to the epithelium (e.g., following viral infections of the tracheobronchial tree, especially influenza, and chemical damage from aspiration or inhalation of corrosive chemicals).

Phagocytic Cells. Nearly a century ago, Metchnikoff[48] argued that phagocytosis is an important defense mechanism against the constant assault on the body by pyogenic microorganisms. The logic of Metchnikoff's deductions has been amply confirmed, and his conclusions have been extended. At present much is known about the cell types involved and the factors that regulate their production, how phagocytes recognize infectious agents and "home in" on them, and how phagocytes engulf and kill microorganisms.[49] There are three types of "professional scavengers" that are constantly on duty in a state of functional readiness. Two types are in the bloodstream (polymorphonuclear leukocytes and monocytes), and one type is in the tissues throughout the body (tissue macrophages, including alveolar macrophages).

Blood Phagocytes. Polymorphonuclear leukocytes and monocytes are the two types of circulating phagocytes. In addition to their presence in the bloodstream, small numbers of both cell types are normally encountered in tissue spaces throughout the body, including the interstitial and alveolar spaces of the lungs (e.g., <1 per cent of cells recovered by bronchoalveolar lavage from normal persons are neutrophils). Furthermore, a dramatic increase in the concentration of either polymorphonuclear neutrophilic leukocytes or monocytes in tissues constitutes one of the histologic hallmarks of differing kinds and durations of inflammatory processes. Both kinds of circulating phagocytes are derived from precursor cells in the bone marrow. Maturation in the marrow of polymorphonuclear neutrophilic leukocytes is slow, but once released into the circulation, they have a short half-life of survival of only six to seven hours; in contrast, monocytes mature faster in the marrow and spend more time in the circulation.[49] Also, as mentioned earlier in the case of alveolar macrophages (Chapter 2), some circulating monocytes enter interstitial tissues of the lung, where they differentiate into alveolar macrophages, which then replicate in the lungs.

Early in the evolution of an inflammatory response, circulating granulocytes and monocytes stick to the endothelium of small blood vessels at the site of injury. If the damage is of sufficient intensity, both cell types migrate into the interstitial space surrounding the vessels. Extravascular emigration occurs by ameboid motion through the intercellular clefts in response to chemotaxis, which can be defined as directed cellular migration along a concentration gradient of a chemoattractant.[50] There are several classes of chemotaxic substances, some of which have already been mentioned: C5a from complement activation, diverse lymphokines from stimulated lymphocytes,

chemoattractants from neutrophils and macrophages, and eosinophil chemotactic factor of anaphylaxis and leukotrienes from mast cells and basophils.

Polymorphonuclear leukocytes emigrate more quickly and in greater numbers than monocytes and so are the principal cell type in the early genesis of an inflammatory response. Although the emigration of mononuclear cells is delayed, it persists for a much longer period than that of granulocytes; therefore, mononuclear cells gradually become the predominant cell type as most inflammatory processes evolve. But the time course and extent of participation by the two types of cells vary greatly with different damaging stimuli. Ordinarily, polymorphonuclear neutrophilic leukocytes degrade substances more effectively than monocytes, and this may be one reason why granulocytes are mobilized first.

It has already been pointed out that the defense mechanisms on the surface of the respiratory tract deal more effectively with relatively insoluble particles than with highly soluble substances. The same disparity exists for materials that penetrate the surface barriers: particulate matter, such as microorganisms, is phagocytosed and detoxified more readily than soluble chemicals. Both types of phagocytes, and other cells as well, take up soluble materials that have not caused a direct chemical injury (such as soluble antigens) by the mechanism of pinocytosis, after which the substances may be detoxified.

The cellular component of the inflammatory response appears to facilitate the isolation and detoxification of the offending agent through particle recognition, phagocytosis, the internalization of the particle through the formation of a phagosome, and particle digestion by lysosomal enzymes.[49] These activities often cause the death of the participating cells, which results in the release of their proteolytic enzymes and further tissue necrosis. In addition, both circulating and tissue phagocytes generate toxic O_2 products that are essential for the killing of bacteria and fungi after they have been phagocytosed. At times, instead of being directed toward microorganisms contained within phagosomes inside the cell, the biologically reactive metabolites of O_2 may escape from the cell and damage neighboring tissue. To protect against tissue injury from unrestrained proteolysis and toxic O_2 radicals, the lungs are equipped with

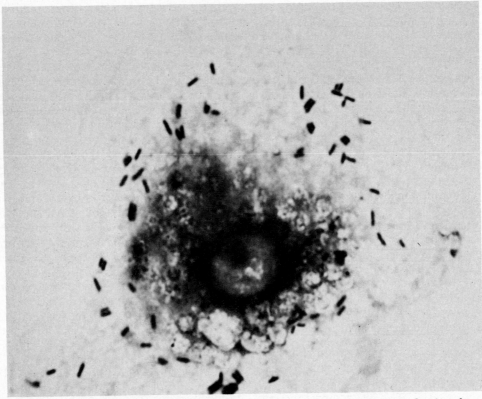

Figure 13–9. Micrograph of cultured human alveolar macrophage, obtained by lung lavage, showing phagocytosed *Listeria monocytogenes.* (× 7000. Courtesy of Dr. Allen B. Cohen.)

antiproteolytic enzymes and antioxidant systems (both described subsequently).

Tissue Macrophages. The resident tissue macrophage in the lung, as discussed earlier, is the alveolar macrophage. These cells are sparse in the interstitium of the lung and common within the liquid film lining the alveolar surface. Alveolar macrophages are avid phagocytes (Fig. 13–9) and are able to dispose of a wide variety of microorganisms by processes similar to that used by neutrophils: recognition, phagocytosis by attachment and ingestion, intracellular killing, and degradation.[51] Thus alveolar macrophages must be regarded as the chief guardians of the extensive surface of the terminal respiratory unit.

However, no one knows how a macrophage locates a microorganism or other particle once it has impacted on the alveolar surface. Presumably, most particles do not exhibit tropism that would attract phagocytes, and macrophages move slowly in random fashion as they scavenge. Although the statistical likelihood of encountering a particle is small, the chance of contact is probably considerably enhanced by the rapid movement of the particles themselves, due to a combination of brownian forces in the alveolus and the slipperiness of the surfactant lining.

It is also unknown how macrophages and occasional unengulfed particles find their way in such a purposeful manner out of the labyrinthine terminal respiratory unit to the mucociliary escalator. A minor pulling force may be imparted to the peripheral surface films by the activity of the more centrally located cilia, and gradients in surface tension have been described. However, the most important force for movement toward the hilus of alveolar secretions, cells, and debris appears to be derived from respiratory movements. Clinical and experimental data clearly demonstrate an impairment of dust clearance with appropriate pathologic sequelae (depending upon the dust) when movement of all or part of a lung is impaired.[6] But how respiratory movements are transmitted to cells and particles on the alveolar surface is unknown.

Besides their role as scavengers of the terminal respiratory units, pulmonary macrophages have many other important bio-

Table 13–2. FUNCTIONS OF PULMONARY
MACROPHAGES*

Defensive Functions
    Microbicidal activity and bacteriostasis
    Phagocytosis of particulate and insoluble substances,
        including antigen-antibody complexes
    Uptake, localization and processing of antigen
    Degradation of antigen and particles
    Synthesis of immunoregulatory substances
    Synthesis of complement components
    Synthesis of interferon
    Synthesis of chemotactic factors
    Synthesis of tumor-inhibiting factors
Nondefensive Functions
    Nonmicrobial scavenging
    Synthesis of arachidonic acid metabolites
    Synthesis of platelet activating factors
    Synthesis of fibroblast activating factor
    Synthesis of enzyme inhibitors
    Synthesis of binding proteins

*Adapted from Nathen, C. F. et al.: Current Concepts. The
macrophage as an effector cell. New Engl. J. Med.,
303:622–626, 1980 and Cohen, A. B.: Lung Cell Biology.
Fed. Proc., 38:2635–2636, 1979.

logic functions. As shown in Table 13–2, these functions are both defensive and nondefensive.[52, 53] The defensive functions involve the humoral and cellular pathways of the immune system (see next section) and many components of the nonimmunologic (innate) system. Through the synthesis of chemotactic factors and mediators, the alveolar macrophage also plays an important role in the pathogenesis of inflammation. Finally, pulmonary macrophages participate in a variety of nondefensive functions involving phagocytosis and, especially, the synthesis of several extraordinarily diverse substances with an equally broad range of biologic activities. These cells must be viewed as remarkable biochemical factories, and we have only just begun to study their synthesizing capabilities.

Biochemical Defenses

The previous discussion has emphasized the important role played by neutrophils and macrophages in the pulmonary defenses against microorganisms. Brief mention was made of the facts that intracellular microbial killing mechanisms involve the synthesis of toxic O_2 radicals and that intracellular degradation requires proteolytic and other enzymes. In recent years it has become clear that, at times, these potent substances may escape from the interior of the cells and injure lung tissue. This sequence has been

postulated to cause pulmonary emphysema[54] and to contribute to acute lung damage of the adult respiratory distress syndrome-type.[55] But it is important to recognize that the lungs are furnished with biochemical systems to defend against enzymes and oxidants. Thus pulmonary injury can only occur when the toxic burden is unusually great or when the biochemical defense capabilities are impaired.

Protease Inhibition. In any inflammatory response, regardless of whether it is of infectious, physicochemical, or immunologic origin, proteolytic enzymes are released by neutrophils and macrophages. Among the proteases are elastase and collagenase, which probably are the major contributors to tissue destruction associated with inflammation. Protease inhibitors are also present in inflammatory exudates, presumably serving to restrain the potentially destructive consequences of inflammation by deactivating newly released proteases.

Of the protease inhibitors present in human serum, alpha-1-antitrypsin is quantitatively the most important and also has been the most carefully studied because of the diseases that are found in association with its deficiency, most notably panlobular emphysema. Models of this form of emphysema have been produced by injecting the plant enzyme papain and, subsequently, enzymes obtained from mammalian leukocytes and macrophages into the lungs of experimental animals. All of these enzymes digest lung tissue and cause typical emphysematous lesions. Emphysema presumably develops in patients with genetically determined decreases in serum levels of alpha-1-antitrypsin because of the unrestrained digestive activity of proteases released in their lungs. A similar imbalance of excessive protease activity relative to available inhibitor capacity may cause the type of emphysema that is found in heavy smokers.

Alpha-1-antitrypsin and other antiproteases also inhibit several other enzymes, including plasmin, plasma thromboplastin antecedent, and kallikrein, that are integral parts of interrelated, cascading enzyme systems that affects coagulation, vascular permeability, kinin generation, fibrinolysis, and complement formation. Thus a deficiency of one or more protease inhibitors could cause emphysema by a variety of indirect mechanisms. Whether alpha-1-antitrypsin and other protease inhibitors act directly or indirectly, it is clear that they should be regarded as circulating substances that contribute in a major way to the defenses of the lungs.

Oxidant Inhibition. In addition to attack by endogenous proteolytic enzymes, the lungs are subject to injury through the local production of powerful oxidants such as superoxide anion, hydrogen peroxide, and the product of these reactants, hydroxyl radical.[56] Oxidants may be generated in the lungs by two distinct mechanisms: (1) by polymorphonuclear leukocytes and other cells involved in local inflammatory reactions, and (2) by the direct effects on lung tissue of high concentrations of inhaled O_2 or toxic substances like paraquat. In either case, the liberated oxidants have potent cytotoxic effects on lung parenchymal cells, although there are variations in susceptibility among different cells. Production of oxidants by the cellular constituents of inflammatory reactions serves as a double-edged sword; one edge is the direct cytotoxicity of the reactants and the other, equally sharp, is their ability to inactivate alpha-1-antitrypsin. Inactivation of the lungs' major defense against proteolysis allows unrestrained activity of neutrophil elastase and other proteolytic enzymes that are also released during inflammation; this sequence is believed to compound lung damage in certain inflammatory disorders such as the adult respiratory distress syndrome. To combat the effects of locally generated oxidants, the lungs are equipped with several intracellular and extracellular protective mechanisms, including the antioxidant enzyme systems superoxide dismutase, catalase, glutathione peroxidase, NADPH, and cytochrome C reductase, and the oxidant-free radical scavengers alpha-tocopherol and ascorbic acid.

SPECIFIC DEFENSE (IMMUNOLOGIC) MECHANISMS

Nonspecific resistance of the respiratory tract depends upon normally functioning clearance mechanisms, antimicrobial substances, anatomic barriers, and circulating and tissue phagocytes. Each of these defenses is present at birth and demonstrates nonselectivity by operating against a wide variety of noxious intruders. In contrast, specific defense mechanisms are latent until actuated by natural exposure to foreign an-

tigenic materials or by artificial induction (vaccination). Thus, specific defenses are acquired (in contrast to innate defenses) and are considered synonymous with immunologic defenses because they involve highly specific stimuli that cause equally specific responses. There are several pathways through which immunologic resistance may be acquired (Table 13–3), but this discussion will consider primarily the contributions of the lungs to the development and expression of naturally acquired immunity.

The immune response begins with the introduction of a foreign molecule—an antigen—into a host capable of reacting to it. Whether or not a substance is antigenic depends on its molecular weight, physical state, and chemical constituents. Furthermore, the capacity to react to a given substance varies considerably from one animal species to another and is genetically determined.

The specialized ability to form antibodies is found only in vertebrates, but the ability is present in all that have been studied, including the most primitive one, the hagfish.[57] Among vertebrates, increasing complexity of immunologic responsiveness correlates with the evolutionary development of lymphoid tissue. It is not yet fully understood why it was essential to develop a system of specific immunity in addition to nonspecific defenses, but undoubtedly part of the explanation lies in the inherent flexibility of the antibody-manufacturing and cell-sensitizing systems. It is clear, also, that immunologic defenses enhance or amplify, both quantitatively and qualitatively, the capacities of nonspecific defense mechanisms (e.g., specific opsonizing antibody increases uptake of microorganisms by phagocytes, and specifically sensitized T cells increase intracellular killing of tubercle bacilli by macrophages through release of lymphokines that activate phagocytosis). Collec-

Table 13–3. PATHWAYS BY WHICH IMMUNOLOGIC DEFENSES MAY BE ACQUIRED: CLASSIFICATION AND CLINICAL EXAMPLES

Acquired naturally
  Active; e.g., following a bout of measles
  Passive; e.g., from placental transfer of immunity to mumps in the newborn

Acquired artificially
  Active; e.g., following immunization with diphtheria toxoid
  Passive; e.g., from injection of tetanus antitoxin

tively, these mechanisms endow vertebrates with the capability of responding to the diverse attacks, such as from infectious agents or cellular mutations, that are likely to be encountered during a lifetime. Certainly, the penalties of multiple infections and a high incidence of neoplasia in immunosuppressed patients are vivid testimony to the importance of acquired immunologic defenses, although it must be appreciated that immunosuppression usually impairs nonspecific defenses as well.

The lymph nodes in the hilus and mediastinum, the lymphoid aggregates, and lymphoepithelial nodules, which compose the bronchus-associated lymphoid tissue, were described in Chapter 3. In addition, small numbers of scattered solitary or aggregated lymphocytes are believed to populate the surface of the terminal respiratory units and the subepithelial tissues of terminal and respiratory bronchioles. Presumably, lymphocytes in each of these areas can participate in immunologic responses, provided a suitable antigenic stimulus reaches them. Figure 13–10 illustrates schematically the sites of lymphoid aggregations in the respiratory tract and the secretions or sampling techniques that provide liquid for analysis of "regional" antibody concentration and lymphocyte subtypes.

The human fetus produces only small amounts of antibodies, and the newborn depends mainly upon passively transferred maternal antibodies for protection during the first few weeks of extrauterine life. The meager production of antibodies by the fetus probably reflects the lack of sufficient antigenic challenge in the sheltered uterine environment to provoke an antibody response, but may also be due to incomplete maturation of the lymphoid system and its control mechanisms. Antibody synthesis increases in the newborn infant a few weeks after delivery and accelerates even further during the first few years of life. The serum concentration of immunoglobulins reaches a near plateau about 15 to 25 years of age and thereafter increases slowly (see Chapter 14 for further details about age-related changes).

The mechanisms by which an antigen provokes an immune response are immensely complex and imperfectly understood. Several general steps are involved: (1) an antigen must be clearly differentiated from a nonantigen, taken up, and "processed" by circulating monocytes or tissue macrophages for presentation to genetically precommitted antigen-reactive lymphocytes; (2) the precursor lymphocytes are then induced to proliferate and differentiate into either sensitized T cells, sensitized B cells, or (usually) both by a process that is controlled by immunoregulatory T cells; (3) the newly sensitized lymphocytes mount ef-

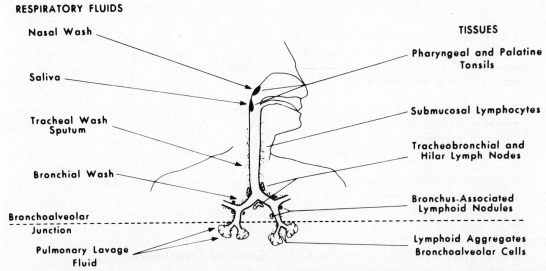

Figure 13–10. Schematic representation of the various fluids and lymphatic tissues associated with the respiratory tract that have been studied experimentally. The bronchoalveolar junction demarcates the airway system from the lung parenchyma. (Reprinted by permission from Kaltreider, H. B.: State of the art. Expression of immune mechanisms in the lung. Am. Rev. Respir. Dis., *113*:347–379, 1976.)

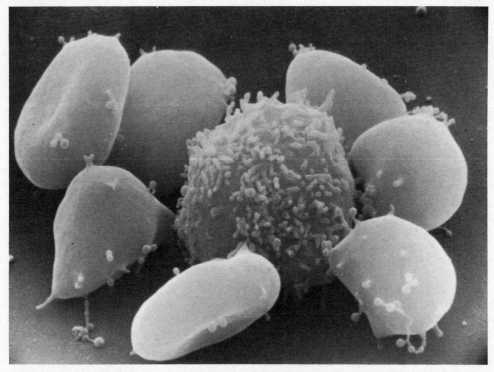

Figure 13–11. Scanning electron micrograph of a human T lymphocyte rosette. The ability of human lymphocytes to bind sheep red blood cells in the absence of antibody and complement has been shown to be a marker for T (thymus-derived) cells; T cells usually have greater than 300 microvilli per cell. (× 9400. Reprinted by permission from Kay, M. M. et al.: Cellular interactions: scanning electron microscopy of human thymus-derived rosette-forming lymphocytes. Clin. Immunol. Immunopathol., 2:301–309, 1974.)

fector responses that include synthesis and release of antibodies by fully differentiated B effector cells or of potent soluble products (lymphokines), and they direct cell-mediated cytotoxicity by completely differentiated T effector cells; and (4) the immune sequence is regulated to ensure that the intended results are attained, but in a limited and controlled manner. Each of these steps is known to occur in the lungs, but the extent to which a *local* pulmonary immune response can be independently generated as distinct from the contribution of *systemic* immune responses to pulmonary immunity is still uncertain.

It is possible to identify T and B cells by testing for specific surface markers, the surface immunoglobulins of B cells, and the ability to form rosettes of T cells (Fig. 13–11).[58] At present it is possible by use of monoclonal antibodies, termed the OKT or T reagents, to define functionally distinct and apparently nonoverlapping T cell subsets. Nearly all peripheral blood T cells from normal persons express the OKT3 marker

and either the OKT4 marker, which defines the functional inducer/helper subset, or the OKT8 marker, which defines the functional cytotoxic/suppressor subset.[59] These functional designations are oversimplifications because the OKT4 population has been shown to contain not only inducer and helper cells but cytotoxic and effector cells as well. Similarly, the OKT8 population contains cells that augment and amplify the interaction of OKT4 cells with B lymphocytes.[59a] Monoclonal antibodies can also be used to subdivide lymphocytes retrieved from the respiratory tract at various levels (see Fig. 13–10); the results presumably reflect the proportions and functional capabilities of the lymphocyte populations throughout the system.

General Considerations

Several general concepts of immunology and local immune responsiveness are considered to play an important role in specific functional immunity in the respiratory tract.[28] First, immune mechanisms are often expressed locally at the site where the antigen contacts the body. Thus, large particles (e.g., rag-weed pollen) that are filtered out of the airstream in the nose are apt to provoke an immunologic reaction in the nose such as allergic rhinitis. Conversely, small inhaled particles (e.g., spores of thermophilic actinomycetes) impact in the terminal respiratory units where they may produce hypersensitivity pneumonitis. Second, local administration by aerosolization or other methods of a large dose of antigen to the lungs will cause *both* respiratory and systemic immune responses, in contrast to the development of only a respiratory reaction when smaller doses are used. In other words, local exposure to large amounts of immunogen overwhelms both local clearance mechanisms and regional exclusivity and "spills over" into the rest of the body. Third, a corollary of the second observation is that the route of exposure to a particular antigen determines the extent of immunologic participation: intravenous administration induces a widespread response, whereas local administration (low dose) evokes a regional response. Finally, it has proved extremely difficult to rigorously separate local and systemic immune responses because, apart from secretory IgA, the same sensitized cells and their products are involved. Thus no one can ever be sure whether a particular immunologic reaction was induced, generated, and expressed autonomously in the respiratory tract or whether the response was merely a local expression of immune effectors that were induced and generated outside the lungs. (The mechanisms that culminate in *expression* of immunity in the respiratory tract have recently been reviewed by Kaltreider[60].)

Local Humoral Immunity

One way of examining the humoral immune reactions occurring in the respiratory tract is to measure the immunoglobulin composition of respiratory liquids. This kind of study has revealed substantial differences among the concentrations of various immunoglobulins at various levels of the respiratory tract and between these values and those in serum (Table 13–4).[61] *Secretory IgA* is the predominant immunoglobulin in samples from the upper respiratory tract, whereas *IgG* is most abundant in bronchoalveolar lavage liquid. These observations are consistent with the finding of cells that stain positively for IgA in the lamina propria and submucosa of the upper airways and bronchi and the virtual absence of these cells in bronchioles.[4] It is likely that locally produced immunoglobulins appearing in mucosal secretions of conducting airways are derived largely from collections of lymphatic tissue that reside in the airway submucosa; in contrast, the immunoglobulins appearing in the terminal respiratory units depend on the influx into parenchymal interstitial tissues of immunoglobulin-secreting cells from systemic sources.

Secretory IgA differs from serum IgA in that the secretory immunoglobulin is a dimer of two IgA molecules linked by a secretory component (SC) and a joining (J) chain. Monomeric IgA and the J chain are synthesized by B cells within the mucous membrane; assembly with SC and transport into external secretions occur in epithelial cells.[62] The secretory IgA complex has a practical advantage over immunoglobulins of other classes in that it is more resistant to proteolysis. Secretory IgA also differs from IgG and IgM in its relative inability to opsonize bacteria or to fix complement.[63]

Table 13–4. CONTENT ($\bar{X} \pm$ S.E.M.) OF CLASS-SPECIFIC IMMUNOGLOBULINS IN SAMPLES FROM THE CANINE RESPIRATORY TRACT AND IN SERUM*

| Fluid | n | Mean Per Cent of the Total Immunoglobulin Concentration | | | Ratio of Concentration |
		IgG	IgA	IgM	IgG/IgA
Stimulated saliva	5	6.3 ± 0.9	83.4 ± 1.4	10.3 ± 0.9	0.1 ± 0.01
Tracheal wash	7	52.7 ± 6.2	33.5 ± 6.2	13.8 ± 3.8	2.1 ± 0.6
Bronchial wash	10	75.0 ± 2.0	19.3 ± 1.9	5.6 ± 0.9	4.1 ± 0.6
Serum	15	77.6 ± 2.7	3.9 ± 0.3	18.6 ± 2.8	23.2 ± 3.0

*Data from Kaltreider, H. B., and Chan, M. K. L.: The class specific immunoglobulin composition of fluids obtained from various levels of the canine respiratory tract. J. Immunol., *116*:423–429, 1976. © (1976) The Williams & Wilkens Co., Baltimore.)

The precise role of secretory IgA in the defense of the lungs is not known. Among its possible activities are complement-independent virus neutralization, and by binding with antigen, agglutination of microorganisms, neutralization of toxins, and reduction of the attachment of bacteria to epithelial surfaces. The latter function may be more generally applicable, thereby limiting absorption of antigen and shielding the body from immunogenic challenge.

IgG appears to be an important immunoglobulin in the lower respiratory tract, judging from its presence in relatively high concentrations in bronchoalveolar lavage liquid. Although not conclusively determined, there is no reason to suspect that alveolar IgG does not exert its classic protective activities: particle agglutination, bacterial opsonization, complement activation, and toxin neutralization.[63]

Because of its high molecular weight, *IgM* is found in relatively low concentrations in respiratory tract secretions (note that the values in Table 13–4 are percentages not concentrations). The role of *IgE* in immediate hypersensitivity reactions that may involve the lungs (e.g., asthma) is well recognized. IgE molecules form a scaffold on the surface of mast cells that when bridged by antigen molecules, causes the mast cells to degranulate and release both preformed and newly formed mediators. But the role of IgE in the defense of healthy lungs remains a mystery.

Thus, the same immunoglobulins that are present in the serum plus secretory IgA are found in respiratory tract secretions. There is reason to believe that these can originate from a resident population of B cells situated in the respiratory tract lymphatic system in response to locally delivered antigen. Although uncertainties remain, it seems logical to postulate that local humoral immunity serves to protect the lungs from viral and bacterial infections and may have other important but unappreciated functions.

Local Cell-Mediated Immunity

When compared with humoral immunity, relatively little is known about the local expression of cell-mediated immunity in the lungs. The information that is available has come chiefly from analysis of the type and functional characteristics of lymphocytes re-

covered from normal persons, patients, or experimental animals by bronchoalveolar lavage. The data of Hunninghake and coworkers[64] show that from 65 to 80 per cent of recoverable lymphocytes from healthy subjects were T-lymphocytes. The fact that these cells could be washed out of the lungs so readily implies that they were on the epithelial surfaces of airways or airspaces or very close to the surface; a corollary of this implication is that the cells did not arise (during the lavage) from the bloodstream.

Thus it is indisputable that the cells that underlie cell-mediated immunity are present in large numbers on or near the respiratory surfaces, but whether they are transient visitors from a blood pool or have been raised in the lungs is open to question. Several investigators have examined the functional capabilities of these "resident" lymphocytes by examining whether or not they can participate in either of the two basic T cell immune effector processes: cell-mediated cytotoxicity and elaboration of lymphokines. To date, there is evidence that T cells recovered from lungs can express both cytotoxicity and lymphokine generation.

Cytotoxic T cells specific for viral antigens that developed in response to induced viral infections have been found in the lungs of mice, hamsters, and rabbits (for further discussion and additional references, see Kaltreider[60]). Sensitized cytolytic T cells appear to contribute to the eradication of viral infection by local containment and lysis of virus-infected cells. Again, these findings substantiate the expression of T-lymphocyte–mediated cytotoxicity in the lungs but do not demonstrate the precise source of the effector cells.

Table 13–5 includes a partial list of lymphokines known to be elaborated by committed T-lymphocytes when stimulated by specific antigen.[65] Several investigators have demonstrated the production by bronchoalveolar cells of macrophage migration inhibitory factor against several microbial antigens such as influenza and mumps viruses, *Streptococcus pneumoniae*, and *Pseudomonas aeruginosa* (see Green and coworkers[28] for review and references). This effect was shown to be transient, which may explain why it has not been possible to document the production of lymphokines by bronchoalveolar lymphocytes from normal

Table 13–5. BIOLOGIC FACTORS ELABORATED BY COMMITTED LYMPHOCYTES STIMULATED BY SPECIFIC ANTIGEN*

Macrophage migration inhibitory factor
Chemotactic factor for macrophages
Chemotactic factor for neutrophilic polymorphonuclear leukocytes
Macrophage-activating factor
Cytotoxic factor
Growth-inhibiting factor
Cloning inhibition factor
Factor preventing DNA synthesis
Mitogenic factor
Skin-reactive factor
Macrophage aggregation factor
Transfer factor
Interferon
Interleukin-2

*Data in part from David, J. R.: Lymphocyte mediators and cellular hypersensitivity. New Engl. J. Med., 288:143–149, 1973.

humans. Of considerable pathogenetic interest is the observation that lavaged lymphocytes from patients with active pulmonary sarcoidosis spontaneously released macrophage migration inhibitory factor[66] and interleukin-2,[67] a substance that causes responsive T cells to proliferate.

Thus there is good evidence that T cells capable of lymphokine production are present in or near bronchoalveolar spaces after suitable means of experimental immunization, and activated T cells are found in patients with certain diseases. However, whether these cells migrate into the lungs from the circulating pool or arise locally from indigenous T cells is unknown. In either case, cell-mediated immune reactions are expressed in the lungs and, presumably, are the major defense against intracellular infections (e.g., tuberculosis). It is important to recognize, however, that the chief effector cell for microbicidal activity is the macrophage, not the T cell; therefore, these cells must communicate with each other.

Interactions

The multiple and diverse roles of macrophages have already been mentioned, but it needs to be emphasized that these members of the nonspecific defense system are essential participants in immune responses. This involves more than casual collaboration between macrophages and lymphocytes: one cell type simply cannot function effectively without the other.

The dual role of macrophages has already been mentioned. By finding and processing antigens for subsequent presentation to immunocompetent lymphocytes, macrophages are the key to the *induction* of an immune reaction. Finally, as just stated, lymphocyte-macrophage interactions are indispensible to the *expression* of cell-mediated immunity.[68] This partnership is beneficial because lymphocytes are not equipped to phagocytose and kill microorganisms whereas macrophages are. Certain lymphokines serve to attract macrophages to a particular site, to keep them at that location and, above all, to activate them. Inactivated macrophages are capable of phagocytosing microorganisms, but they are not normally able to kill them (e.g., tubercle bacilli). However, the release of lymphokines by sensitized T cells has profound effects on macrophages: their intracellular metabolism is greatly increased, which augments their capacity to migrate, phagocytose, and dispose of offending pathogens. Moreover, these phagocytic activities can be directed at microorganisms besides those to which the activated T cells are sensitized. In other words, immunologically committed lymphocytes induced by contact with tubercle bacillus antigen will react and release lymphokines only on subsequent contact with that particular antigen and to no other antigen; however, the macrophages activated in the process will demonstrate increased microbicidal effectiveness against not only tubercle bacilli but other microorganisms as well.[69]

Thus it is clear that both B cell- and T cell-mediated immunologic reactions occur in the lungs, although there is still some uncertainty about the extent of local autonomy, particularly of cell-mediated responses. But whether antibodies or lymphokines are the final immunologic effector, participation by phagocytes is necessary both to initiate the response and to carry out phagocytosis, killing, and degradation. Protection of the lungs can be characterized by close interdependency among the components of the specific and nonspecific defense systems. Future work will be aimed at harnessing and manipulating these systems to provide even more effective responses against potential pathogens in the respiratory tract.[70]

REFERENCES

1. Muir, D. C. F.: Deposition and clearance of inhaled particles. In Muir, D. C. F. (ed.): Clinical Aspects of Inhaled Particles. London, Heinemann, 1972, pp. 1–20.
2. Brain, J. D., and Volberg, P. A.: State of the art. Deposition of aerosol in the respiratory tract. Am. Rev. Respir. Dis., 120:1325–1373, 1979.
3. Hoffman, R. A., and Billingham, J.: Effect of altered G levels on deposition of particulates in the human respiratory tract. J. Appl. Physiol., 38:955–960, 1975.
4. Newhouse, M., Sanchis, J., and Bienenstock, J.: Lung defense mechanisms. New Engl. J. Med., 295:990–995, 1045–1052, 1976.
5. Task Group on Lung Dynamics: Deposition and retention models for internal dosimetry of the human respiratory tract. Health Phys., 12:173–207, 1966.
6. Hatch, T. F., and Gross, P.: Pulmonary Deposition and Retention of Inhaled Aerosols. New York, Academic Press, 1964, pp. 67–85.
7. Oberst, F. W.: Factors affecting inhalation and retention of toxic vapours. In Davies, C. N. (ed.): Inhaled Particles and Vapours. New York, Pergamon Press, 1961, pp. 249–266.
8. Forster, R. E.: Diffusion of gases. In Fenn, W. O., and Rahn, H. (eds.): Handbook of Physiology, Section 3. Respiration. Vol. I. Washington, D.C., American Physiology Society, 1964, pp. 839–872.
9. Farhi, L. E.: Elimination of inert gas by the lung. Respir. Physiol., 3:1–11, 1967.
10. Richardson, P. S., and Peatfield, A. C.: Reflexes concerned in the defense of the lungs. Bull. Eur. Physiopathol. Respir., 17:979–1012, 1981.
11. Szereda-Przestaszewska, M., and Widdicombe, J. G.: Reflex effects of chemical irritation of the upper airways on the laryngeal lumen in cat. Respir. Physiol., 18:107–115, 1973.
12. Widdicombe, J. G., and Sterling, G. M.: The autonomic nervous system and breathing. Arch. Intern. Med., 126:311–329, 1970.
13. Mills, J. E., Sellick, H., and Widdicombe, J. G.: Activity of lung irritant receptors in pulmonary microembolism, anaphylaxis and drug-induced bronchoconstrictions. J. Physiol. (Lond.), 203:337–357, 1969.
14. Nadel, J. A., Salem, H., Tamplin, B., and Tokiwa, Y.: Mechanism of bronchoconstriction during inhalation of sulfur dioxide. J. Appl. Physiol., 20:164–167, 1965.
15. Speizer, F. E., and Frank, N. R.: A comparison of changes in pulmonary flow resistance in healthy volunteers acutely exposed to SO_2 by mouth and by nose. Brit. J. Industr. Med., 23:75–79, 1966.
16. Ingelstedt, S.: Studies on the conditioning of air in the respiratory tract. Acta Otolaryngol. (Suppl.), 131:1–80, 1956.
17. McFadden, E. R., Jr.: Respiratory heat and water exchange: physiological and clinical implications. J. Appl. Physiol., 54:331–336, 1983.
18. Proctor, D. F.: State of the art. The upper airways. I. Nasal physiology and defense of the lungs. Am. Rev. Respir. Dis., 115:97–129, 1977.
19. Proctor, D. F., and Lundqvist, G.: Clearance of inhaled particles from the human nose. Arch. Intern. Med., 131:132–139, 1973.
20. Rhodin, J. A. G.: Ultrastructure and function of the human tracheal mucosa. Am. Rev. Respir. Dis., 93(Suppl.):1–15, 1966.
21. Palmblad, J., Mossberg, B., and Afzelius, B. A.: Ultrastructural, cellular, and clinical features of the immotile-cilia syndrome. Annu. Rev. Med., 35:481–492, 1984.
22. Mygind, N., Nielsen, M. H., and Pederson, M. (eds.): Kartagener's syndrome and abnormal cilia. Eur. J. Respir. Dis., 64(Suppl. 127):1–167, 1983.
23. Yoneda, K.: Mucous blanket of the rat bronchus. An ultrastructural study. Am. Rev. Respir. Dis., 114:837–842, 1976.
24. Camner, P.: Editorial review. Clearance of particles from the human tracheobronchial tree. Clin. Sci., 59:79–84, 1980.
25. Dalhamn, T.: Mucus flow and ciliary activity in the trachea of healthy rats and rats exposed to respiratory irritant gases (SO_2, H_3N, HCHO); functional and morphologic (light microscopic and electron microscopic) study, with special reference to technique. Acta Physiol. Scand. 36(Suppl. 123):1–161, 1956.
26. Santa Cruz, R., Landa, J., Hirsch, J., and Sackner, M. A.: Tracheal mucous velocity in normal man and patients with obstructive lung disease; effects of terbutaline. Am. Rev. Respir. Dis., 109:458–463, 1974.
27. Albert, R. E., Lippmann, M., Peterson, H. T., Jr., Berger, J., Sanborn, K., and Bohning, D.: Bronchial deposition and clearance of aerosols. Arch. Intern. Med., 131:115–127, 1973.
28. Green, G. M., Jakab, G. J., Low, R. B., and Davis, G. S.: State of the art. Defense mechanisms of the respiratory membrane. Am. Rev. Respir. Dis., 115:479–514, 1977.
29. La Belle, C. W., and Brieger, H.: The fate of inhaled particles in the early postexposure period. Arch. Environ. Health, 1:432–437, 1960.
30. Masson, P. L., and Heremans, J. F.: Sputum proteins. In Dulfano, M. (ed.): Sputum, Fundamentals and Clinical Pathology. Springfield, Charles C Thomas, 1973, pp. 412–475.
31. Litt, M.: Basic concepts of mucus rheology. Bull. Eur. Physiopathol. Respir., 9:33–46, 1973.
32. Wanner, A.: State of the art. Clinical aspects of mucociliary transport. Am. Rev. Respir. Dis., 116:73–125, 1977.
33. Olver, R. E., Davis, B., Marin, M. G., and Nadel, J. A.: Active transport of Na^+ and Cl^- across the canine tracheal epithelium in vitro. Am. Rev. Respir. Dis., 112:811–815, 1975.
34. Nadel, J. A., Davis, B., and Phipps, R. J.: Control of mucus secretion and ion transport in airways. Annu. Rev. Physiol., 41:369–381, 1979.
35. Welsh, M. J.: Intracellular chloride activities in canine tracheal epithelium. Direct evidence for sodium-coupled intracellular chloride accumulation in a chloride-secreting epithelium. J. Clin. Invest., 71:1392–1401, 1983.
36. Barton, A. D., and Lourenco, R. V.: Bronchial secretions and mucociliary clearance. Arch. Intern. Med., 131:140–144, 1973.
37. Johnason, W. G., Jr., Jay, S. J., and Pierce, A. K.: Bacterial growth in vivo. An important determinant of the pulmonary clearance of Diplococcus pneumoniae in rats. J. Clin. Invest., 53:1320–1325, 1974.
38. Green, G. M., and Kass, E. H.: The influence of

bacterial species on pulmonary resistance to infection in mice subjected to hypoxia, cold stress, and ethanolic intoxication. Brit. J. Exp. Pathol., 46:360–366, 1965.

39. O'Neill, S., Lesperance, E., and Klass, D. J.: Rat lung lavage surfactant enhances bacterial phagocytosis and intracellular killing by alveolar macrophages. Am. Rev. Respir. Dis., 130:225–230, 1984.

40. Weiser, R. S., Myrvik, Q. N., and Pearsall, N. N.: Fundamentals of Immunology for Students of Medicine and Related Sciences. Philadelphia, Lea & Febiger, 1969, p. 363.

41. Isaacs, A., and Lindenmann, J.: Virus interference: I. The interferon. Proc. R. Soc. Lond. (Biol.), 147:258–267, 1957.

42. Cesario, T. C.: The clinical implications of human interferon. Med. Clin. North Am., 67:1147–1162, 1983.

43. Epstein, L. B.: Interferon as a model lymphokine. Fed. Proc., 40:56–61, 1981.

44. Acton, J. D., and Myrvik, Q. N.: Production of interferon by alveolar macrophages. J. Bacteriol., 91:2300–2304, 1966.

45. Epstein, L. B., Cline, M. J., and Merigan, T. C.: The interaction of human macrophages and lymphocytes in the phytohemagglutinin-stimulated production of interferon. J. Clin. Invest., 50:744–753, 1971.

46. Colten, H. R., Alper, C. A., and Rosen, F. S.: Current concepts in immunology. Genetics and biosynthesis of complement proteins. New Engl. J. Med., 304:653–656, 1981.

47. Perez, H. D.: Biologically active complement (C5)-derived peptides and their relevance to disease. CRC Rev. Oncol. Hematol., 1:199–225, 1984.

48. Metchnikoff, E.: Immunity in Infective Diseases. London, Cambridge University Press, 1905, p. 591.

49. Stossel, T. P.: Phagocytosis. New Engl. J. Med., 290:717–723, 774–780, 833–839, 1974.

50. Snyderman, R., and Goetzl, E. J.: Molecular and cellular mechanisms of leukocyte chemotaxis. Science, 213:830–837, 1981.

51. Hocking, W. G., and Golde, D. W.: Medical progress. The pulmonary-alveolar macrophage. New Engl. J. Med., 301:580–587, 639–645, 1979.

52. Nathan, C. F., Murray, H. W., and Cohn, Z. A.: Current concepts. The macrophage as an effector cell. New Engl. J. Med., 303:622–626, 1980.

53. Cohen, A. B.: Lung cell biology. Fed. Proc., 38:2635–2636, 1979.

54. Cohen, A. B.: Potential adverse effects of lung macrophages and neutrophils. Fed. Proc., 38:2644–2647, 1979.

55. Tate, R. M., and Repine, J. E.: State of the art. Neutrophils and the adult respiratory distress syndrome. Am. Rev. Respir. Dis., 128:552–559, 1983.

56. Klebanoff, S. J.: Basic review. Oxygen metabolism

and the toxic properties of phagocytes. Ann. Int. Med., 93:480–489, 1980.

57. Grey, H. M.: Phylogeny of immunoglobulins. Adv. Immunol., 10:51–104, 1969.

58. Kay, M. M., Belohradsky, B., Yee, K., Vogel, J., Butcher, D., Wybran, J., and Fudenberg, H. H.: Cellular interactions: scanning electron microscopy of human thymus-derived rosette-forming lymphocytes. Clin. Immunol. Immunopathol., 2:301–309, 1974.

59. Fauci, A. S., Lane, H. C., and Volkman, D. J.: Activation and regulation of human immune responses: implications in normal and disease states. Ann. Int. Med., 99:61–75, 1983.

59a. Seligmann, M., Chess, L., Fahey, J. L., Fauci, A. S., Lachmann, P. J., L'Age-Stehr, J., Ngu, J., Pinching, A. J., Rosen, F. S., Spira, T. J., and Wybran, J.: AIDS—an immunologic reevaluation. New Engl. J. Med., 311:1286–1292, 1984.

60. Kaltreider, H. B.: Local immunity. In Bienenstock, J. (ed.): Immunology of the Lung and Upper Respiratory Tract. New York, McGraw-Hill Co., 1984, pp. 191–215.

61. Kaltreider, H. B., and Chan, M. K. L.: The class-specific immunoglobulin composition of fluids obtained from various levels of the canine respiratory tract. J. Immunol., 116:423–429, 1976.

62. Tomasi, T. B., Jr.: Secretory immunoglobulins. New Engl. J. Med., 287:500–506, 1972.

63. Kaltreider, H. B.: State of the art. Expression of immune mechanisms in the lung. Am. Rev. Respir. Dis., 113:347–379, 1976.

64. Hunninghake, G. W., Gadek, J. E., Kawanami, O., Ferrans, V. J., and Crystal, R. G.: Inflammatory and immune processes in the human lung in health and disease: evaluation by bronchoalveolar lavage. Am. J. Pathol., 97:149–205, 1979.

65. David, J. R.: Lymphocyte mediators and cellular hypersensitivity. New Engl. J. Med., 288:143–149, 1973.

66. Crystal, R. G., Roberts, W. C., Hunninghake, G. W., Gadek, J. E., Fulmer, J. D., and Line, B. R.: Pulmonary sarcoidosis: a disease characterized and perpetuated by activated lung T-lymphocytes. Ann. Int. Med., 94:73–94, 1981.

67. Pinkston, P., Bitterman, P. B., and Crystal, R. G.: Spontaneous release of interleukin-2 by lung T-lymphocytes in active pulmonary sarcoidosis. New Engl. J. Med., 308:793–800, 1983.

68. Unanue, E. R.: Cooperation between mononuclear phagocytes and lymphocytes in immunity. New Engl. J. Med., 303:977–985, 1980.

69. Mackaness, G. B.: The immunological basis of acquired cellular resistance. J. Exp. Med., 120:105–120, 1964.

70. Bienenstock, J.: The lung as an immunologic organ. Annu. Rev. Med., 35:49–62, 1984.

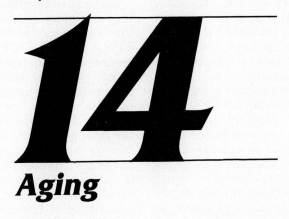

Aging

INTRODUCTION

Most people recognize that improvements in socioeconomic conditions and in health care during the last several decades have extended the average life span of human beings by many years, but it is not so well known that the maximum duration of life in modern times is nearly the same as it was in antiquity.[1] Thus, every person is mortal, and contrary to popular belief, there is no foreseeable practical way of extending maximum life span. If the two leading causes of death in the United States—heart disease and stroke—were successfully eliminated, the average life span would increase by approximately 18 years.[2] If the third biggest killer, cancer, were eliminated, two more years would accrue. Eradication of diseases that cause early death allows life expectancy to approach more closely its biologically determined maximum, which for humans is 100 to 110 years.

Development from fertilization to maturity and then to death is clearly a time-dependent process and thus related to aging. These processes differ, however, because growth is characterized by the elaboration of cells, tissues, and organs with new structures or functions, whereas senescence is associated with loss of adaptation and increased vulnerability to disease.[3] Embryogenesis and early postnatal structural development of the lungs are considered in

Chapters 1 and 2. In this chapter the effects of aging on respiratory and nonrespiratory functions of the lungs during both growth and senescence will be discussed; the structural basis for these changes will be included when information is available.

The mechanisms responsible for the cellular effects of aging are unknown, but most theories involve alterations, either genetically programmed or acquired, in genetic machinery.[2, 3] A useful update on the theoretical and experimental approaches to aging has recently been published.[4] Some organs (e.g., thymus and ovaries) usually involute and cease to function long before death occurs. However, the lungs appear to be relatively durable and, even though important alterations in their structure and function develop with age, unless affected by disease they are capable of maintaining adequate gas exchange for the maximum life span.

It is important to document the effects of growth and senescence on pulmonary function in order to establish the limits of "normal" development and aging; this is obviously necessary before functional impairment from pulmonary diseases can be identified. New and useful information about pulmonary function in newborn babies, infants, and children has become available during the last two decades, although there is still an important gap in knowledge between the newborn period and five to six years of age; much of this data has been collated in recent reviews.[5, 6] In addition, the effects of senescence on respiratory function have attracted increased attention lately, and these findings have also been summarized.[7, 8] The boundary between normality and disease is often ill-defined and presents a problem of definition that is especially troublesome in the aged, in whom it is difficult to sort out the subtle effects of acquired insults. Therefore, some of the data from which conclusions about the effects of senescence on respiration have been reached must be accepted with reservations because of uncertainties about smoking habits, environmental exposure, and physical activity.

STATIC PROPERTIES

As discussed in Chapter 4, the determinants of static lung volumes are the elastic properties of the lungs and chest wall and the forces that can be generated by the muscles of respiration to inflate and deflate the respiratory system. It is well established that respiratory muscle strength increases during the period of somatic growth and for several years thereafter, and that senescence, especially after 55 years of age, is accompanied by progressive weakening of maximal inspiratory and expiratory pressures in both men and women.[9, 10] However, the chief physiologic effects of aging on pulmonary function are attributable to changes in the compliance of both the lungs and the chest wall. Data from several studies have supplied much needed information about the compliance of human lungs in relation to age,[11, 12] and knowledge about existing gaps in the continuum of information can be inferred with reasonable confidence. In contrast, studies about the age-related behavior of the chest wall are still extremely limited, especially in infants and children; these data are needed because they are necessary to allow examination of the entire respiratory system and because they may explain the serious clinical consequences of lower respiratory tract infections in infants. For example, it was mentioned in Chapter 4 that children younger than five years of age may be at a disadvantage compared with adults because their small airways are disproportionately smaller; however, changes in the functional capabilities of the chest wall could either compound or minimize the effects of differences in airway caliber.

Compliance

Figure 14–1 summarizes the relationship between static elastic recoil at 60 per cent of TLC and age, based on separate studies of different age groups.[11–15] Static elastic recoil increases from birth until growth ceases and then gradually diminishes. Although it is difficult to compare volume-pressure curves of children of different ages because of marked changes in body size and lung volume (Fig. 14–2A), when related to TLC or to a pressure that approximates TLC, age-related differences from 6 to 18 years are still observed (Fig. 14–2B).[16] However, these differences are not striking in their magnitude, presumably because much of the maturation of the elastic tissue elements, which continues to young adulthood, is already completed before eight years of

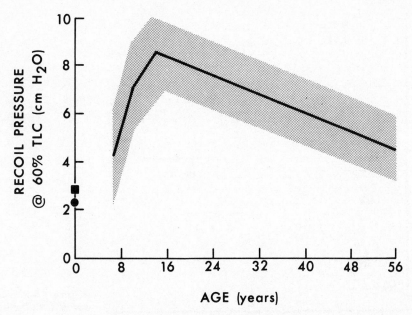

Figure 14–1. Static elastic recoil at 60 per cent total lung capacity (TLC) as a function of age. (Data of Turner, Mead, and Wohl[12] and Zapletal, Misur, and Samanek.[13]) Shaded area represents ± one standard deviation of mean values. Mean values in newborn period (■ ●) from Gribetz, Frank, and Avery[14] and Nelson.[15] (Adapted and reprinted by permission from Mansell, A. et al.: Airway closure in children. J. Appl. Physiol., *33*:711–714, 1972.)

age.[17] Similarly, the decrease in recoil that occurs during senescence, although real and readily detectable, is most apparent at high lung volumes. Indeed, in one large study of the effects of age on the mechanical properties of the lungs, a decrease in recoil was evident in elderly persons only at lung volumes greater than 40 per cent of TLC (Fig. 14–3).[18] However, the progressive loss of pulmonary elasticity, albeit small and well-tolerated, accounts in large part for the age-related changes in lung volumes, expiratory flow rates, and arterial blood gas values.

In the final analysis, the elastic properties of the lung can be separated into two components: surface forces and tissue forces. There is no evidence that the surface-active lining of terminal respiratory units alters its basic mechanical behavior with age. Thus, changes in surface forces do not appear to contribute to age-related changes, with the exception that variations in elastic recoil from surface forces may occur secondary to the influence of tissue forces on alveolar dimensions and geometry.[12] The lungs grow by both the formation of new alveoli and the expansion of existing alveoli (see Chapter 2). The enlargement of the

lungs from birth to maturity is associated with increases in both surface and tissue forces, the former from simple expansion of the surface of individual alveoli and the latter from changing connective tissue composition. Presumably the most important structural development that affects the mechanical properties of growing lungs is the increased content and complexity of the fibrous tissue meshwork.[17] It is also possible that changes in the collagen framework of the lung parenchyma may contribute to an increase in tissue forces during growth.

The diminution in static elastic recoil of the lung that occurs during senescence is more difficult to account for on a structural basis than the increase that occurs during growth, although connective tissue elements have also been implicated. It was originally believed that there was a progressive increase in elastin content of the lung with age after maturity;[19] subsequent data indicated that the increase was confined to an increase in the elastin content of the pleura whereas that of the parenchyma remained constant.[20] However, neither report provides a satisfactory explanation for the consistent reduction in elastic recoil of the lungs dur-

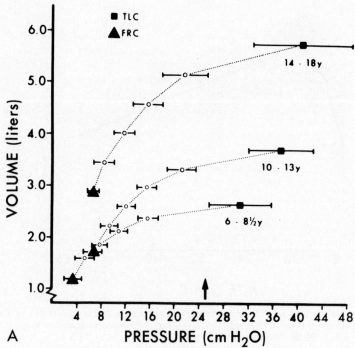

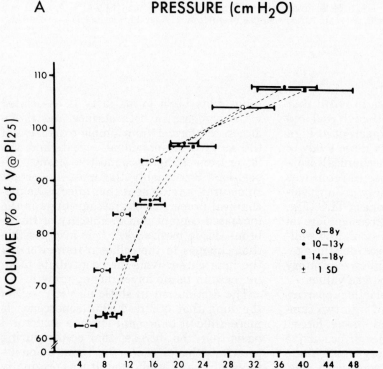

Figure 14–2. Volume-pressure curves from three groups of children of different ages. *A*, Results expressed in absolute volume. *B*, Results expressed as per cent of volume at a distending pressure of 25 cm H_2O (% of V @ Pl 25). (Reprinted from Bryan, A. C., et al.: Development of the mechanical properties of the respiratory system. *In* Hodson, W. A. (ed.): Development of the Lung. New York, 1977, pp. 445–468 by courtesy of Marcel Dekker, Inc.)

ing senescence, which changes in a highly predictable manner.[21] Even careful morphometric studies of the total length and diameter of elastic fibers failed to reveal changes in the lungs during senescence.[22] However, because the elasticity of a complex meshwork is a function not only of the elastic properties of the individual fibers themselves but also of their spatial arrangement, remodeling of the delicate parenchymal elastic fiber network may account for the findings. This notion is supported by the morphologic changes that occur during the course of aging in terminal respiratory units: alveolar ducts increase in diameter, and the alveoli arising from them become wider and shallower. It is also possible that pseudoelastin is present in aging human lungs and speciously increases the total elastin content as measured by the usual chemical analyses.[23] If this were the case, the actual amount of elastin would decrease during senescence and provide, in turn, a straightforward explanation for the age-related decrease in distensibility.

Studies in newborns and young infants demonstrated that the compliance of the lung and chest wall combined[24] is nearly the same as that of the lung alone.[25] This means that compliance of the chest wall must be high in the neonatal period. Similar conclusions from direct measurements were reported for dogs[26] and for goats.[27] The similarities of chest wall mechanics among newborns of several mammalian species probably relate to the requirements of passage through the birth canal.

Chest wall compliance presumably decreases during childhood to the values found in young adults, although only the sequence of changes in the early postnatal years has been documented.[28] In adulthood, a progressive reduction in compliance was demonstrated in men 24 to 78 years of age.[29] The stiffening of the chest wall is presumably related to ossification and other structural changes within the rib cage and its articulations.

Data on both chest wall compliance and lung elastic recoil have been coupled in Figure 14–4 to depict the volume-pressure diagrams for an "ideal" newborn, and "ideal" 20 and 60 year old persons. (For further discussion of how these diagrams are constructed, see Chapter 4, Fig. 4–7). The curves were compiled using data from studies previously cited.[12, 15, 24, 29] However, these do not provide all the necessary information and so parts of the curves are conjectural, particularly the lowermost 50 per

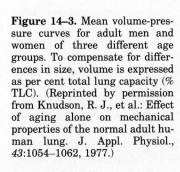

Figure 14–3. Mean volume-pressure curves for adult men and women of three different age groups. To compensate for differences in size, volume is expressed as per cent total lung capacity (% TLC). (Reprinted by permission from Knudson, R. J., et al.: Effect of aging alone on mechanical properties of the normal adult human lung. J. Appl. Physiol., 43:1054–1062, 1977.)

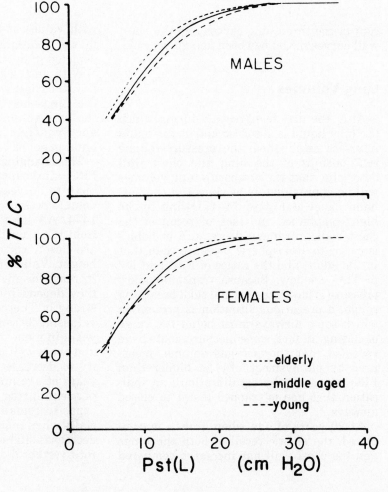

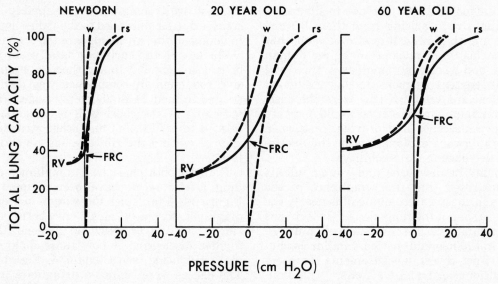

Figure 14–4. Static volume-pressure relationships of lungs (l), chest wall (w), and total respiratory system (rs) for a normal newborn and 20 and 60 year old adults. RV = residual volume; FRC = functional residual capacity. (Data from Turner, J. M. et al.: Elasticity of human lungs in relation to age. J. Appl. Physiol., *25*:664–671, 1968; Nelson, N. M.: Neonatal pulmonary function. Pediatr. Clin. North Am., *13*:769–799, 1966; Richards, C. C., and Bachman, L.: Lung and chest wall compliance of apneic paralyzed infants. J. Clin. Invest., *40*:273–278, 1961; and Mittman, C. et al.: Relationship between chest wall and pulmonary compliance and age. J. Appl. Physiol., *20*:1211–1216, 1965.)

cent of the three lung curves and the chest wall curves in the newborn and 20 year old.

Lung Volumes

After the first few breaths, during which the lung liquid is absorbed and an air-liquid interface established, the pressure-volume relationships of the lung and chest wall determine that the newborn's lung volumes will be approximately as shown in the left-hand panel of Figure 14–4. Owing to the high compliance and lack of recoil of the chest wall, intrapleural pressure in babies is closer to atmospheric pressure than that in the adult, and the ratios of FRC and RV to TLC are low. Because transpulmonary pressure is low in the normal tidal breathing range, a precarious situation is present in which some airways must be on the verge of closing. In fact, some measurements have revealed that thoracic gas volume (measured by plethysmography) is higher than FRC (measured by equilibration), an indication that gas is trapped distal to closed airways.[15]

At 20 years of age when growth is completed, the elastic recoil of both the lungs and the chest wall has increased compared

with values at birth. These changes result in the relationships among lung volumes depicted in the middle panel of Figure 14–4.

With increasing senescence after maturity, the chest wall becomes even stiffer, but the lungs become more distensible. Thus, the lung volumes of a 60 year old man are approximately those shown in the right-hand panel of Figure 14–4.

The changing relationships between RV, FRC, vital capacity, and TLC and age from birth to 80 years can be inferred from the volume-pressure curves shown in Figure 14–4. All lung volumes typically increase from birth until somatic growth stops and are closely correlated with increasing body height. Values for VC and TLC continue to increase for another 10 to 15 years, because they depend in part on respiratory muscle strength. Thereafter, compared with "best" values at 20 years of age in women and 27 years in men, the effects of changes in lung and chest wall mechanics cause vital capacity to decrease to about 75 per cent at 70 years of age and RV to increase nearly 50 per cent during the same period. Total lung capacity remains virtually constant, especially when related to height, which actually decreases slightly owing to flattening of the intervertebral disks.

DYNAMIC PROPERTIES

Growth is associated with an increase in forced expiratory volume in 1 sec (Fig. 14–5) and with related measurements of resistance to airflow such as peak expiratory flow rate and specific airway conductance.[6] Expired airflow velocity increases during growth because the lungs' elastic recoil increases, and the tracheobronchial system enlarges. Thus both the caliber of the airways and the driving force for maximal airflow change in the direction that augments expiratory flow rates. After maturity, in addition to the decrease in slow and forced vital capacity values, a consistent decline with age has been demonstrated for several indexes of expired airflow velocity: forced expiratory volume in 1 sec (see Fig. 14–5), maximal expiratory flow rate, maximal midexpiratory flow, and maximal expiratory flow rate at a given lung volume.

Airflow Rates

As already indicated, body height ceases to increase during adolescence, but as shown in Figure 14–5, ventilatory function continues to develop until the age of 20 years in women and 27 years in men;[30] much of this improvement can be related to increasing respiratory muscle strength. After these ages, the inevitable decline begins. But the results of recent studies suggest that at least until 40 years of age, most of the age-related decreases in forced vital capacity and maximal expiratory flow rates can be attributed to changes in body weight and strength and may not necessarily indicate attrition of tissues.[31] It has been traditional to express the decline in pulmonary function variables such as the forced vital capacity and forced expiratory volume in 1 sec as a constant quantity per year (linear function).[32] Knudson and coworkers[33] recently reaffirmed the usefulness of this approach, but when they looked at the same data another way (Table 14–1), they found that the decline in forced expiratory volume in 1 sec is small at first and then increases progressively with increasing age. Similar results have been noted by others.[34]

Several studies of the effects of age on maximum expiratory flow volume relationships have revealed a decrease in mean

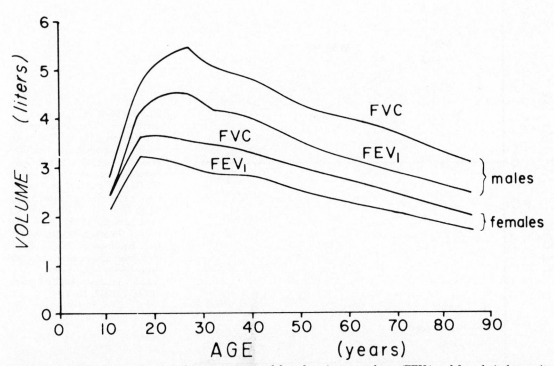

Figure 14–5. Mean values showing changes in 1 second forced expiratory volume (FEV$_1$) and forced vital capacity (FVC) with age in normal men and women. (Reprinted by permission from Knudson, R. J., et al.: The maximal expiratory flow-volume curve. Normal standards, variability and the effects of age. Am. Rev. Respir. Dis., *113*:587–600, 1976.)

Table 14–1. MEAN RATE OF CHANGE OF FORCED EXPIRATORY VOLUME IN 1 SEC (ML/YR) IN HEALTHY NONSMOKERS ACCORDING TO AGE (YEARS)*

Sex	Overall	25–39 (men) 20–39 (women)	40–64	65 and over
Men	−29.7	−19.7	−31.0	−37.9
Women	−22.9	−10.7	−23.9	−31.0

*Data from Knudson, R. J. et al.: Changes in the normal maximal expiratory flow-volume curve with growth and aging. Am. Rev. Respir. Dis., *127*:725–734, 1983.

maximal flow rates within the effort-independent range of the forced vital capacity maneuver, particularly at low lung volumes;[18, 35] this change causes a curvilinear appearance of the maximal expiratory flow-volume curve (Fig. 14–6) that simulates the abnormalities produced by chronic cigarette smoking. The preservation of maximal expiratory airflow at high lung volumes and the decrease at low lung volumes are exactly opposite to the findings that would be predicted from the age-related changes in elastic recoil.[18] This paradox, especially when coupled with the striking variations in maximal expiratory flow rates among persons of a given age group, indicates that factors besides elastic recoil, which may or may not be related to age, are important determinants of airway geometry and resistance.[36] Some of these variations have been attributed to differences between the development of lung volume and airway size, the so-called dysanapsis.[37] It should also be pointed out that body build, and hence lung development and pulmonary function, vary among persons of different racial backgrounds. For this reason, it is unwise to extrapolate findings from one ethnic group to another.

Distribution of Ventilation

Newborn infants may exhibit uniform ventilation when tested by the usual relatively insensitive multiple breath N_2 washout test.[38] However, the plethysmographic

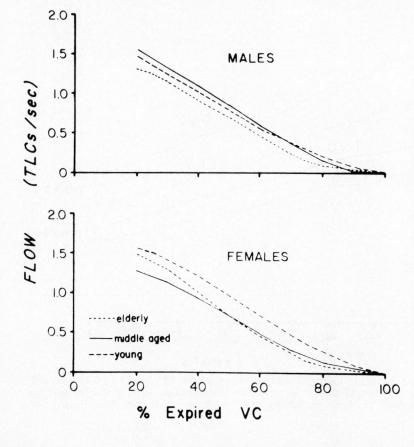

Figure 14–6. Maximum expiratory flow-volume curves for men and women of three different age groups. To compensate for differences in size, flow is expressed as total lung capacity per second (TLCs/sec) and volume as per cent expired vital capacity (% VC). Only the effort-independent portions of the curves are shown. (Reprinted by permission from Knudson, R. J. et al.: Effect of aging alone on mechanical properties of the normal adult human lung. J. Appl. Physiol., *43*:1054–1062, 1977.)

demonstration of air trapping is convincing evidence that inspired air is distributed unevenly. Furthermore, recent studies of closing volume in children demonstrated regional inequalities that are similar to those of aged adults, and presumably the disturbances in both age groups can be related to changes in pulmonary elastic recoil.[11, 39] The low elastic recoil that characterizes the lungs of children and aged adults (see Fig. 14–1) means that airways in the dependent regions, where transpulmonary distending pressure is normally lower than in the uppermost regions, will close at higher lung volumes than when elastic recoil is increased (see Chapter 4). Gas distal to the sites of closure will be either trapped or poorly communicating, and thus nonuniformity of the mixing of inspired air must result. As stated, young children and aged adults have high closing volumes; moreover, some young adults may have no closing

volume at all. During senescence, closing capacity, which equals closing volume plus residual volume, increases more rapidly than FRC, and when the two are equal, some dependent airways may be closed and the terminal respiratory units they supply will not be ventilated continuously during normal tidal breathing. When in the seated position, closing capacity begins to exceed FRC at approximately 65 years of age (Fig. 14–7) and when in the supine position, this occurs at about 44 years of age.[40] Under these conditions, the abnormalities in the distribution of ventilation should be corrected by breathing with a large tidal volume so that FRC plus tidal volume greatly exceeds closing volume; in a study of old men, breathing deeply did improve the uniformity of ventilation compared with breathing normally. The relationship between closing capacity with respect to FRC (see Fig. 14–7) not only affects the distri-

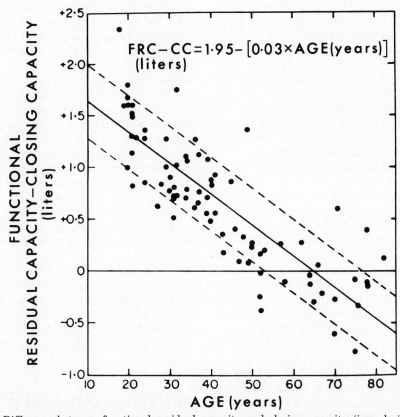

Figure 14–7. Difference between functional residual capacity and closing capacity (i.e., closing volume plus residual volume), in liters, as a function of age in 80 seated subjects, with regression line (solid line) ± 1 SD (dashed lines). Negative values indicate that airway closure is present during normal tidal breathing. (Modified and reprinted by permission from Leblanc, P. et al.: Effects of age and body position on "airway closure" in man. J. Appl. Physiol., *28*:448–451, 1970.)

Table 14–2. POSTNATAL CHANGES IN NUMBER OF ALVEOLI, ALVEOLAR SURFACE AREA (SA), BODY SURFACE AREA (SB), AND ALVEOLAR SURFACE TO BODY SURFACE RATIO (SA/SB)*

Age	Number of Aveoli, × 10^6	Alveolar Surface Area, m^2	Body Surface Area, m^2	SA/SB
Newborn	24	2.8	0.21	13.3
3 months	77	7.2	0.29	24.8
7 months	112	8.4	0.38	22.1
13 months	129	12.2	0.45	27.1
4 years	257	22.2	0.67	33.1
8 years	280	32.0	0.92	34.8
Adult	296	75.0	1.90	39.5

*Data from Dunnill, M. S.: Postnatal growth of the lung. Thorax, *17*:329–333, 1962.

bution of ventilation but, as will be discussed, is an important determinant of age-related changes in arterial Po_2.

DIFFUSING CAPACITY

Most investigations of diffusing capacity in children have examined the age range from 5 to 15 years and ignored the period from infancy to preschool. The interval from birth to five years of age is of particular interest because, as shown in Table 14–2, the ratio of alveolar surface area to body surface area increases during the first four years of life from 13.3 to 33.1; thereafter, the changes are much less remarkable, the adult values reaching only 39.5.[41] The increase in alveolar surface area during the first few years of life is explained by the explosive proliferation of new alveoli and pulmonary capillaries (see Chapter 2).

Detailed morphometric studies in growing rats by Weibel[42] revealed a steady increase of all variables that characterize pulmonary diffusing capacity during the first five days of life (Phase II); thereafter, there is again a steady increase that is proportional to lung volume (Phase III). The diffusing capacity per square meter of body surface of human newborns is about half that of normal adults.[15] Whether the maturation of diffusing capacity in humans occurs in three phases similar to those observed in rats is not known; however, there does appear to be a phase of extremely rapid increase in diffusion surface (comparable to Phase II) sometime during infancy or early childhood because by the time the child is about five to six years of age diffusing capacity per square meter of body surface has increased practically to adult values. During the remainder of the growth period, diffusing ca-

pacity increases nearly in proportion to increases in height (comparable to Phase III). There is no reason to suspect that simple enlargement of alveoli, once they are formed, should increase diffusing capacity. The change is probably explained by the additional development of pulmonary capillaries so that capillary blood volume increases proportionately as airspaces enlarge.

Virtually all studies of the effects of senescence on single breath diffusing capacity for CO agree that there is a progressive reduction ranging from 0.20 to 0.32 ml/min × mm Hg per year of adulthood for men and 0.06 to 0.18 ml/min × mm Hg per year for women.[32] As was found with measurements of forced expiratory volume in 1 sec (see Table 14–1), the decline during senescence in diffusing capacity of CO and its subdivisions is not linear, although linear regression lines are shown in Figure 14–8. Decreases in total pulmonary diffusing capacity and membrane diffusing capacity are more evident after 40 years of age than before, and pulmonary capillary blood volume changes even later.[44] It is uncertain whether these age-related decreases are determined by morphologic changes in the alveolar-capillary membrane or by increasing inhomogeneities in ventilation or blood flow. The fact that the overall reduction in diffusing capacity is proportionately about the same as morphometric estimates of the loss of surface area[45] argues for the former explanation.

ARTERIAL BLOOD GASES

The effects of age on arterial blood gases and pH are reasonably well documented. After the early newborn period, arterial Po_2

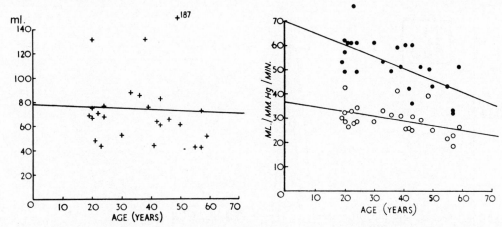

Figure 14–8. Relation between pulmonary diffusing capacity (DL = ○), membrane diffusing capacity (DM = ●), and pulmonary capillary blood volume (Vc = +), and age. DL and DM decrease with age but Vc does not. (Reprinted by permission from Hamer, N. A. J.: The effect of age on the components of the pulmonary diffusing capacity. Clin. Sci., *23*:85–93, 1962.)

varies much more with age than either arterial P_{CO_2} or pH.

Arterial Oxygen Tension

Sequential changes in arterial P_{O_2} from birth to old age are summarized in Figure 14–9.[11, 15, 46] The pattern of a rise in arterial P_{O_2} from birth to maturity followed by a gradual decline with advancing age is exactly the same as that of the changes in elastic recoil during growth and senescence (see Fig. 14–1). Moreover, these two varia-

bles are believed to be related through the effects of elastic recoil on airway caliber and hence on the distribution of ventilation and on airway closure. Computer analysis of 2233 studies of presumed normal adults (20 years of age or older) in which age and arterial P_{O_2} (Pa_{O_2}) were reported yielded the following regression equation:[47]

$$Pa_{O_2} = 100.1 - 0.323 \, (age). \qquad (1)$$

As indicated earlier and also in Chapter 4, dependent airways are exposed to a lower distending pressure than those located more

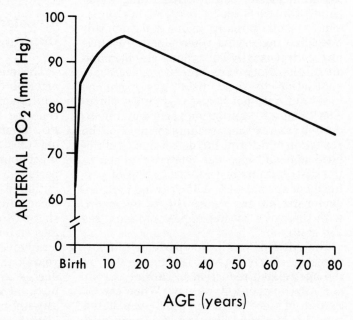

Figure 14–9. Arterial P_{O_2} as a function of age from birth to 80 years. (Data from Mansell, A. et al.: Airway closure in children. J. Appl. Physiol., *33*:711–714, 1972; Nelson, N. M.: Neonatal pulmonary function. Pediatr. Clin. North Am., *13*:769–799, 1966; and Sorbini, C. A., et al.: Arterial oxygen tension in relation to age in healthy subjects. Respiration, *25*:3–13, 1968.)

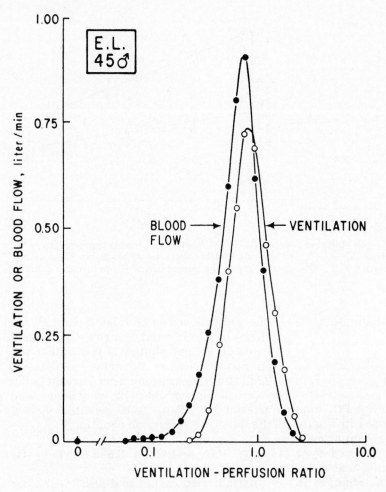

Figure 14–10. *See legend on opposite page.*

superiorly, because of the vertical gradient of pleural pressure (more negative at the top than at the bottom). Accordingly, dependent airways tend to close or narrow as elastic recoil decreases during deflation; this effect is exaggerated when elastic recoil is low, as it normally is in young children and old adults. Narrowing of airways decreases ventilation to their distal gas exchange units but does not necessarily affect perfusion. Thus, a ventilation-perfusion imbalance is created that accounts for most of the reduction of arterial Po_2 detectable in childhood and old age. Age-related changes in the distributions of ventilation and of perfusion of normal 44 and 45 year old men are demonstrated in Figure 14–10 (compare with those of a normal 22 year old man; see Fig. 8–6).

The effect of ventilation-perfusion imbalances in elderly persons is compounded by the age-related reduction in cardiac output and mixed venous O_2 content. When the O_2 content of blood perfusing poorly ventilated spaces is lowered, the effect of a given ven-

tilation-perfusion in equality on arterial Po_2 is magnified (see Fig. 8–10).

Alveolar-Arterial Oxygen Tension Difference

The mechanisms that cause the reduced arterial Po_2 in infants, children, and old adults—compared with mature adults—are reflected by an increased alveolar-arterial Po_2 difference in the very young and very old. Most, but not all, of the Po_2 difference is attributable to the presence of ventilation-perfusion abnormalities. The other contribution is from right-to-left shunting of blood. In infants, the usual right-to-left shunt through the foramen ovale ceases almost immediately after birth (although the foramen may remain patent for many years); the right-to-left shunt through the ductus arteriosus ordinarily reverses after birth, and the new shunt becomes functionally unimportant within a few days.

With senescence, in addition to widening

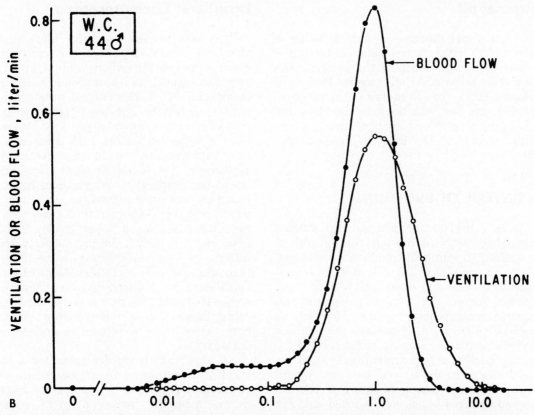

Figure 14–10. The distributions of ventilation and blood flow in a 45 year old man *(A)* and a 44 year old man *(B)*. Compared with a younger subject (see Fig. 8–6), there is more dispersion and less symmetry in ventilation and perfusion curves. Both older subjects demonstrate blood flow to low ventilation-perfusion regions, but the effect is greater in W. C. than in E. L. (Reprinted by permission from Wagner, P. D. et al.: Continuous distributions of ventilation-perfusion ratios in normal subjects breathing air and 100 per cent O_2. J. Clin. Invest., *54*:54–68, 1974.)

of the alveolar-arterial Po_2 difference from ventilation-perfusion inequalities, there is evidence of an increased right-to-left shunt of blood;[49] this most likely reflects the effect of a reduction in mixed venous O_2 content, attributable to the age-related decrease in cardiac output; another possible cause is an increase in postpulmonary shunting (e.g., through thebesian or bronchial veins). It should be mentioned that even though diffusing capacity decreases with old age and may be relatively low during infancy, the reduction does not contribute measurably to the alveolar-arterial Po_2 differences observed in resting subjects at sea level.

Arterial Carbon Dioxide Tension

Within one to four hours, normal newborn infants lower their arterial Pco_2 values from about 76 mm Hg at birth to about 38 mm Hg, and by 24 hours after birth to about 33 mm Hg (for serial measurements see reference 6). No one knows why arterial Pco_2 values are "low" in infants, but because they are similar to those found in pregnant women at the time of delivery it is possible that the maternal environment "sets" the buffering capacity of the newborn's body. After birth, increases in arterial Pco_2 cannot take place until the infant has developed its own systems for generating and conserving HCO_3^-; any increase in Pco_2 evokes a brisk ventilatory response, owing to the presence of well-developed CO_2 sensitivity in infants. It is not known precisely how long these adjustments take, but one review cites "several months."[15]

Once arterial Pco_2 reaches 40 mm Hg in the newborn period (or values appropriate for residence at high altitude), it remains virtually constant for the rest of the person's life. This constancy occurs despite the reduction in CO_2 sensitivity that occurs during senescence.

Arterial pH

Arterial pH reaches its normal value of about 7.40 within a few hours of birth and tends to remain constant thereafter.[15] The stability of arterial pH while PCO_2 and plasma HCO_3^- are changing in the newborn period signifies that the two variables are changing proportionately to maintain a constant ratio of HCO_3^- to H_2CO_3 (see Chapter 9).

CONTROL OF BREATHING

During the last decade, several studies have been carried out on the control of breathing in young and old healthy subjects. From the results of these studies, it is possible to provide a general outline of the age-related changes that occur in peripheral and central chemoreceptor function. However, as will be pointed out, important gaps in our knowledge exist in many other related aspects, particularly concerning integrative mechanisms in the central nervous system. Also, the time course of many of the observed changes is not well worked out. For example, it is known that the Hering-Breuer inflation reflex is present in the newborn and increases in intensity from 10 to 35 days after delivery;[50] the Hering-Breuer reflex is also known to be weak or absent in adults.[51] But when the change occurs from one state to the other has not been determined.

Peripheral Chemoreceptors

It is now widely accepted, after many years of uncertainty, that the peripheral chemoreceptors of newborn infants, presumably the carotid bodies, respond to changes in arterial PO_2.[52] The normal newborn human responds to induced hypoxia with a biphasic ventilatory response, first by transiently hyperventilating and, after one to two minutes, by exhibiting ventilatory depression. By seven to eight days after birth, the ventilatory response to hypoxia becomes sustained. However, the age at which peripheral chemoreceptor function is maximally developed is not known. It may take up to a month for prematurely born infants to lose their biphasic ventilatory response and demonstrate sustained hyperventilation to induced hypoxia. There is suggestive evidence that some of the respiratory depression exhibited during the newborn period may be related to endogenous opiates.[53]

An important study demonstrated a substantial attentuation in the heart rate and ventilatory responses to hypoxia and hypercapnia in healthy persons 64 to 73 years of age compared with those in subjects 22 to 30 years of age;[54] data from this study are presented in Table 14-3. Although the reasons for the suppression of breathing are unknown and undoubtedly complex, the data indicate that aging is associated with diminution of an important protective mechanism. Moreover, elderly persons, who are

Table 14-3. HEART RATE AND VENTILATORY RESPONSES TO HYPOXIA AND HYPERCAPNIA IN YOUNG AND OLD NORMAL SUBJECTS*

Age Range† (Years)	Young Subjects 22-30 Years		Old Subjects 64-73 Years		P Value
	Mean	SEM	Mean	SEM	
Ventilatory response					
Hypoxia ($\Delta V40$, L/min)	40.1	4.7	10.2	1.2	<0.001
Hypercapnia (L/min/mm Hg)	3.4	0.5	2.0	0.2	<0.025
Heart rate response					
Hypoxia (% change control to PA_{O_2} 40 mm Hg)	34.1	5.2	11.5	2.2	<0.005
Hypercapnia (% change control to PA_{CO_2} 55 mm Hg)	15.0	2.8	-0.9	1.0	<0.001

*Data from Kronenberg, R. S., and Drage, C. W.: Attenuation of the ventilatory and heart rate responses to hypoxia and hypercapnia with aging in normal men. J. Clin. Invest., 52:1812–1819, 1973.
†$\Delta V40$ = change in ventilation (L/min) from initial value breathing room air to that during hypoxia when alveolar PO_2 = 40 mm Hg; PA_{O_2} = alveolar PO_2; PA_{CO_2} = alveolar PCO_2.

most likely to be afflicted with chronic pulmonary diseases, are least able to respond to changes in arterial blood Po_2 and Pco_2.

Central Chemoreceptors

Sensitivity to inhaled CO_2 increases during gestation, judging from the responses in premature infants, and also increases during the postnatal period following term or premature delivery.[55] Part of the brisk stimulus to breathe from increased CO_2 can be attributed to the reduced $[HCO_3^-]$ in the baby's plasma and CSF. Thus, for any incremental increase in Pco_2, a greater pH change will occur with consequent stimulation of both central and peripheral chemoreceptors. The contributions of these two sites have not been differentiated, although the central effect is undoubtedly the more profound, owing to the lower buffering capacity of CSF compared with that of plasma (see Chapter 10).

The data shown in Table 14–3 indicate that the ventilatory response to CO_2 is diminished in old compared with young healthy adult men.[54] Whether this is caused by suppression of central or peripheral receptor systems or both has not been established. However, because the amount of reduction of CO_2 sensitivity in the old men (41 per cent) was greater than the demonstrable total contribution of carotid chemoreceptors to the normal hypercapneic response (30 per cent), central mechanisms were probably involved.

Integrated Responses

Peterson and coworkers[56] recently reported the results of studies on the effects of aging on the ventilatory and occlusion pressure responses to hypoxia and hypercapnia. Older subjects had a decreased ventilatory response to both hypoxia and hypercapnia of approximately 50 per cent that was related to a decrease in occlusion pressure, a measure of total neuromuscular drive to breathe. Accordingly, either the respiratory muscles are faulty, which seems unlikely, or central neural inspiratory output decreases with age. Other studies on the ability of old and young adults to perceive added resistive loads during breathing also suggest a decrease in central nervous system integrative functions during senescence.[57]

EXERCISE CAPACITY

The complex interrelations among the factors that govern maximal O_2 uptake are discussed in Chapter 11. It is generally agreed that genetic influences are the chief determinants of the physical dimensions of the O_2 transport system, including blood volume, red blood cell mass, heart volume, vital capacity, pulmonary diffusing capacity, and skeletal muscle mass. Physical training is decisive in developing the functional capabilities inherent in the respiratory and circulatory systems. To a large extent this happens during the ordinary physical activities of childhood, but purposeful athletic training during youth appears essential for persons to develop championship capability. In a study of "ordinary" boys and girls 6 to 17 years of age, it was observed that several variables that reflect O_2 transport during exercise were proportionately related to body weight.[58] This means that cardiac output is closely tied to the size of the muscles and that the cardiorespiratory systems of growing children and adolescents are capable of delivering a steadily increasing quantity of O_2 during exercise.

Figure 14–11 shows the relationship between maximal O_2 uptake and age in normal Swedish men who were in good physical condition. It is clear that in groups with comparable amounts of athletic conditioning, age is a significant factor in defining maximal O_2 uptake. In a study of several of the principal components of the O_2 transport system, it was demonstrated that significant age-related decreases occurred only in forced vital capacity and maximal heart rate; the effect of age on maximal O_2 uptake, therefore, is a loss of functional capabilities despite maintenance of the dimensional capacity of youth.[59]

This conclusion is supported by serial studies of young women who were highly trained competitive swimmers. Follow-up measurements several years after they had ceased training (average five years) revealed no change in their dimensional characteristics but a striking decrease in maximal O_2 uptake.[60] Similar effects were noted when

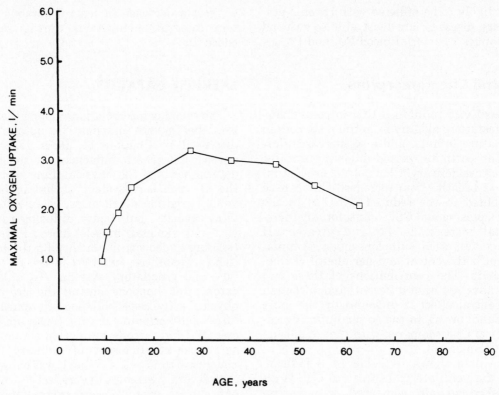

Figure 14–11. Maximal O_2 uptake as a function of age in Swedish men. (Adapted and reprinted by permission from Grimby, G., and Saltin, B.: Physiological effects of physical training. Scand. J. Rehab. Med., *3*:6–14, 1971.)

former successful cross-country runners and skiers were examined 10 to 30 years after they had given up competition and training.[61] However, the athletically inclined can be reassured by the evidence that regular physical training markedly retards the rate of decrease in maximal O_2 uptake with age.

The decrease in O_2 transport capacity during senescence is tightly linked to an age-related decrease in cardiac output. The other determinant of O_2 delivery, arterial O_2 content, changes very little. The results of recent studies of myocardial aging do not support the concept of a general decline in function, but they indicate instead that there are changes in certain specific aspects of cardiac biochemistry and metabolism, such as decreases in maximal myocardial O_2 consumption and substrate oxidation rates.[62] The molecular basis for these changes has not been precisely defined.

Pulmonary Hemodynamics

Pulmonary arterial systolic, diastolic, and mean pressures increase steadily during exercise (see Fig. 11–12). Furthermore, as shown in Figure 14–12, there is an age-related increase in pulmonary vascular resistance.[63] The physiologic axiom that the effects of a given increase in resistance are more profound when flow across the resistance is increased is evident in Figure 14–12. At rest when cardiac output is relatively low, pulmonary vascular pressures are similar in all age groups except the oldest (60 to 69 years). In contrast, during exercise when blood flow is augmented, the trend for all pulmonary intravascular pressures to increase progressively with increasing age is very clear.[63] No quantitative information is available on the anatomic basis for these functional changes.

Peripheral Factors

There is a decrease in total muscle mass with increasing age, which is accounted for by a reduction in the total number of muscle fibers. These changes provide a straightforward explanation for the decrease in muscle strength that characterizes old age. The

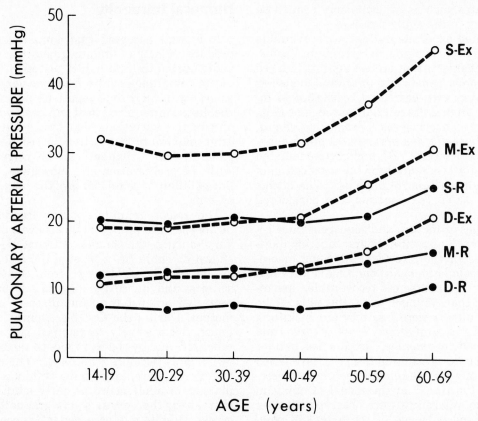

Figure 14–12. Systolic, mean, and diastolic pulmonary arterial pressures at rest (solid symbols and lines) and during exercise (open symbols, dashed lines) in healthy subjects of different ages. S-Ex = systolic pressure during exercise; M-Ex = mean pressure during exercise; S-R = systolic pressure at rest; D-Ex = diastolic pressure during exercise; M-R = mean pressure at rest; D-R = diastolic pressure at rest. (Data from Ehrsam, R. E., et al.: Influence of age on pulmonary haemodynamics at rest and during supine exercise. Clin. Sci., 65:653–660, 1983. Copyright © 1983 The Biochemical Society, London.)

metabolic capacity, enzymatic profile, and capillary density of the muscle fibers that remain present during senescence appear to be the same as those in younger persons.[64] Thus, the age-related decreases in strength and aerobic exercise capacity are quantitatively linked to attrition of muscle mass, and functional derangements of the remaining fibers are much less evident. Whether central or peripheral factors are more important in limiting maximal exercise capacity in old age is still an unsettled question. Striking changes occur in both components.

DEFENSE MECHANISMS

The intricate regional and systemic defense mechanisms that protect the lungs and the rest of the body against inhaled microorganisms, toxins, allergens, and the development of malignancies are described in Chapter 13. Numerous clinical observations

indicate that the very young and the very old have a high incidence of infections and malignancies; one can infer from these data that there are likely to be age-related changes in the functional capabilities of the pulmonary clearance and the immune systems that normally prevent such occurrences. This section briefly reviews what is known about the effects of growth and senescence on the defense mechanisms of the lung.

Clearance Mechanisms

There are few systematic studies of the effect of age on mucociliary transport. The results of those that have been carried out indicate that, on average, older persons have a slower rate of transport than younger persons.[65] The mechanisms responsible for this change have not been identified, and it is difficult to sort out the effects of acquired influences such as air pollution from those inherent to the aging process.

Limited experimental data are available on the effects of aging on certain antibacterial mechanisms that protect against induced pneumonia. Senescence in animal models is associated with decreased resistance to infection from intracellular pathogens (e.g., *Listeria monocytogenes, Toxoplasma gondii,* or *Salmonella typhimurium*), presumably because effective T-lymphocyte–mediated immunity is essential for the eradication of these intracellular organisms.[66] The effects of age on T cell function are considered subsequently.

Studies of mature and senescent mice revealed both quantitative and functional differences in their resident alveolar macrophage populations: although aged mice had greater numbers of recoverable macrophages than younger mice, the cells of the older animals were less efficient in killing clinical strains of *Staphylococcus aureus* and *Klebsiella pneumoniae*.[67] In contrast, studies of monocyte function in humans have failed to identify an age-related decline in macrophage function.[68] In the model of aging in mice no differences were observed between young and old mice in the extent of polymorphoneutrophil recruitment into the lungs after a large inoculation of either *Staphylococcus* or *Klebsiella*, and the senescent mice actually cleared viable organisms faster than their younger counterparts.[67] The opposite effect was observed with small inoculations in which the predominant recoverable cell was the alveolar macrophage. Obviously, there is a great need for further studies of the effects of aging on innate pulmonary defense mechanisms.

Humoral Immunity

It is well accepted that human fetuses produce selective immunoglobulins, especially during the last half of gestation.[69] The various immunoglobulin fractions vary considerably in their concentrations at birth, in the duration required to attain peak values, and in the variations that occur with age after maximum production is reached. In general, these changes can be correlated with the proliferation and subsequent atrophy of different components of the lymphatic system.

The major immunoglobulin fraction of newborns, like adults, is IgG. Levels of IgG vary during the human lifetime,[70, 71] as shown in Table 14–4. Most of the IgG present at birth is derived from maternal sources, and hence the newborn is briefly protected against the same diseases as its mother. During the first few months of infancy, the passively transferred IgG is catabolized, and by the third month the baby's own supply becomes dominant.[69] The quantity increases rapidly during childhood to a plateau in adolescence or early adulthood; thereafter, the serum levels gradually increase. Despite the increased IgG concentrations, the antibody response to extrinsic antigens, such as pneumococcal constituents, is reduced considerably in old age; presumably, the increased circulating immunoglobulin reflects increased production of antibody to various intrinsic antigens (i.e., autoantibodies), which replaces production of specific antibodies.[72]

Immunoglobulin IgM, which does not cross the placental barrier, is normally synthesized by the fetus after the 14th week,

Table 14–4. LEVELS OF IMMUNOGLOBULINS IN SERUM OF NORMAL SUBJECTS AT DIFFERENT AGES*

Age Groups	IgG		IgM		IgA	
	Mean	*SD*	*Mean*	*SD*	*Mean*	*SD*
Newborn	1031	200	11	5	2	3
1–3 months	430	119	30	11	21	13
7–12 months	661	219	54	23	37	18
3–5 years	929	228	56	18	93	27
12–16 years	946	124	59	20	148	63
20–29 years	865	459	—	—	—	—
40–49 years	979	739	—	—	—	—
60–69 years	1393	541	—	—	—	—
Adults, all ages	1158	305	99	27	200	61

*Data from Stiehm, E. R., and Fundenberg, H. H.: Serum levels of immune globulins in health and disease: a survey. Pediatrics, *37*:715–727, 1966 and Das, B. C., and Bhattacharya, S. K.: Changes in human serum protein fractions with age and weight. Can. J. Biochem. Physiol., *39*:569–579, 1961.

and small amounts are measurable at birth (11 ± 5 mg/100ml); in cases of antenatal infection, larger amounts may be demonstrable and, if present, may serve as a guide to the detection of intrauterine infectious complications.[69] Levels of IgM in the serum increase rapidly during infancy and childhood, although the exact sequence has not been agreed upon. During senescence, serum values of IgM tend to decrease dramatically.

There is virtually no IgA in the serum of human infants at birth, but small amounts are detectable shortly afterward, and the concentration increases steadily, reaching adult levels after puberty. In contrast, the secretory IgA system reaches maturity within one or two months of age, at least judging from the quantities of IgA present in saliva.[73] It is of interest that secretory component (see Chapter 13) appears in human lungs during fetal development long before immunoglobulin-containing cells are evident. This observation led to the speculation that secretory component may have additional functions besides the selective transport of IgA.[73a]

The levels of immunoglobulins in the bloodstream are only a rough guide to humoral immune competence. As emphasized in Chapter 13, the ability to generate an effective humoral response depends on the interaction among helper T cells, suppressor T cells, macrophages, and B cells. Thus, the impairment of humoral responsiveness that accompanies senescence could be accounted for by an abnormality in the number or function of one or more of these cell types. The results of several studies (summarized by Weksler[72]) indicate that the chief defect is an alteration in the function of helper T cells, although minor changes in suppressor T cell or B cell activity may contribute to the overall disturbance. It should be pointed out, however, that in contrast to the decline in functional capabilities that occurs in the remainder of the humoral immune system, little or no age-related change was observed in the mucosa-associated lymph nodes of the secretory system.[74]

Cellular Immunity

Until recently, the effects of age on humoral immunity have received more intensive study than the effects on cellular immunity. During the last decade, however, given the importance of the thymus gland and T cells as controllers of immune responsiveness, considerable attention has been directed toward the mechanisms that underlie the development of various cellular aspects of immunity during growth and their attenuation during senescence. It has been recognized for many years that normal newborn experimental animals are capable of expressing the presence of cellular immunity by rejecting transplants of foreign tissues. In addition, it is now known that three cellular immune functions are well developed in human fetuses and newborns: (1) the blastogenic response of lymphocytes to phytohemagglutinin, (2) the nonspecific ability of cord lymphocytes to destroy target cells (chicken erythrocytes), and (3) the development of rosette-forming cells in several different human fetal lymphoid organs.[75] Although it is difficult to compare the results of these experiments with results from comparable studies in the adult, it can be concluded that many important aspects of cellular immunity are fully developed in human beings at birth. The blastogenic response to plant mitogens (phytohemagglutinin and pokeweed mitogen) has also been used to demonstrate a functional depression in the lymphocytes from elderly (75 to 96 years) compared with young (25 to 50 years) adults.[76] Similarly, the number of positive delayed hypersensitivity skin reactions to five common antigens was significantly lower in the aged than in the young; furthermore, the mortality rate of old persons (>80 years of age) who were hyporesponsive to the battery of skin tests was significantly higher than that of old persons who were responsive.[77]

Thus, cell-mediated immunity appears to be reasonably well developed at birth but clearly declines during senescence; these findings correlate roughly with the presence of the thymus gland in the newborn and its subsequent involution during adulthood. Because atrophy of the thymus affects the functioning capabilities of T-lymphocytes, during senescence the total number of circulating T cells remains constant but fewer of them are capable either of responding to an immune challenge or of proliferating. Heightened suppressor T cell activity appears also to contribute to the impaired proliferative response.[72]

Summary

The effects of age on the nonspecific and particularly on the specific components of the defense systems of the lungs and body are responsible for the vulnerability to infections of the newborn and to both infections and malignancy of aged adults. It is also possible that inherent immunologic attrition may underlie the aging process itself. The poorly protected aged host has increasing difficulty withstanding both the continuous onslaught of hostile microorganisms and other noxious agents from the external environment and the cellular mischief constantly taking place in his own body; it is also possible that immunologic failure may accelerate the ravages of degenerative diseases. Thus, attenuation of defense mechanisms, especially immunologically mediated defenses, sets the stage for the inevitable clinical consequences that terminate in death.

REFERENCES

1. Comfort, A.: Ageing: The Biology of Senescence. New York, Holt, Rinehart & Winston, 1964, p. 5.
2. Hayflick, L.: The cell biology of human aging. New Engl. J. Med., 295:1302–1308, 1976.
3. Goldstein, S.: The biology of aging. New Engl. J. Med., 285:1120–1129, 1971.
4. Fuich, C. E., and Hayflick, L. (eds.): The handbook of the biology of aging. Van Nostrand Reinhold Co., New York, 1977, pp. 1–771.
5. Scarpelli, E. M. (ed.): Pulmonary physiology of the fetus, newborn and child. Lea & Febiger, Philadelphia, 1975, pp. 1–369.
6. Polgar, G., and Weng, T. R.: State of the art. The functional development of the respiratory system: from the period of gestation to adulthood. Am. Rev. Respir. Dis., 120:625–695, 1979.
7. Ohar, S., Shaski, S. R., and Lenora, R. A.: Aging and the respiratory system. Med. Clin. North Am., 50:1121–1139, 1976.
8. Wahba, W. M.: Influence of aging on lung function—clinical significance of changes from age twenty. Anesth. Analg., 62:764–776, 1983.
9. Cook, C. D., Mead, J., and Orzalesi, M. M.: Static volume-pressure characteristics of the respiratory system during maximal efforts. J. Appl. Physiol., 19:1016–1022, 1964.
10. Black, L. F., and Hyatt, R. E.: Maximal respiratory pressures: normal values and relationships to age and sex. Am. Rev. Respir. Dis., 99:696–702, 1969.
11. Mansell, A., Bryan, C., and Levison, H.: Airway closure in children. J. Appl. Physiol., 33:711–714, 1972.
12. Turner, J. M., Mead, J., and Wohl, M. D.: Elasticity of human lungs in relation to age. J. Appl. Physiol., 25:664–671, 1968.
13. Zapletal, A., Misur, A., and Samanek, M.: Static recoil pressure of the lungs in children. Bull. Physiopathol. Respir., 7:139–143, 1971.
14. Gribetz, I., Frank, N. R., and Avery, M. E.: Static volume-pressure relations of excised lungs of infants with hyaline membrane disease, newborn and stillborn infants. J. Clin. Invest., 38:2168–2175, 1959.
15. Nelson, N. M.: Neonatal pulmonary function. Pediatr. Clin. North Am., 13:769–799, 1966.
16. Bryan, A. C., Mansell, A. L., and Levison, H.: Development of the mechanical properties of the respiratory system. In Hodson, W. A. (ed.): Development of the Lung. New York, Marcel Dekker, Inc., 1977, pp. 445–468.
17. Loosli, C. G., and Potter, E. L.: Pre- and postnatal development of the respiratory portion of the human lung with special reference to the elastic fibers. Am. Rev. Respir. Dis., 80(Suppl. 1):5–23, 1959.
18. Knudson, R. J., Clark, D. F., Kennedy, T. C., and Knudson, D. E.: Effect of aging alone on mechanical properties of the normal adult human lung. J. Appl. Physiol., 43:1054–1062, 1977.
19. Pierce, J. A.: Age-related changes in the fibrous proteins in the lungs. Arch. Environ. Health, 6:50–54, 1963.
20. John, R., and Thomas, J.: Chemical compositions of elastins isolated from aortas and pulmonary tissues of humans of different ages. Biochem. J., 127:261–269, 1972.
21. Niewoehner, D. E., Kleinerman, J., and Liotta, L.: Elastic behavior of postmortem human lungs—effects of aging and mild emphysema. J. Appl. Physiol., 39:943–949, 1975.
22. Niewoehner, D. E., and Kleinerman, J.: Morphometric study of elastic fibers in normal and emphysematous human lungs. Am. Rev. Respir. Dis., 115:15–21, 1977.
23. Ranga, V., Kleinerman, J., Ip, M. P. C., and Sorensen, J.: Age-related changes in elastic fibers and elastin of lung. Am. Rev. Respir. Dis., 119:369–376, 1979.
24. Richards, C. C., and Bachman, L.: Lung and chest wall compliance of apneic paralyzed infants. J. Clin. Invest., 40:273–278, 1961.
25. Cook, C. D., Sutherland, J. M., Segal, S., Cherry, R. B., Mead, J., McIlroy, M. B., and Smith, C. A.: Studies of respiratory physiology in the newborn infant. III. Measurements of mechanics of respiration. J. Clin. Invest., 36:440–448, 1957.
26. Agostoni, E.: Volume-pressure relationships of the thorax and lung in the newborn. J. Appl. Physiol., 14:909–913, 1959.
27. Avery, M. E., and Cook, C. D.: Volume-pressure relationships of lungs and thorax in fetal, newborn, and adult goats. J. Appl. Physiol., 16:1034–1038, 1961.
28. Motoyama, E. K.: Pulmonary mechanics during early postnatal years. Pediatr. Res., 11:220–223, 1977.
29. Mittman, C., Edelman, N. H., Norris, A. H., and Shock, N. W.: Relationship between chest wall and pulmonary compliance and age. J. Appl. Physiol., 20:1211–1216, 1965.
30. Knudson, R. J., Slatin, R. C., Lebowitz, M. D., and Burrows, B.: The maximal expiratory flow-volume curve. Normal standards, variability and the effects of age. Am. Rev. Respir. Dis., 113:587–600, 1976.

31. Rea, H., Becklake, M. R., and Ghezzo, H.: Lung function changes as a reflection of tissue aging in young adults. Bull. Eur. Physiopathol. Respir., 18:5–19, 1982.

32. Muiesan, G., Sorbini, C. A., and Grassi, V.: Respiratory function in the aged. Bull. Eur. Physiopathol. Respir., 7:973–1009, 1971.

33. Knudson, R. J., Lebowitz, M. D., Holberg, C. J., and Burrows, B.: Changes in the normal maximal expiratory flow-volume curve with growth and aging. Am. Rev. Respir. Dis., 127:725–734, 1983.

34. Schoenberg, J. B., Beck, G. J., and Bouhuys, A.: Growth and decay of pulmonary function in healthy blacks and whites. Respir. Physiol., 33:367–393, 1978.

35. Black, L. F., Offord, K., and Hyatt, R. E.: Variability in the maximal expiratory flow volume curve in asymptomatic smokers and in nonsmokers. Am. Rev. Respir. Dis., 110:282–292, 1974.

36. Green, M., Mead, J., and Turner, J. M.: Variability of maximum expiratory flow-volume curves. J. Appl. Physiol., 37:67–74, 1974.

37. Mead, J.: Dysanapsis in normal lungs assessed by the relationship between maximal flow, static recoil, and vital capacity. Am. Rev. Respir. Dis., 121:339–342, 1980.

38. Strang, L. B., and McGrath, M. W.: Alveolar ventilation in normal newborn infants studied by air wash-in after oxygen breathing. Clin. Sci., 23:129–139, 1962.

39. Holland, J., Milic-Emili, J., Macklem, P. T., and Bates, D. V.: Regional distribution of pulmonary ventilation and perfusion in elderly subjects. J. Clin. Invest., 47:81–92, 1968.

40. Leblanc, P., Ruff, F., and Milic-Emili, J.: Effects of age and body position on "airway closure" in man. J. Appl. Physiol., 28:448–451, 1970.

41. Dunnill, M. S.: Postnatal growth of the lung. Thorax, 17:329–333, 1962.

42. Weibel, E. R.: Morphological basis of alveolar-capillary gas exchange. Physiol. Rev., 53:419–495, 1973.

43. Hamer, N. A. J.: The effect of age on the components of the pulmonary diffusing capacity. Clin. Sci., 23:85–93, 1962.

44. Georges, R., Saumon, G., and Loiseau, A.: The relationship of age to pulmonary membrane conductance and capillary blood volume. Am. Rev. Respir. Dis., 117:1069–1078, 1978.

45. Thurlbeck, W. M.: The internal surface area of nonemphysematous lungs. Am. Rev. Respir. Dis., 95:765–773, 1967.

46. Sorbini, C. A., Brassi, V., Solinas, E., and Muiesan, G.: Arterial oxygen tension in relation to age in healthy subjects. Respiration, 25:3–13, 1968.

47. Mays, E. E.: Unpublished observations, 1974.

48. Wagner, P. D., Laravuso, R. B., Uhl, R. R., and West, J. B.: Continuous distributions of ventilation-perfusion ratios in normal subjects breathing air and 100 per cent O_2. J. Clin. Invest., 54:54–68, 1974.

49. Kanber, G. J., King, F. W., Eshchar, Y. R., and Sharp, J. T.: The alveolar-arterial oxygen gradient in young and elderly men during air and oxygen breathing. Am. Rev. Respir. Dis., 97:376–381, 1968.

50. Thach, B. T., Frantz, I. D., III, Adler, S. M., and Taeutsch, H. W., Jr.: Maturation of reflexes influencing inspiratory duration in human infants. J. Appl. Physiol., 45:203–211, 1978.

51. Guz, A., Noble, M. I. M., Widdicombe, J. G., Trenchard, D., Mushin, W. W., and Makey, A. R.: The role of vagal and glossopharyngeal afferent nerves in respiratory sensation, control of breathing and arterial pressure regulation in conscious man. Clin. Sci., 30:161–170, 1966.

52. Haddad, G. G., and Mellins, R. B.: Hypoxia and respiratory control in early life. Ann. Rev. Physiol., 46:629–643, 1984.

53. Jansen, A. H., and Chernick, V.: Development of respiratory control. Physiol. Rev., 63:437–483, 1983.

54. Kronenberg, R. S., and Drage, C. W.: Attenuation of the ventilatory and heart rate responses to hypoxia and hypercapnia with aging in normal men. J. Clin. Invest., 52:1812–1819, 1973.

55. Rigatto, H., Brady, J. P., Verduzco, R. T.: Chemoreceptor reflexes in preterm infants. II. The effect of gestational and postnatal age on the ventilatory response to inhaled carbon dioxide. Pediatrics, 55:614–620, 1975.

56. Peterson, D. D., Pack, A. I., Silage, D. A., and Fishman, A. P.: Effects of aging on ventilatory and occlusion pressure responses to hypoxia and hypercapnia. Am. Rev. Respir. Dis., 124:387–391, 1981.

57. Tack, M., Altose, M., and Cherniack, N. S.: Effect of aging on the perception of resistive ventilatory loads. Am. Rev. Respir. Dis., 126:463–467, 1982.

58. Cooper, D. M., Weiler-Ravell, D., Whipp, B. J., and Wasserman, K.: Growth-related changes in oxygen uptake and heart rate during progressive exercise in children. Pediatr. Res., 18:845–851, 1984.

59. Davies, C. T. M.: The oxygen-transporting system in relation to age. Clin. Sci., 42:1–13, 1972.

60. Eriksson, B. O., Engstrom, I., Karlberg, P., Saltin, B., and Thoren, C.: A physiological analysis of former girl swimmers. Acta Paediatr. Scand. (Suppl.), 217:68–72, 1971.

61. Saltin, B., and Grimby, G.: Physiological analysis of middle-aged and old former athletes: comparison with still active athletes of the same ages. Circulation, 38:1104–1115, 1968.

62. Lakatta, E. G., and Yin, F. P.: Myocardial aging: functional alterations and related cellular mechanisms. Am. J. Physiol., 242:H927–H941, 1982.

63. Ehrsam, R. E., Perruchoud, A., Oberholzer, M., Burkart, F., and Herzog, H.: Influence of age on pulmonary haemodynamics at rest and during supine exercise. Clin. Sci., 65:653–660, 1983.

64. Grimby, G., Danneskiold-Samsoe, B., and Saltin, B.: Morphology and enzymatic capacity in arm and leg muscles in 78–81 year old men and women. Acta Physiol. Scand., 115:125–134, 1982.

65. Camner, P.: Editorial review. Clearance of particles from the human tracheobronchial tree. Clin. Sci., 59:79–84, 1980.

66. Gardner, I. D., and Remington, J. S.: Age-related decline in resistance of mice to infection with intracellular pathogens. Infect. Immun., 16:593–598, 1977.

67. Esposito, A. L., and Pennington, J. E.: Effects of aging on antibacterial mechanisms in experimental pneumonia. Am. Rev. Respir. Dis., 128:662–667, 1983.

68. Gardner, N. D., Lim, S. T. K., and Lawton, J. W. M.: Monocyte function in ageing humans. Mech. Ageing Dev., 16:233–239, 1981.

69. Frommel, D., and Good, R. A.: Immunological mechanisms. *In* Gairdner, D., and Hull, E. (eds.): Recent Advances in Paediatrics, 4th Ed. London, J. & A. Churchill, 1971, pp. 401–427.

70. Stiehm, E. R., and Fundenberg, H. H.: Serum levels of immune globulins in health and disease: a survey. Pediatrics, *37*:715–727, 1966.

71. Das, B. C., and Bhattacharya, S. K.: Changes in human serum protein fractions with age and weight. Can. J. Biochem. Physiol., *39*:569–579, 1961.

72. Weksler, M. E.: Senescence of the immune system. Med. Clin. North Am., *19*:73–82, 1983.

73. Selner, J. C., Merrill, D. A., and Claman, H. N.: Salivary immunoglobulin and albumin: development during the newborn period. J. Pediatr., *72*:685–689, 1968.

73a. Takemura, T., and Eishi, Y.: Distribution of secretory component and immunoglobulins in the developing lung. Am. Rev. Respir. Dis., *131*:125–130, 1985.

74. Szewczuk, M. R., and Wade, A. W.: Aging and the mucosal-associated lymphoid system. Ann. N.Y. Acad. Sci., *409*:333–344, 1983.

75. Sites, D. P., Wybran, J., Carr, M. C., and Fundenberg, H. H.: Development of cellular immunocompetence in man. *In* Ontogeny of Acquired Immunity. New York, Associated Scientific Publishers, 1972, pp. 113–132.

76. Weksler, M. E., and Hutteroth, T. H.: Impaired lymphocyte function in aged humans. J. Clin. Invest., *53*:99–104, 1974.

77. Roberts-Thomson, I. C., Whittingham, S., Youngchaiyud, U., and Mackay, I. R.: Ageing, immune response and mortality. Lancet, *2*:368–370, 1974.

Index

Note: Numbers in *italics* refer to illustrations; numbers followed by (t) indicate tables.

Enzyme, angiotensin-converting, 295, *296*
Epithelial cell(s), ciliated, *319*
Epithelium, *300*
  airway, 25–26, *76*
    cells of, 25–26, *26*
    "ciliary escalator" of, 26
  alveolar, *301*
    composition of, 48, *49*
  bronchial, 25–28, *26, 27*
  tracheobronchial, lymphocytes in, 32
Equal pressure point, 102
Equal pressure point theory, 101–103, *102*
  alveolar pressure in, *102*
  pleural pressure in, *102*
  static recoil pressure in, *102*
Equation, Bohr, 199
  buffer mixture, 214
  carbon dioxide, carbonic acid, 215
  for airway resistance, 94
  for alveolar air, 186
  for alveolar CO_2 pressure, 187
  for alveolar ventilation, 199
  for arterial CO_2 pressure, 187, 215
  for arterial oxygen tension regression, 349
  for bicarbonate dissociation, 215
  for bicarbonate formation, 178
  for bicarbonate in blood, 215
  for blood oxygen capacity, 173
  for chest wall compliance, 85
  for chest wall distending pressure, 84
  for chest wall tissue resistance, 94
  for compliance, 84
  for diffusing capacity, 167
    of carbon monoxide, 167
  for diffusion resistance, 168
  for frictional resistance of lung tissue, 94
  for gas pressure in right-to-left shunts, 194
  for hemoglobin saturation, 173
  for liquid flow across endothelial barrier, 303
  for lung compliance, 85
  for lung distending pressure, 84
  for net liquid flow, 303
  for physiologic dead space, 199
  for plasma carbon dioxide, 216
  for pulmonary resistance, 94
  for pulmonary vascular resistance, 150
  for resistance, 94
  for respiratory system compliance, 85
  for respiratory system distending pressure, 84
  for systemic oxygen transport, 202
  for total carbon dioxide, 216
  for total interstitial pressure, 146
  for total renal acid, 223
  for urinary hydrogen ion, 223
  for ventilation, 251
  for wasted ventilation, 199
  Henderson-Hasselbalch, 216
  hydration-dehydration, 178
  Laplace, 90
  pH, 213
  shunt, 195
  Starling, 303
Equilibrium, acid-base, 211–230. See also *Acid-base equilibrium.*
  of carbon dioxide, 178–180
  of gases, mechanisms of, 165
  of oxyhemoglobin, 172–178
    factors affecting, 175–178
  total interstitial pressure and, 147

Erythrocyte(s), *300*
  2,3 diphosphoglycerate in, 177
  oxygen saturation of, 208, *208*
  survival of, 204
Erythropoiesis, disturbances of, 205–207
Erythropoietin, 207
Exercise, 261–281
  aging and, 353–355, *354*
  alveolar-arterial carbon dioxide tension and, 268
  alveolar-arterial oxygen tension and, 267–268, *267*
  blood volume and, 274–275
  body temperature and, 277–278, *277*
  circulation and, 272–277, *271, 272, 273, 275, 276, 277*(t)
  diffusing capacity and, 266–267
  efficiency of, 280
  energetics of, 262–263, *262*
  gas exchange in, 263–268, *264–267*
  J receptors in, 73(t), 74–75
  heart rate and, 273–274, *273*
  hematocrit and, 274–275
  normal response to, 262
  peripheral blood flow and, 276–277, 277(t)
  pH and, 268
  regulation of ventilation and, 264–265
  stroke volume and, 273–274, *273*
  training and, 278–280
    on cardiac output, 278, 278(t), 279
    on peripheral factors, 278, 278(t), 279–280
    on respiratory factors, 278, 278(t), 280
  vascular pressures and, 275–276, *275, 276*
  ventilation and, 264–265, *264, 265*
Expiratory flow limitation, 99
Expiratory flow-volume curve, *101, 105*
Extraalveolar blood vessel(s), perivascular pressure and, 147–148
  pressure determinants of, 147, *147*
Extracellular pH, 218–219, *220*

Fatigue, cause of, 132
  central, 131
  diaphragm and, *133*
  measurement of, 132, *133*
  peripheral, 131, 132
Fetus, airways and terminal respiratory units of, 3–7
  breathing in, 16
  lung development in, 11
    canalicular period of, 5, *6*
    embryonic period of, 5, *6*
    pseudoglandular period of, 5, *6*
    terminal sac period of, 5, *6*
Fiber(s), axial, *53*
  collagen, in elastic recoil, 90
  elastin, in elastic recoil, 90
  peripheral, *53*
Fibrinopeptides, 159
Fibroblast, *77*
Fibrosis, pulmonary, volume-pressure curve in, 87
Film, surface, 52, 54, *541*
Filopodia, *52*
First breath, 16–20
  circulatory adjustments in, 19–20
  lung expansion in, 17–18
  lung liquid removal in, 18–19
  pulmonary vascular resistance changes in, 19
Flooding, alveolar, 307
Flow-pressure curve(s), isovolumic, 99–101, *99, 100, 101*